Applied Respiratory Physiology

Applied Respiratory Physiology

Third edition

J. F. Nunn

MD, PhD, FRCS, FFARCS, FFARACS (Hon), FFARCSI (Hon.)
Head of Division of Anaesthesia, Medical Research Council Clinical Research Centre; Honorary
Consultant Anaesthetist, Northwick Park Hospital, Middlesex
Formerly Professor of Anaesthesia, University of Leeds; Dean of Faculty of Anaesthetists, Royal
College of Surgeons of England

Butterworths
London Boston Durban Singapore Sydney Toronto Wellington

© Butterworth & Co. (Publishers) Ltd. 1987

First published, 1969
Reprinted 1971 (twice), 1972, 1975
Second edition, 1977
Reprinted 1978, 1981
Third edition, 1987

British Library Cataloguing in Publication Data
Nunn, J.F.
  Applied respiratory physiology.—3rd ed.
  1. Respiratory organs 2. Anaesthesia
  I. Title
  612′.2′024617   QP121

  ISBN 0–407–00342–8

Library of Congress Cataloging-in-Publication Data
Nunn, J.F. (John Francis)
  Applied respiratory physiology.

  Bibliography: p.
  Includes index.
  1. Respiration. 2. Anesthesia. I. Title.
  [DNLM: 1. Anesthesia. 2. Respiration. WF 102 N972a]
  QP121.N75 1987   612.2′024′617   86–31019
  ISBN 0–407–00342–8

Photoset by Page Bros. Ltd. Norwich, Norfolk, and TecSet Ltd, Wallington, Surrey
Printed in Great Britain at the University Press, Cambridge

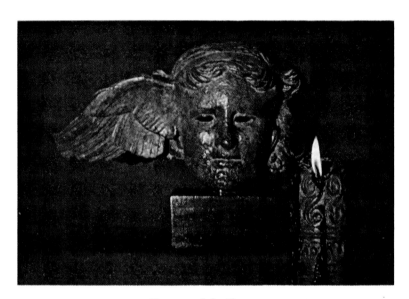

Hypnos and the Flame
(original photograph courtesy of Dr John W. Severinghaus)

Foreword to the First Edition

A Flame for Hypnos

The lighted candle respires and we call it flame. The body respires and we call it life. Neither flame nor life is substance, but process. The flame is as different from the wick and wax as life from the body, as gravitation from the falling apple, or love from a hormone. Newton taught science to have faith in processes as well as substances—to compute, predict and depend upon an irrational attraction. Caught up in enlightenment, man began to regard himself as a part of nature, a subject for investigation. The web of self-knowledge, woven so slowly between process and substance, still weaves physiology, the process, and anatomy, the substance, into the whole cloth of clinical medicine. Within this multihued fabric, the warp fibres of process shine most clearly in the newest patterns, among which must be numbered anaesthesiology. The tailors who wove the sciences into the clinical practice of anaesthetics are men of our time such as Ralph Waters and Chauncey Leake who knit together respiratory physiology and pharmacology to cloak the first medical school Department of Anesthesiology, at Wisconsin, scarcely 45 years ago. Both of them still delight in watching the fashion parade they set in motion. Their partnership lasted only five years, but anaesthesiology and respiratory physiology remain as intimately interwoven as any pair of clinical and basic sciences. In this volume stands the evidence: references to more than 100 anaesthetists who have substantially contributed to respiratory physiology and John Francis Nunn's superb text which, for the first time, comprehensively binds the two together.

Man's interest in his own reaction to his environment constituted a further leap of the intellect. From substance to process to self-examination, and then full circle to the processes of interaction. 1969 may be considered the centenary of environmental or applied physiology. One hundred years ago Paul Bert, in a series of lectures to the Academie de Science in Paris, proposed to investigate the role of the low partial pressure of oxygen upon the distress experienced at high altitudes. Applying Dalton's law of partial pressures to physiology for the first time, he thus launched his monumental research of the barometric pressure, surely the cornerstone of applied physiology. The demands of military aviation during World War II generated a quantum jump of interest in applied physiology, exemplified by the founding 21 years ago of the *Journal of Applied Physiology*. This youngster, having just come of age, provides well over 100 references in Nunn's text, many of them written by anaesthetists. Anaesthesia may justly claim its birthright share of *Applied Respiratory Physiology*. Three years hence will be celebrated the bicentenary of N_2O, noting that Joseph Priestley reported N_2O two years before O_2!

And what of the god of sleep, patron of anaesthesia? The centuries themselves number more than 21 since Hypnos wrapped his cloak of sleep over Hellas. Now before Hypnos, the artisan, is set the respiring flame--that he may, by knowing the process, better the art.

San Francisco   JOHN W. SEVERINGHAUS

Preface to the First Edition

Clinicians in many branches of medicine find that their work demands an extensive knowledge of respiratory physiology. This applies particularly to anaesthetists working in the operating theatre or in the intensive care unit. It is unfortunately common experience that respiratory physiology learned in the preclinical years proves to be an incomplete preparation for the clinical field. Indeed, the emphasis of the preclinical course seems, in many cases, to be out of tune with the practical problems to be faced after qualification and specialization. Much that is taught does not apply to man in the clinical environment while, on the other hand, a great many physiological problems highly relevant to the survival of patients find no place in the curriculum. It is to be hoped that new approaches to the teaching of medicine may overcome this dichotomy and that, in particular, much will be gained from the integration of physiology with clinical teaching.

This book is designed to bridge the gap between pure respiratory physiology and the treatment of patients. It is neither a primer of respiratory physiology nor is it a practical manual for use in the wards and operating theatres. It has two aims. Firstly, I have tried to explain those aspects of respiratory physiology which seem most relevant to patient care, particularly in the field of anaesthesia. Secondly, I have brought together in review those studies which seem to me to be most relevant to clinical work. Inevitably there has been a preference for studies of man and particular stress has been laid on those functions in which man appears to differ from laboratory animals. There is an unashamed emphasis on anaesthesia because I am an anaesthetist. However, the work in this specialty spreads freely into the territory of our neighbours.

References have been a problem. It is clearly impracticable to quote every work which deserves mention. In general I have cited the most informative and the most accessible works, but this rule has been broken on numerous occasions when the distinction of prior discovery calls for recognition. Reviews are freely cited since a book of this length can include only a fraction of the relevant material. I must apologize to the writers of multi-author papers. No one likes to be cited as a colleague, but considerations of space have precluded naming more than three authors for any paper.

Chapters are designed to be read separately and this has required some repetition. There are also frequent cross-references between the chapters. The principles of methods of measurement are considered together at the end of each chapter or section.

In spite of optimistic hopes, the book has taken six years to write. Its form, however, has evolved over the last twelve years from a series of lectures and tutorials given at the Royal College of Surgeons, the Royal Postgraduate Medical School, the University of Leeds and in numerous institutions in Europe and the United States which I have been privileged to visit. Blackboard sketches have gradually taken the form of the figures which appear in this book.

The greater part of this book is distilled from the work of teachers and colleagues. Professor W. Melville Arnott and Professor K. W. Donald introduced me to the study of clinical respiratory physiology and I worked under the late Professor Ronald Woolmer for a further six years. My debt to them is very great. I have also had the good fortune to work in close contact with many gifted colleagues who have not hesitated to share the fruits of their experience. The list of references will indicate how much I have learned from Dr John Severinghaus, Professor Moran Campbell, Dr John Butler and Dr John West. For my own studies, I acknowledge with gratitude the part played by a long series of research fellows and assistants. Some fifteen are cited herein and they come from eleven different countries. Figures 2, 3, 6, 11 and 15 [Figures 1.5. 4.3, 2.4, and 2.1 in the third edition] which are clearly not my blackboard sketches, were drawn by Mr H. Grayshon Lumby. I have had unstinted help from librarians, Miss M. P. Russell, Mr W. R. LeFanu and Miss E. M. Reed. Numerous colleagues have given invaluable help in reading and criticizing the manuscript.

Finally I must thank my wife who has not only borne the inevitable preoccupation of a husband writing a book but has also carried the burden of the paper work and prepared the manuscript.

J.F.N.

Preface to the Third Edition

It is now a quarter of a century since the first edition of *Applied Respiratory Physiology* was conceived, although its gestation period was lengthy and it was not published until 1969. The original purpose of the book was to bring the scientific basis of respiratory physiology into the practice of anaesthesia and, on re-reading the first edition, I detect a missionary zeal which was perhaps appropriate to those years. The second edition was a stage in an evolutionary process which saw the book's coverage widened to include other applications of respiratory physiology, particularly intensive care which was then a major interest of many anaesthetists.

The third edition of a book is well known to be an important milestone and this seemed to be the appropriate time to make major changes. Firstly I have rearranged the contents into two parts. The first is confined to general principles, while the second deals separately with the various applied situations, the whole being linked by numerous page references. The purpose of this change is to make it easier to find material: even the author has often found this to be quite difficult in the second edition. The second major change is an expansion of the applications which have been considered.

The first part can now be read as a general introduction to human respiratory physiology in preparation for consideration of the various applied fields. The text is no longer interrupted by lengthy digressions into particular applications which may not be of interest to every reader.

The second part is intended to provide a series of compact reviews of discrete topics with a listing of the key references. These chapters are intended to be read in relation to the corresponding sections in Part I, and cross-references are provided for this purpose. However, the expansion of this part of the book is not at the expense of anaesthesia which is, in fact, given greater prominence, particularly in the control of breathing and the relative distribution of ventilation and perfusion. The section on artificial ventilation has been extended to cover the new techniques of ventilation, and extracorporeal gas exchange now merits a separate chapter. Special forms of lung pathology which have a major effect on lung function have also been accorded their own chapters, and these include the adult respiratory distress syndrome, pulmonary oedema, embolus and collapse. Sleep, smoking, diving and drowning are virtually new chapters and there has been a substantial increase in the coverage of exercise, high altitude, children and neonates. I am well aware of the open-ended nature of the applications of respiratory physiology, and complete coverage must be an illusion. Nevertheless, I hope that the most important fields are now included.

The inclusion of new topics has been much influenced by the work within my own Division at the Clinical Research Centre. I never cease to be astonished that a Division of Anaesthesia should have a Group (led by Michael Halsey) undertaking dives to pressures of 100 atmospheres and that James Milledge should have explored the human response to life at extremes of high altitude. Other members of the Division have worked in the fields of smoking, sleep and, more recently, in exercise and drowning. I am deeply indebted to my colleagues in the Division of Anaesthesia at the Clinical Research Centre who have given freely of their advice and have kindly read my manuscripts. In particular I want to thank Michael Barrowcliffe, Ronald Cormack, Michael Halsey, Mark Harries, Gareth Jones, Christopher Jordan, James Milledge, Barbara Royston, David Royston, Christine Thornton and Nigel Webster.

Outside the Clinical Research Centre, many friends have given permission to include their own material, have kindly drawn my attention to work I had overlooked and have read drafts of chapters. Without their help my task would have been impossible and it is with great pleasure that I express my gratitude, and not for the first time, to Siggaard-Andersen, Mick Bakhle, William Barker, Judy Donegan, Edmond Eger, David Flenley, Thomas Hornbein, Richard Knill, Hans Loeschcke, Bryan Marshall, Frank Preston, Kai Rehder, John Severinghaus, Norman Staub, Keith Sykes, Erwald Weibel, John West and James Whitwam. I am particularly indebted to Erwald Weibel for the magnificent scanning electron micrograph (*Figure 1.10*) which graces the cover of this edition.

In the preparation of the manuscript I am deeply indebted for all the help I have received from Brenda Dobson and Norma Saunders. My dear wife has borne the burden with her accustomed fortitude and support, without which the work would never have been completed.

J.F.N.

Contents

PART II   THE APPLICATIONS

Part I

Basic principles

Chapter 1

Functional anatomy of the respiratory tract

A clear understanding of structure is a sure foundation on which to base a study of function. This chapter is not a comprehensive account of the structure of the respiratory tract but concentrates on those aspects which are most relevant to an understanding of function.

Mouth and pharynx

Structural aspects of the function of the muscles of the mouth and pharynx are best considered in relation to a paramedian sagittal section (*Figure 1.1*). Part (a) shows the relaxed position with mouth slightly open and a clear airway through both mouth and nose. Part (b) shows the mouth closed with occlusion of the oral airway by approximation of tongue and palate, this being the preferred position during normal quiet breathing for all except mouth breathers. Part (c) shows forced mouth breathing, as for instance when blowing through the mouth, without pinching the nose. Note that the soft palate is arched upwards and is approximated against a band of the superior constrictor of the pharynx known as Passavant's ridge which, together with the soft palate, forms the palatopharyngeal sphincter (Passavant, 1869; Whillis, 1930). These fibres of the superior constrictor are hypertrophied in cases of cleft palate. Note also that the orifice of the eustachian tube lies above the palatopharyngeal sphincter and the tubes can be inflated only by the subject himself when the nose is pinched.

Part (d) shows the occlusion of the respiratory tract during swallowing when the bolus is just passing over the back of the tongue. The larynx is elevated by contraction of the infrahyoid muscles and the epiglottis folds backwards, causing total occlusion of the entrance to the larynx (Fink and Demarest, 1978). This extremely effective protection of the larynx is capable of withstanding pharyngeal pressure as high as 80 kPa (600 mmHg) which may be generated during swallowing.

Figure 1.2 is concerned with respiratory obstruction caused by the tongue. Part (a) shows the normal position, which is substantially the same as in *Figure 1.1a*. The continuous lines in the body of the tongue represent the fibres of genioglossus extending from the superior genial tubercle at the symphysis menti into the body of the tongue. It is now known that this muscle has a high resting tension in the normal conscious subject and this tone shows phasic activity during the inspiratory part of the respiratory cycle (Remmers et al., 1978).

3

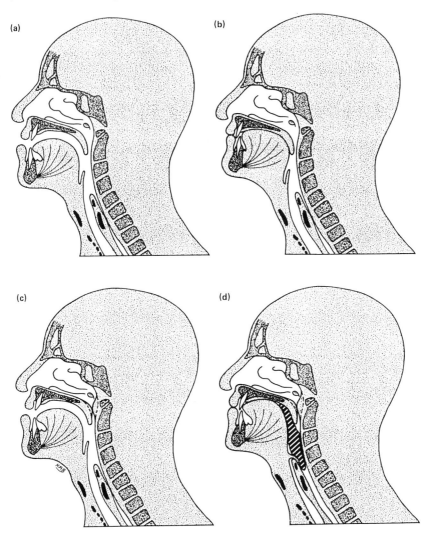

Figure 1.1 Factors in the patency of the mouth and pharynx. (a) The relaxed position with both oral and nasal airways open. (b) Oral airway occluded by the tongue, as in normal nasal breathing. (c) Nasal airway occluded at the palatopharyngeal sphincter. (d) Occlusion of the larynx and nasopharynx during swallowing. Note down-folding of the epiglottis.

The tone in the genioglossus may be lost under certain conditions, including obstructive sleep apnoea (page 306) and almost invariably during anaesthesia (page 375). The result of this is that the relaxed tongue collapses against the posterior pharyngeal wall opposite the 2nd and 3rd cervical vertebrae, causing partial or total obstruction (*Figure 1.2b*).

During anaesthesia and in the comatose patient the pharyngeal airway can usually but not always be cleared by one of two manoeuvres. The simplest method, advocated for emergency resuscitation, is extension of the neck at the atlanto-occipital joint (*Figure 1.2c*). The effect of this has been considered in detail by

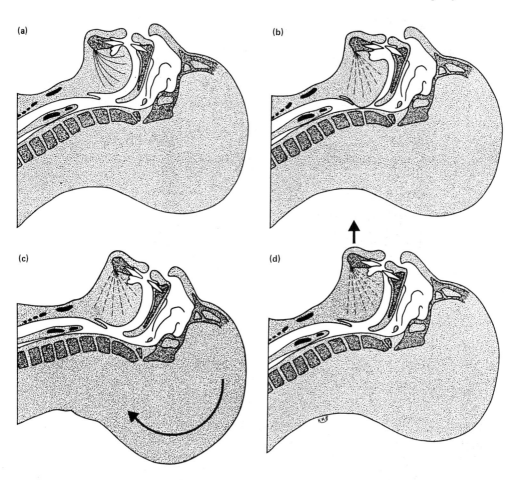

Figure 1.2 Supine position. (a) Normal relaxed position with both oral and nasal airways open. (b) Genioglossus muscle relaxed (as in coma or anaesthesia), causing obstruction between tongue and posterior pharyngeal wall. (c) Airway restored by extension of the atlanto-occipital junction. (d) Airway restored by protrusion of the mandible.

Safar, Escarraga and Chang (1959). In the position shown in *Figure 1.2c*, the distance between the genial tubercle and the posterior pharyngeal wall is increased by about 25 per cent. The other manoeuvre to compensate for a relaxed genioglossus is protrusion of the jaw (*Figure 1.2d*). This is considerably more difficult and tiring to achieve but it is commonly practised by anaesthetists in patients without tracheal intubation. By this means the tongue is lifted bodily forward with the intention of clearing a passage between it and the posterior pharyngeal wall. Jaw protrusion can be combined with extension of the neck, and one or the other or both will almost always clear the airway in an unconscious patient.

Since this type of respiratory obstruction most commonly occurs in the supine position, *Figure 1.2* has been drawn in that position, but it must be emphasized that gravity cannot be relied upon to solve the problem and the prone position does not usually clear a passage between tongue and posterior pharyngeal wall. It does, nevertheless, have important advantages in the clearing of secretions.

The larynx

A full account of the larynx is beyond the scope of this book and the reader is referred to Fink and Demarest (1978) for much new information on this often neglected and misunderstood organ.

Occlusion of the larynx is achieved in various stages ranging from whisper to speech with varying degrees of approximation of the vocal folds. Tighter occlusion can, however, be achieved for the purpose of making expulsive efforts. Further to simple apposition of the vocal folds and arytenoid cartilages, there is apposition of the cuneiform cartilages and vestibular folds and approximation of the thyroid cartilage and hyoid bone, with infolding of the aryepiglottic folds and apposition of the median thyrohyoid fold to the lower part of the adducted vestibular folds (Fink and Demarest, 1978). The full procedure constitutes effort closure and is able to withstand the highest pressures which can be generated in the thorax, usually at least 12 kPa (90 mmHg) and often more. Sudden release of the obstruction is essential for effective coughing, when the linear velocity of air through the larynx is said to approach the speed of sound. Effort closure is also involved in the protection of the larynx during swallowing and it is suggested that it has an important role in locking the thorax to provide a firm origin for the muscles which control the movements of the upper limbs.

The tracheobronchial tree

Classic accounts of the structure of the lung have been presented by Miller (1947) and von Hayek (1960). The most useful approach to understanding the tracheobronchial tree is that of Weibel (1963) who numbered successive generations of air passages from the trachea (generation 0) down to alveolar sacs (generation 23). *Table 1.1* traces their essential characteristics progressively down the respiratory tract. As a rough approximation it may be assumed that the number of passages in each generation is double that in the previous generation and the number of passages in each generation is 2 raised to the power of the generation number. This formula indicates one trachea, two main bronchi, four lobar bronchi, sixteen segmental bronchi, etc.

Trachea (generation 0)

The trachea has a mean diameter of 1.8 cm and length of 11 cm. It is supported by U-shaped cartilages which are joined posteriorly by smooth muscle bands. In spite of the cartilaginous support, the trachea is fairly easy to occlude by external pressure of the order of 5–7 kPa (50–70 cmH$_2$O).

The part of the trachea in the neck is not subjected to intrathoracic pressure changes but it is subject to pressures arising in the neck due, for example, to haematoma formation after thyroidectomy. Within the chest, the trachea can be compressed by raised intrathoracic pressure during, for example, a cough, when the decreased diameter increases the efficiency of removal of secretions.

The mucosa is columnar ciliated epithelium containing numerous mucus-secreting goblet cells. The cilia beat in a co-ordinated manner, causing an upward stream of mucus and foreign bodies. Cilial beat is rendered ineffective by clinical concentrations of anaesthetics (Nunn et al., 1974) and also by drying which is prone to occur when patients breathe dry gas through a tracheostomy.

Table 1.1 Structural characteristics of the air passages

	Generation (mean)	Number	Mean diameter (mm)	Area supplied	Cartilage	Muscle	Nutrition	Emplacement	Epithelium
Trachea	0	1	18	Both lungs	U-shaped	Links open end of cartilage			
Main bronchi	1	2	13	Individual lungs					
Lobar bronchi	2 → 3	4 → 8	7 → 5	Lobes	Irregular shaped and helical plates	Helical bands	From the bronchial circulation	Within connective tissue sheath alongside arterial vessels	Columnar ciliated
Segmental bronchi	4	16	4	Segments					
Small bronchi	5 → 11	32 → 2 000	3 → 1	Secondary lobules					
Bronchioles Terminal bronchioles	12 → 16	4 000 → 65 000	1 → 0.5		Absent	Strong helical muscle bands		Embedded directly in the lung parenchyma	Cuboidal
Respiratory bronchioles	17 → 19	130 000 → 500 000	0.5	Primary lobules		Muscle bands between alveoli	From the pulmonary circulation		Cuboidal to flat between the alveoli
Alveolar ducts	20 → 22	1 000 000 → 4 000 000	0.3	Alveoli		Thin bands in alveolar septa		Form the lung parenchyma	Alveolar epithelium
Alveolar sacs	23	8 000 000	0.3						

(After Weibel, 1963)

Main, lobar and segmental bronchi (generations 1–4)

The trachea bifurcates asymmetrically, with the right bronchus being wider and making a smaller angle with the long axis of the trachea. It is thus more likely to receive foreign bodies. Main, lobar and segmental bronchi have firm cartilaginous support in their walls, U-shaped in the main bronchi but in the form of irregularly shaped and helical plates lower down. Where the cartilage is in the form of irregular plates, the bronchial muscle takes the form of helical bands which form a geodesic network. The bronchial epithelium is similar to that in the trachea although the height of the cells gradually diminishes in the more peripheral passages until it becomes cuboidal in the bronchioles. Bronchi in this group (down to generation 4) are sufficiently regular to be be individually named (*Figure 1.3*). Total cross-sectional area of the respiratory tract is minimal at the third generation (*Figure 1.4*).

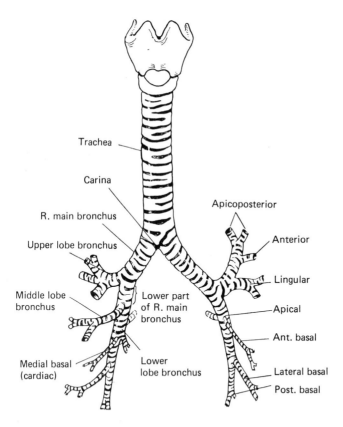

Figure 1.3 Named branches of the tracheobronchial tree, viewed from the front. (Reproduced from Ellis and Feldman (1983) with permission of the authors and the publishers)

These bronchi are subjected to the full effect of changes in intrathoracic pressure and will collapse when the intrathoracic pressure exceeds the intraluminar pressure by about 5 kPa (50 cmH$_2$O). This occurs in the larger bronchi during a forced expiration since the greater part of the alveolar-to-mouth pressure difference is

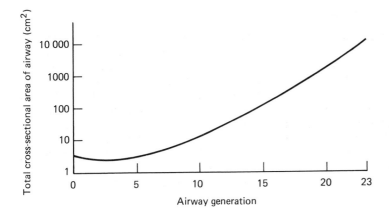

Figure 1.4 The total cross-sectional area of the air passages at different generations of the airways. Note that the minimal cross-sectional area is at generation 3 (lobar to segmental bronchi). The total cross-sectional area becomes very large in the smaller air passages. It approaches a square metre in the alveolar ducts. (Redrawn from data of Weibel, 1964)

taken up in the segmental bronchi under these circumstances. Therefore the intraluminar pressure, particularly within the larger bronchi, remains well below the intrathoracic pressure, particularly in patients with emphysema (Macklem, Fraser and Bates, 1963; Macklem and Wilson, 1965). Collapse of the larger bronchi limits the peak expiratory flow rate in the normal subject and gives rise to the brassy note of a 'voluntary wheeze' produced in this way.

Small bronchi (generations 5–11)

The small bronchi extend through about seven generations with their diameter progressively falling from 3.5 to 1 mm. Since their number approximately doubles with each generation, the total cross-sectional area increases markedly with each generation to a value (at generation 11) which is about seven times the total cross-sectional area at the level of the lobar bronchi.

Down to the level of the true bronchi, air passages lie in close proximity to branches of the pulmonary artery in a sheath containing pulmonary lymphatics which can be distended with oedema fluid giving rise to the characteristic 'cuffing' (*Plates 1* and *2*). This is responsible for the earliest radiographical changes in pulmonary oedema.

Since these air passages are not directly attached to the lung parenchyma, they are not subject to direct traction and rely for their patency on cartilage within their walls and on the transmural pressure gradient which is normally positive from lumen to intrathoracic space. It now appears that this pressure gradient is seldom reversed since the pressure gradient between the alveoli and the small bronchi is less than had formerly been deduced from postmortem studies in which the lungs had been fixed without inflation. It is now believed that, even during a forced expiration, the intraluminar pressure in the small bronchi rapidly rises to more than 80 per cent of the alveolar pressure. This is sufficient to withstand the collapsing pressure of the high extramural intrathoracic pressure.

Secondary lobule. The area supplied by a small bronchus immediately before the change to a bronchiole is sometimes referred to as a secondary lobule, each of which has a volume of about 2 ml and is defined by connective tissue septa.

Bronchioles (generations 12–16)

An important change occurs at about the eleventh generation where the diameter is about 1 mm. Cartilage disappears from the wall below this level and structural rigidity ceases to be a factor in maintaining patency. However, beyond this level the air passages are directly embedded in the lung parenchyma, the elastic recoil of which holds the air passages open like the guy ropes of a bell tent. Therefore the calibre of the airways below the eleventh generation is mainly influenced by lung volume, since the forces holding their lumina open are stronger at higher lung volumes. Calibre is thus primarily a function of lung volume and it is this effect which leads to airway closure at reduced long volume (see page 62).

In succeeding generations, the number of bronchioles increases far more rapidly than the calibre diminishes (*Table 1.1*). Therefore the total cross-sectional area increases until, in the terminal bronchioles, it is about 30 times the area at the level of the large bronchi (*Figure 1.4*). Thus the flow resistance of the smaller air passages (less than 2 mm) is only about one-tenth of the total (Macklem and Mead, 1967).

Bronchioles have strong helical muscular bands and cuboidal epithelium. Contraction of the muscle bands is able to wrinkle the mucosa into longitudinal folds. This increases flow resistance and, in extreme cases, results in total airway obstruction.

Down to the terminal bronchiole, the air passages derive their nutrition from the bronchial circulation and are thus influenced by systemic arterial blood gas levels. Beyond this point the smaller air passages rely upon the pulmonary circulation for their nutrition.

Respiratory bronchioles (generations 17–19)

Down to the smallest bronchioles, the functions of the air passages are solely conduction and humidification. Beyond this point there is a gradual transition from conduction to gas exchange. In the three generations of respiratory bronchioles there is a gradual increase in the number of alveoli in their walls (*Figure 1.5* and *Plate 3*). The epithelium is cuboidal between the mouths of the mural alveoli in the earlier generations of respiratory bronchioles but becomes progressively flatter until it is entirely alveolar epithelium in the alveolar ducts. Like the bronchioles, the respiratory bronchioles are embedded in lung parenchyma. However, they have well a marked muscle layer with bands which loop over the opening of the alveolar ducts and the mouths of the mural alveoli. There is no significant change in calibre of advancing generations of respiratory bronchioles and the total cross-sectional area at this level is of the order of hundreds of square centimetres.

Primary lobule or terminal respiratory unit. This is probably the equivalent of the alveolus when it is considered from the functional standpoint. The primary lobule is usually defined as the zone supplied by a first order respiratory bronchiole (*Figure 1.5*). According to this definition, there are about 130 000 primary lobules, each with a diameter of about 3.5 mm and containing about 2000 alveoli (*Table 1.2*).

They probably correspond to the small zones which are seen to pop open when a collapsed lung is inflated at thoracotomy.

Alveolar ducts (generations 20–22)

Alveolar ducts arise from the terminal respiratory bronchiole, from which they differ by having no walls other than the mouths of mural alveoli (about 20 in number). The alveolar septa form a series of rings forming the walls of the alveolar ducts and containing smooth muscle. About half of the alveoli arise from ducts, and some 35 per cent of the alveolar gas resides in the alveolar ducts and the alveoli which arise directly from them.

Alveolar sacs (generation 23)

The last generation of the air passages differ from alveolar ducts solely in the fact that they are blind. About 17 alveoli arise from each alveolar sac and account for about half of the total number of alveoli.

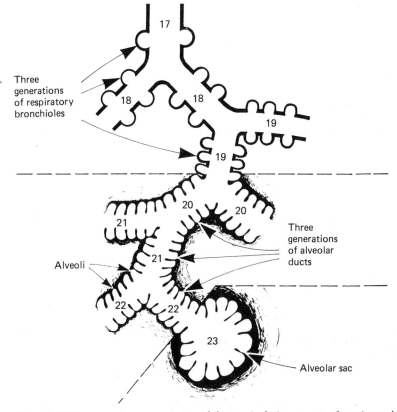

Figure 1.5 Diagrammatic representation of the terminal air passages of a primary lobule or functional unit. Successive generations are numbered and correspond to Table 1.1. The strict bifurcation at each generation affords an adequate model for explanation of function, but the actual structure is less regular. Different authors have variously defined the primary lobules as the area of lung supplied by the first, second or third generation of respiratory bronchiole.

Table 1.2 Distribution of alveoli in a primary lobule or acinus (syn. terminal respiratory unit)

	Generation (as in Table 1.1)	Number of alveoli per unit (mean)	Number of units per generation (mean)	Number of alveoli per generation (mean)
Respiratory bronchioles:				
1st order	16	5	1	5
2nd order	18	8	2	16
3rd order	19	12	4	48
Alveolar ducts:				
1st order	20	20	8	160
2nd order	21	20	16	320
3rd order	22	20	32	640
Alveolar sacs	23	17	64	1088
Total number of alveoli in primary lobule				2277

Diameter of primary lobule at FRC, 3.5 mm; volume of primary lobule at FRC, 23 μl; number of primary lobules in average lung, 130 000; total number of alveoli in average lung, 300 000 000; diameter of alveolus at FRC, 0.2mm.
(After Weibel, 1963)

The alveoli

The mean total number of alveoli is usually given as 300 million but ranges from about 200 million to 600 million, correlating with the height of the subject (Angus and Thurlbeck, 1972). The size of the alveoli is proportional to lung volume but they are larger in the upper part of the lung except at maximal inflation when the vertical gradient in size disappears (Glazier et al., 1967). The vertical gradient is dependent on gravity and presumably disappears in space. The reduction in size of alveoli and the corresponding reduction in calibre of the smaller airways in the dependent parts of the lung has most important implications in gas exchange)which are considered below (pages 62, 142, 153). At functional residual capacity the mean diameter is 0.2 mm, astonishingly close to the estimate of 1/100 inch made by the Reverend Stephen Hales in 1731.

Electron microscopy is essential to an understanding of the detailed structure at the alveolar level, and reference may be made to Weibel (1984, 1985).

Alveolar walls which separate two adjacent alveoli consist of two layers of alveolar epithelium on separate basement membranes enclosing the interstitial space. This contains the pulmonary capillaries, elastin and collagen fibres, nerve endings and occasional migrant polymorphs and macrophages. The interstitial space is asymmetrically disposed in relation to the capillaries (*Figures 1.6* and *1.7*). On one side the capillary endothelium and the alveolar epithelium are closely apposed and the

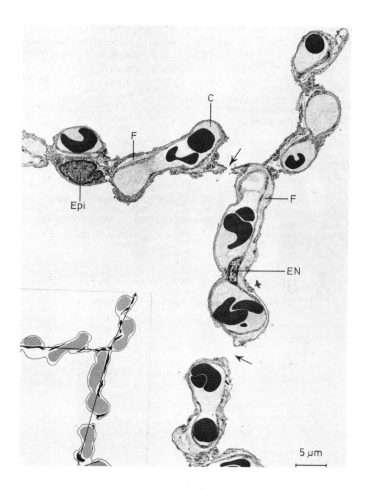

Figure 1.6 Electron micrograph of the junction of three alveolar septa of inflated lung of dog, showing the form of the continuous network of collagen fibrils, into which the capillary network is interwoven. C, capillary; EN, endothelial nucleus: Epi, epithelial nucleus (type I); F, collagen fibrils; arrows point to pores of Kohn. (Reproduced from Weibel (1973) by permission of the author and the Editors of Physiological Reviews)

total thickness from gas to blood is usually less than 0.4 μm (*Figure 1.8*). This may be considered the active side of the capillary and the gas exchange must be more efficient on this side. The other side of the capillary is usually more than 1–2 μm thick and contains abundant collagen and elastin fibres in an expanded tissue space. This side may be considered the service side of the capillary and it provides the connective tissue framework which maintains the geometry of the lung. The distinction between the two sides of the capillary is clearly shown in *Figure 1.6* and it has considerable physiological significance. The active side tends to be spared in the accumulation of both oedema fluid (*Figure 1.9* and page 431) and fibrous tissue in fibrosing alveolitis or Hamman–Rich syndrome (page 194). *Figure 1.8* shows a rare depiction of the alveolar lining fluid, but it has been proposed that the lining of the alveoli is, in fact, largely dry (Hills, 1982).

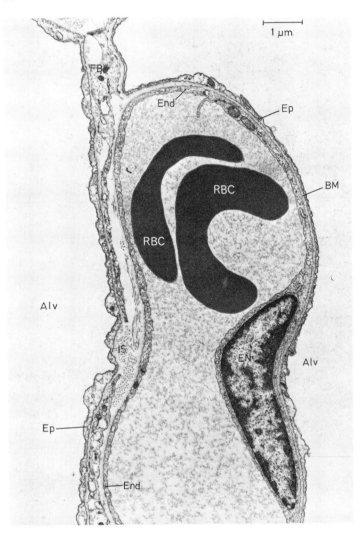

Figure 1.7 Details of the interstitial space, the capillary endothelium and alveolar epithelium. Note that the thickening of the interstitial space is confined to the left of the capillary) (the 'service side') while the total alveolar/capillary membrane remains thin on the right (the 'active side') except where it is thickened by the endothelial nucleus.

Alv, alveolus; BM, basement membrane; EN, endothelial nucleus; End, endothelium; Ep, epithelium; IS, interstitial space; RBC, erythrocyte; FB, fibroblast process. (Electron micrograph kindly supplied by Professor E.R. Weibel)

The alveolar septa are generally flat (*Figure 1.6*) due to tension generated partly by elastic fibres but more by surface tension at the air/fluid interface. As explained below (page 24), the surface tension of the alveolar lining fluid is considerably modified by the presence of surfactant. The septa are perforated by small fenestrations known as the pores of Kohn (*Figure 1.6* and *Plate 4*). These pores provide collateral ventilation which can be demonstrated between air spaces supplied by

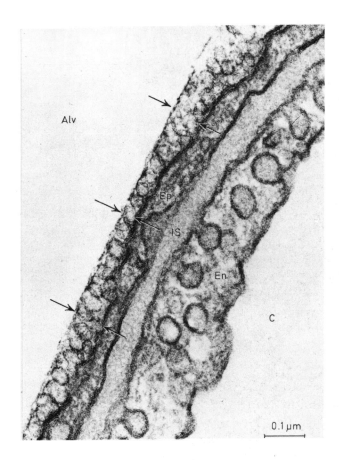

Figure 1.8 High powered electron micrograph showing detailed structure of the alveolar/capillary membrane of the rat. Alv, alveolus; C, capillary; En, endothelium; Ep, epithelium; IS, interstitial space. The material between the arrows appears to be the alveolar lining fluid as shown by the method described by Weibel and Gil (1968). (Reproduced from Weibel (1973) by permission of the author and the Editors of Physiological Reviews)

fairly large bronchi (Leibow, 1962). Direct communications have also been found between small bronchioles and neighbouring alveoli (Lambert, 1955).

Special cell types at the alveolar and bronchial level

A number of structurally distinct cells may be identified as follows (see general reviews by Ryan, 1982; Gail and Lenfant, 1983; Weibel, 1984, 1985).

1. *Capillary endothelial cells.* These cells are continuous with the endothelium of the general circulation and, in the pulmonary capillary bed, have a thickness of only 0.1 μm except where expanded to contain nuclei (see *Figures 1.6* and *1.7*). Scanning electron microscopy shows the surface to be covered with projections resembling coral (Ryan, 1982). Transmission electron microscopy shows the flat parts of the cytoplasm to be devoid of all organelles except for small vacuoles

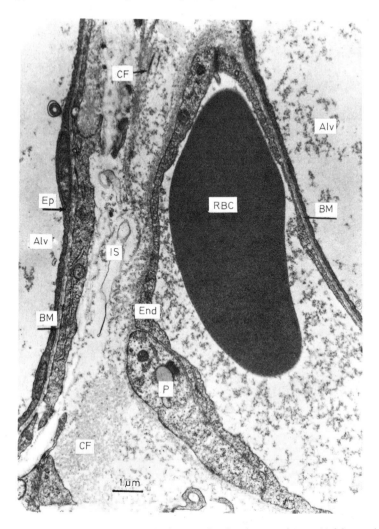

Figure 1.9 Electron micrograph showing the distribution of interstitial haemodynamic pulmonary oe-dema. Note that the interstitial space on the 'service side' of the pulmonary capillary has been considerably thickened by oedema fluid while the 'active side' remains unchanged in thickness. Alv, alveolus; BM, basement membrane; CF, collagen fibres; End, endothelium; Ep, epithelium; IS, interstitial space; P, pericyte; RBC,red blood corpuscle. (Reproduced from Fishman (1972) by permission of the author and the Editors of Circulation)

(caveolae) which may open onto the basement membrane or the lumen of the capillary or be entirely contained within the cytoplasm (see *Figure 1.8*). It is not clear whether they are engaged in pinocytosis or whether they are static. The lining of the caveolae acts as an extension of the cell membrane beyond its already vast size of about 126 m^2 (Weibel, 1983). Surface enzymes are located on the lining of the caveolae as well as on membrane lining the capillaries (Ryan, 1982). The pulmonary capillary endothelium has a metabolic activity approaching that of the liver (Chapter 11). The total volume of capillary endothelium in the human lung is estimated to be 49 ml (Weibel, 1984).

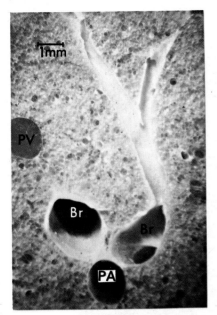

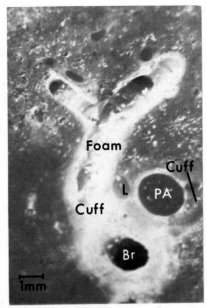

Plate 1

Plate 2

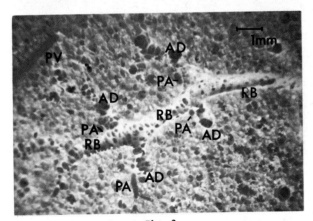

Plate 3

Plate 1. Branchings of cartilaginous bronchi (BR), together with associated pulmonary artery (PA). The corresponding pulmonary vein (PV) is separate. Rapidly frozen normal cat lung showing natural colours. (Photograph by courtesy of Dr N. A. Staub)

Plate 2. Severe pulmonary oedema in freshly frozen dog lung. The bronchi (BR) contain oedema fluid foam and are surrounded by free fluid cuffs. The pulmonary artery and its branches (PA) are also surrounded by cuffs. Note the presence of a distended lymph vessel (L). Lung parenchyma in the background is severely waterlogged. (Reproduced from Staub (1963b) by courtesy of the author and the Editor of Anesthesiology)

Plate 3. Branchings of respiratory bronchioles (RB) showing transition to alveolar ducts (AD). Each airway branch is accompanied by its associated branch of the pulmonary artery (PA). The pulmonary vein (PV) lies separate. Fresh frozen cat lung. (Photograph by courtesy of Dr N. A. Staub)

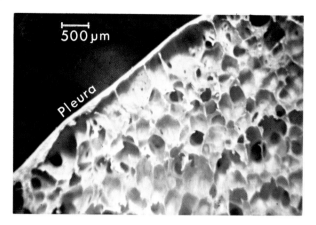

Plate 4

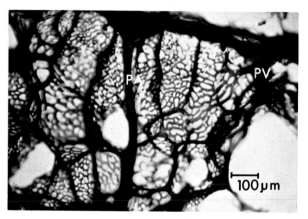

Plate 5

Plate 4. *Fresh frozen human lung showing size and shape of alveoli close to the pleura. Note numerous fenestrations between adjacent alveoli. (Photograph by courtesy of Dr N. A. Staub)*

Plate 5. *Maximally congested pulmonary capillary network in alveolar septum of fresh frozen dog lung. Average length of capillaries from pulmonary artery (PA) to pulmonary vein (PV) is 600–800 µm and crosses several adjacent alveoli. Note capillaries leaving and entering larger blood vessels at right angles. (Photograph by courtesy of Dr N. A. Staub)*

The endothelial cells abut against one another at fairly loose junctions which are of the order of 5 nm wide (DeFouw, 1983). These junctions permit the passage of quite large molecules, and the pulmonary lymph contains albumin at about half the concentration in plasma. Macrophages pass freely through these junctions under normal conditions, and polymorphs can also pass in response to chemotaxis.

Endothelial cells can be grown in culture but only with cells derived from larger vessels and not from the pulmonary capillaries. Nevertheless, cells in these cultures possess most of the metabolic activities known to be present in the pulmonary microcirculation (Ryan, 1982).

2. Alveolar epithelial cells—type I. These cells line the alveoli and also exist as a thin sheet approximately 0.1 µm in thickness except where expanded to contain nuclei (*Figures 1.6 and 1.7*). Like the endothelium, the flat part of the cytoplasm is devoid of organelles except for small vacuoles.

Epithelial cells cover several alveoli as a continuous sheet and meet at tight junctions with a gap of only about 1 nm (DeFouw, 1983). These junctions may be seen as narrow lines snaking across the septa in the elegant scanning electron micrograph (*Figure 1.10*) from Weibel (1984). The tightness of these junctions is crucial for prevention of the escape of large molecules, such as albumin, into the alveoli, thus preserving the oncotic pressure gradient essential for the avoidance of pulmonary oedema (see page 432). Nevertheless, these junctions permit the free passage of macrophages. Polymorphs may also pass in response to a chemotactic stimulus.

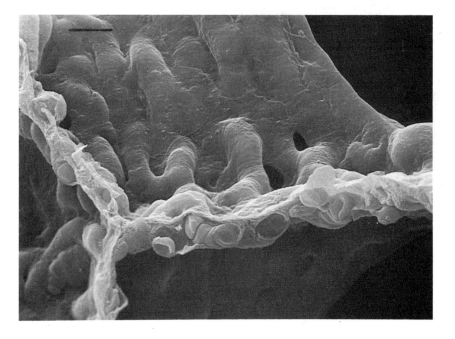

Figure 1.10 Scanning electron micrograph of the junction of three alveolar septa which are shown in both surface view and section. Two pores of Kohn are seen to the right of centre. Erythrocytes are seen in the cut ends of the capillaries. The scale bar (top left) is 10 µm. (Reproduced from Weibel (1984) by permission of the author and the publishers)

Type I cells do not divide and cannot be grown in culture. Their total volume in the human lung is estimated to be 23 ml (Weibel, 1984). They are particularly sensitive to damage from high concentrations of oxygen (page 492).

3. *Alveolar epithelial cells—type II.* These are the stem cells from which type I cells arise. They do not function as gas exchange membranes, and are rounded in shape and situated at the junction of septa. They have large nuclei and microvilli (*Figure 1.11*). The cytoplasm contains characteristic striated osmiophilic organelles which seem to contain stored surfactant.

Type II cells are easily grown in culture and tend to proliferate in lung explant tissue cultures. They are resistant to oxygen toxicity, tending to replace type I cells after prolonged exposure to high concentrations of oxygen (page 492).

4. *Alveolar brush cells—type III.* Brush cells are seen only rarely and their function is not established. It is possible that they may have a receptor function but neuronal connections have not been demonstrated.

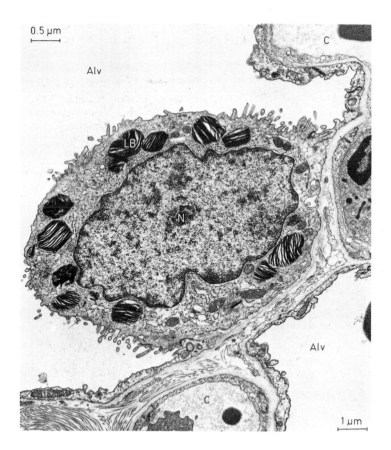

Figure 1.11 Electron micrograph of an alveolar epithelial cell of type II of dog. Note the large nucleus, the microvilli and the osmiophilic lamellar bodies thought to release the surfactant. Alv, alveolus; C, capillary; LB, lamellar bodies; N, nucleus. (Reproduced from Weibel (1973) by permission of the author and the Editors of Physiological Reviews)

5. *Alveolar macrophages.* The lung is richly endowed with these phagocytes which pass freely from the circulation, through the interstitial space and thence through the gaps between alveolar epithelial cells to lie on their surface within the alveolar lining fluid (*Figure 1.12*). They can re-enter the body but are remarkable for their ability to live and function outside the body. The macrophages are active in combatting infection and scavenging foreign bodies such as dust particles. They contain a variety of destructive enzymes but are also capable of generating oxygen-derived free radicals (page 487). These are highly effective bactericidal agents but may also rebound to damage the host. Dead macrophages may also release the enzyme trypsin which may cause tissue damage in patients who are deficient in the protein α_1-antitrypsin (page 286).

6. *Neutrophils.* These cells are not normally present within the alveoli but may appear in response to a neutrophil chemotactic factor released from the alveolar macrophages. They are usually present in the alveoli of smokers (page 340).

7. *Mast cells.* In common with other organs, the lungs contain numerous mast cells which are located in the walls of airways and alveoli. Some also lie free in the lumen of the airways and may be recovered by bronchial lavage. Their important role in bronchoconstriction is described on pages 54 et seq.

8. *Non-ciliated bronchiolar epithelial (Clara) cells.* These cells are found in the mucosa of the terminal bronchioles. They are metabolically active and secretory but their role is not yet established (Gail and Lenfant, 1983). It now seems unlikely

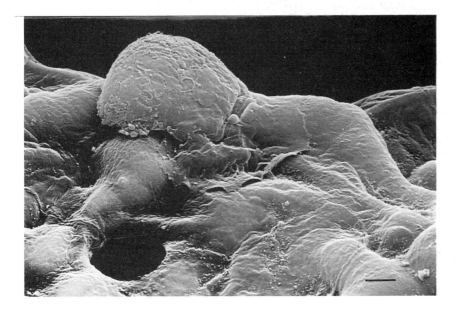

Figure 1.12 Scanning electron micrograph of an alveolar macrophage advancing to the right over epithelial type I cells, preceded by its lamella. The scale bar is 3 μm. (Reproduced from Weibel (1984) by permission of the author and the publishers)

that they play any significant role in the production of surfactant as was once believed.

9. *APUD cells.* These cells occur in bronchial epithelium and, from morphological considerations, are believed to be a part of the APUD series, so named because of their ability to undertake amine and amine-precursor uptake and decarboxylation. APUD cells elsewhere are known to produce a range of hormones including ACTH, insulin, calcitonin and gastrin.

The pulmonary vasculature

Pulmonary arteries

Although the pulmonary circulation carries roughly the same flow as the systemic circulation, the arterial pressure and the vascular resistance are normally only one-sixth as great. The media of the pulmonary arteries is about half as thick as in systemic arteries of corresponding size. In the larger vessels it consists mainly of elastic tissue but in the smaller vessels it is mainly muscular, the transition being in vessels of about 1 mm diameter. Pulmonary arteries lie close to the corresponding air passages in connective tissue sheaths.

Pulmonary arterioles

The transition to arterioles occurs at an internal diameter of 100 μm. These vessels differ radically from their counterparts in the systemic circulation, being virtually devoid of muscular tissue. There is a thin media of elastic tissue separated from the blood by endothelium. Structurally there is no real difference between pulmonary arterioles and venules.

Pulmonary capillaries

Pulmonary capillaries tend to rise abruptly from much larger vessels, the pulmonary metarterioles (Staub, 1963b). The capillaries form a dense network over the walls of one or more alveoli and the spaces between the capillaries are similar in size to the capillaries themselves (*Plate 5*). In the resting state, about 75 per cent of the capillary bed is filled but the percentage is higher in the dependent parts of the lungs. This gravity-dependent effect is the basis of the vertical gradient of ventilation/perfusion ratios in the lung (page 153). Inflation of the alveoli reduces the cross-sectional area of the capillary bed and increases resistance to blood flow. One capillary network is not confined to one alveolus but passes from one alveolus to another (see *Figure 1.10*) and blood traverses a number of alveolar septa before reaching a venule. This clearly has a bearing on the concept of 'capillary transit time' (page 191).

From the functional standpoint it is often more convenient to consider the pulmonary microcirculation rather than just the capillaries. The microcirculation is defined as the vessels which are devoid of a muscular layer and it commences with arterioles of diameter 75 μm and continues through the capillary bed as far as venules of diameter 200 μm. Special roles of the microcirculation are considered in chapters 11 and 23.

Pulmonary venules and veins

Pulmonary capillary blood is collected into venules which are structurally almost identical to the arterioles. In fact, Duke (1954) obtained satisfactory gas exchange when an isolated cat lung was perfused in reverse. The pulmonary veins do not run alongside the pulmonary arteries but lie some distance away, close to the septa which separate the segments of the lung (see *Plate 1*).

Bronchial circulation

Down to the terminal bronchioles, the air passages and the accompanying blood vessels receive their nutrition from the bronchial vessels which arise from the systemic circulation. Part of the bronchial circulation returns to the systemic venous system but part mingles with the pulmonary venous drainage, thereby contributing a shunt (pages 199 and 172).

Bronchopulmonary arterial anastomoses

It is well known that in pulmonary arterial stenosis, blood flows through a pre-capillary anastomosis from the bronchial circulation to reach the pulmonary capil-laries. It is less certain whether this can occur in normal lungs (page 119).

Pulmonary arteriovenous anastomoses

It has been established that, when the pulmonary arterial pressure of the dog is raised by massive pulmonary embolization, pulmonary arterial blood is able to reach the pulmonary veins without apparently having traversed a capillary bed (page 173). The nature of this communication and whether it occurs in man are discussed in Chapter 7, since it offers a possible explanation of some abnormalities of gas exchange during anaesthesia.

Pulmonary lymphatics (see review by Staub, 1974)

There are no lymphatics visible in the interalveolar septa but small lymph vessels commence at the junction between alveolar and extra-alveolar spaces. There is a well developed lymphatic system around the bronchi and pulmonary vessels, capable of containing up to 500 ml, and draining towards the hilum. Down to airway generation 11 the lymphatics lie in a potential space around the air passages and vessels, separating them from the lung parenchyma. This space becomes distended with lymph in pulmonary oedema (see *Plate 2*) and accounts for the characteristic butterfly shadow of the chest radiograph. It is uncertain whether lymphatics are present at the alveolar level.

In the hilum of the lung, the lymphatic drainage passes through several groups of tracheobronchial lymph glands, where they receive tributaries from the superficial subpleural plexus. Most of the lymph from the left lung usually enters the thoracic duct, where it can be conveniently sampled in the sheep. The right side drains into the right lymphatic duct. However, the pulmonary lymphatics often cross the midline and pass independently into the junction of internal jugular and subclavian veins on the corresponding sides of the body. Studies in dogs have indicated that approximately 15 per cent of the flow in the thoracic duct derives from the lungs (Meyer and Ottaviano, 1972).

Pulmonary lymphatics are intimately concerned in the pathogenesis of pulmonary oedema (page 431) and in the transport system for inactivated proteases (page 286).

Chapter 2

Elastic forces and lung volumes

The movements of the lungs are entirely passive and respond to forces external to the lungs. In the case of spontaneous breathing the external forces are the respiratory muscles, whilst artificial ventilation is usually in response to a pressure gradient which is developed between the airway and the environment. In each case, the pattern of response by the lung is governed by the physical impedance of the chest wall system. This impedance, or hindrance, falls mainly into two categories:

1. Elastic resistance of tissue and alveolar gas/liquid interface.
2. Frictional resistance to gas flow.

Additional minor sources of impedance are the inertia of gas and tissue and the friction of tissue deformation. Work performed in overcoming elastic resistance is dissipated as heat and lost. Work performed in overcoming elastic resistance is stored as potential energy, and elastic deformation during inspiration is the usual source of energy for expiration during both spontaneous and artificial breathing.

This chapter is concerned with the elastic resistance afforded by lungs and chest wall, which will be considered separately and then together. These factors govern the resting end-expiratory lung volume or functional residual capacity (FRC), and therefore lung volumes will be considered later in this chapter.

Elastic recoil of the lungs

The lungs can be considered as an elastic structure, with transmural pressure gradient corresponding to stress and lung volume corresponding to strain. Over a limited range these variables obey Hooke's law, and the change in lung volume per unit change in transmural pressure gradient (the compliance) corresponds to Young's modulus. Elastance is the reciprocal of compliance. It is perhaps unfortunate that two different terms are used to quantify the degrees of stiffness of the lungs. Compliance is usually expressed in litres (or millilitres) per kilopascal (or centimetre of water). Stiff lungs have a low compliance. Elastance is expressed in kilopascals (or centimetres of water) per litre. Stiff lungs have a high elastance.

The nature of the forces causing recoil of the lung

For many years it was thought that the recoil of the lung was due entirely to stretching of the yellow elastin fibres present in the lung parenchyma. However, in

1929, von Neergaard showed that a lung completely filled with and immersed in water, had an elastance which was less than the normal value obtained when the lung was filled with air. He correctly concluded that much of the 'elastic recoil' was due to surface tension acting throughout the vast air/water interface lining the alveoli.

Surface tension at an air/water interface produces forces which tend to reduce the area of the interface. Thus the gas pressure within a bubble is always higher than the surrounding gas pressure because the surface of the bubble is in a state of tension. Alveoli resemble bubbles in this respect, although the alveolar gas is connected to the exterior by the air passages.

The pressure inside a bubble is higher than the surrounding pressure by an amount depending on the surface tension of the liquid and the radius of curvature of the bubble according to the Laplace equation:

$$P = 2T/R$$

where P is the pressure within the bubble (dyn/cm^2), T is the surface tension of the liquid (dyn/cm) and R is the radius of the bubble (cm).

In coherent SI units (see Appendix A), the appropriate units would be pressure in pascals (Pa), surface tension in newtons/metre (N/m) and radius in metres (m). Note that mN/m is identical to the old dyn/cm.

On the left of *Figure 2.1a* is shown a typical alveolus of radius 0.1 mm. Assuming that the alveolar lining fluid has a normal surface tension of 20 mN/m (or dyn/cm), the pressure within the alveolus will be 0.4 kPa (4 cmH$_2$O), which is rather less than the normal transmural pressure at FRC. If the alveolar lining fluid had the same surface tension as water (72 mN/m), the lungs would be very stiff.

The alveolus on the right of *Figure 2.1a* has a radius of only 0.05 mmHg and the Laplace equation indicates that, if the surface tension of the alveolus is the same, its pressure should be double the pressure in the left-hand alveolus. Thus gas would tend to flow from smaller alveoli into larger alveoli and the lung would be unstable which, of course, is not the case. Similarly, the retractive forces of the alveolar lining fluid would increase at low lung volumes and decrease at high lung volumes—exactly the reverse of what is observed.

These paradoxes were clear to von Neergaard in 1929 and he concluded that the surface tension of the alveolar lining fluid must be considerably less than would be expected from the properties of simple liquids and, furthermore, that its value must be variable. Observations on bubbles in lung froth (Pattle, 1955) and later on alveolar extracts (Brown, Johnson and Clements, 1959) have demonstrated that the surface tension of alveolar lining fluid is indeed much lower than water. Furthermore, its value is not constant but changes in proportion to the area of the interface. *Figure 2.1b* shows an experiment in which a floating bar is moved in a trough containing an alveolar extract. As the bar is moved to the right, the surface film is concentrated and the surface tension changes as shown in the graph on the right of the Figure. During expansion, the surface tension increases to 40 mN/m, a value which is close to that of plasma but, during contraction, the surface tension falls to 19 mN/m, a lower value than any other body fluid. The relationship between pressure and area is different during expansion and contraction, and a typical hysteresis loop is described.

The consequences of these changes are very important. In contrast to a bubble, the pressure within an alveolus tends to decrease as the radius of curvature is decreased. This is illustrated in *Figure 2.1c* where the right-hand alveolus has a

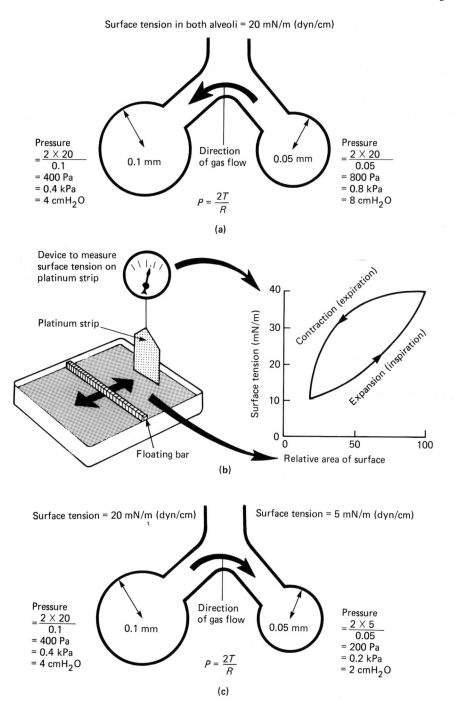

Surface tension in both alveoli = 20 mN/m (dyn/cm)

Pressure
$= \dfrac{2 \times 20}{0.1}$
= 400 Pa
= 0.4 kPa
= 4 cmH$_2$O

0.1 mm

Direction of gas flow

0.05 mm

$P = \dfrac{2T}{R}$

Pressure
$= \dfrac{2 \times 20}{0.05}$
= 800 Pa
= 0.8 kPa
= 8 cmH$_2$O

(a)

Device to measure surface tension on platinum strip

Platinum strip

Floating bar

(b)

40

30

20

10

0

Surface tension (mN/m)

Contraction (expiration)

Expansion (inspiration)

0   50   100

Relative area of surface

Surface tension = 20 mN/m (dyn/cm)

Surface tension = 5 mN/m (dyn/cm)

Pressure
$= \dfrac{2 \times 20}{0.1}$
= 400 Pa
= 0.4 kPa
= 4 cmH$_2$O

0.1 mm

Direction of gas flow

0.05 mm

$P = \dfrac{2T}{R}$

Pressure
$= \dfrac{2 \times 5}{0.05}$
= 200 Pa
= 0.2 kPa
= 2 cmH$_2$O

(c)

Figure 2.1 Surface tension and alveolar transmural pressure. (a) The pressure relations in two alveoli of different size but with the same surface tension of their lining fluids. (b) The changes in surface tension in relation to the area of the alveolar lining film. (c) The pressure relations of two alveoli of different size when allowance is made for the probable changes in surface tension.

smaller diameter and a much lower surface tension than the left-hand alveolus. Its transmural pressure is therefore less than in the left-hand alveolus. Gas tends to flow from the larger to the smaller alveolus and stability is maintained. Similarly, the recoil pressure of the lung decreases with decreasing lung volume, thus giving the appearance of being an elastic body and obeying Hooke's law.

The alveolar surfactant. The low surface tension of the alveolar lining fluid and its dependence on its area (*Figure 2.1b*) are due to the presence of a surface active material. Generally known as the surfactant, it consists of phospholipids which have the general structure shown in *Figure 2.2*. The fatty acids are hydrophobic and project into the gas phase. The other end of the molecule is hydrophilic and lies within the alveolar lining fluid. The molecule is thus confined to the surface where, being detergents, they lower surface tension in proportion to the concentration at the interface. During expiration, as the area of the alveoli diminishes, the surfactant molecules are packed more densely and so the surface tension decreases as shown in *Figure 2.1b*.

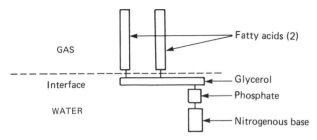

Figure 2.2 General structure of phospholipids.

The lung is known to be active in the synthesis of fatty acids, esterification of lipids, hydrolysis of lipid–ester bonds and oxidation of fatty acids (King and Clements, 1985). The main site of release of surfactants is the type II alveolar cell (page 18), and the lamellar bodies (see *Figure 1.11*) are believed to be stored surfactant.

The most important constituent of these phospholipids is dipalmitoyl lecithin. The base is choline and the palmitic fatty acid chains are saturated and therefore straight. Harlan and Said (1969) have advanced the attractive theory that straight fatty acids will pack together in a more satisfactory manner during expiration than would unsaturated fatty acids such as oleic acid which are bent at the double bond. Other constituents of the surfactant include sphingomyelin, phosphatidyl inositol and phosphatidyl dimethylethanolamine (Gluck, 1971).

Surfactant levels increase in the late stages of gestation and are low in babies with the respiratory distress syndrome (RDS) (Avery and Mead, 1959; Pattle et al., 1962). Before birth, amniocentesis gives some indication of surfactant development in the lung (Gluck et al., 1971). The level of sphingomyelin remains fairly constant while the lecithin content rises sharply late in gestation. Absolute levels in the amniotic fluid do not give a reliable estimate of concentrations in the lung, but the lecithin/sphingomyelin (L/S) ratio is a useful measure of maturity of the surfactant system. There is still no clear resolution of the extent to which reductions in surfactant concentrations contribute to various clinical conditions in which compliance is reduced. Evidence for this is considered in the appropriate chapters in the second part of this book. Classic reviews of surfactant activity were contributed during the heyday of the subject by Clements (1970) and King (1974).

Pulmonary transudation is also affected by surface forces. Surface tension causes the pressure within the alveolar lining fluid to be less than the alveolar pressure. Since the pulmonary capillary pressure in most of the lung is greater than the alveolar pressure (page 122), both factors encourage transudation, a tendency which is checked by the oncotic pressure of the plasma proteins (page 432). Thus the surfactant, by reducing surface tension, diminishes one component of the pressure gradient and helps to prevent transudation. A deficiency of surfactant might tip the balance in favour of the development of pulmonary oedema.

Surface forces also influence the rate of alveolar collapse. The disappearance of very small bubbles in water is accelerated by the rapidly increasing pressure gradient as the bubbles get smaller, due to the Laplace relationship. This may be observed in bubbles in water under the coverslip of a microscope. The rate of shrinkage of the bubbles increases progressively until they vanish abruptly when the radius of curvature has reached a critical value. At this stage, the pressure within the bubble has become so high that the gas is rapidly driven into solution. This does not occur if surfactant is present when there is an indefinite delay in the final disappearance of very small gas bubbles. The same effect would delay the absorption of gas from obstructed alveoli of small size.

There has been a suggestion that the alveolar lining is, in fact, largely dry with the surfactant acting as an anti-wetting agent (Hills, 1982). This would have implications which would run counter to much that has been written above.

The transmural pressure gradient and intrathoracic pressure

The transmural pressure gradient is the difference between intrathoracic (or 'intrapleural') and alveolar pressure. The pressure within an alveolus is always greater than the pressure to the surrounding interstitial tissue except when the volume has been reduced to zero. With increasing lung volume, the transmural pressure gradient steadily increases as shown for the whole lung in *Figure 2.3*. If an appreciable pneumothorax is present, the pressure gradient from alveolus to pleural cavity provides a measure of the overall transmural pressure gradient. Otherwise, the oesophageal pressure may be used to indicate the pleural pressure but there are conceptual and technical difficulties. The technical difficulties are considered at the end of the chapter while some of the conceptual difficulties are indicated in *Figure 2.4*.

The alveoli in the upper part of the lung have a larger volume than those in the dependent parts except at total lung capacity. The greater degree of expansion of the alveoli in the upper parts results in a greater transmural pressure gradient which decreases steadily down the lung at about 0.1 kPa or 1 cmH₂O) per 3 cm of vertical height; such a difference is indicated in *Figure 2.4a*. Since the pleural cavity is normally empty, it is not strictly correct to speak of an intrapleural pressure and, furthermore, it would not be constant throughout the pleural 'cavity'. One should think rather of the relationship shown in *Figure 2.3* as applying to various horizontal strata of the lung, each with its own volume and therefore its own transmural pressure gradient on which its own 'intrapleural' pressure would depend. The transmural pressure gradient has an important influence on many aspects of pulmonary function and so its horizontal stratification confers a regional difference on many features of pulmonary function, including airway closure, ventilation/per-

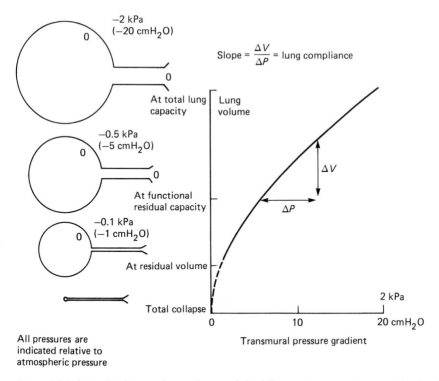

Figure 2.3 Relationship between lung volume and the difference in pressure between the alveoli and the intrathoracic space (transmural pressure gradient). The relationship approximates to linear over the normal tidal volume range. The calibre of the small air passage decreases in parallel with alveolar volume. Airways begin to close at the closing capacity (Figure 2.12) and there is widespread airway closure at residual volume, particularly in older subjects. Values in the diagram relate to the upright position.

fusion ratios and therefore gas exchange. These matters are considered in detail in the appropriate chapters of this book.

At first sight it might be thought that the subatmospheric intrapleural pressure would result in the accumulation of gas evolved from solution in blood and tissues. In fact, the total of the partial pressures of gases dissolved in blood, and therefore tissues, is always less than atmospheric (see *Table 29.2*), and this factor keeps the pleural cavity free of gas.

Time dependence of pulmonary elastic behaviour

In common with other bodies which obey Hooke's law, the lungs exhibit hysteresis. If an excised lung is rapidly inflated and then held at the new volume, the inflation pressure falls exponentially from its initial value to reach a lower level which is attained after a few seconds. This also occurs in the intact subject. Following inflation to a sustained lung volume, the pulmonary transmural pressure falls from its initial value to a new value some 20–30 per cent less than the original pressure, over the course of about a minute (Marshall and Widdicombe, 1961). It is broadly true to say that the volume change divided by the initial change in transmural pressure gradient corresponds to the dynamic compliance while the volume change

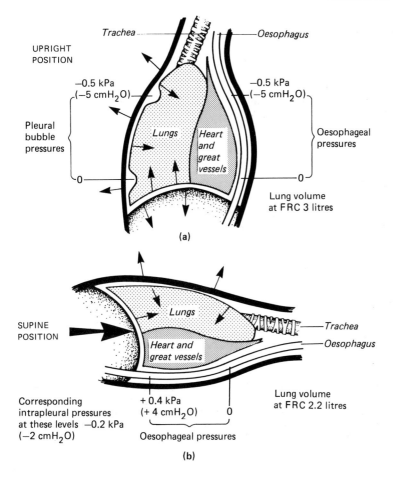

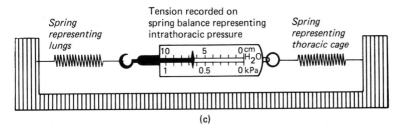

Figure 2.4 Intrathoracic pressures: static relationships in the resting end-expiratory position. The lung volume corresponds to the functional residual capacity (FRC). The figures in (a) and (b) indicate the pressure relative to ambient (atmospheric). The arrows show the direction of elastic forces. The heavy arrow in (b) indicates displacement of the abdominal viscera. In (c) the tension in the two springs is the same and will be indicated on the spring balance. In the supine position: (1) the FRC is reduced; (2) the intrathoracic pressure is raised; (3) the weight of the heart raises the oesophageal pressure above the intrapleural pressure.

divided by the ultimate change in transmural pressure gradient (i.e. measured after it has become steady) corresponds to the static compliance. Static compliance will thus be larger than the dynamic compliance by an amount determined by the degree of time-dependence in the elastic behaviour of a particular lung.

In practice static compliance is measured after a lung volume has been held for as long as is practicable, while dynamic compliance is usually measured in the course of normal rhythmic breathing. The rate of inflation usually depends on the respiratory frequency, which has been shown to influence dynamic pulmonary compliance in the normal subject (Mills, Cumming and Harris, 1963) but frequency dependence is much more pronounced in the presence of pulmonary disease (Otis et al., 1956; Channin and Tyler, 1962; Woolcock, Vincent and Macklem, 1969). The effect may be demonstrated during artificial ventilation of patients with respiratory paralysis, and Watson (1962a) found a marked increase in compliance when inspiration was prolonged from 0.5 to 1.7 seconds, but with a less marked increase on further extension to 3 seconds. Changes in the waveform of inflation pressure, on the other hand, had no detectable effect on compliance.

Hysteresis. If the lungs are slowly inflated and then slowly deflated, the pressure/ volume curve for static points during inflation differs from that obtained during deflation. The two curves form a loop which becomes progressively broader as the tidal volume is increased (*Figure 2.5*). Expressed in words, the loop in *Figure 2.5* means that rather more than the expected pressure is required during inflation and rather less than the expected recoil pressure is available during deflation. This resembles the behaviour of perished rubber or polyvinyl chloride which are reluctant to accept deformation under stress and, once deformed, are again reluctant to assume their original shape. This phenomenon is present to a greater or less extent in all elastic bodies and is known as elastic hysteresis.

Effect of recent ventilatory history. The compliance of the lung is maintained by recent rhythmic cycling with the effect being dependent on the tidal volume. Thus a period of hypoventilation without periodic deep breaths may lead to a reduction of compliance, particularly in pathological states; compliance may then be restored by one or more large breaths corresponding to sighs. This was first observed during artificial ventilation of patients with respiratory paralysis (Butler and Smith, 1957) and later during anaesthesia with artificial ventilation at rather low tidal volumes (Bendixen, Hedley-Whyte and Laver, 1963). These observations led to the introduction of artificial ventilators which periodically administer 'sighs'. There can be no doubt of the importance of periodic expansion of the lungs during prolonged artificial ventilation of diseased lungs but the case for 'sighs' during anaesthesia is less convincing, since it has no demonstrable effect on arterial Po_2 in an uncomplicated anaesthetic.

There is good evidence that compliance is reduced if the lung volume is restricted. Caro, Butler and DuBois, in 1960, demonstrated a reduction in compliance following a period of breathing within the expiratory reserve as a result of elastic strapping of the rib cage.

Causes of time dependence of pulmonary elastic behaviour

There are many possible explanations of the time dependence of pulmonary elastic behaviour, the relative importance of which may vary in different circumstances.

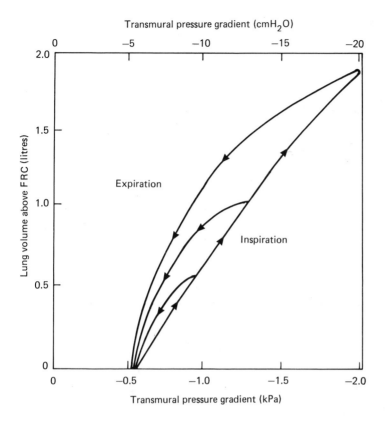

Transmural pressure gradient (cmH$_2$O)

Figure 2.5 Static plot of lung volume against transmural pressure gradient (intraoesophageal pressure relative to atmosphere at zero air flow). Note that inspiratory and expiratory curves form a loop which gets wider the greater the tidal volume. These loops are typical of elastic hysteresis. For a particular lung volume, the elastic recoil of the lung during expiration is always less than the distending transmural pressure gradient required during inspiration at the same lung volume.

Redistribution of gas. In a lung consisting of functional units with identical time constants of inflation, the distribution of gas should be independent of the rate of inflation, and there should be no redistribution when inflation is held. However, if different parts of the lungs have different time constants, the distribution of inspired gas will be dependent on the rate of inflation and redistribution will occur when inflation is held. This problem is discussed in greater detail on page 143 but for the time being we can distinguish 'fast' and 'slow' alveoli (the term 'alveoli' here referring to functional units rather than the anatomical entity). The 'fast' alveolus has a low airway resistance or low compliance (or both) while the 'slow' alveolus has a high airway resistance and/or a high compliance (*Figure 2.6b*). These properties give the fast alveolus a shorter time constant (see Appendix F) and are preferentially filled during a short inflation. This preferential filling of alveoli with low compliance gives an overall higher pulmonary transmural pressure gradient. A slow or sustained inflation permits increased distribution of gas to slow alveoli and so tends to distribute gas in accord with the compliance of the different functional units. There should then be a lower overall transmural pressure and no redistribution of gas when inflation is held. The extreme difference between fast and slow alveoli shown in *Figure 2.6b* applies to diseased lungs and no such differences exist in normal lungs. Gas redistribution is therefore unlikely to be a major factor in healthy subjects but it can be important in patients with increased airway obstruction, particularly in emphysema, asthma and chronic bronchitis. In such patients, the demonstration of frequency-dependent compliance is one of the earliest signs of an abnormality of gas distribution (Woolcock, Vincent and Macklem, 1969).

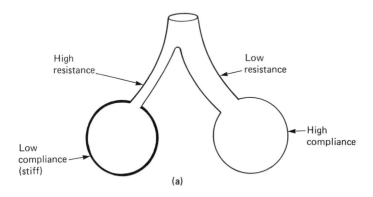

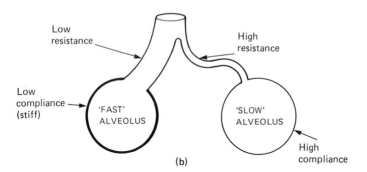

Figure 2.6 Schematic diagrams of alveoli to illustrate conditions under which static and dynamic compliances may differ. (a) Represents an idealized state which is probably not realized even in the normal subject. the reciprocal relationship between resistance and compliance results in gas flow being preferentially delivered to the most compliant regions, regardless of the rate of inflation. Static and dynamic compliance are equal. (b) Illustrates a state which is typical of many patients with respiratory disease. The alveoli can conveniently be divided into fast and slow groups. The direct relationship between compliance and resistance results in inspired gas being preferentially delivered to the stiff alveoli if the rate of inflation is rapid. An end-inspiratory pause then permits redistribution from the fast alveoli to the slow alveoli.

Recruitment of alveoli. Below a certain lung volume, some alveoli tend to close and only reopen at a considerably greater lung volume, in response to a much higher transmural pressure gradient than that at which they closed (Mead, 1961). Reopening of collapsed functional units (probably primary lobules) may be seen during re-expansion of the lung at thoracotomy.

Recruitment of closed alveoli appears at first sight to be a plausible explanation of all the time-dependent phenomena described above but there are two reasons why this is unlikely. Firstly, the pressure required for reopening a closed unit is very high and is unlikely to be achieved during normal breathing. Secondly, there is no histological evidence for collapsed alveoli in normal lungs at functional residual capacity. In the presence of pathological lung collapse, a sustained deep inflation may well cause re-expansion and an increased compliance. This is likely to occur during 'bagging' of patients on prolonged artificial ventilation, but opening and closing of alveoli during a respiratory cycle is now considered unlikely.

Changes in surfactant activity. It has been explained above that the surface tension of the alveolar lining fluid is greater at larger lung volume and also during inspiration than at the same lung volume during expiration (see *Figure 2.1b*). This is probably the most important cause of the observed hysteresis in the intact lung (see *Figure 2.5*).

Stress relaxation. If a spring is pulled out to a fixed increase in its length, the resultant tension is maximal at first and then declines exponentially to a constant value. This is an inherent property of elastic bodies, known as stress relaxation. Like hysteresis, it is minimal with metals, detectable with rubber (particularly aged rubber) and very marked with many synthetic materials such as polyvinyl chloride. Stress relaxation is also dependent on the form of the material and is, for example, present in woven nylon but scarcely detectable in monofilament nylon thread. The crinkled structure of collagen in the lung is likely to favour stress relaxation and excised strips of human lung show stress relaxation when stretched (Sugihara, Hildebrandt and Martin, 1972). The time course is of the same order as the observed changes in pressure when lungs are held inflated at constant volume, and Marshall and Widdicombe (1961) concluded that the effect was due to stress relaxation.

Influence of alveolar muscle. It is possible that sustained inflation might cause reduction in the tone of muscle fibres within the terminal airways and alveolar wall, resulting in changes similar to those of stress relaxation. Alveolar muscle is present in the alveolar wall of the cat but there is difference of opinion as to the importance of alveolar muscle in man.

Displacement of pulmonary blood. A sustained inflation might be expected to displace blood from the lungs and so to increase compliance by reducing the splinting effect of the pulmonary vasculature. The importance of this factor is not known but experiments with excised lung indicate that all the major time-dependent phenomena are present when the pulmonary vasculature is empty.

Factors affecting lung compliance

Lung volume. It is important to remember that compliance is related to lung volume (Marshall, 1957). An elephant has a much higher compliance than a mouse. This factor is most conveniently related to FRC to yield the specific compliance (i.e. compliance/FRC) which is almost constant for both sexes and all ages down to neonatal.

Posture. Lung volume changes with posture (page 39) and there are also problems in the measurement of intrapleural pressure in the supine position (page 42) When these factors are taken into account, it seems unlikely that changes of posture have any significant effect on the specific compliance.

Pulmonary blood volume. The pulmonary blood vessels probably make an appreciable contribution to the stiffness of the lung. Pulmonary venous congestion from whatever cause is associated with reduced compliance.

Age. One would have expected age to influence the elasticity of the lung as of other tissues in the body. However, Butler, White and Arnott (1957) were unable to detect any correlation between age and compliance, even after allowing for predicted changes in lung volume. This accords with the concept of lung 'elasticity' being largely determined by surface forces.

Restriction of chest expansion. Elastic strapping of the chest reduces both lung volume and compliance. However, when lung volume is returned to normal, either by removal of the restriction or by a more forceful inspiration, the compliance remains reduced. Normal compliance can be restored by taking a single deep breath (Caro, Butler and DuBois, 1960).

Recent ventilatory history. This important factor has been considered above (page 28) in relation to the time dependence of pulmonary elastic behaviour.

Disease. Important changes in lung pressure/volume relationships are found in certain lung diseases. Emphysema is unique in that *static* pulmonary compliance is increased, as a result of destruction of pulmonary tissue and loss of both elastin and surface retraction. The FRC is increased. However, distribution of inspired gas may be grossly disordered, as shown in *Figure 2.6*, and therefore the *dynamic* compliance is commonly reduced. In asthma the pressure/volume curve is displaced upwards without a change in compliance (Finucane and Colebatch, 1969). The elastic recoil is nevertheless reduced at normal transmural pressure and the FRC is therefore increased.

Most other types of pulmonary pathology result in decreased lung compliance, both static and dynamic. In particular, all forms of pulmonary fibrosis (e.g. fibrosing alveolitis), consolidation, collapse, vascular engorgement, fibrous pleurisy and especially adult respiratory distress syndrome will all reduce compliance and FRC.

Elastic recoil of the thoracic cage

An excised lung will always tend to contract until all the contained air is expelled. In contrast, when the thoracic cage is opened it tends to expand to a volume about 1 litre greater than FRC. The FRC in a paralysed patient is the volume at which the inward elastic recoil of the lungs is balanced by the outward recoil of the thoracic cage.

The thoracic cage comprises the rib cage and the diaphragm. Each is a muscular structure and can be considered as an elastic structure only when the muscles are relaxed, and that is not easy to achieve except under the conditions of paralysis. Relaxation curves have been prepared relating pressure and volumes in the supposedly relaxed subject but it is now doubtful whether true relaxation could be achieved. For example, it is now clear that the diaphragm is not fully relaxed at the end of expiration but maintains a resting tone which is abolished by anaesthesia (Muller et al., 1979). This maintains the FRC about 400 ml above the value in the paralysed or anaesthetized patient.

Compliance of the thoracic cage is defined as change in lung volume per unit change in the pressure gradient between atmosphere and the intrapleural space. The units are the same as for pulmonary compliance. The measurement is seldom made but the value is of the order of 2 l/kPa (200 ml/cmH$_2$O).

Factors influencing compliance of the thoracic cage

Anatomical factors. These factors include the ribs and the state of ossification of the costal cartilages. Obesity and even pathological skin conditions may have an appreciable effect. In particular, scarring of the skin overlying the front of the chest may result from scalding in children and this may actually embarrass the breathing.

In terms of compliance, the diaphragm simply transmits pressure from the abdomen which may be increased in obesity, abdominal distension and venous congestion. Posture clearly has a major effect and this is considered below in relation to FRC. Ferris (1952) suggested that thoracic cage compliance was 30 per cent greater in the seated subject. Lynch, Brand and Levy (1959) found the total static compliance of the respiratory system to be 60 per cent less when the subject was turned from the supine into the prone position: much of this difference is likely to be due to the diminished elasticity of the rib cage and diaphragm in the prone position.

Pressure/volume relationships of the lung plus thoracic cage

Compliance is analogous to electrical capacitance, and in the respiratory system the compliances of lungs and thoracic cage are in series. Therefore the total compliance of the system obeys the same relationship as for capacitances in series, in which reciprocals are added to obtain the reciprocal of the total value, thus:

$$\frac{1}{\text{total compliance}} = \frac{1}{\text{lung compliance}} + \frac{1}{\text{thoracic cage compliance}}$$

$$\frac{1}{0.85} = \frac{1}{1.5} + \frac{1}{2}$$

(static values for the supine paralysed patient—l/kPa)

The alternative measure of elasticity, the elastance, is far more convenient as total elastance is obtained simply by adding elastances in series:

$$\text{total elastance} = \text{lung elastance} + \text{thoracic cage elastance}$$
$$1.17 = 0.67 + 0.5$$

(corresponding values, kPa/l)

Relationship between alveolar, intrathoracic and ambient pressures

At all times the alveolar/ambient pressure gradient is the algebraic sum of the alveolar/intrathoracic (or transmural) and intrathoracic/ambient pressure gradients. This relationship is independent of whether the patient is breathing spontaneously or whether he is being ventilated by intermittent positive pressure. Actual values depend upon compliances, lung volume and posture and typical values are shown for the upright conscious relaxed subject in *Figure 2.7*, and for the supine anaesthetized and paralysed patient in *Figure 2.8*. The values in these two illustrations are static and relate to conditions when no gas is flowing.

Lung volumes

Certain lung volumes, particularly the functional residual capacity, are determined by elastic forces and this is therefore a convenient point at which to consider the various lung volumes and their subdivision (*Figure 2.9*).

Total lung capacity (TLC). This is the volume of gas in the lungs at the end of a maximal inspiration. TLC is achieved when the maximal force generated by the inspiratory muscles is balanced by the forces opposing expansion. It is rather surprising that *expiratory* muscles are contracting strongly at the end of a maximal inspiration.

Residual volume (RV). This is the volume remaining after a maximal expiration. In the young, RV is governed by the balance between the maximal force generated by expiratory muscles and the elastic forces opposing reduction of lung volume. However, in older subjects total closure of small airways may prevent further expiration.

Functional residual capacity (FRC). This is the volume at the end of a normal expiration. Within the framework of TLC, RV and FRC, other capacities and volumes shown in *Figure 2.9* are self-explanatory.

Factors affecting the FRC

So many factors affect the FRC that they require a special section of this chapter. The actual volume of the FRC has particular importance because of its relationship to the closing capacity (page 41).

Body size. FRC is linearly related to height. Estimates range from an increase in FRC of 32 ml/cm (Cotes, 1975) to 51 ml/cm (Bates, Macklem and Christie, 1971). Obesity causes a marked reduction in FRC compared with lean subjects of the same height.

Sex. For the same body height, females have an FRC about 10 per cent less than in males (Bates, Macklem and Christie, 1971).

Age. Bates, Macklem and Christie (1971) regard FRC as independent of age in the adult while Needham, Rogan and McDonald (1954) observed a slight increase in FRC with age. The nomogram of Cotes (1975) allows for a slight increase with age.

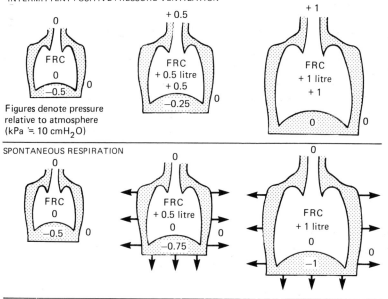

INTERMITTENT POSITIVE PRESSURE VENTILATION

Figures denote pressure
relative to atmosphere
(kPa ≈ 10 cmH₂O)

SPONTANEOUS RESPIRATION

PRESSURE/VOLUME CURVES FOR THE RELAXED OR PARALYSED SUBJECT

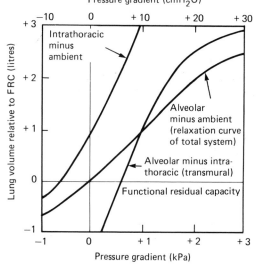

Figure 2.7 Static pressure/volume relations for the intact thorax for the conscious subject in the upright position. The transmural pressure gradient bears the same relationship to lung volume during both intermittent positive pressure ventilation and spontaneous breathing. The intrathoracic-to-ambient pressure difference, however, differs in the two types of ventilation due to muscle action during spontaneous respiration. At all times:

$$\text{alveolar/ambient pressure difference} = \text{alveolar/intrathoracic pressure difference} + \text{intrathoracic/ambient pressure difference}$$

(due attention being paid to the sign of the pressure difference). Lung compliance, 2 l/kPa (200 ml/cmH₂O); thoracic cage compliance, 2 l/kPa (200 ml/cmH₂O); total compliance, 1 l/kPa (100 ml/cmH₂O.

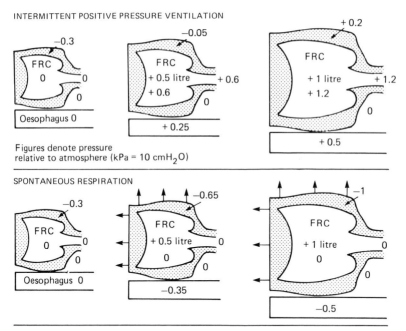

INTERMITTENT POSITIVE PRESSURE VENTILATION

−0.3

FRC
0   0
                0

Oesophagus 0

Figures denote pressure
relative to atmosphere (kPa = 10 cmH₂O)

−0.05

FRC
+ 0.5 litre   + 0.6
+ 0.6
                0

+ 0.25

+ 0.2

FRC
+ 1 litre   + 1.2
+ 1.2
                0

+ 0.5

SPONTANEOUS RESPIRATION

−0.3

FRC
0   0
                0

Oesophagus 0

−0.65

FRC
+ 0.5 litre   0
0
                0

−0.35

−1

FRC
+ 1 litre   0
0
                0

−0.5

PRESSURE/VOLUME CURVES FOR THE PARALYSED SUBJECT

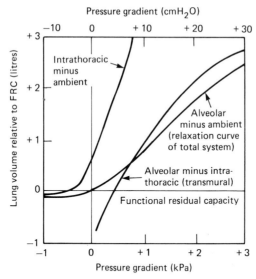

Figure 2.8 Static pressure/volume relations for the intact thorax for the anaesthetized patent in the supine position. The transmural pressure gradient bears the same relationship to lung volume during both intermittent positive pressure ventilation and spontaneous breathing. The intrathoracic-to-ambient pressure difference, however, differs in the two types of respiration due to muscle action during spontaneous respiration. At all times:

$$\frac{alveolar/ambient}{pressure~difference} = \frac{alveolar/intrathoracic}{pressure~difference} + \frac{intrathoracic/ambient}{pressure~difference}$$

(due attention being paid to the sign of the pressure difference). The oesophageal pressure is assumed to be 0.3 kPa (3 cmH₂O) higher than intrathoracic at all times. Lung compliance, 1.5 l/kPa (150 ml/cmH₂O); thoracic cage compliance, 2 l/kPa (200 ml/cmH₂O); total compliance, 0.85 l/kPa (85 ml/cmH₂O).

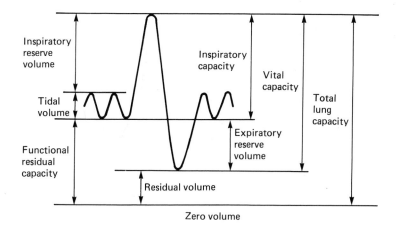

Figure 2.9 Static lung volumes. The 'spirometer curve' indicates the lung volumes which can be measured by simple spirometry. These are the tidal volume, inspiratory reserve volume, expiratory reserve volume, inspiratory capacity and vital capacity. The residual volume cannot be measured by observation of a simple spirometer trace and it is therefore impossible to measure the functional residual capacity or the total lung capacity without further elaboration of methods.

The author has pooled preoperative observations of FRC in the supine position derived from many studies (page 358) and these values indicate no correlation with age.

Diaphragmatic muscle tone. FRC has in the past been considered to be the volume at which there is a balance between the elastic forces represented by the inward retraction of the lungs and the outward expansion of the thoracic cage (pages 34 et seq.). However, as explained above, it is now clear that residual end-expiratory muscle tone is a major factor maintaining the FRC about 400 ml above the volume in the totally relaxed subject, which in practice means paralysed or anaesthetized.

Posture. Figures 2.4 and 2.10 show the reduction in FRC in the supine position, which may be attributed to the increased pressure of the abdominal contents on the diaphragm. Values of FRC in the Figures are typical for a subject of 168–170 cm height and reported mean differences between supine and upright positions range from 500 to 1000 ml. Our own observations indicate a difference of about a litre, and *Figure 2.10* shows that most of the change takes place between horizontal and 60 degrees head-up.

Lung disease. The FRC will be reduced by increased elastic recoil of the lungs, chest wall or both. Possible causes include fibrosing alveolitis, organized fibrinous pleurisy, kyphoscoliosis, obesity and scarring of the thorax following burns. Conversely, elastic recoil of the lungs is diminished in emphysema and asthma and the FRC is usually increased. This is beneficial since airway resistance decreases as the lung volume increases. In emphysema, there is an actual increase in static compliance due to loss of lung tissue. In asthma, the compliance is only marginally increased but there is an upward displacement of the transmural pressure/lung volume curve (*Figure 2.11*).

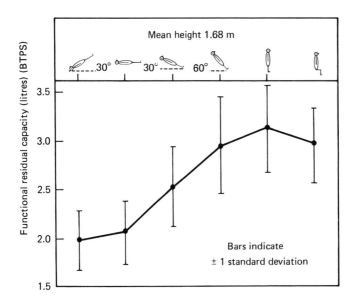

Figure 2.10 Studies by the author and his co-workers of the functional residual capacity in various body positions.

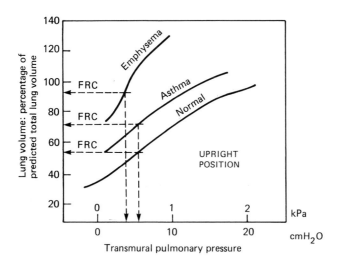

Figure 2.11 Pulmonary transmural pressure/volume plots for normal subjects, patients with asthma in bronchospasm and patients with emphysema. The broken horizontal lines indicate the FRC in each of the three groups and the corresponding point on the abscissa indicates the resting intrathoracic pressure at FRC. (Redrawn from Finucane and Colebatch, 1969)

FRC in relation to closing capacity

In Chapter 3 (page 62) it is explained how reduction in lung volume below a certain level results in airway closure with relative or total underventilation in the dependent parts of the lung. The lung volume below which this effect becomes apparent is known as the closing capacity (CC). With increasing age, CC rises until it equals FRC at about 66 years in the upright position but only 44 in the supine position (*Figure 2.12*). This is a major factor in the decrease of arterial Po_2 with age (page 270).

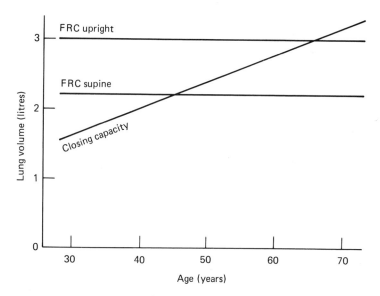

Figure 2.12 Functional residual capacity (FRC) and closing capacity as a function of age. (Redrawn from data of Leblanc et al., 1970)

Principles of measurement of compliance

Compliance is measured as the change in lung volume divided by the corresponding change in the appropriate pressure gradient, there being no gas flow when the two measurements are made. For the lung the appropriate pressure gradient is alveolar/ intrapleural (or intrathoracic) and for the total compliance alveolar/ambient. Measurement of compliance of the thoracic cage is seldom undertaken.

Volume may be measured with a spirometer, a body plethysmograph or by integration of a pneumotachogram. Points of zero air flow are best indicated by a pneumotachogram. Static pressures can be measured with a simple water manometer but electrical transducers are more usual today. Intrathoracic pressure is usually measured as oesophageal pressure which, in the upright subject, is different at different levels. The pressure rises as the balloon descends, the change being roughly in accord with the specific gravity of the lung (0.3 g/ml). It is usual to measure the pressure 32–35 cm beyond the nares, the highest point at which the measurement is free from artefacts due to mouth pressure and tracheal and neck movements (Milic-Emili et al., 1964). In the supine position the weight of the heart may introduce an artefact (see *Figure 2.4*) but there is usually a zone some 32–40 cm beyond the nares where the oesophageal pressure is close to atmospheric and probably only about 0.2 kPa (2 cmH$_2$O) above the neighbouring intrathoracic pressure. Alveolar pressure equals mouth pressure when no gas is flowing and it cannot be measured directly.

Static compliance. In the conscious subject, a known volume of air is inhaled from FRC and the subject then relaxes against a closed airway. The various pressure gradients are then measured and compared with the resting values at FRC. It is, in fact, very difficult to ensure that the respiratory muscles are relaxed, but the measurement of lung compliance is valid since the static alveolar/intrathoracic pressure difference is unaffected by any muscle activity.

In the paralysed subject there are no difficulties about muscular relaxation and it is very easy to measure static compliance of the whole respiratory system. However, due to the uncertainties about interpretation of the oesophageal pressure in the supine position (*Figure 2.4*), there is usually some uncertainty about the pulmonary compliance. Measurement of total respiratory static compliance in the paralysed patient may be made with nothing more complicated than a spirometer and a water manometer (Nims, Connor and Comroe, 1955), as shown in *Figure 2.13*.

Dynamic compliance

These measurements are made during rhythmic breathing, but compliance is calculated from pressure and volume measurements made when no gas is flowing, usually at end-inspiratory and end-expiratory 'no-flow' points. Two methods are in general use.

Loops. The required pressure gradient and the respired volume are displayed simultaneously as X and Y co-ordinates. The resultant trace forms a loop as in *Figure 2.14a*, the 'no-flow' points being where the trace is horizontal. The dynamic lung compliance is the slope of the line joining these points when the pressure gradient is ambient/intrathoracic. The area of the loop is mainly a function of airway resistance (page 69).

Multichannel recording of volume, pressure gradient and flow rate. This method differs from the one described above only in the manner of display; the principles are the same. Volume and pressure are displayed separately (*Figure 2.14b*). The volume change is derived from the volume trace and is divided by the difference in pressure at the two 'no-flow' points. In *Figure 2.14b*, these points are identified as the horizontal part of the volume trace but are more precisely indicated by a pneumotachogram which may be integrated to give volume and thereby dispense with a spirometer. This method was introduced in 1927 by von Neergaard and Wirz (1927a) and may be used for both spontaneous and artificial breathing. The calculations may conveniently be undertaken on-line with a microcomputer interfaced to the volume and pressure transducers.

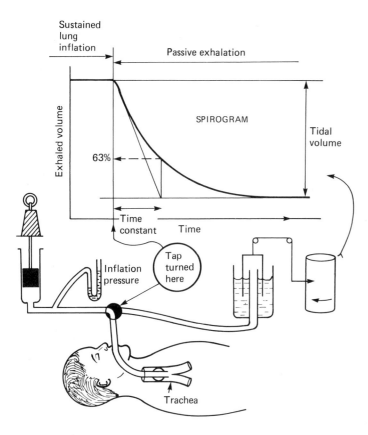

Figure 2.13 Measurement of resistance and compliance by analysis of the passive spirogram. This method is applicable only to the paralysed patient. Only a water manometer and a spirometer are required.

$$Static\ compliance = \frac{tidal\ volume}{inflation\ pressure}$$

$$Compliance \times resistance = time\ constant$$

$$Initial\ resistance = \frac{initial\ pressure\ gradient}{initial\ flow\ rate} = \frac{inflation\ pressure}{tidal\ vol./time\ constant}$$

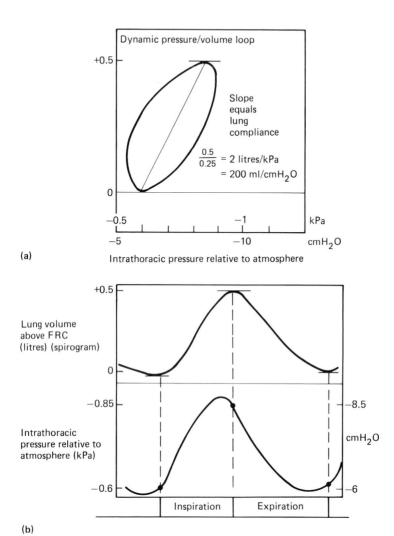

Figure 2.14 Measurement of dynamic compliance of lung by simultaneous measurement of tidal excursion (lung volume relative to FRC) and intrathoracic pressure (relative to atmosphere). In (a) these variables are displayed as the Y and X co-ordinates on a two-dimensional plotting device (e.g. cathode ray oscillograph). In (b) they are displayed simultaneously against time on a two-channel oscillograph. In each case, lung compliance is derived as lung volume change divided by transmural pressure gradient change. The transmural pressure gradient is indicated by the intrathoracic pressure (relative to atmosphere) when the lung volume is not changing. At these times the alveolar pressure must equal the atmospheric pressure since no gas is flowing. End-expiratory and end-inspiratory 'no-flow' points are indicated in (b). They correspond to horizontal parts of the loop in (a).

Principles of measurement of lung volumes

Vital capacity, tidal volume, inspiratory reserve and expiratory reserve can all be measured with a simple spirometer (see *Figure 2.9*). Total lung capacity, functional residual capacity and residual volume all contain a fraction (the residual volume) which cannot be measured by simple spirometry. However, if one of these volumes is measured (most commonly the FRC), the others can easily be derived.

Measurement of FRC

Three techniques are available. The first employs nitrogen wash-out by breathing 100% oxygen. Total quantity of nitrogen eliminated is measured as the product of the expired volume collected and the concentration of nitrogen. If, for example, 4 litres of nitrogen was collected and the initial alveolar nitrogen concentration was 80%, then the initial lung volume was 5 litres.

The second method uses the wash-in of a tracer gas such as helium, the concentration of which may be conveniently measured by catharometry (Hewlett et al., 1974a). If, for example, 50 ml of helium is introduced into the lungs and the helium concentration is then found to be 1%, the lung volume is 5 litres.

The third method uses the body plethysmograph (DuBois et al., 1956). The subject is totally contained within a gas-tight box and he attempts to breathe against an occluded airway. Changes in alveolar pressure are recorded at the mouth and compared with the small changes in lung volume, derived from pressure changes within the plethysmograph. Application of Boyle's law then permits calculation of lung volume. This method would include trapped gas which might not be registered by the two previous methods.

Measurement of closing capacity is considered on page 71.

$$4L = EV \times 80$$

Chapter 3

Resistance to gas flow and airway closure

Excessive resistance to gas flow is the commonest and most important cause of ventilatory failure. Severe obstruction to breathing is life threatening and may arise anywhere from the smallest airways, through the tracheobronchial tree, larynx and pharynx to include external factors and any apparatus through which the patient may be breathing.

Gas flows from a region of high pressure to one of lower pressure. The rate at which it does so is a function of the pressure difference and the resistance to gas flow (*Figure 3.1*). The precise relationship between pressure difference and flow rate depends on the nature of the flow which may be laminar, turbulent or a mixture of the two. It is useful to consider laminar and turbulent flow as two separate entities but mixed patterns of flow usually occur in the respiratory tract.

Laminar flow

Characteristics of laminar flow

Below its critical flow rate, gas flows along a straight unbranched tube as a series of concentric cylinders which slide over one another, with the peripheral cylinder stationary and the central cylinder moving fastest (*Figure 3.2*). This is also termed streamline flow and is characteristically inaudible. Gas sampled from the periphery of a tube during laminar flow may not be representative of gas of a different composition advancing down the centre of the tube.

The advancing cone front means that some fresh gas will reach the end of a tube while the volume entering the tube is still less than the volume of the tube. In the context of the respiratory tract, this is to say that there may be a significant alveolar ventilation when the tidal volume is less than the anatomical dead space, a fact which was noted by Rohrer in 1915 and is very relevant to high frequency ventilation (page 406). For the same reason, laminar flow is relatively inefficient for purging the contents of a tube.

Quantitative relationships during laminar flow

With laminar flow, the gas flow rate is directly proportional to the driving pressure (*Figure 3.2*), the constant being resistance to gas flow, thus:

$$\text{pressure difference} = \text{flow rate} \times \text{resistance}$$

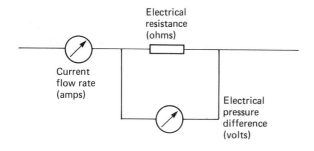

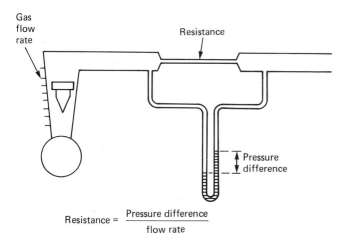

$$Resistance = \frac{Pressure\ difference}{flow\ rate}$$

Figure 3.1 Electrical analogy of gas flow. Resistance is pressure difference per unit flow rate. Resistance to gas flow is analogous to electrical resistance (provided that flow is laminar). Gas flow corresponds to electrical current (amps); gas pressure corresponds to potential (volts); gas flow resistance corresponds to electrical resistance (ohms); Poiseuille's law corresponds to Ohm's law.

Note the parallel with Ohm's law (see *Figure 3.1*):

$$potential\ difference = current \times resistance$$

For gas flow in a straight unbranched tube, the value for resistance is:

$$\frac{8 \times length \times viscosity}{\pi \times (radius)^4}$$

In this rearrangement of the Hagen–Poiseuille equation, the direct relationship between flow and the fourth power of the radius of the tube explains the critical importance of narrowing of air passages, as well as in the choice of an appropriate cannula for an intravenous infusion.

Viscosity is the only property of a gas which is relevant under conditions of laminar flow. Helium has a low density but a viscosity close to that of air. Helium will not therefore improve gas flow if the flow is laminar. This is not a practical problem since flow is usually turbulent when resistance to breathing becomes a problem.

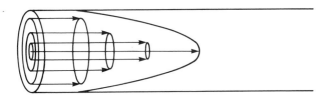

(a)

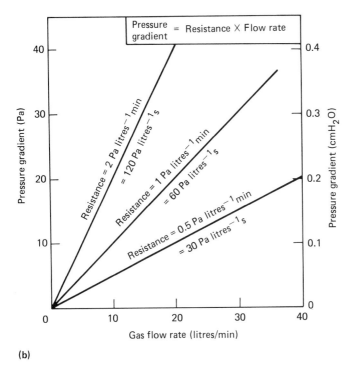

(b)

Figure 3.2 Laminar flow. (a) Laminar gas flow down a straight tube as a series of concentric cylinders of gas with the central cylinder moving fastest. This gives rise to a 'cone front' when the composition of the gas is abruptly changed as it enters the tube. (b) The linear relationship between gas flow rate and pressure gradient. The slope of the lines indicates the resistance (1 Pa $\doteqdot$ 0.01 cmH$_2$O).

In the Hagen–Poiseuille equation, the units must be coherent. In CGS units, dyn/cm^2 (pressure), ml/s (flow) and cm (length and radius) are compatible with the unit of poise for viscosity (dyn sec cm^{-2}). In SI units, with pressure in kilopascals, the unit of viscosity is newton second metre^{-2} (see Appendix A).

It is sometimes convenient to refer to conductance, which is the reciprocal of resistance and might, for example, be expressed as l/s per cmH$_2$O. Specific airway conductance (s.G$_{aw}$) is the conductance of the lower airways divided by the lung volume (Lehane, Jordan and Jones, 1980). Since it takes into account the effect of lung volume (page 64) it is a convenient measure of bronchomotor tone.

Turbulent flow

Characteristics of turbulent flow

High flow rates, particularly through branched or irregular tubes, result in a breakdown of the orderly flow of gas described above as laminar. An irregular movement is superimposed on the general progression along the tube (*Figure 3.3*),

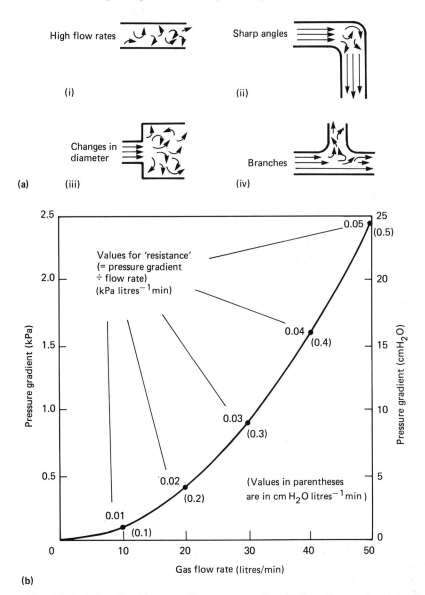

Figure 3.3 Turbulent flow. (a) Four circumstances under which gas flow tends to be turbulent. (b) The square law relationship between gas flow rate and pressure gradient when flow is turbulent. Note that the value for 'resistance', calculated as for laminar flow, is quite meaningless during turbulent flow.

with a square front replacing the cone front of laminar flow. Turbulent flow is often audible and is almost invariably present when high resistance to gas flow is a problem.

The square front means that no fresh gas can reach the end of a tube until the amount of gas entering the tube is almost equal to the volume of the tube. Conversely, turbulent flow is more effective than laminar flow in purging the contents of a tube. Turbulent flow provides the best conditions for drawing a representative sample of gas from the periphery of a tube.

Quantitative relationships during turbulent flow

The relationship between driving pressure and flow rate differs from the relationship described above for laminar flow in three important respects:

1. The driving pressure is proportional to the square of the required gas flow rate.
2. The driving pressure is proportional to the density of the gas and is independent of its viscosity.
3. The required driving pressure is, in theory, inversely proportional to the fifth power of the radius of the tube (Fanning equation).

The square law relating driving pressure and flow rate is shown in *Figure 3.3*. Resistance, defined as pressure gradient divided by flow rate, is not constant as in laminar flow but increases in proportion to the flow rate. It is thus meaningless to use the Ohm's law concept of resistance when flow is turbulent or partly turbulent, and units such as cmH_2O per l/s should be used only when flow is entirely laminar. The following methods of quantification of 'resistance' should be used when flow is totally or partially turbulent.

Two constants. This method considers resistance as comprising two components, one for laminar flow and the other for turbulent flow. The simple relationship for laminar flow given above would then be extended as follows:

$$\text{pressure difference} = k_1 \text{ (flow)} + k_2 \text{ (flow)}^2$$

k_1 contains the factors of the Hagen–Poiseuille equation while k_2 includes factors in the corresponding equation for turbulent flow. Mead and Agostoni (1964) summarized studies of normal human subjects in the following equation:

$$\text{pressure gradient (kPa)} = 0.24 \text{ (flow)} + 0.03 \text{ (flow)}^2$$

or

$$\text{pressure gradient (cmH}_2\text{O)} = 2.4 \text{ (flow)} + 0.3 \text{ (flow)}^2$$

The exponent ^{n}. Over a surprisingly wide range of flow rates, the equation above may be condensed into the following single-term expression with little loss of precision:

$$\text{pressure gradient} = K \text{ (flow)}^n$$

The exponent ^{n} has a value ranging from 1 with purely laminar flow to 2 with purely turbulent flow, the value of ^{n} being a useful indication of the nature of the flow. The constants for the normal human respiratory tract are:

$$\text{pressure gradient (kPa)} = 0.24 \text{ (flow)}^{1.3}$$

or

$$\text{pressure gradient (cmH}_2\text{O)} = 2.4 \, (\text{flow})^{1.3}$$

The graphical method. It is often most convenient to represent 'resistance' as a graph of pressure difference against gas low rate, on either linear or logarithmic co-ordinates. Logarithmic co-ordinates have the advantage that the plot is usually a straight line whether flow is laminar, turbulent or mixed, and the slope of the line indicates the value of ^{n} in the equation above.

Reynolds' number

In the case of long straight unbranched tubes, the nature of the gas flow may be predicted from the value of Reynolds' number, which is a non-dimensional quantity derived from the following expression:

$$\frac{\text{linear velocity of gas} \times \text{tube diameter} \times \text{gas density}}{\text{gas viscosity}}$$

When Reynolds' number is less than 1000, flow is laminar. Above a value of 1500, flow is entirely turbulent. Between these values, both types of flow coexist. *Figure 3.4* shows the nature of the gas flow for three different gas mixtures in terms of gas flow rate and diameter of tube. It will be seen that mixed flow patterns will often be present under conditions which are likely to occur in the clinical situation.

The property of the gas which affects Reynolds' number is the ratio of density to viscosity. Values for some gas mixtures that a patient may inhale are shown relative to air in *Table 3.1*. Viscosities of respirable gases do not differ greatly but there may be very large differences in density. Note that use of a less dense gas such as helium not only reduces resistance during turbulent flow but also renders turbulent flow less likely to occur.

Table 3.1 Physical properties of anaesthetic gas mixtures relating to gas flow

	Viscosity relative to air	Vapour density relative to air	Vapour density / Viscosity relative to air
Oxygen	1.11	1.11	1.00
70% N_2O/30% O_2	0.89	1.41	1.59
80% He/20% O_2	1.08	0.33	0.31

Threshold resistors

Certain resistors are designed to allow no gas to pass until a threshold pressure is reached. Once that pressure is reached, gas passes freely with little further rise in pressure as the flow rate increases.

The classic prototype threshold resistor is the Starling valve (*Figure 3.5*). Gas will flow only when the upstream pressure exceeds the threshold pressure. A similar effect may be obtained with a properly designed spring-loaded valve or by exhalation

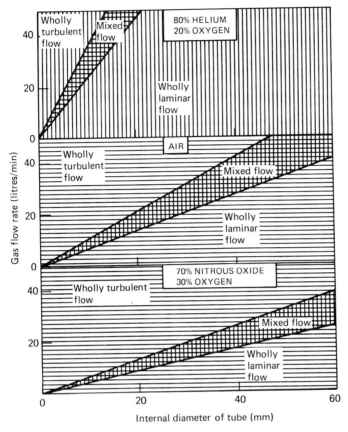

Figure 3.4 Graphs to show the nature of the gas flow through tubes of various diameters for three different gas mixtures; 25 l/min is a typical peak flow rate during spontaneous respiration. It will be seen that the nature of flow in the trachea and in endotracheal tubes will be markedly dependent on the composition of the gas mixture.

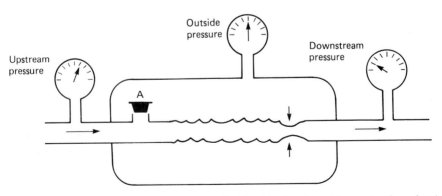

Figure 3.5 The Starling resistor consists of a length of flaccid collapsible tubing passing through a rigid box. When the pressure outside the collapsible tubing exceeds the upstream pressure, the tubing collapses where shown by the arrows. No gas can flow, whatever the level of the downstream pressure. If the orifice A is opened, the outside pressure rises with the upstream pressure and so limits flow rate to a level which is independent of the magnitude of the upstream pressure. The relevance of this to effort-independent expiratory flow rate is considered on page 59. The relevance of the Starling resistor to the pulmonary capillary circulation is considered on page 130.

through a prescribed depth of water. Although such valves are now extensively used for application of positive end-expiratory pressure (PEEP), they are not new and have long been used as safety valves for boilers and pressure cookers.

Besides acting as a simple threshold resistor, the Starling valve has other special properties. Once gas is flowing, an increase in downstream pressure will distend the tubing and so decrease the resistance of the device. However, a decreased downstream pressure cannot initiate flow. These properties make the Starling resistor a model for important aspects of the behaviour of pulmonary blood vessels (page 130) and the air passages, the latter being considered later in this chapter under flow-related airway collapse.

Minor sources of resistance to gas flow

The major non-elastic component of the total resistance to breathing is the airway resistance to gas flow described above. However, with special methods of measurement, it is also possible to detect certain additional minor sources of resistance. Lung tissue offers a small frictional resistance to deformation. This is probably less than a fifth of the airway resistance in the normal subject but may be increased in pathological conditions such as pulmonary oedema, hyaline membrane disease and pulmonary fibrosis. The thoracic cage and abdominal contents offer a further frictional resistance to deformation but this is difficult to measure. Respired gases, the lungs and the thoracic cage all have inertia and therefore offer an impedance to change in direction of gas flow, analogous to electrical inductance. This component, which is termed 'inertance', is usually negligible.

When the components listed in the last paragraph are included, the total resistance is generally termed the *pulmonary resistance*, to distinguish it from *airway resistance* which is the quantity most commonly measured.

Increased airway resistance

Four grades of increased airway resistance may be identified.

Grade 1. Slight resistance is that against which the patient can indefinitely sustain a normal alveolar ventilation.

Grade 2. Moderate resistance is that against which a considerable increase in work of breathing is required to avoid a decrease in alveolar ventilation, with deterioration of arterial gas tensions. Patients vary in their response. Some increase their work of breathing, exhibiting obvious dyspnoea but maintaining normal arterial blood gas tensions. Others do not increase their work of breathing sufficiently to avoid an increase in arterial P_{CO_2} and a decrease in arterial P_{O_2}. They may not appear dyspnoeic and their hypercapnia may be overlooked. In the case of chronic obstructive lung disease the former group are known as 'pink puffers' and the latter as 'blue bloaters' (page 384).

Grade 3. Severe resistance is that against which no patient is able to preserve his alveolar ventilation. The increase in the arterial P_{CO_2} is the best indication of the gravity of the situation (see Chapter 20).

Grade 4. Respiratory obstruction may be defined as an increase in airway resistance which is incompatible with life.

Causes of increased airway resistance

As in obstruction of other biological systems, it is helpful to think in terms of conducting tubes being blocked by:

1. Material within the lumen.
2. Thickening or contraction of the wall of the passage.
3. Pressure from outside the air passage.

External apparatus

Severe or lethal increases in airway resistance may arise in apparatus through which a patient is breathing. Tracheal tubes or tracheostomies usually offer resistance which is higher than that of the normal respiratory tract. During artificial ventilation this is of little consequence as the work of breathing is undertaken by either the anaesthetist or a machine. Furthermore, during spontaneous breathing it appears that the anaesthetized patient can usually increase his work of breathing to overcome quite large increases in resistance (Nunn and Ezi-Ashi, 1961). The position is very different when massive increase in resistance arises due, for example, to kinked endotracheal tubes or blocked valves. The situation is then extremely serious and fatalities have occurred.

The pharynx and larynx

The lumen may be blocked with foreign material such as gastric contents or blood. The walls may contract as in laryngeal spasm or the tongue may fall back onto the posterior pharyngeal wall as a result of relaxation of the genioglossus muscle (see *Figure 1.2*). This usually occurs during anaesthesia (page 357) and coma, and often in REM sleep in elderly patients (page 306) in whom it may result in hypoventilation and periods of hypoxaemia, often severe.

Apart from laryngospasm, obstruction may occur in the larynx from carcinoma, diphtheria, and cricoid and subcricoid oedema. Provided the patient remains calm, he can withstand surprisingly high resistance. However, once he is alarmed and starts to struggle, he may enter a vicious cycle of raised oxygen consumption, increased ventilatory demand and increased work of breathing leading to a further increase in oxygen consumption which cannot be met.

Bronchospasm

In this section it is convenient to include other aspects of bronchial hyper-reactivity, including mucosal oedema, mucus plugging and epithelial desquamation. Increased airway obstruction from these causes is a major feature of asthma and other conditions featuring airway hyper-reactivity as well as the response to various drugs, toxic substances and irritants. The section is summarized in *Figure 3.6*.

Parasympathetic system. This system is of major importance in the control of bronchomotor tone (see review by Boushey et al., 1980). Afferents arise from

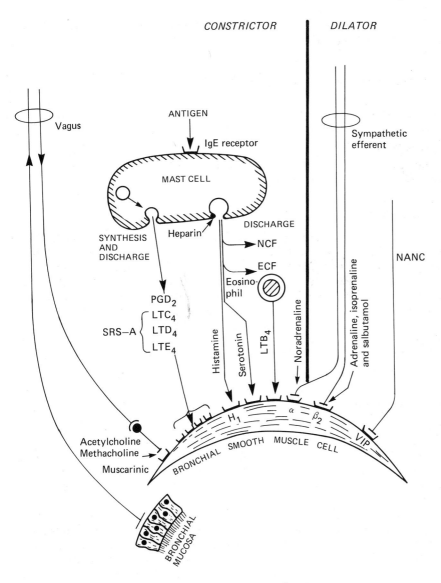

Figure 3.6 Factors influencing bronchomotor tone. For explanation, see text.

receptors under the tight junctions of the bronchial epithelium and pass centrally in the vagus. The system responds to a great number of noxious stimuli, and histamine also acts directly on the parasympathetic afferents in addition to its direct action on airway smooth muscle. Efferent preganglionic fibres also run in the vagus to ganglia located in the walls of the small bronchi. Thence, short postganglionic fibres lead to nerve endings which release acetylcholine to act at muscarinic receptors in the bronchial smooth muscle. This system is functionally very important. Stimulation of any part of the reflex arc results in bronchoconstriction, and some degree of resting tone is normally present. The muscarinic receptors can be stimulated with methacholine and blocked with atropine. The parasympathetic reflex arc plays a major part in the bronchoconstrictor response to inhaled irritants.

Sympathetic system. In contrast to the parasympathetic system, the sympathetic system is poorly represented in the lung and not yet proven to be of major importance in man (Boushey et al., 1980). Bronchial smooth muscle has β_2-adrenergic receptors on which noradrenaline has little effect. Beta blockers may cause mild bronchoconstriction in healthy subjects but most investigators have found little effect. However, they may cause severe bronchoconstriction in asthmatics and some bronchitics, also resulting in insensitivity to beta stimulators.

Non-adrenergic non-cholinergic (NANC) system. It has recently become apparent that the airways are provided with a third autonomic nerve system which is neither adrenergic nor cholinergic. The efferent fibres run in the vagus and pass to the smooth muscle of the airway where the neurotransmitter is probably vasoactive intestinal polypeptide (VIP). Stimulation of NANC efferents or administration of VIP will both cause prolonged relaxation of bronchi but the clinical significance of this system is not yet fully established (Barnes, 1984).

The mast cell. Mast cells are plentiful in the walls of airways and alveoli and also lie free in the lumen of the airways where they may be recovered by bronchial lavage. The surface of the mast cell contains a very large number of binding sites for the Fc portion of the immunoglobulin IgE. Activation of the cell results from antigen bridging only a small number of these antibodies. The triggering mechanism is thus extremely sensitive. Activation may also be initiated by a wide range of compounds, including the complement fractions C3a, C4a and C5a and many drugs and other organic molecules.

In many respects basophils behave like mast cells, both in their activation and in the pattern of their response. However, it is not certain that all aspects of the response occur in all mast cells and there may be different cell types with specialized functions.

The earliest events after activation are probably increases in cyclic AMP (cAMP) and in intracellular calcium ions. Activation increases the activity of the membrane-bound enzyme adenylate cyclase which converts ATP into cAMP, which is thought to act as a second messenger although its precise role is still unclear (Robinson and Holgate, 1985).

The rise in intracellular calcium is due to the opening of calcium channels resulting in a rapid entry of calcium into the cell. This effect can be inhibited by calcium channel blockers, and nifedipine and verapamil have been found to diminish bronchoconstriction in certain circumstances, although these drugs may also be acting at other sites, including the bronchial smooth muscle itself (Fanta and Drazen, 1983). However, these authors conclude that, on present evidence, it seems unlikely that the currently available calcium channel blockers will have a major role in the treatment of acute bronchospasm.

The next stage in mast cell activation is unclear although it is probable that it depends upon the interaction of calcium and the protein calmodulin. Whatever the mechanism, two separate events follow the calcium entry. Firstly, within 30 seconds of activation, there is discharge of a range of preformed mediators associated with the granules (*Table 3.2*). These granules are in effect phagolysosomes containing a a wide array of inflammatory mediators (Robinson and Holgate, 1985). The most

Table 3.2 Mediators released from mast cells

Preformed mediators
Histamine
Heparin (probably not released)
Serotonin
Lysosomal enzymes:
  Tryptase
  Arylsulphatase
  Galactosidase
  Glucuronidase
  Hexosaminidase
  Carboxypeptidase
Neutrophil chemotactic factor
Eosinophil chemotactic factor

Mediators synthesized after activation
Prostaglandin D_2
Slow-reacting substance, comprising:
  LTC_4
  LTD_4
  LTE_4
Platelet-activating factor

---

widely studied constituent is histamine, which acts directly on H_1 receptors in the bronchial smooth muscle fibres to cause contraction. It also stimulates mucus secretion and increases vascular permeability, causing mucosal oedema. The histamine is associated with heparin but the heparin in the granules is not released and remains associated with the membrane of the mast cell. The granules also contain proteases, mainly tryptase, which detach epithelium from the basement membrane resulting in desquamation. Amongst other constitutents are serotonin and chemotactic factors for both neutrophils and eosinophils.

The second major event after mast cell activation is the initiation of synthesis of arachidonic acid derivatives. This begins with progressive methylation of phosphatidyl ethanolamine by S-adenosyl methionine. This yields arachidonic acid which is then metabolized along two main pathways, catalysed respectively by cyclooxygenase and lipoxygenase. In the mast cell, the most important derivative of the former pathway is prostaglandin PGD_2, which is a bronchoconstrictor, although its clinical significance is not yet clear. The lipoxygenase pathway results in the formation of three leukotrienes, LTC_4, LTD_4 and LTE_4, formerly known collectively as slow-reacting substance (SRS-A) until the constituents were identified (Morris et al., 1980). These leukotrienes cause a slow but sustained contraction of bronchial muscle, which can be inhibited by indomethacin.

Neutrophil and eosinophil. Mast cell granules contain chemotactic factors for both these cells (NCF and ECF in *Figure 3.6*), and this effect is reinforced by histamine. As these cells accumulate in the vicinity of the bronchial musculature, they make their own contribution to bronchoconstriction, particularly through LTB_4 from eosinophils, while neutrophils contribute to proteolytic damage. Neutrophils may also release oxygen-derived free radicals (page 487) and it may be noted that mast cell granules contain superoxide dismutase. It will be clear that the full mast cell response has much in common with the inflammatory reaction.

Bronchial muscle receptors (see *Figure 3.6*). The main bronchodilator receptor is the β_2-adrenergic receptor, which is sensitive to circulating adrenaline and also to therapeutically administered isoprenaline and salbutamol. Activation of this receptor results in conversion of ATP to cAMP by the membrane-bound and coupled enzyme adenylate cyclase. The level of cAMP controls the degree of relaxation of the bronchial smooth muscle. Cyclic AMP is converted to 5'AMP by the enzyme phosphodiesterase which is inhibited by theophylline, the active component of the well tried preparation aminophylline. However, inhibition of phosphodiesterase occurs only at concentrations greatly in excess of those at which theophylline is an effective bronchodilator. Mackay, Baldwin and Tattersfield (1983) have presented evidence for believing that theophylline causes bronchodilatation by more than one mechanism, of which catecholamine release is one. In addition, it may block histamine release from the mast cell and it may also affect calcium entry. Furthermore, theophylline probably blocks the bronchoconstrictor effect of adenosine in asthmatics (Cushley, Tattersfield and Holgate, 1984) and also appears to drive the diaphragm, even in the long term (Murciano et al., 1984).

There are numerous bronchoconstrictor receptors, of which the H_1 histamine receptor and the muscarinic receptors are the most important, the latter being sensitive not only to the neurotransmitter acetylcholine but also to parasympathomimetic drugs such as methacholine. Serotonin and α-adrenergic receptors are also bronchoconstrictor. The former can be blocked with ketanserin.

External factors. Many external factors can initiate bronchoconstriction by stimulation of vagal afferents. Some of these are physical and include mechanical stimulation of the upper air passages by laryngoscopy or the presence of foreign bodies in the trachea. Inhalation of cold air is a potent stimulus and can be used as a provocation test (Heaton, Henderson and Costello, 1984). Inhalation of particulate matter or even an aerosol of water will cause bronchoconstriction. An aerosol of histamine produces part of its effect by stimulation of vagal afferents.

Many chemical stimuli result in bronchoconstriction. Gases include suphur dioxide, ozone and nitrogen dioxide. Liquids with a pH of less than about 2.5 provoke Mendelson's syndrome (1946), of which bronchoconstriction is a prominent feature in the early stages.

A great many drugs will activate the mast cell. This may follow sensitization of the cell but may also occur when a drug is first administered. Several drugs used by anaesthetists have this effect as a rare though frightening complication. Particular problems have occurred with *d*-tubocurarine, suxamethonium and Althesin (this last now withdrawn). In some cases the drug responsible for the reaction may be identified by skin testing, undertaken with care since this procedure may initiate bronchospasm. Splitting of complement C3 into C3a and C3b may be demonstrated soon after injection and the peripheral leucocyte count may decrease because of margination. The reaction usually occurs within a minute of administration and there is sometimes a temporary loss of pulsation in major vessels. This is usually transient and is presumably due to sudden vasodilation. Alarming though this response may be, the mortality is apparently low and not a single case features in the report of Lunn and Mushin (1982) on anaesthetic mortality.

Hyper-reactive airways. Asthmatics, some patients with chronic bronchitis and others exhibit exaggerated responses to a wide variety of the factors which can cause bronchoconstriction (Boushey et al., 1980). This may be demonstrated with provocation tests using histamine, methacholine or cold air. There is no single cause of the condition and possible factors include a reduction in resting airway calibre (considered below), autonomic imbalance, increased sensitivity of the mast cell and an increased responsiveness of the airway smooth muscle. Hyper-reactive airways may be considered an essential precursor and feature of asthma.

Resting calibre of the airways. In the healthy subject, the small airways make only a small contribution to total airway resistance because their aggregate cross-sectional area increases to very large values after about the eighth generation (see *Figure 1.4*). However, they are the site of most of the important causes of obstruction in a range of pathological conditions, including chronic bronchitis, emphysema, bronchiectasis, cystic fibrosis, asthma and bronchiolitis (Macklem, 1971). These airways have been termed the 'quiet zone' because they must undergo a considerable increase in their resistance before the change can be detected by tests of overall airway resistance which is dominated by the resistance of the larger airways. Once their calibre is reduced sufficiently to exert a significant effect on airway resistance, then further small changes in calibre have a major effect due to the relationship between flow and fourth or fifth power of the radius (pages 47 et seq.).

Flow-related airway collapse

All the airways can be compressed by reversal of the normal transmural pressure gradient to a sufficiently high level. The cartilaginous airways have considerable structural resistance to collapse but even the trachea may be compressed with an external pressure in the range 5–7 kPa (50–70 cmH_2O) and this may result from neoplasm or haemorrhage. Airways beyond generation 11 have no structural rigidity (see *Table 1.1*) and rely instead on the traction on their walls which arises from elastic recoil of the lung tissue in which they are embedded. They can be collapsed by a reversed transmural pressure gradient which is considerably less than that which closes the cartilaginous airways.

Reversal of the transmural pressure gradient may be caused by high levels of air flow during expiration. The mechanism is shown in *Figure 3.7*. During expiration, the resistance to gas flow in the smaller air passages results in a pressure gradient between the alveoli and the larger air passages. However, during normal breathing (*Figure 3.7b* and *c*), the pressure in the lumen of the air passages should always remain well above the subatmospheric pressure in the thorax, and the positive transmural pressure gradient should ensure that all the airways remain patent.

During a maximal forced expiration (*Figure 3.7d*), the intrathoracic pressure will be raised well above atmospheric. This pressure will be transmitted to the alveoli which preserve their normal transmural pressure gradient due to their own elastic recoil. However, at high gas flow rates, the pressure drop down the airways is increased and there will be a point at which airway pressure equals the intrathoracic pressure. At that point (the equal pressure point) the smaller air passages are held open only by the elastic recoil of the lung parenchyma in which they are embedded or, if it occurs in the larger airways, by their structural rigidity. Downstream of the equal pressure point, the transmural pressure gradient is reversed and at some point may overcome the forces holding the airways open, resulting in airway collapse. This effect is also influenced by lung volume (see below) and the equal pressure point moves progressively down towards the smaller airways as lung volume is decreased.

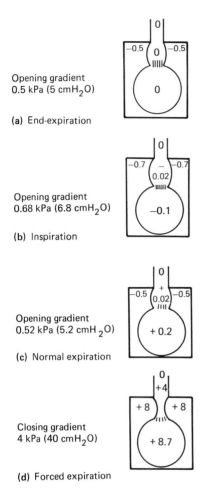

Opening gradient
0.5 kPa (5 cmH₂O)

(a) End-expiration

Opening gradient
0.68 kPa (6.8 cmH₂O)

(b) Inspiration

Opening gradient
0.52 kPa (5.2 cmH₂O)

(c) Normal expiration

Closing gradient
4 kPa (40 cmH₂O)

(d) Forced expiration

Figure 3.7 Typical transmural pressure gradients of the intrathoracic air passages under various conditions of ventilation. Note the pressure drop occurring in the smallest air passages, leading to a pressure difference between the alveoli and the larger air passages. (a) Static pressures at the end of expiration (upright, conscious subject). (b) Pressures at the middle of a normal inspiration. Note the increased favourable transmural pressure gradient of the intrathoracic airway. (c) Pressures at the middle of a normal expiration. Note the decreased (but still favourable) transmural pressure gradient of the intrathoracic airway. (d) Typical pressures during a forced expiration. Note the unfavourable transmural pressure gradient of the intrathoracic airway—leading to collapse.

Flow-related collapse occurs in the larger bronchi during a forced expiration and limits the flow rate. It also accounts for the brassy note which is heard. During coughing, the reduction in calibre of the bronchi increases the velocity of air flow, thereby improving the scavenging of secretions from the walls of the air passages (Clarke, Jones and Oliver, 1970). Expiratory narrowing of the bronchi can be clearly seen at bronchoscopy.

Flow-related collapse of the smaller air passages occurs more easily in certain pathological states, particularly emphysema and asthma, in which it accounts for the phenomenon known as trapping. In emphysema, this is mainly due to destruction of lung parenchyma, resulting in loss of the elastic recoil which normally holds these airways open. Loss of parenchyma occurs particularly in patients with α_1-antitrypsin deficiency. In asthma, there is high bronchomotor tone and mucosal oedema which augments forces tending to collapse the air passages. Furthermore, the increased airway resistance augments the pressure drop along the airways, so facilitating the reversal of the transmural pressure gradient (*Figure 3.7*).

These effects are best demonstrated on a flow/volume plot. *Figure 3.8* shows

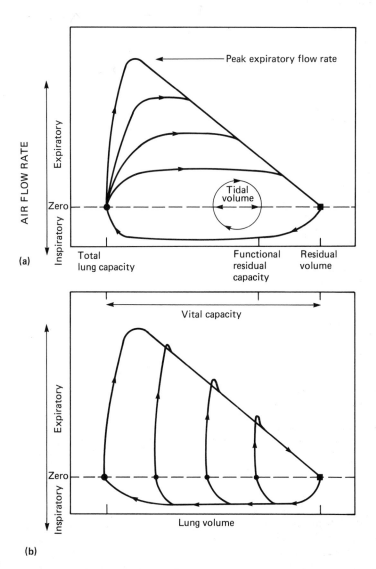

Figure 3.8 Normal flow/volume curves. Instantaneous air flow rate (ordinate) is plotted against lung volume (abscissa). (a) The normal tidal excursion is shown as the small loop. In addition, expirations from total lung capacity at four levels of expiratory effort are shown. Within limits, peak expiratory flow rate is dependent on effort but, during the latter part of expiration, all curves converge on an effort-independent section where flow rate is limited by airway collapse. (b) The effect of forced expirations from different lung volumes. The pips above the effort-independent section probably represent air expelled from collapsed airways.

the normal relationship between lung volume on the abscissa and instantaneous respiratory flow rate on the ordinate. Time is not directly indicated. In part (a) of the Figure the small loop shows a normal tidal excursion above FRC and with air flow rate either side of zero. Arrows show the direction of the trace. At the end of a maximal expiration the black square indicates residual volume. The lower part of the large curve then shows the course of a maximal inspiration to TLC (black circle). There follow four expiratory curves, each with different expiratory effort and each attaining a different peak expiratory flow rate. Within limits, the greater the effort, the greater is the resultant peak flow rate. However, all the expiratory curves terminate in a final common pathway which is independent of effort. In this part of the curves, the flow rate is limited by airway collapse and the maximal air flow rate is governed by the lung volume (abscissa). The greater the effort the greater the degree of airway collapse and the resultant gas flow rate remains the same. The relationship between inspiratory lung volume and peak flow rate is shown in *Figure 3.8b*. It clearly shows the importance of a maximal inspiration before measurement of peak expiratory flow rate.

Figure 3.9a shows the typical appearance of the flow volume curve in a patient with obstructive airway disease. Residual volume is commonly increased, for reasons explained in the following section, and vital capacity is decreased. Inspiration is relatively normal but a forced expiration is characterized by a peak flow which is diminished in both rate and duration, giving rise to a typically boot-shaped curve. Various simple bedside tests indicate this state of affairs. The forced expiratory volume in 1 second (FEV_1) is the most reliable of the simple tests but the peak flow rate is more convenient to measure. Large airway obstruction (due, for example, to carcinoma of the larynx) also results in a reduced FEV_1 and peak flow rate but the shape of the flow/volume curve is quite different (*Figure 3.9b*).

Volume-related airway collapse

It has already been pointed out in relation to *Figure 3.8* that expiratory flow rate is, under some circumstances, related to lung volume. When the lung volume is reduced, there is a proportional reduction in the volume of all air-containing components, including the air passages. Thus, if other factors such as bronchomotor tone remain constant, airway resistance is an inverse function of lung volume (*Figure 3.10*).

The closing capacity. In addition to the overall effect on airway resistance shown in *Figure 3.10*, there are most important regional differences. This is because the airways and alveoli in the dependent parts of the lungs are always smaller than those at the top of the lung except at total lung capacity when all are the same size (*Figure 3.11*). As the lung volume is reduced towards residual volume, there is a point at which dependent airways begin to close, and the lung volume at which this occurs is known as the closing capacity (CC) (*Figure 3.12*). The alternative term, 'closing volume' (CV), equals the closing capacity minus the residual volume (RV).

Closing capacity is less than FRC in young adults but increases with age to become equal to FRC at a mean age of 44 years in the supine position and 66 years in the upright position (see *Figure 2.12*). When the tidal range is wholly or partly within the closing capacity, some of the pulmonary blood flow will be distributed to inadequately ventilated parts of the lung. The closing capacity appears to be

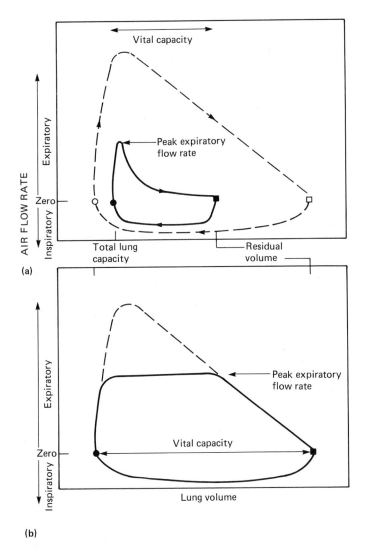

Figure 3.9 (a) A flow/volume curve which is typical of a patient with obstructive airway disease of the smaller air passages. Note the diminished vital capacity and flattening of the effort-independent sector of the curve (compared with the broken curve which shows the normal). The expiratory curve is characteristically concave upwards. (b) The cut-off of high flow rates which is characteristic of upper airway obstruction (e.g. due to carcinoma of the larynx). The plateau is highly effort-dependent.

independent of body position but the FRC changes markedly with position (see *Figure 2.10*).

Shunting of blood through areas of the lung with closed airways is an important cause of decreasing arterial PO_2 with increasing age (page 270) and changes of position (page 360).

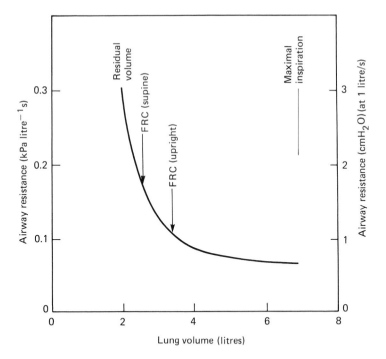

Figure 3.10 Airway resistance is a function of lung volume. This curve is a hyperbola and conductance (reciprocal of resistance) is linearly related to lung volume. Note that a reduction of FRC of about 0.4 litre, which is known to occur during anaesthesia, would itself increase the airway resistance sufficiently to account for most of the actual increase in resistance which has been reported under these circumstances. (This curve is compounded of curves reported by Mead and Agostoni (1964) and Zamel et al. (1974).)

Effect of lung volume on resistance to breathing. Figure 3.10 shows the inverse effect of lung volume on airway resistance, and there is a direct relationship between lung volume and the maximum expiratory flow rate which can be attained (see *Figure 3.8)*. Furthermore, flow-dependent airway collapse (see above) occurs more readily at low lung volume when the initial airway calibre and the transmural pressure are less. There are thus certain situations where increasing lung volume may reduce airway resistance and prevent trapping. This is most conveniently achieved by the application of continuous positive airway pressure (CPAP) to the spontaneously breathing subject or positive end-expiratory pressure (PEEP) to the paralysed ventilated patient. PEEP is, however, most commonly used not for decreasing airway resistance but for improving oxygenation of the arterial blood (page 414). The circulatory effects of PEEP are complex and are considered on pages 417 et seq. Many patients with obstructive airway disease acquire the habit of increasing their expiratory resistance by exhaling through pursed lips. This has the effect of preserving their airway transmural pressure gradient and so reducing airway resistance and preventing trapping.

Relationship between minute volume and instantaneous respiratory flow rates

Some of the more important effects of increased resistance to breathing are due to abnormal pressure gradients resulting from tidal flow of gas past the elevated

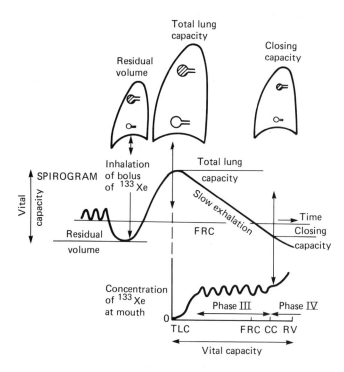

Figure 3.11 Measurement of closing capacity by the use of a tracer gas such as ^{133}Xe. The bolus of tracer gas is inhaled near residual volume and, due to airway closure, is distributed only to those alveoli whose air passages are still open (shown shaded in the diagram). During expiration, the concentration of the tracer gas becomes constant after the dead space is washed out. This plateau (phase III) gives way to a rising concentration of tracer gas (phase IV) when there is closure of airways leading to alveoli which did not receive the tracer gas.

resistance. It is therefore important to appreciate the relationships between instantaneous flow rates and the minute volume of respiration. *Figure 3.13* sets out the relationships for various respiratory waveforms. The triangular waveform gives the lowest ratio (2.0:1) between peak flow rates and minute volume. The sine waveform is approximated in spontaneous hyperventilation and the peak flow is π times the minute volume. In the more usual types of breathing the peak flow/minute volume ratios tend to be in the range 3.5:1–5:1.

Compensation for increased resistance to breathing

Inspiratory resistance

The normal response to increased inspiratory resistance is increased inspiratory muscle effort with little change in the FRC (Fink, Ngai and Holaday, 1958). Accessory muscles are brought into play according to the degree of resistance. There is generally a remarkable ability to preserve an adequate alveolar ventilation even with gross airway obstruction in emphysema. In a study of patients presenting

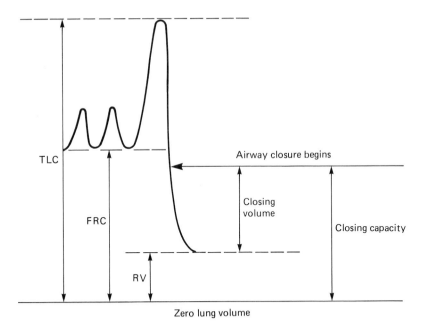

Figure 3.12 Spirogram to illustrate the relationship between closing volume and closing capacity. The example would be in a young adult with closing capacity less than functional residual capacity (FRC). TLC, total lung capacity; RV, residual volume.

for surgery with FEV_1 values of less than 1 litre, there was no correlation between FEV_1 and arterial PCO_2 which was normal in many patients with an FEV_1 of less than 0.5 litre (Nunn et al., 1986).

Asthmatic patients also show a remarkable capacity to compensate for increased resistance. Twenty patients in status asthmaticus studied by Palmer and Diament (1967) were found to have a mean arterial PCO_2 in the lower reaches of the normal range. An increased arterial PCO_2 in the presence of increased airway resistance is always serious.

Mechanisms of compensation. There are two principal mechanisms of compensation for high inspiratory resistance. The first operates immediately and even during the first breath in which resistance is applied. It seems probable that the muscle spindles indicate that the inspiratory muscles have failed to shorten by the intended amount and their afferent discharge then augments the activity in the motoneurone pool of the anterior horn. This is, in fact, typical of the servo operation of the spindle system. The conscious subject can detect very small increments in inspiratory resistance (Campbell et al., 1961).

A second compensatory mechanism develops over about 90 seconds and overacts for a similar period when the resistance is removed (Nunn and Ezi-Ashi, 1961). The time course suggests that this second mechanism is driven by elevation of arterial PCO_2. A similar two-phase response has been demonstrated in dogs (Bendixen and Bunker, 1962).

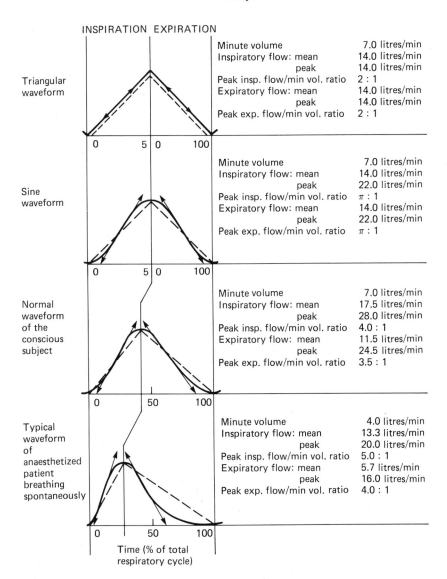

INSPIRATION EXPIRATION

Triangular waveform

Minute volume	7.0 litres/min
Inspiratory flow: mean	14.0 litres/min
peak	14.0 litres/min
Peak insp. flow/min vol. ratio	2 : 1
Expiratory flow: mean	14.0 litres/min
peak	14.0 litres/min
Peak exp. flow/min vol. ratio	2 : 1

0   5 0   100

Sine waveform

Minute volume	7.0 litres/min
Inspiratory flow: mean	14.0 litres/min
peak	22.0 litres/min
Peak insp. flow/min vol. ratio	π : 1
Expiratory flow: mean	14.0 litres/min
peak	22.0 litres/min
Peak exp. flow/min vol. ratio	π : 1

0   5 0   100

Normal waveform of the conscious subject

Minute volume	7.0 litres/min
Inspiratory flow: mean	17.5 litres/min
peak	28.0 litres/min
Peak insp. flow/min vol. ratio	4.0 : 1
Expiratory flow: mean	11.5 litres/min
peak	24.5 litres/min
Peak exp. flow/min vol. ratio	3.5 : 1

0   50   100

Typical waveform of anaesthetized patient breathing spontaneously

Minute volume	4.0 litres/min
Inspiratory flow: mean	13.3 litres/min
peak	20.0 litres/min
Peak insp. flow/min vol. ratio	5.0 : 1
Expiratory flow: mean	5.7 litres/min
peak	16.0 litres/min
Peak exp. flow/min vol. ratio	4.0 : 1

0   50   100

Time (% of total respiratory cycle)

Figure 3.13 Respiratory waveforms showing the relationship between minute volume, mean flow rates (broken lines) and peak flow rates (indicated by arrows). The normal waveform of the conscious subject is taken from Cain and Otis (1949). The waveform of the anaesthetized patient is derived from 44 spirograms of patients during surgery.

Expiratory resistance

Expiration against 1 kPa (10 cmH$_2$O) does not usually result in activation of the expiratory muscles in conscious or anaesthetized subjects. The additional work to overcome this resistance is, in fact, performed by the inspiratory muscles. The subject augments his inspiratory force until he achieves a lung volume at which the elastic recoil is sufficient to overcome the expiratory resistance (Campbell, 1957). The pattern of this extraordinary response in the anaesthetized patient is shown in *Figure 3.14*; it has been demonstrated by Campbell, Howell and Peckett (1957) and Nunn and Ezi-Ashi (1961). The response is clearly counter to what might be expected from application of the Hering–Breuer reflex. However, this reflex is weak in man (page 92). The mechanism for resetting the FRC at a higher level probably requires accommodation of the intrafusal fibres of the spindles to allow for an altered length of diaphragmatic muscle fibres due to the obstructed expiration. This would reset the developed inspiratory tension in accord with the increased FRC (Nunn and Ezi-Ashi, 1961). The conscious subject normally uses his expiratory muscles to overcome expiratory pressures in excess of about 1 kPa (10 cmH$_2$O).

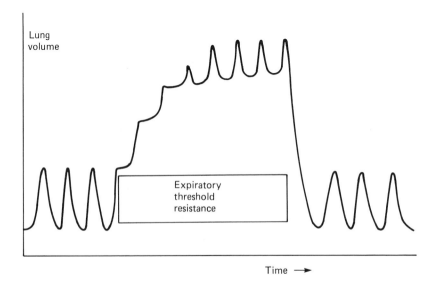

Figure 3.14 Spirogram showing response of an anaesthetized patient to the sudden imposition of an expiratory threshold resistor. Note that there is immediate augmentation of the force of contraction of the inspiratory muscles. This continues with successive breaths until the elastic recoil is sufficient to overcome the expiratory resistor (Nunn and Ezi-Ashi, 1961).

Studies of the response of the conscious subject to external resistance have been reported by Cain and Otis (1949), MacIlroy et al. (1956) and Zechman, Hall and Hull (1957). Immediate effects of excessive resistance may be less important than the long-term response of the patient. In common with other muscles, the respiratory muscles can become fatigued (see review by Moxham, 1984). This is a major factor in the onset of respiratory failure (page 383).

Principles of measurement of flow resistance

Flow resistance is determined by the simultaneous measurement of gas flow rate and the driving pressure gradient. In the case of the respiratory tract, the difficulty centres around the measurement of alveolar pressure. Methods of presentation of results are discussed earlier in this chapter.

Apparatus resistance

Measurement of driving pressure during continuous flow of gas offers the simplest method and the approach shown in *Figure 3.1* will usually suffice. Reciprocating gas flow has the advantage of testing under actual conditions of use and a sine wave pump may be used in conjunction with manometers having a rapid response.

Nasal resistance

Similar principles may be used for measuring nasal resistance. The subject breathes through his nose with his mouth closed round a tube leading to a manometer. Either continuous or reciprocating flow may be used, powered either by the subject himself or by some external device (Seebohm and Hamilton, 1958; Butler, 1960).

Airway and pulmonary resistance

Simultaneous measurement of air flow rate and intrathoracic-to-mouth pressure gradient. In Chapter 2 it was shown how simultaneous measurement of tidal volume and intrathoracic pressure yielded the dynamic compliance of the lung (see *Figure 2.14*). For this purpose, pressures were selected at the times of zero air flow when pressures were uninfluenced by air flow resistance. The same apparatus may be employed for the determination of flow resistance by eliminating the pressure component used in overcoming elastic forces (*Figure 3.15*). The shaded areas in the pressure trace indicate the components of the pressure required to overcome flow resistance and these may be related to the concurrent gas flow rates.

Alternatively, the intrathoracic-to-mouth pressure gradient and respired volume may be displayed as X and Y co-ordinates of a loop. *Figure 2.14* showed how dynamic compliance could be derived from the no-flow points of such a loop. The area of the loop is a function of the work performed against flow resistance.

The interrupter technique. A single manometer may be used to measure both mouth and alveolar pressure if the air passages distal to the manometer are momentarily interrupted with a shutter. The method is based on the assumption that, while the airway is interrupted, the mouth pressure comes to equal the alveolar pressure, a concept open to some doubt. Resistance is then determined from the relationship between flow rate (measured before interruption) and the pressure difference between mouth (measured before interruption) and alveoli (measured during interruption). Both this and the preceding methods were first described by von Neergaard and Wirz (1927b).

Oscillating air flow. In this technique, a high frequency oscillating air flow is applied to the airways, with measurement of the resultant pressure and air flow changes. By application of alternating current theory it is possible to derive a continuous measurement of airway resistance (Goldman et al., 1970; Hyatt et al., 1970). The technique has recently been developed to function during a vital capacity manoeuvre and so to display airway resistance as a function of lung volume and derive specific airway conductance (Lehane, Jordan and Jones, 1980).

The body plethysmograph. During inspiration, alveolar pressure falls below ambient as a function of airway resistance and the alveolar gas expands in accord with Boyle's law. The increased displacement of the body is then recorded as an

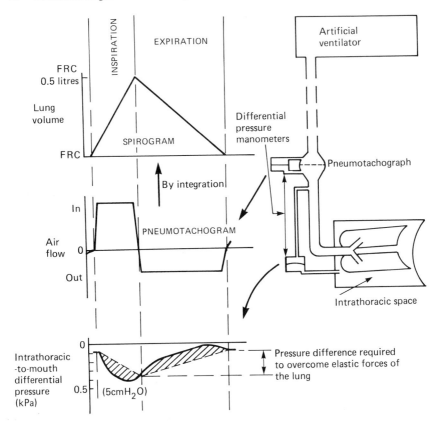

Figure 3.15 The measurement of pulmonary resistance and dynamic compliance by simultaneous measurement of air flow and intrathoracic-to-mouth differential pressure (von Neergaard and Wirz, 1927b). The spirogram is conveniently obtained by integration of the pneumotachogram. In the pressure trace, the dotted line shows the pressure changes which would be expected in a hypothetical patient with no pulmonary resistance. Compliance is derived as shown in Figure 2.14. Pulmonary resistance is derived as the difference between the measured pressure differential and that which is required for elastic forces (shaded area) compared with the flow rate shown in the pneumotachogram. Note that the pneumotachogram is a much more sensitive indicator of the no-flow points than the spirogram.

increase in pressure in the body plethysmograph. Airway (as opposed to respiratory) resistance may be derived directly from measurements of air flow and pressure changes (DuBois, Botelho and Comroe, 1956). The method is non-invasive and FRC may be measured at the same time.

Analysis of the passive spirogram. An entirely different approach, applicable only to the paralysed patient, is based on analysis of a passive spirogram. This may be either a passive expiration into an ordinary spirometer (Comroe, Nisell and Nims, 1954) or the inflation of a patient by a weighted spirometer. The first of these methods is shown in *Figure 2.13*. It is based on the fact that the time constant of the exponential discharge equals the product of static compliance and airway resistance (see Appendix F). Static compliance is the expired tidal volume/inflation pressure and so the airway resistance may be very simply derived on the assumption that flow is mainly laminar.

Tests of ventilatory capacity

It is rather unusual to undertake formal measurement of airway resistance in the clinical situation. The more usual procedure is to infer airway resistance from impairment of ventilatory capacity, since this is most commonly reduced as a result of increased airway resistance due either to bronchospasm or to flow-related airway collapse, or both. It must, however, be remembered that there are many other causes of reduction of ventilatory capacity which are nothing to do with airway resistance. Tests of ventilatory capacity and their interpretation are described at the end of Chapter 5.

Measurement of closing capacity

This is perhaps the most convenient place to outline the measurement of closing capacity. This is the maximal lung volume at which airway closure can be detected in the dependent parts of the lungs (page 62). The measurement is made during expiration and is based on having different concentrations of a tracer gas in the upper and lower parts of the lung. This may be achieved by inspiration of a bolus of tracer gas at the commencement of an inspiration from residual volume, at which time airways are closed in the dependent part of the lungs (see *Figure 3.11*). The tracer gas will then be preferentially distributed to the upper parts of the lungs. After a maximal inspiration to total lung capacity, the patient slowly exhales while the concentration of the tracer gas is measured at the mouth. When lung volume reaches the closing volume and airways begin to close in the dependent parts, the concentration of the tracer gas will rise (phase IV) above the alveolar plateau (phase III). Suitable tracers are [133]Xe (Dollfuss, Milic-Emili and Bates, 1967), 100% oxygen, measured as a fall in nitrogen concentration (Anthonisen et al., 1969) or sulphur hexafluoride enhancement of the nitrogen method (Newberg and Jones, 1974). The technique can be undertaken in the conscious subject who performs the ventilatory manoeuvres spontaneously or in the paralysed subject in whom ventilation is artificially controlled.

Chapter 4

Control of breathing

Breathing results from rhythmic contraction and relaxation of voluntary striated muscles under automatic control. The subject is normally unaware of this action, which continues during sleep or light anaesthesia, although it may, within limits, be over-ridden by voluntary cortical control or interrupted by involuntary non-rhythmic acts such as sneezing or coughing. Elucidation of respiratory control has proved to be a formidable problem since many different mechanisms can be shown to influence breathing under particular circumstances, although not all are in play at any one time. It appears, for example, that during exercise the mechanisms which control the minute volume are not those which are most important in the resting state.

This chapter starts with a discussion of the origin of the rhythmicity of breathing in the neurones of the hindbrain which appear to subserve respiration ('respiratory centres'). The efferent path is then traced to the muscles of respiration with an account of the peripheral control systems. The next section is concerned with the chemical control of respiration and this is followed by a discussion of the influence of respiratory reflexes and mechanical factors.

The origin of the respiratory rhythm

In 1812, Legallois published reports showing that rhythmic inspiratory movements persisted after removal of the cerebellum and all parts of the brain above the medulla, but ceased when the medulla was removed. During the next 150 years a long series of distinguished investigators carried out more detailed localization of the neurones concerned in the control of respiration and studied their interaction. Marckwald and Kronecker (1880) differentiated between inspiratory and expiratory neurones, and Ramon y Cajal, as early as 1909, concluded from histological studies that the respiratory rhythm was generated in the nucleus of the tractus solitarius in the medulla. This view, which is so close to modern thinking, was eclipsed in the next few decades (see review by Mitchell and Berger, 1981).

Lumsden (1923a–d) described and named the pneumotaxic and apneustic pontine centres. He also advanced the concept of an internal feedback mechanism by which a tonic inspiration was inhibited at the end of inspiration by discharge of the pneumotaxic centre acting through the expiratory centre, the whole loop functioning as an internal pacemaker. These observations were based on ablation experiments which are now recognized to result in rather unpredictable functional loss due to trauma and interference with blood supply. Pitts, Magoun and Ranson (1939a) described the anatomical localization of the overlapping inspiratory and expiratory neurones in the medulla, dispelling any idea of discrete 'inspiratory and expiratory centres'. In a later paper (1939b), they advanced the concept of the inhibition of one centre by another, or by vagal afferents from stretch sensors in the lungs. In a third paper Pitts, Magoun and Ranson (1939c) concluded that respiratory rhythmicity is caused by two separate and alternative feedback loops, one based on the pneumotaxic centre and the other on the vagal reflex sensitive to lung stretch, the two mechanisms being similar and mutually replaceable. When removal of the pneumotaxic areas was combined with bilateral vagotomy, a sustained inspiration, or apneusis, was found to result. The suggestion of self-limitation of inspiration by vagal impulses arising from inflation of the lung was not new and had first been made in the classic studies of Breuer (1868), previously reported by his chief, Professor Hering (1868).

The next landmark in the long series of studies of the interaction of the various respiratory centres was the paper by Wang, Ngai and Frumin (1957), stressing the pontile apneustic centre as the site of the inspiratory tonicity and also as the site of rhythmic inhibition by both the pneumotaxic centre and the vagus. The general plan of the respiratory centres and the concepts illustrated in diagrams such as *Figure 4.1* have been widely accepted for a number of years. However, the essential

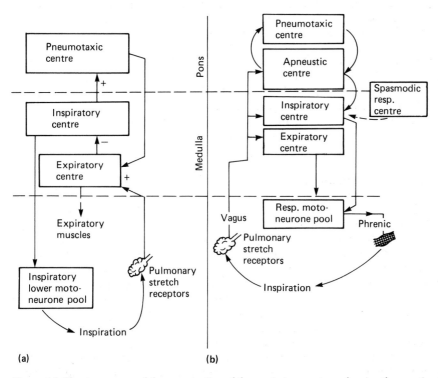

Figure 4.1 Classic concepts of the organization of the respiratory centres, showing the negative feedback loops believed to maintain the rhythmicity of breathing (see text). Expiratory muscles are not active during quiet breathing in conscious man, and the role of the expiratory neurones is primarily that of inhibition of the inspiratory neurones. ((a) according to Pitts (1946); (b) from Wang, Ngai and Frumin (1957) by permission of the authors and the American Physiological Society)

roles of the pneumotaxic centre and the vagus have been strongly challenged on the basis of new experiments and new interpretations of old experiments.

Inherent rhythmicity of the respiratory neurones in the pons and medulla

Eupnoea was demonstrated with an isolated medulla by Wang, Ngai and Frumin (1957) and following bilateral destruction of the pneumotaxic centre in vagotomized cat (St John, Glasser and King, 1972; Gautier and Bertrand, 1975). Further evidence for a medullary origin of the respiratory rhythm is provided by the studies of Hoff and Breckenridge (1949), Salmoiraghi and Burns (1960) and Salmoiraghi (1963). Guz et al. (1964, 1966b) demonstrated that bilateral vagal block had no obvious effect upon the pattern of respiration in man. There is now overwhelming evidence that the respiratory rhythm can be generated within the medulla without input from the lungs or elsewhere in the body (Mitchell and Berger, 1981; Berger and Hornbein, 1987).

There is no doubt of the existence of pontile neurones firing in synchrony with different phases of respiration but this is not to say that they are essential for the generation of the respiratory rhythm. Bertrand, Hugelin and Vibert (1974) described discrete temporal and spatial distributions of three types of neurones in the pneumotaxic region. According to their firing patterns the three types were defined as inspiratory, expiratory and phase-spanning. Although the pontile pneumotaxic centre is no longer thought to be the dominant controller of the respiratory rhythm, the pattern of firing of these neurones suggests a role in modification and fine control of the respiratory rhythm, as, for example, in setting the lung volume at which inspiration is terminated.

Spatial organization of the medullary neurones

Respiratory neurones in the medulla are concentrated in two groups, the ventral and dorsal respiratory groups (Mitchell and Berger, 1981). The ventral group contains both inspiratory and expiratory neurones in each of two nuclei (*Figure 4.2*). The nucleus ambiguus (located rostrally) has inspiratory and expiratory efferents passing mainly to the larynx, where abductor muscles are active in inspiration and adductor in expiration. The nucleus retroambigualis (located more laterally and caudally) has efferents from both inspiratory and expiratory neurones passing to the spinal cord of the other side. There are numerous interconnections between the two nuclei of the ventral group and also to the contralateral nuclei.

The dorsal group lies in close relation to the tractus solitarius, where visceral afferents from cranial nerves IX and X terminate. It is predominantly composed of inspiratory neurones which pass to the spinal phrenic nuclei of the other side. The dorsal group is probably of paramount importance in driving the inspiratory muscles.

Mechanism of the generation of the respiratory rhythm

Single pacemaker cells are probably responsible for generation of the respiratory rhythm in molluscs and crustaceans. However, in mammals, it seems likely that the rhythm is generated within a neural network by feedback loops between inspiratory and expiratory neurones (Salmoiraghi and Burns, 1960; Salmoiraghi, 1963; Robson, 1967; Berger and Hornbein, 1987). The concept is based on a bistable system with alternating predominant activity of either the inspiratory or the expiratory neurones.

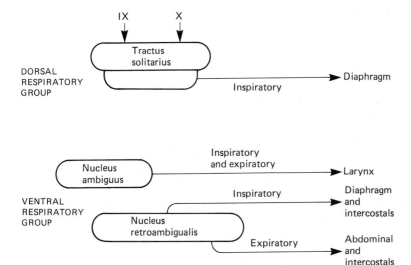

Figure 4.2 Organization of respiratory neurones in the medulla, shown in parasagittal section. Cephalad to the left, caudad to the right. Input of cranial nerves IX and X is shown at the top.

The system thus rests in either inspiration or expiration, normally cycling between the two phases in a rhythmic manner. This contrasts with Pitts' concept which is of a unistable system with only one resting position, that of inspiration of apneusis, which is rhythmically interrupted by negative feedback from either the pneumotaxic centre or the pulmonary stretch receptors (see *Figure 4.1*).

In the bistable system, the inspiratory and expiratory neurones are believed to be separately arranged in two groups of self-re-excitatory chains, capable of raising their activity by internal positive feedback loops. As the burst proceeds, there is a progressive rise in the firing threshold of the group which soon terminates its activity (Salmoiraghi and von Baumgarten, 1969). However, the inspiratory and expiratory groups of neurones are linked by mutually inhibitory pathways which enforce reciprocal activity. Therefore, as the activity dies away in one group, it grows in the other, only to be terminated in due course by the development of a raised threshold in that group. Activity then recommences in the original group and so the cycle continues. It should be stressed that cyclical activity in the expiratory neurones does not necessarily imply activity of expiratory muscles and, indeed, under resting conditions the expiratory neurones are exclusively anti-inspiratory in their action.

Influence of volition and wakefulness

Douglas and Haldane (1909) observed appreciable periods of apnoea following voluntary hyperventilation, in studies which closely followed the classic paper of Haldane and Priestley (1905) describing the major role of carbon dioxide in the regulation of breathing. Since ventilation is so easily influenced by voluntary control under experimental conditions, when the subject's attention is focused on his breathing, it seemed worth repeating this study with subjects who had no preconceived ideas on the role of carbon dioxide.

Fink (1961) found that 13 naive conscious subjects all continued to breathe rhythmically during recovery from reduction of end-expiratory P_{CO_2} to 3.3 kPa (25 mmHg) or less, induced by 5–10 minutes of mechanical hyperventilation. However, Fink's results were not confirmed by Bainton and Mitchell (1965) or Moser, Rhodes and Kwaan (1965), who were able to obtain apnoea after hyperventilation in some, but not all, of their conscious subjects. Whatever the uncertainty which seems to exist in conscious man, there is no doubt of the ease with which apnoea may be produced by moderate hypocapnia in anaesthetized patients (Hanks, Ngai and Fink, 1961), and these studies have a most important practical bearing on the restoration of spontaneous respiration in anaesthetized patients who have been subjected to a period of artificial hyperventilation.

St John, Glasser and King (1972) have reported an important effect of wakefulness on the breathing of cats with long-term bilateral pneumotaxic lesions and vagotomy. Relatively normal rhythmic breathing was changed to apneustic breathing during anaesthesia, thus confirming the observations of many investigators working with anaesthetized or decerebrate animals.

Breathing can be voluntarily interrupted and the pattern of respiratory movements altered within limits determined mainly by changes in arterial blood gas tensions. This is essential for such acts as speech, singing, sniffing, coughing and expulsive efforts. There are numerous reports of alteration in the pattern of breathing when various cortical areas are stimulated (Berger and Hornbein, 1987). In addition to volitional changes in the pattern of breathing, there are numerous suprapontine reflex interferences with respiration such as sneezing, swallowing and reflex coughing.

Ondine's curse and primary alveolar hypoventilation

This is perhaps the best place to mention the condition which Severinghaus and Mitchell (1962) have aptly called 'Ondine's curse' from its first description in German legend. The water nymph, Ondine, having been jilted by her mortal husband, took from him all automatic functions, requiring him to remember to breathe. When he finally fell asleep he died. These authors describe three patients who exhibited long periods of apnoea even when awake but who breathed on command. These patients had become apnoeic during surgery involving the high cervical cord or brain stem, but a somewhat similar situation exists in patients with primary alveolar hypoventilation occurring as a feature of many different diseases, including chronic poliomyelitis and the pickwickian syndrome, although upper airway obstruction is now recognized as an important cause of apnoea in these patients (page 306). Characteristics include a raised P_{CO_2} in the absence of pulmonary pathology, a flat CO_2/ventilation response curve and periods of apnoea which may be central or obstructive. A similar condition is also produced by overdosage with opiates. The influence of sleep is discussed further in Chapter 13.

Motor pathways concerned in breathing

Three groups of upper motoneurones converge on the anterior horn cells from which arise the lower motoneurones supplying the respiratory muscles. Final integration of respiratory control takes place at the level of the anterior horn cell (Mitchell and Berger, 1975, 1981). This does not exclude the possibility of some co-ordination taking place at the level of the pontomedullary centres (Berger and Hornbein, 1987).

The first group of upper motoneurones is mainly concerned with involuntary rhythmic breathing. Efferent fibres from the inspiratory and expiratory medullary neurones cross the midline in the region of the obex and descend in the ventrolateral quadrant of the spinal cord. The second group is concerned with voluntary control of breathing (speech, respiratory gymnastics, etc.) and lies in the dorsolateral and ventrolateral quadrants of the cord. The third group is concerned with involuntary non-rhythmic respiratory control (swallowing, cough, hiccup, etc.). This group does not occupy a single compact location in the cord but appears to be separate from the tracts concerned with rhythmic input to the diaphragm (Newsom Davis and Plum, 1972). Selective cordotomies can interfere with rhythmic but not voluntary respiration, particularly during sleep, while Newsom Davis (1974) has described a patient with partial transverse cervical myelitis who had normal rhythmic breathing but could not voluntarily alter his ventilation.

The respiratory muscles, in common with other skeletal muscles, have their tension controlled by a servo mechanism mediated by muscle spindles. They appear to play a more important role in the intercostal muscles than in the diaphragm (Corda, von Euler and Lennerstrand, 1965). There was, in fact, some doubt about the existence of spindles in the human diaphragm until a small number were demonstrated by Muller et al. (1979). Their function is largely inferred from knowledge of their well established role in other skeletal muscles not concerned with respiration (Granit, 1955).

Two types of cell can be distinguished in the motoneurone pool of the anterior horn cell. The alpha motoneurone has a thick efferent fibre (12–20 μm diameter) and passes by the ventral root directly to the neuromuscular junction of the muscle fibre (*Figure 4.3*). The gamma motoneurone has a thin efferent fibre (2–8 μm) which also passes by the ventral root but terminates in the intrafusal fibres of the muscle spindle. Contraction of the intrafusal fibres increases the tension in the central part of the spindle (the nuclear bag), causing stimulation of the annulospiral endings. Impulses so generated are then transmitted via fibres which lie in the dorsal root to reach the anterior horn where they have an excitatory effect on the alpha motoneurones. It will be seen that an efferent impulse transmitted by the gamma system may cause reflex contraction of the main muscle mass by means of an arc through the annulospiral afferent and the alpha motoneurone. Thus contraction of the whole muscle may be controlled entirely by efferents travelling in the gamma fibres and this has been suggested in relation to breathing (Robson, 1967).

Alternatively, muscle contraction may in the first instance result from discharge of the alpha and gamma motoneurones. If the shortening of the muscle is unopposed, main (extrafusal) and intrafusal fibres will contract together and the tension in the nuclear bag of the spindle will be unchanged (*Figure 4.3*). If, however, the shortening of the muscle is opposed, the intrafusal fibres will shorten more than the extrafusal fibres, causing the nuclear bag to be stretched. The consequent stimulation of the annulospiral endings results in afferents which raise the excitatory state of the motoneurones, causing the main muscle fibres to increase their tension until the resistance is overcome, allowing the muscle to shorten and the tension in the nuclear bag of the spindle to be reduced.

By this mechanism, fine control of muscle contraction is possible. The message from the upper motoneurone is in the form: 'muscles should contract with whatever

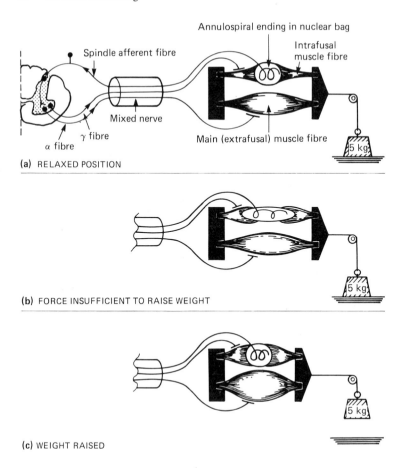

Figure 4.3 Diagrammatic representation of the servo mechanism mediated by the muscle spindles. (a) The resting state with muscle and intrafusal fibres of spindle relaxed. (b) The muscle is attempting to lift the weight following discharge of both alpha and gamma systems. The force developed by the muscle is insufficient: the weight is not lifted and the muscle cannot shorten. However, the intrafusal fibres are able to shorten and stretch the annulospiral endings in the nuclear bag of the spindle. Afferent discharge causes increased excitation of the motoneurone pool in the anterior horn. (c) Alpha discharge is augmented and the weight is finally lifted by the more powerful contraction of the muscle. When the weight is lifted, the tension on the nuclear bag is relieved and the afferent discharge from the spindle ceases. This series of diagrams relates to the lifting of a weight but it is thought that similar action of spindles is brought into play when the inspiratory muscles contract against augmented airway resistance.

force may be found necessary to effect such and such a shortening', and not simply: 'muscles should contract with such and such a force'. Clearly the former message is far more satisfactory for such a task as lifting up a suitcase, the precise weight of which is not known until an attempt is made to lift it. It is common experience that, provided the weight is not grossly different from the anticipated weight, we can, in fact, raise a suitcase to a predetermined distance from the floor with considerable precision without knowing the exact weight in advance. This feat can be achieved only by means of an efficient servo system which the spindles appear able to provide. The workings of the system are probably relayed to the cortex and provide information of 'length–tension' relationships which enable us to assess the weight of an object or the elasticity of a piece of rubber.

Campbell and Howell (1962) presented evidence for believing that a similar mechanism governs the action of the respiratory muscles. According to this belief, the message conveyed by the efferent tract from the inspiratory neurones of the medulla would be in the form: 'inspiratory muscles should contract with whatever force may be necessary to effect such and such a change in length (corresponding to a certain tidal volume)' and not simply: 'inspiratory muscles should contract with such and such a force'.

The use of the servo loop implies that the action of the respiratory muscles must be dependent upon the integrity of the dorsal roots which contain the efferents from the annulospiral endings. This appears to be the case, and dorsal root section at the appropriate level causes temporary paralysis of the respiratory muscles in man (Nathan and Sears, 1960).

The spindle servo mechanism provides an excellent mechanism for dealing with sudden changes in airway resistance. The compensation is made at spinal level and operates within the duration of a single inspiration, long before changes in arterial blood gas tensions are able to exert their effect. The nature and magnitude of the response to resistance is described in Chapter 3 (page 65). Inspiratory resistance causes an augmentation of tension developed in the inspiratory muscles, while expiratory resistance also causes an augmentation of inspiratory effort resulting in an increase in lung volume, until the increased elastic recoil is sufficient to overcome the expiratory resistance. These changes are explicable in the light of the function of the spindles but cannot be explained in terms of the Hering–Breuer reflexes. Relay to cortical levels is probably the mechanism of detection of external changes in compliance (Campbell et al., 1961) or resistance (Bennett et al., 1962).

Chemical control of breathing

Pflüger in his classic paper of 1868 gave the first convincing evidence that breathing could be stimulated either by a reduction of oxygen content or by an increase of carbon dioxide content of the arterial blood. However, the importance of the role of carbon dioxide was not fully established until the work of Haldane and Priestley (1905). In one paper they presented their technique for sampling alveolar gas, showed the constancy of the alveolar Pco_2 under a wide range of circumstances and also demonstrated the great sensitivity of ventilation to small changes in alveolar Pco_2.

Until 1926 it was thought that changes in the chemical composition of the blood, mainly the Pco_2 influenced ventilation solely by direct action on the respiratory centre, which was presumed to be sensitive to these influences although direct experimental proof was lacking. However, between 1926 and 1930 there occurred a major revision following the histological studies of de Castro (1926) which led him to suggest a chemoreceptor function for the carotid bodies. These receptors were found to be sensitive to hypoxia and the role of the carotid bodies in the control of breathing was clearly established (Heymans and Heymans, 1927; Heymans, Bouckaert and Dautrebande, 1930). A similar function for the aortic bodies was reported in 1939 by Comroe and C. Heymans received a Nobel prize for his work in 1938.

Division of the afferent nerves from the peripheral chemoreceptors does not greatly diminish the ventilatory response to elevation of the arterial P_{CO_2} and until recently it was generally believed that the respiratory centre itself was sensitive to carbon dioxide. However, it is now known that the central chemoreceptors, as they have come to be called, are actually separate from the respiratory neurones of the medulla although located only a short distance away.

The chemical control of breathing is shown schematically in *Figure 4.4*. The plan of this section of the chapter is first to give a separate account of the peripheral and central chemoreceptors and then to consider the quantitative aspects of their function in combination.

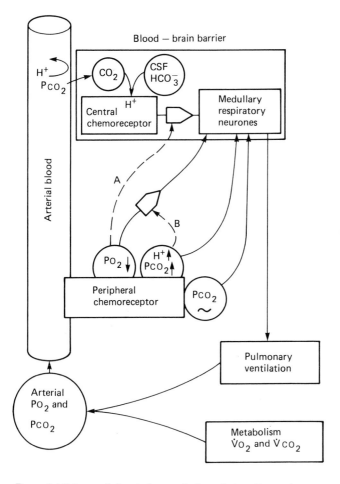

Figure 4.4 Scheme of chemical control of ventilation. For explanation, see text.

The peripheral chemoreceptors
(reviews by McDonald, 1981; McQueen and Pallot, 1983)

The peripheral chemoreceptors are fast-responding monitors of the arterial blood, responding to a fall in Po_2, a rise in Pco_2 or H^+ concentration, or a fall in their perfusion rate. Of the peripheral chemoreceptors, the bilaterally paired carotid bodies are almost exclusively responsible for the respiratory response. Their structure/function relationships have been exhaustively reviewed by McDonald (1981). Each is only about 6 mm^3 in volume and they are located close to the bifurcation of the common carotid artery. The carotid bodies undergo hypertrophy and hyperplasia under conditions of chronic hypoxia and are usually lost in the operation of carotid endarterectomy.

The carotid bodies contain large sinusoids with a very high rate of perfusion which is about ten times the level which would be proportional to their metabolic rate, which is itself very high. Therefore the arterial/venous Po_2 difference is small. This accords with their role as a sensor of arterial blood gas tensions, and their rapid response which is within the range 1–3 seconds (Ponte and Purves, 1974).

At the cellular level, the main feature is the glomus or type I cell, which is in synaptic contact with nerve endings derived from an axon with its cell body in the petrosal ganglion of the glossopharyngeal nerve (*Figure 4.5*). These endings are mainly postsynaptic to the glomus cell. Type I cells are partly encircled by type II or sheath cells whose function is still obscure. Efferent nerves, which are known to modulate receptor afferent discharge, include preganglionic sympathetic fibres from the superior cervical ganglion, amounting to 5 per cent of the nerve endings on the glomus cell. In addition, the glossopharyngeal terminations on the glomus cell are partly presynaptic. Glomus cells secrete dopamine, which is known to alter chemoreceptor sensitivity, and possibly also noradrenaline, serotonin, acetylcholine and polypeptides.

It is still not clear which structure is the actual chemoreceptor. The contenders are the glomus cell itself and the afferent nerve endings, with the type I cells functioning as dopaminergic interneurones which modulate the sensitivity of the chemoreceptive nerve endings (McDonald and Mitchell, 1975; McDonald, 1981).

Types of stimulant. Discharge in the afferent nerves increases in the following circumstances:

1. *Decrease of arterial Po_2.* Reduced oxygen content does not stimulate the bodies, provided that Po_2 remains normal, and there is little stimulation in anaemia, carboxyhaemoglobinaemia or methaemoglobinaemia (Comroe and Schmidt, 1938). The response of ventilation to reduction of arterial Po_2 approximates to a rectangular hyperbola asymptotic to a Po_2 of about 4.3 kPa (32 mmHg) and to the level of ventilation at high Po_2 (*Figure 4.6*). Withdrawal of the carotid chemoreceptor response to normal Po_2 by the inhalation of 100% oxygen reduces the ventilatory response of the central chemoreceptors to Pco_2 by about 15 per cent (Cunningham, 1974). This would be represented by interruption of the broken line 'A' in *Figure 4.4*. Quantitative aspects of the response to Po_2 are considered in greater detail below.

   A small number of otherwise normal subjects lack a measurable ventilatory response to hypoxia when studied at normal Pco_2 (see data of subjects 4 and 5 reported by Cormack, Cunningham and Gee, 1957). This is of little importance

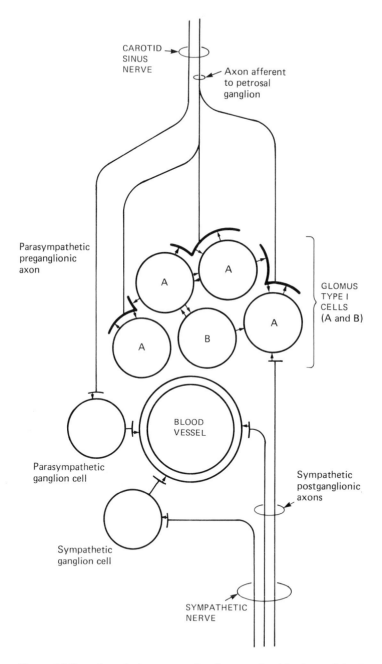

Figure 4.5 Grouping of glomus type I cells around a blood vessel in the carotid body, showing innervation. This grouping would be surrounded by a sheath cell which is not shown, and is sometimes termed a glomoid.

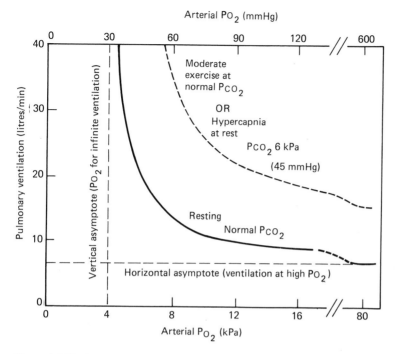

Figure 4.6 The heavy curve represents the normal P_{O_2}/ventilation response curve at constant (normal) P_{CO_2}. It has the form of a rectangular hyperbola asymptotic to the ventilation at high P_{O_2} and the P_{O_2} at which ventilation becomes infinite. The curve is displaced upwards by both hypercapnia and exercise at normal P_{CO_2}. The curve is depressed by anaesthetics. See text for references.

under normal circumstances because the P_{CO_2} drive from the central chemoreceptors will normally ensure a safe level of P_{O_2}. However, in certain therapeutic and abnormal environmental circumstances, it could be dangerous. Such people would do badly at high altitude.

2. *Decrease of arterial pH.* Acidaemia of perfusing blood causes stimulation, the magnitude of which is the same whether it is due to carbonic or to 'non-respiratory' acids such as lactic (Hornbein and Roos, 1963). Quantitatively, the change produced by elevated P_{CO_2} on the peripheral chemoreceptors is only about one-sixth of that caused by the action on the central chemosensitive areas.

3. *Respiratory oscillations of P_{CO_2}.* The P_{CO_2} (and consequently the pH) of arterial blood shows small oscillations in phase with respiration (see *Figure 9.6*), but the oscillations are greatly increased during exercise when the venous/arterial P_{CO_2} difference is increased. The mechanism of the stimulation of the central chemoreceptors is too slow to respond to these changes but the output of the peripheral chemoreceptor in the sinus nerve has been found to vary during the respiratory cycle (Hornbein, Griffo and Roos, 1961). The timing of the nerve discharge suggests that the response is to the rate of rise of P_{CO_2} as well as to its magnitude. A series of square waves of raised P_{CO_2} in the carotid artery of the dog results in a higher level of ventilation than is obtained when the P_{CO_2} is maintained steady at the same mean value (Dutton, Fitzgerald and Gross, 1968), but respiratory oscillations in P_{O_2} do not appear to have this effect.

The effect of oscillations of PCO_2 has been demonstrated in the dog, cat and rat, but in man direct investigation is not possible and recourse has to be made to elaborate experiments involving artificially imposed changes in the composition of the inspired gas (Cunningham and Ward, 1975a, b). In contrast to animal experiments, there is no evidence that the overall ventilation in man is higher than it would be with the same mean PCO_2 held at a steady level, and this applies even to hypoxic conditions. However, if the PCO_2 is made to rise sharply during inspiration then an augmentation of ventilation occurs (Cunningham, Howson and Pearson, 1973). This mechanism may have relevance to hyperventilation of exercise when the increased mixed venous/arterial PCO_2 difference causes a more abrupt rise in arterial PCO_2 during expiration. Phase change between the respiratory cycle and the arterial PCO_2 cycle may also have an effect on ventilation and play a part in the production of the hyperventilation of exercise (Black and Torrance, 1971).

4. *Hypoperfusion of peripheral chemoreceptors* causes stimulation, possibly by causing a 'stagnant hypoxia' of the chemoreceptor cells. Hypoperfusion may result from hypotension.
5. *Blood temperature elevation* causes stimulation of breathing.
6. *Chemical stimulation* by a wide range of substances is known to cause increased ventilation through the medium of the peripheral chemoreceptors. These substances fall into two groups. The first comprises agents such as nicotine and acetylcholine which stimulate sympathetic ganglia. Action of this group of drugs can be blocked with ganglion-blocking agents (e.g. hexamethonium). The second group of chemical stimulants comprises substances such as cyanide and carbon monoxide which block the cytochrome system and so prevent oxidative metabolism. Respiration is also stimulated through the carotid bodies by the drugs doxapram and almitrine.

The gain of the carotid bodies is under nervous control. There is an efferent pathway in the sinus nerve which, on excitation, decreases chemoreceptor activity. Excitation of the sympathetic nerve supply to the carotid body causes an increase in activity (Biscoe and Willshaw, 1981).

Mechanism of action. It would be attractive to offer a unified theory which would explain how this wide range of stimuli can excite the chemoreceptors by a common mechanism. Thought has been given to the possibility that the chemoreceptor cells might be uniquely sensitive to a fall in intracellular pH. It would then be possible to postulate their stimulation by a rise in PCO_2 (which lowers intracellular pH by diffusion of carbon dioxide into the cell), or by reduction of PO_2 (which, if sufficiently severe, would cause the cell to utilize anaerobic metabolic pathways). Hypoperfusion or poisoning of cytochrome a3 would also prevent or diminish aerobic metabolism, and so could cause intracellular acidosis from the production of lactic acid. Alternatively, hypoxia might be expected to change electrochemical gradients within the cell, as a result of relatively anaerobic conditions interfering with the sodium pump (Biscoe, 1971).

An entirely different mechanism has been proposed by Mills and Jobsis (1972) who reported the presence of a different type of cytochrome a3 in the carotid body. Unlike the usual cytochrome a3 (page 237), which is also present in the carotid body, the special type is 50 per cent reduced at the very high level of PO_2 of 12 kPa (90 mmHg) and they suggest that it is the PO_2 sensor. It has also been suggested by

Neil and Joels (1963) that certain stimuli (e.g. acidosis) may shunt blood past the sinusoids and so cause stagnant hypoxia in the vicinity of the chemoreceptor calls, which can then be considered to respond only to hypoxia. These theories remain conjectural and there is no firm evidence for the mechanism of action.

Other effects of stimulation. Apart from the well known increase in depth and rate of breathing, chemoreceptor stimulation causes a number of other effects, including bradycardia, hypertension, increase in bronchiolar tone and adrenal secretion. Stimulation of the carotid bodies has predominantly respiratory effects, while the aortic bodies have a greater influence on circulation.

Glossopharyngeal block and loss of carotid bodies. Reference has been made above to the studies of bilateral vagal block in man (Guz et al., 1964, 1966a, b). The technique employed also blocked the glossopharyngeal nerve and so denervated the carotid bodies. Apart from the loss of swallowing and phonation, and the development of hypertension, there was no change in the pattern or sensation of breathing. End-tidal P_{CO_2} and respiratory rate were unchanged but there was a substantial increase in the duration of breath holding. Loss of ventilatory response to hypoxia produced by inhaling 8% oxygen in nitrogen was also reported in another publication by the same team (Guz et al., 1966a). Bilateral vagal block was not found to influence ventilation in five anaesthetized patients (Guz et al., 1964). Interpretation of these studies is complicated by the fact that afferents from pulmonary stretch receptors were unavoidably blocked at the same time as those from the peripheral chemoreceptors.

Studies of patients who have lost their carotid bodies as a result of bilateral carotid endarterectomy (Wade et al., 1970) together with the work of Guz's group, referred to above, clearly show that the carotid bodies are not essential for the maintenance of reasonably normal breathing under conditions of rest and mild exercise. However, patients without peripheral chemoreceptors would be dangerously at risk if exposed to low partial pressures of oxygen in their inspired gas. They would also lose the augmented response to hypoxia in the presence of hypercapnia or exercise, which is considered below in relation to *Figure 4.6*. There are, in addition, the circulatory responses to chemoreceptor stimulation which generally have the effect of diverting blood flow to vital organs under adverse conditions.

The central chemoreceptors
(reviews by Bledsoe and Hornbein, 1981; Loeschcke, 1983)

About 80 per cent of the total respiratory response to inhaled carbon dioxide originates in the central medullary chemoreceptors (Mitchell, 1966). The central response is thus the major factor in the regulation of breathing by carbon dioxide and it had long been thought that the actual neurones of the 'respiratory centre' were themselves sensitive either to P_{CO_2} (Haldane and Priestley, 1905) or to pH (Winterstein, 1911; Gessell, 1923).

More recently attention has been turned to the role of the cerebrospinal fluid (CSF) in the control of breathing. This followed the important studies of Leusen (1950, 1954) who showed that the ventilation of anaesthetized dogs was stimulated by perfusion of the ventriculo-cisternal system with mock CSF of elevated P_{CO_2} and reduced pH.

Localization of the central chemoreceptors. Leusen's work touched off a long series of studies aimed at localizing central chemoreceptors. They were thought to lie superficially and in contact with one or other of the reservoirs of CSF, since it seemed unlikely that changes in the composition of the CSF could influence the respiratory neurones within the substance of the medulla in the few minutes required for full development of the ventilatory response to inhaled carbon dioxide.

It now appears likely that the central respiratory response to carbon dioxide is mediated mainly through superficial chemosensitive areas lying within 0.2 mm of the anterolateral surfaces of the medulla, close to the origins of the glossopharyngeal and vagus nerves, and crossed by the anterior inferior cerebellar arteries. In the cat, there are, on each side, rostral and caudal areas which are sensitive to pH (*Figure 4.7*). It seems likely that their connections pass through a third intermediate area and all chemosensitivity is lost if the intermediate areas are destroyed (Berger and Hornbein, 1986).

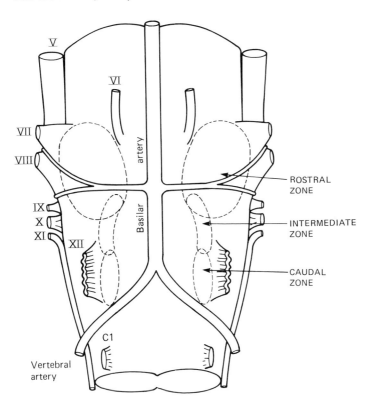

Figure 4.7 Location of the chemoreceptor zones on the anterolateral surface of the medulla of the cat. (Redrawn after Schläfke et al. (1975) with permission of the Editors of the Bulletin de Physio-Pathologie Respiratoire)

Mechanism of action. An elevation of arterial P_{CO_2} causes an approximately equal rise of CSF, cerebral tissue and jugular venous P_{CO_2}, all of which are approximately equal and about 1.3 kPa (10 mmHg) higher than the arterial P_{CO_2}. Over the short term, and without change in CSF bicarbonate, a rise in CSF P_{CO_2} causes a fall in

CSF pH, and it was postulated by Mitchell and his colleagues (1963) that the reduction in pH stimulated the respiratory neurones indirectly through receptors in the chemosensitive area. The theory was especially attractive because the time course of change in CSF pH accorded with the well known delay in the ventilatory response to a change in arterial P_{CO_2} (Lambertsen, 1963; Loeschcke, 1965).

The blood/brain barrier (operative between blood and CSF) is permeable to carbon dioxide but not hydrogen ions, and in this respect resembles the membrane of a P_{CO_2}-sensitive electrode (page 232). In both cases, carbon dioxide crosses the barrier and hydrates to carbonic acid which then ionizes to give a pH which is inversely proportional to the log of the P_{CO_2}. A hydrogen ion sensor is thus made to respond to P_{CO_2}. This accords with the old observation that the ventilatory response to a respiratory acidosis is greater than to a metabolic acidosis with the same change in blood pH. Ventilation is, in fact, a single function of CSF pH in both conditions (Fencl, Miller and Pappenheimer, 1966).

If the P_{CO_2} is maintained at an abnormal level, the CSF pH gradually returns towards normal over the course of a few days as a result of changes in the CSF bicarbonate level. This is analogous to and proceeds in parallel with the partial restoration of blood pH in patients with chronic hyper- or hypocapnia. The mechanism of the shift in bicarbonate was originally thought to be due to active transport of bicarbonate ion (Severinghaus et al., 1963). It was later shown that CSF pH was not completely restored to normal (Dempsey, Forster and doPico, 1974; Forster, Dempsey and Chosy, 1975) and compensatory changes were found to be similar in CSF and blood, suggesting that changes were due to passive ion distribution. Further studies by Pavlin and Hornbein (1975a, b, c) and Hornbein and Pavlin (1975) also indicated that the bicarbonate shift could be explained by passive distribution although the possibility of active ion transfer could not be excluded.

High altitude. A shift in CSF bicarbonate is a major factor in early acclimatization to altitude and is discussed on page 316.

Effect of passive hyperventilation. Changes in CSF bicarbonate occur during prolonged periods of artificial ventilation with high minute volumes. Semple (1965) pointed out that CSF bicarbonate would be significantly reduced after 1 hour of hyperventilation, and Christensen (1974) reported that CSF pH had returned to normal 30 hours after commencing passive hyperventilation. Hornbein and Pavlin (1975) found substantial resetting of the CSF pH within $4\frac{1}{2}$ hours of a step increase in the ventilation of an anaesthetized paralysed dog. This offers one reason why patients subjected to this treatment may demand high minute volumes, and often continue to hyperventilate after resumption of spontaneous breathing.

Response to metabolic acidosis. The stability of the CSF pH is not confined to the circumstances of respiratory alkalosis of altitude but is also found in chronic respiratory acidosis and metabolic acidosis and alkalosis (Mitchell et al., 1965). Mean values of CSF pH in Mitchell's study did not differ by more than 0.011 units from the normal value (7.326) in spite of mean arterial pH values ranging from 7.334 to 7.523. The constancy of CSF pH cannot be explained either by diffusion of bicarbonate between blood and CSF or by renal compensation.

If the bicarbonate of the CSF is altered by pathological factors, the pH is changed and ventilatory disturbances follow. Froman and Crampton-Smith (1966) described three patients who hyperventilated after intracranial haemorrhages. In each case the CSF pH and bicarbonate were persistently below the normal values and it was postulated that this was due to the metabolic breakdown products of blood which contaminated the CSF. In a later communication, Froman (1966) reported correction of hyperventilation by intrathecal administration of 3–5 mmol of bicarbonate.

Effect of hypoxia. Unlike the peripheral chemoreceptors, the central chemoreceptors are not stimulated by hypoxia. In fact, the central respiratory neurones are depressed by hypoxia, and apnoea follows severe medullary hypoxia whether due to ischaemia or to hypoxaemia.

Quantitative aspects of the chemical control of breathing

Integration of the chemical factors controlling breathing has been a recurrent and challenging problem of respiratory physiology. It was at one time thought that the various factors interacted so that the resultant ventilation depended on the algebraic sum of the individual factors caused by changes of P_{CO_2}, P_{O_2}, pH, etc. Hypoxia and hypercapnia were, for example, thought to be simply additive in their effect. It is now realized that the interactions between P_{CO_2} and P_{O_2} are far more complex (Lloyd and Cunningham, 1963), and exercise complicates the position further. The P_{O_2}/ventilation response curve will now be considered, together with factors which modify it. The P_{CO_2}/ventilation response curve will then receive similar treatment. The methods of presentation and measurement of ventilatory responses to both P_{CO_2} and P_{O_2} have been reviewed by Rebuck and Slutsky (1981).

The P_{O_2}/ventilation response curve has already been mentioned above. The thick continuous line in *Figure 4.6* represents a typical normal response, but it must be stressed that there are very wide individual variations, including absence of response to low P_{O_2}. The curve may conveniently be considered as a rectangular hyperbola which is asymptotic to the ventilation at high P_{O_2} and to the P_{O_2} at which ventilation theoretically becomes infinite, a parameter known as 'C' and usually about 4.3 kPa (32 mmHg), this being the approach developed by Lloyd, Jukes and Cunningham in 1958. The ventilatory response to P_{O_2} may then be expressed as $W/(P_{O_2} - C)$, where W is a multiplier (i.e. the gain of the system) and partly dependent upon the P_{CO_2}. The ventilatory response would be the difference between the actual ventilation and the ventilation at high P_{O_2}, the P_{CO_2} being unchanged. Others have suggested that the P_{O_2}/ventilation response curve be considered as an exponential function but curve-fitting to available data will not give a clear-cut answer as to which model is the better.

The inconvenience of the non-linear relationship between ventilation and P_{O_2} may be overcome by plotting ventilation against oxygen saturation. It so happens that the relationship between these two variables is linear (with a negative slope), at least down to a saturation of 70% (Rebuck and Campbell, 1974). Saturation may be measured simply and non-invasively (page 281), and this provides an attractive alternative to the traditional approach.

The ventilatory response to hypoxia may be enhanced under either of two circumstances, and the upper broken line in *Figure 4.6* is typical of the enhanced response which may be obtained in man. The first factor causing enhancement is elevated P_{CO_2} (Cormack, Cunningham and Gee, 1957). This effect is well marked and the line in *Figure 4.6* would correspond to a P_{CO_2} of about 6 kPa (45 mmHg). This interaction (shown by the broken line 'B' in *Figure 4.4*) contributes to the ventilatory response in asphyxia being greater than the sum of the response to be expected from the rise in P_{CO_2} and the fall in P_{O_2} considered separately.

Simple elicitation of the ventilatory response to hypoxia will normally result in hypocapnia and the response is then a combination of the hypoxic drive and the resultant hypocapnic depression of breathing. Precise measurement of the hypoxic drive *per se* requires that the P_{CO_2} be maintained at a constant level.

The response to hypoxia is also enhanced by exercise even if the P_{CO_2} is not raised (Weil et al., 1972). This may be due to lactacidosis, oscillations of P_{CO_2} or perhaps to catecholamine secretion. The upper broken line in *Figure 4.6* would also correspond to the response during exercise at an oxygen consumption of about 800 ml/min. Insufficient data exist to define the difference in the form of the curves obtained during hypercapnia and exercise but the general shapes appear roughly similar. It is important to note that the slope of the curve at normal P_{O_2} is considerably increased under both these circumstances and thus there will be appreciable 'hypoxic' drive to ventilation. Enhanced response to P_{O_2} during exercise appears to be an important component in the overall ventilatory response to exercise which is considered further below. The P_{O_2}/ventilation response is virtually abolished during anaesthesia (page 353).

The P_{CO_2}/ventilation response curve is linear over the range which is usually studied. It may therefore be defined in terms of the parameters slope and intercept (see Lloyd, Jukes and Cunningham, 1958):

$$\text{ventilation} = S(P_{CO_2} - B)$$

where S is the slope ($1 \text{ min}^{-1} \text{ kPa}^{-1}$ or $1 \text{ min}^{-1} \text{ mm Hg}^{-1}$) and B is the intercept at zero ventilation (kPa or mmHg). The heavy continuous line in *Figure 4.8* is a typical normal curve with an intercept (B) of about 4.8 kPa (36 mmHg) and a slope (S) of about $15 \text{ l min}^{-1} \text{ kPa}^{-1}$ (2 l/min/mmHg). There is in fact a very wide individual variation in P_{CO_2}/ventilation response curves and the response may be decreased by disease or drugs. Actual values of P_{CO_2} and ventilation depend on the inspired carbon dioxide concentration and the metabolic rate. The broken line in *Figure 4.8* shows the relationship between arterial P_{CO_2} and ventilation in the resting state when the inspired carbon dioxide concentration is negligible. It is, in fact, the P_{CO_2} in response to changing ventilation (as in *Figure 5.8*) and is a section of a rectangular hyperbola. The normal resting P_{CO_2} and ventilation are indicated by the intersection of this curve with the normal P_{CO_2}/ventilation response curve, which is obtained by varying the carbon dioxide concentration in the inspired gas.

The P_{CO_2}/ventilation response curve is the response of the entire respiratory system to the challenge of a raised P_{CO_2}. Apart from reduced sensitivity of the central chemoreceptors, the overall response may be blunted by neuromuscular blockade or by obstructive or restrictive lung disease (see *Figure 20.2*). These factors must be taken into account in drawing conclusions from a reduced response, and diffuse airway obstruction is a most important consideration (Clark, Clarke and Hughes, 1966). Nevertheless the slope of the P_{CO_2}/ventilation response curve remains one of the most valuable parameters in the assessment of the responsiveness of the respiratory system to carbon dioxide and its depression by drugs.

Extensions to the response curves are shown in *Figure 4.8* below the dotted curve which defines the effect of ventilation on P_{CO_2}. These extensions are of two types.

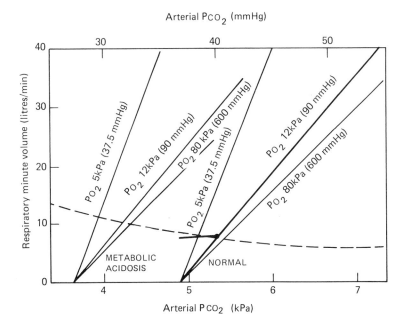

Figure 4.8 Two fans of P_{CO_2}/ventilation response curves at different values of P_{O_2}. The right-hand fan is at normal metabolic acid–base state (zero base excess). The left-hand fan represents metabolic acidosis. The broken line represents the P_{CO_2} produced by the indicated ventilation for zero inspired P_{CO_2}, at basal metabolic rate. The intersection of the broken curve and any response curve indicates the resting P_{CO_2} and ventilation for the relevant metabolic acid–base state and P_{O_2}. The heavy curve is the normal curve. For details, see text.

Slopes and intercepts of P_{CO_2}/ ventilation response curves are subject to very wide individual variation. The curves in this diagram are only intended to indicate general principles and considerable deviations may be found in healthy subjects

The first is an extrapolation of the curve to intersect the X axis (zero ventilation) at a P_{CO_2} sometimes known as the apnoeic threshold P_{CO_2}. If P_{CO_2} is depressed below this point, apnoea may result, particularly in the anaesthetized patient, and the extension of the curve is a graphical representation of Haldane's post-hyperventilation apnoea. The second type of extension is shown on the middle line of the right hand fan. It is horizontal and to the left, like a golf club, representing the response of a subject who continues to breathe regardless of the fact that his P_{CO_2} has been reduced. This has been discussed above in relation to wakefulness, but persistent breathing is much more likely to occur in hypoxia.

If P_{CO_2} is raised above about 10.7 kPa (80 mmHg), the linear relationship between P_{CO_2} and ventilation is lost. As P_{CO_2} is raised a point of maximal ventilatory stimulation is reached (probably within the range 13.3–26.7 kPa or 100–200 mmHg). Thereafter the ventilatory stimulation is reduced until, at very high P_{CO_2}, the ventilation is actually depressed below control value and finally apnoea results, at least in the dog and almost certainly in man as well. It does not appear to be possible to arrest breathing in the cat by this means in spite of elevation of P_{CO_2} to more than 67 kPa or 500 mmHg (Hornbein, personal communication; Raymond and Standaert, 1967). The full P_{CO_2}/ventilation curve is thus something like a parabola rising from the apnoeic threshold P_{CO_2} (4.9 kPa or 37 mmHg), reaching a peak at about 20 kPa (150 mmHg) and returning to base line at a P_{CO_2} of the order of 40 kPa (300 mmHg) (Graham, Hill and Nunn, 1960).

The response curves above have been described in relation to arterial P_{CO_2}. It seems likely that internal jugular or CSF P_{CO_2} might be more appropriate and these have been shown to give particularly straight curves. Alternatively, in the clinical environment it may be more convenient to use end-expiratory P_{CO_2} as a substitute for arterial P_{CO_2} although this is not satisfactory in conditions such as chronic bronchitis which are associated with a marked arterial/end-expiratory P_{CO_2} difference (see Chapter 9). Methods of obtaining response curves are summarized at the end of this chapter.

Interaction of P_{CO_2}, P_{O_2} and metabolic acidosis. Reference has been made above to the influence of the chemoreceptor drive from P_{O_2} on the central ventilatory response to P_{CO_2} (broken line 'A' in *Figure 4.4*). Typical quantitative relationships are shown in *Figure 4.8*, with hypoxia at the left of the fan and hyperoxia on the right. The curve marked P_{O_2} 80 kPa represents total abolition of chemoreceptor drive obtained by the inhalation of 100% oxygen. A similar result follows carotid endarterectomy, which usually results in destruction of the carotid bodies (Mitchell et al., 1964; Wade et al., 1970). This provides important evidence that the respiratory drive from the peripheral chemoreceptors is almost entirely from the carotid bodies, with the aortic bodies having little respiratory effect.

Metabolic acidosis displaces the whole fan of curves to the left as shown in *Figure 4.8*. The intercept (*B*) is reduced but the slope of the curves at each value of P_{O_2} is virtually unaltered. Display of the fan of P_{CO_2}/ventilation response curves at different P_{O_2} is a particularly complete method of representing the state of respiratory control in a patient but it is unfortunately laborious to determine.

Reflex control of breathing

We have already considered the reflex arcs with afferent limbs arising in the peripheral chemoreceptors in relation to chemical control. In addition, there are the ventilatory reflexes in response to pain, which are similar in many respects to the arousal state. There remain, however, a number of neural control mechanisms which are more appropriately considered specifically under the heading of reflexes.

Baroreceptor reflexes

The most important groups of arterial baroreceptors are in the carotid sinus and around the aortic arch. These receptors are primarily concerned with regulation of the circulation but a decrease in pressure produces hyperventilation, while a rise in pressure causes respiratory depression and, ultimately, apnoea (Heymans and Neil, 1958). This is the likely cause of apnoea produced by a massive dose of catecholamines. Baroreceptors are sensitized by diethyl ether (Robertson, Swan and Whitteridge, 1956), cyclopropane (Price and Widdicombe, 1962) and halothane (Biscoe and Millar, 1964). This effect has been considered mainly in relation to circulatory control during anaesthesia and the respiratory implications are not yet established.

Pulmonary stretch reflexes

There are a large number of different types of receptors in the lungs (see review by Widdicombe, 1981) sensitive to inflation, deflation, mechanical and chemical stimulation. Afferents from all are conducted by the vagus, although some fibres may be additionally carried in the sympathetic. The stretch receptors are predominantly in the airways rather than in the alveoli and are probably located in the airway smooth muscle. These receptors have attracted much attention since the associated inflation and deflation reflexes were described by Hering (1868) and Breuer (1868).

It is perhaps appropriate at this point to explain the relationship between these two authors who produced two papers of identical title in the same journal from the same department in the same year. Breuer was a clinical assistant and apparently the work was at his own instigation. However, Hering, who was a corresponding member of the Vienna Academy of Science, published Breuer's work under his own name, in accord with the custom of the time. Breuer's role was clearly stated in Hering's paper but he was not a co-author. Later the same year, Breuer was able to publish a much fuller account of his work under his own name. The extent of the individual contributions of Hering and Breuer has been discussed by Ullmann (1970), who also appended an English translation of the original papers.

The inflation reflex consists of inhibition of inspiration in response to a sustained inflation of the lung. An exactly similar effect may be obtained by obstructing expiration so that an inspiration is retained in the lungs. At least in animals, rhythmic breathing may be modified by a negative feedback loop from the pulmonary stretch receptors via the vagus and the expiratory neurones of the medulla (see *Figure 4.1*).

Generations of medical students have been brought up with the unquestioned belief in the role of the Hering–Breuer reflex in man. This appears to have resulted from an unwarranted extrapolation of animal findings to man without regard for species difference. Widdicombe (1961) compared the strength of the inflation reflex in eight species and found the reflex weakest in man. His method for the human subjects was to weight the bell of a spirometer connected to spontaneously breathing, lightly anaesthetized patients. Inflation to transpulmonary pressures of 0.7–1.1 kPa (7–11 cm H_2O) did not produce apnoea lasting longer than 10 seconds, in contrast to the rabbit in which increases of transpulmonary pressure of 0.5–0.7 kPa (5–7 cm H_2O) on two occasions killed rabbits by asphyxia during the prolonged apnoea that followed. Widdicombe's traces show some reduction of tidal volume in the human subjects but the movement of a weighted spirometer bell at an increased lung volume is a very indirect measure of inspiratory effort.

The view that the Hering–Breuer inflation reflex is weak if not absent in man is supported by the response of anaesthetized patients to expiratory resistance. This is discussed on page 355, but the essential feature is that patients respond by an increased inspiratory force until the lung volume is increased to the point at which the increased elastic recoil is sufficient to overcome the expiratory resistance (Campbell, Howell and Peckett, 1957). In the face of high expiratory resistance, the lung volume increases in a series of steps, with ever-increasing end-inspiratory pressure associated with increasing inspiratory effort (Nunn and Ezi-Ashi, 1961). This remarkable series of changes, which can be confirmed by any anaesthetist, provides clear evidence that lung inflation in the anaesthetized human subject augments the force of contraction of the inspiratory muscles in complete contrast to what might be expected if the effect of the Hering–Breuer inflation reflex were dominant. This provides no proof of the absence of the inflation reflex, and its effect, if present, might be overcome by other mechanisms producing an opposite effect. The role of the spindles has been discused earlier in this chapter and on page 356.

The pulmonary stretch receptors are stimulated by a decrease of P_{CO_2}, but it is unlikely that this effect is of great practical importance (Widdicombe, 1981). The receptors are unaffected by changes in P_{O_2}. An increase in pulmonary venous pressure of 4 kPa (30 mmHg) causes an augmentation of stretch receptor activity of about 20 per cent (Marshall and Widdicombe, 1958).

The deflation reflex consists of an augmentation of inspiration in response to deflation of the lung. Guz et al. (1971) studied the effect of sudden unilateral lung deflation in four patients with spontaneous pneumothorax. This was painless, but all patients developed tachypnoea and arterial P_{O_2} decreased. Breath-holding times were decreased and the ventilatory response to carbon dioxide was increased in two patients. Guz concluded that the results were consistent with the hypothesis that lung deflation has a reflex excitatory effect on breathing but that the threshold is higher than for other mammalian species. The deflation reflex in the rabbit is blocked by breathing a local anaesthetic aerosol (Jain et al., 1973).

The inflation and deflation reflexes were the basis of the *Selbststeuerung* (self-steering) hypothesis of Hering and Breuer. This concept has played a major role in theories of the control of breathing and, even though its role in man may be questionable, it remains a classic example of a physiological autoregulating mechanism.

Head's paradoxical reflex. Head (1889), working in Professor Hering's laboratory, described a reversal of the inflation reflex, which could be elicited during partial block of the vagus nerves in the course of thawing after cold block. Under these conditions, inflation of the lung of the rabbit causes strong maintained contractions of an isolated diaphragmatic slip (curve VI, Plate I in Head, 1889). Many authors have reported that, with normal vagal conduction, sudden inflation of the lungs of many species may cause a transient inspiratory effort before the onset of apnoea due to the inflation reflex (Widdicombe, 1961). A similar response may also be elicited in newborn infants (Cross et al., 1960), but it has not been established whether this 'gasp reflex' is analogous to Head's paradoxical reflex. Widdicombe was unable to detect the response in patients anaesthetized with thiopentone but many anaesthetists will know that the response may be elicited in patients who receive opiates (particularly pethidine) in dosage sufficient to reduce the respiratory frequency to less than about five breaths per minute. Transient compression of the reservoir bag often causes an immediate deep gasping type of inspiration and the respiratory frequency may be conveniently raised by manual triggering. This response does not appear to have been studied in detail in anaesthetized man. There is a possible relationship between the reflex and the mechanism of sighing which may be considered a normal feature of breathing (Bendixen, Smith and Mead, 1964).

The cough reflex

The cough reflex may be elicited by mechanical stimuli arising in the larynx, trachea, carina and main bronchi. Chemical stimuli are effective further down the respiratory tract (Widdicombe, 1964). The cough reflex is complex and comprises three main stages:

1. An inspiration, which takes into the lungs a volume of air sufficient for the expiratory activity.
2. Build-up of pressure in the lungs by contraction of expiratory muscles against a closed glottis.
3. Forceful expiration through narrowed airways with high linear velocity of gas flow which sweeps irritant material up towards the pharynx.

Irritant receptors have been reviewed by Mills, Sellick and Widdicombe (1970) and Widdicombe (1981).

The mechanism of the narrowing of the airways is discussed in Chapter 3 (page 59). Transient changes of pressure up to 40 kPa (300 mmHg) may occur in the thorax, arterial blood and the CSF during the act of coughing (Sharpey-Schafer, 1953).

Other pulmonary afferents

Pulmonary embolization and pneumothorax may each cause rapid shallow breathing by a reflex arc with afferents carried in the vagi. Changes in blood gas tensions may also produce secondary changes in ventilation. The pattern of discharge of medullary neurones in these conditions was reported by Katz and Horres (1972). More recent work suggests the stretch receptors are sensitized after microembolism.

C-fibre endings (J receptors). These endings lie in close relationship to the capillaries. One group is in relation to the bronchial circulation and the other to the pulmonary microcirculation. The latter correspond to Paintal's juxtapulmonary capillary receptors (J receptors, for short) which were reviewed by him in 1983 and by Coleridge and Coleridge in 1984. Afferent unmyelinated fibres are in the vagus.

These receptors are relatively silent during normal breathing but appear to be stimulated under various pathological conditions. They appear to be nociceptive and activated by tissue damage, accumulation of interstitial fluid and release of various mediators (Widdicombe, 1981). In the laboratory they can be activated by intravascular injection of capsaicin to produce the so-called pulmonary chemoreflex which comprises bradycardia, hypotension, apnoea or shallow breathing, bronchoconstriction and increased mucus secretion. They may well be concerned in the dyspnoea of pulmonary vascular congestion and the ventilatory response to exercise and pulmonary embolization. C-fibre endings have been characterized in physiological studies but have never been identified histologically although non-myelinated nerve fibres have been seen in the alveolar walls.

Lung chemoreceptors. Various phenomena such as the hyperventilation of exercise could be very conveniently explained by the existence of chemoreceptors on the arterial side of the pulmonary circulation, which would be sensitive to mixed venous blood gas tensions. Widdicombe (1981) has reviewed the evidence for believing their existence to be unlikely.

Afferents from the musculoskeletal system. Kalia et al. (1972) have shown that a variety of mechanical stimuli applied to the gastrocnemius muscle of the dog can produce a reflex increase in ventilation. This occurred when afferents from the pressure–pain receptors were blocked by antidromic stimulation. The afferents causing stimulation of ventilation were carried by non-medullated fibres. Afferents from the musculoskeletal system probably have an important role in the hyperventilation of exercise (Chapter 12).

Breath holding

Blood gas tensions

When the breath is held after air breathing, the arterial and alveolar P_{CO_2} are remarkably constant at the breaking point and values are normally close to 6.7 kPa (50 mmHg). This does not mean that P_{CO_2} is the sole or dominant factor and concomitant hypoxia is probably more important. Preliminary oxygen breathing delays the onset of hypoxia, and breath-holding times may be greatly prolonged with consequent elevation of P_{CO_2} at the breaking point. The relationship between P_{CO_2} and P_{O_2} at breaking point, after varying degrees of preoxygenation, is shown in *Figure 4.9*. The breaking point curve is displaced upwards and to the left by

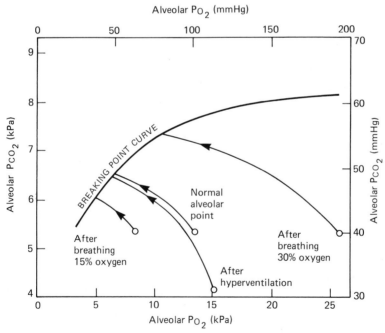

Figure 4.9 The 'breaking point' curve defines the coexisting values of alveolar P_{O_2} and P_{CO_2}, at the breaking point of breath holding, starting from various states. The normal alveolar point is shown (P_{O_2}, 13.3 kPa or 100 mmHg; P_{CO_2}, 5.3 kPa or 40 mmHg) and the curved arrow shows the changes in alveolar gas tensions which occur during breath holding. Starting points are displaced to the right by preliminary breathing of oxygen-enriched gas mixtures, and to the left by breathing mixtures containing less than 21% oxygen. Hyperventilation displaces the point representing the alveolar gas tensions to the right and downwards. The length of the arrows from starting point to the 'breaking point' curve gives an approximate indication of the possible duration of breath holding. This can clearly be prolonged by oxygen breathing or by hyperventilation, maximal prolongation occurring after hyperventilation with 100% oxygen. (Data for construction of the 'breaking point' curve have been taken from Ferris et al. (1946) and Otis, Rahn and Fenn (1948))

carotid body resection (Davidson et al., 1974). Guz et al. (1966b) observed marked prolongation of breath holding after vagal and glossopharyngeal block but advanced cogent reasons for believing that this was not due primarily to block of the chemoreceptors. Oxygen breathing would also prevent the chemoreceptor drive but this did not prolong breath holding to the same extent as the nerve block.

Lung volume

Breath-holding time is directly proportional to the lung volume at the onset of breath holding, other factors being constant. In part this is related to the onset of hypoxia, since an appreciable part of the total body oxygen store is in the alveolar gas (page 271). There are, however, other effects of lung volume and its change, which are mediated by afferents arising from both chest wall and the lung itself. Following the experiments of Guz mentioned above, Campbell et al. (1967, 1969) reported an equally impressive prolongation of breath-holding time following curarization of conscious subjects. Their explanation was that the distress leading to the termination of breath holding is caused by frustration of reflex motor response from pulmonary afferents blocked in the experiment of Guz. The motor response consists of involuntary contractions of the respiratory muscles, including the diaphragm, which have been found to increase progressively during breath holding (Agostoni, 1963). These contractions should produce movement which would be detected by joint and tendon receptors in the chest wall. However, in breath holding, movement is prevented by closure of the glottis and there is an 'inappropriateness' between the muscle activity and the (lack of) movement which results. This accords with the idea of 'inappropriateness' advanced as a general hypothesis to explain the sensation of dyspnoea (Campbell and Howell, 1963). The discomfort of breath holding would then be regarded as an extreme form of inappropriateness, differing only quantitatively from that of mechanically hindered breathing.

According to this hypothesis, the discomfort of breathing could be alleviated at the following points:

1. Block of pulmonary afferents causing the involuntary contraction of the respiratory muscles (Guz et al., 1966b).
2. Prevention of the involuntary contraction of the respiratory muscles (Campbell et al., 1967, 1969).
3. Prevention of the frustration of the contractions of the respiratory muscles by permitting chest movement without alleviating the changes in alveolar P_{CO_2} and P_{O_2}.

Eisele et al. (1968) showed that spinal analgesia (affecting intercostal muscles but not the diaphragm) had no effect on breath holding. In contrast, Noble et al. (1971) showed that phrenic nerve block increased breath-holding time. It thus appears that the inappropriateness arises in the diaphragm rather than in the intercostals, in spite of the paucity of afferents from the former (Corda, von Euler and Lennerstrand, 1965).

Prolongation of breath-holding time by prevention of frustration of contraction of respiratory muscles may be convincingly demonstrated by Fowler's experiment (1954). After normal air breathing, the breath is held until breaking point, which is usually about 60 seconds. If the expirate is then taken in a bag and immediately reinhaled, there is a marked sense of relief although it may be shown that the rise of P_{CO_2} and fall of P_{O_2} are quite uninfluenced by the manoeuvre.

Extreme durations of breath holding may be attained after hyperventilation and preoxygenation. Times of 14 minutes have been reached and the limiting factor is then reduction of lung volume to residual volume, as oxygen is removed from the alveolar gas by the circulating pulmonary blood (Klocke and Rahn, 1959).

Ventilatory response to loaded breathing

This important subject is considered in Chapter 3, pages 65 et seq.

Outline of methods of assessment of factors in control of breathing

Sensitivity to carbon dioxide

For clinical purposes, ventilatory failure is detected by measurement of P_{CO_2} but, by itself, this measurement does not identify any particular factor in the control of breathing. However, if the measurement of P_{CO_2} is combined with simultaneous measurement of ventilation, over a range of values of P_{CO_2} (obtained by increasing the carbon dioxide concentration of the inspired gas), this gives a useful indication of the ability of the ventilatory mechanism to respond to elevation of P_{CO_2}. However, it is important to note that the response may be be reduced as a result of impaired function anywhere between the medullary neurones and the mechanical properties of the lung (*Figure 20.2*). Thus it cannot be assumed that a decreased ventilation/P_{CO_2} response is necessarily due to failure of the central chemoreceptor mechanism.

The steady state method requires the simultaneous measurement of minute volume and P_{CO_2} after P_{CO_2} has been raised by increasing the concentration of carbon dioxide in the inspired gas. The ventilation is usually reasonably stable after 5 minutes of inhaling a fixed concentration of carbon dioxide. P_{CO_2} may be measured in arterial blood but end-expiratory gas is more usual. Several points are needed to define the P_{CO_2}/ventilation response curve and it is a time-consuming process which may be distressing to some patients. Methods of measurement of ventilation are outlined on page 112 and P_{CO_2} on page 230.

The rebreathing method introduced by Read (1967) has greatly simplified determination of the slope of the P_{CO_2}/ventilation response curve. The subject rebreathes for up to four minutes from a 6-litre bag originally containing 7% carbon dioxide and about 50% oxygen, the remainder being nitrogen. The carbon dioxide concentration rises steadily during rebreathing while the oxygen concentration should remain above 30%. Thus there should be no appreciable hypoxic drive and ventilation is driven solely by the rising arterial P_{CO_2}, which should be very close to the P_{CO_2} of the gas in the bag. Ventilation is measured by any convenient means and plotted against the P_{CO_2} of the gas in the bag. Milledge, Minty and Duncalf (1974) described an automated technique by which the P_{CO_2}/ventilation response curve is automatically determined and presented on an X–Y plotter.

The P_{CO_2}/ventilation response curve measured by the rebreathing technique is displaced to the right by about 0.7 kPa (5 mmHg) compared with the steady state method, but there is good evidence that the slope of normal subjects and patients with obstructive airway disease as measured by the rebreathing technique is the same as the slope measured by the conventional steady state method (Read, 1967; Clark, 1968).

It was suggested by Whitelaw, Derenne and Milic-Emili (1975) that a better indication of the output of the respiratory centre may be obtained by measuring the subatmospheric pressure developed in the airways when obstructed for 0.1 second at the beginning of inspiration ($P_{0.1}$). This eliminates any effect due to increased airway resistance or reduced compliance, and the $Pco_2/P_{0.1}$ response curve is thus a better index of central sensitivity to carbon dioxide. Nevertheless, it will still be influenced by impaired performance in the lower motoneurones or respiratory muscles.

The ventilatory response to Pco_2 may be separated into rib cage and abdominal components. The former is considerably greater than the latter (Tusiewicz, Bryan and Froese, 1977), suggesting that the major response is in the intercostals rather than the diaphragm.

Sensitivity to hypoxia

There is generally more reluctance to test sensitivity to hypoxia because of the reduction in Po_2 to which the patient is exposed. Various approaches to the problem have been reviewed by Rebuck and Slutsky (1981).

Intermittent inhalation of high oxygen concentration will cause a temporary withdrawal of peripheral chemoreceptor drive. Ventilation should then be reduced by about 15 per cent. This may be used as an indication of the existence of carotid body activity (Dejours, 1962) but clearly it cannot be a very sensitive indicator of the level of activity. Alternatively, chemoreceptor response may be assessed by the inhalation of four vital capacity breaths of 15% carbon dioxide in nitrogen. This should be instantly followed by two or three large breaths before there is time for central chemoreceptor response.

The steady state method for oxygen is best undertaken by preparing Pco_2/ventilation response curves at different levels of Po_2, which are presented as a fan (see *Figure 4.8*). The spread of the fan is an indication of peripheral chemoreceptor sensitivity but it is also possible to present the data in the form of the rectangular hyperbola (see *Figure 4.6*) by plotting the ventilatory response for different values of Po_2 at the same Pco_2 (intercepts of components of the fan with a vertical line drawn through a particular value of Pco_2). The parameters of the hyperbola may then be derived as outlined above.

A minimum of 5 minutes is required to reach a steady state although it is possible to speed up the process by varying Po_2 while keeping Pco_2 constant, the response to a change in Po_2 being far quicker than for Pco_2 (Weil et al., 1970). Alternatively, the ventilation may be kept approximately constant while Pco_2 and Po_2 are both raised by appropriate amounts so that the Pco_2 stimulus increases by the same amount as the hypoxic drive diminishes (Lloyd and Cunningham, 1963). Nevertheless, it is a laborious undertaking to determine the oxygen response by these methods and patients may be distressed, particularly by the run at low Po_2 and high Pco_2.

The rebreathing method has been adapted to measure the response to hypoxia (Rebuck and Campbell, 1974). The oxygen concentration of the rebreathed gas is reduced by the oxygen consumption of the subject but active steps have to be taken to maintain the P_{CO_2} at a constant level. Calculation of the response is greatly simplified by measuring the oxygen saturation (usually non-invasively by means of an ear oximeter) and plotting the response as ventilation against saturation. This normally approximates to a straight line and the slope is a function of the chemoreceptor sensitivity. However, even if P_{CO_2} is held constant, the response is directly influenced by the patient's sensitivity to P_{CO_2}.

Chapter 5

Pulmonary ventilation

Mechanisms of breathing

The movements of the lung in breathing are purely passive and may be produced either by use of the respiratory muscles or by the development of a pressure gradient between the airways and the space surrounding the chest. An adequate alveolar ventilation may be obtained by either means but there are subtle differences between the two types of ventilation. This chapter is concerned solely with pulmonary ventilation achieved by use of the respiratory muscles. Passive ventilation by means of the generation of pressure gradients is considered in Chapter 21.

Figure 2.9 shows the volume changes which may be produced by use of the respiratory muscles. Expiration normally proceeds to the functional residual capacity (FRC). Inspiration encroaches on the inspiratory capacity but normally leaves a substantial volume, the inspiratory reserve volume, before total lung capacity is reached. Similarly, there is a substantial volume, the expiratory reserve volume, between FRC and the residual volume. By voluntary effort it is possible to change the lung volume to any level within the vital capacity but the work of breathing is minimal from the FRC. When attention is distracted from breathing, it is usual to resume the pattern described at the beginning of this paragraph. The radiographic appearance of some of these volumes is shown in *Figure 5.1*.

Inspiration is active and depends upon contraction of the inspiratory muscles. In quiet breathing, expiration is normally passive and is powered by the elastic recoil of the tissue deformation which occurred during expiration. Thus the work of both inspiration and expiration is performed by the inspiratory muscles. Expiratory muscles may reinforce the normally passive expiration, and the circumstances under which this happens are considered below.

The respiratory muscles

The inspiratory muscles are not easy of access for electromyographic or other methods of study and this has greatly complicated elucidation of their pattern of contraction. Measurement of pressures within the thorax and abdomen is particularly useful to distinguish between active and passive movements of the diaphragm. Radiographic and a wide range of other imaging and stethographic methods will indicate the change in shape of the confines of thorax, abdomen and lungs but do not necessarily indicate the muscle groups responsible. Inspiratory muscle activity does not terminate abruptly at the end of inspiration. There is a

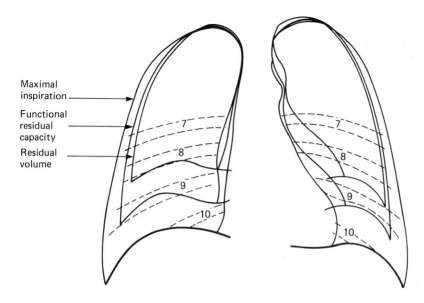

Maximal inspiration

Functional residual capacity

Residual volume

7

8

9

10

7

8

9

10

Figure 5.1 Outlines of chest radiographs of a normal subject at various levels of lung inflation. The numbers refer to ribs as seen in the position of maximal inspiration. (I am indebted to Dr R.L. Marks who was the subject)

gradual let-down of their tone during early expiration which does not therefore assume the pattern of an exponential decay as seen in the paralysed patient.

The diaphragm. The diaphragm is the most important inspiratory muscle. During inspiration, the origins and insertions into the central tendon are approximated, resulting both in descent of the domes of the diaphragm and elevation and rotation of the ribs. The normal excursion of the domes is 1.5 cm, increasing to 6–7 cm during deep breathing (Wade and Gilson, 1951). The diaphragm has considerable reserve of function, and unilateral paralysis (which was formerly used as a thera-peutic procedure for pulmonary tuberculosis) causes little decrement of overall ventilatory capacity. Although the diaphragm is the most important inspiratory muscle, other muscle groups have a remarkable ability to compensate, and, sur-prisingly, bilateral phrenic interruption is compatible with good ventilatory function (Dowman, 1927; Eisele et al., 1972).

Electromyographic activity in the crura may be recorded with a bipolar oeso-phageal lead (Agostoni, Sant'Ambrogio and Carrasco, 1960; Agostoni, 1962). Other parts of the diaphragm are less accessible and the use of surface leads is complicated by activity in the overlying intercostal muscles. This difficulty was ingeniously overcome by Muller and his colleagues (1979) by intercostal nerve block. This silenced the intercostal muscle activity and permitted surface recordings of diaphragmatic activity.

The intercostal muscles. These muscles are divided into the external group (deficient anteriorly), the less powerful internal group (deficient posteriorly) and the feeble strands of intercostalis intima, with vessels and nerves lying between the internal intercostals and the intercostalis intima. Distinction between these muscles by electromyography is difficult and there has been much controversy about their function. It has even been suggested that they are vestigial remnants without any important function, but this seems unlikely since the intercostal muscles acting alone are able to maintain a high level of ventilation (Otis, Fenn and Rahn, 1950). Campbell (1955) found them to contract during inspiration in most but not all subjects. However, he was unable to demonstrate in man the expiratory activity which has been reported in animals. It is generally taught that the internal inter-costals are expiratory and the externals inspiratory.

Other inspiratory muscles. Pectoralis minor and the scalenes may be active in quiet breathing.

The expiratory muscles

The expiratory muscles are normally silent during quiet breathing but become active when the minute volume exceeds about 40 l/min, in the face of substantial expiratory resistance, during phonation and when making expulsive efforts. However, their use in breathing is complicated by their role in the maintenance of posture. Thus the abdominal muscles are normally active in the upright position but silent during quiet breathing in the supine position.

The most important expiratory muscles are rectus abdominis, external and internal obliques, and tranversalis. The muscles of the pelvic floor have a supportive role. External oblique is usually monitored as an indication of expiratory muscle activity but gastric pressure is a valuable index of their activity since they cannot contract without causing an increase in intra-abdominal pressure.

Active hyperventilation

As ventilation is increased, the inspiratory muscles contract more vigorously and accessory muscles are recruited. The first group to be recruited is usually the scalenes but considerable hyperventilation (about 50 l/min) is usually attained before the sternomastoids and extensors of the vertebral column are brought into play (Campbell, 1958). Maximal hyperventilation requires the use of many groups of muscles. The pectorals, for example, reverse their usual origin/insertion and help to expand the chest provided the arms are fixed by grasping a suitable support. Expiratory muscle activity is evident only when the minute volume exceeds about 40 l/min (Campbell, 1952). Thereafter it becomes progressively more important until ventilation assumes a quasi sine wave push–pull pattern in extreme hyperventilation (Cooper, 1961).

Effect of posture

The effect of posture on lung volumes is considered on page 39. The diaphragm tends to lie some 4 cm higher in the supine position (Wade and Gilson, 1951) and this accords with the reduction in FRC (see *Figure 2.4*). The dimensions of the rib cage are probably little altered. Although there is a greater tendency to airway closure at the reduced FRC, the diaphragm is able to contract more effectively the higher it rises into the chest. In the lateral position (*Figure 5.2*), the lower dome of the diaphragm is pushed higher into the chest by the weight of the abdominal

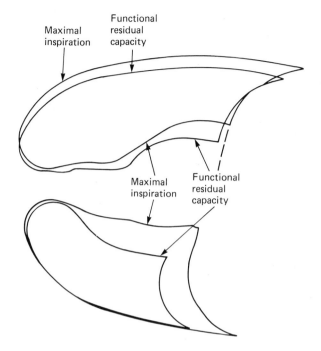

Figure 5.2 Radiographic outlines of the lungs at two levels of lung volume in a conscious subject during spontaneous breathing in the lateral position (right side down). This is the same subject as in Figure 5.1: comparison will show that, in the lateral position at FRC, the lower lung is close to residual volume while the upper lung is close to inspiratory capacity. The diaphragm therefore lies much higher in the lower half of the chest. Both these factors contribute to the greater volume changes which occur in the lower lung during inspiration. The mediastinum seems to rest on a pneumatic cushion at FRC and rises during inspiration.

contents while the upper dome is flattened. It follows that the lower dome can contract more effectively than the upper, and the ventilation of the lower lung is about twice that of the upper. This is fortunate since gravity causes a preferential perfusion of the lower lung. Thus the ventilation/perfusion ratio of each lung remains approximately constant regardless of position (Svanberg, 1957). This subject is discussed more fully in Chapters 6 and 7.

Dyscoordinated breathing

Under a wide range of pathological circumstances, there may occur a type of breathing in which there is lack of co-ordination between thoracic and diaphragmatic components. In its extreme form there is failure to synchronize, and the chest wall moves inwards during inspiration. Pontoppidan, Geffin and Lowenstein (1972) discussed this problem in their review of acute respiratory failure, and pointed out that it is relatively common and may exist between the two sides of the diaphragm which is difficult to diagnose without recourse to imaging techniques. Respiratory muscle dyscoordination increases the work of breathing and reduces the effective tidal volume. It may delay successful weaning from artificial ventilation.

Failure of ventilation is considered in Chapter 20.

The work of breathing

As described above, expiration is passive during quiet breathing and the work of breathing is performed entirely by the inspiratory muscles. Approximately half of this work is dissipated during inspiration as heat in overcoming the frictional forces opposing inspiration. The other half is stored as potential energy in the deformed elastic tissues of lung and chest wall. This potential energy is thus available as the source of energy for expiration and is then dissipated as heat in overcoming the frictional forces resisting expiration. The whole of the work of breathing is dissipated as heat by the end of expiration (upper section of *Figure 5.3*). Energy stored in deformed elastic tissue thus permits the work of *expiration* to be transferred to the *inspiratory* muscles.

If there is increased inspiratory resistance, the work performed during inspiration is increased (middle section of *Figure 5.3*). Potential energy stored for expiration is unchanged. If, however, there is a moderate level of expiratory resistance, this is still overcome by use of potential energy stored during inspiration. The inspiratory muscles contract more forcefully by a mechanism considered on page 67 and increase the end-inspiratory lung volume within the inspiratory reserve. There is then greater deformation of elastic tissue and a higher recoil pressure (see *Figure 2.3*) which is available to overcome the increased expiratory resistance (lower section of *Figure 5.3*). This mechanism suffices for fairly high levels of expiratory resistance, but with very high levels the expiratory muscles are brought into play as described above.

The actual rate of work performed by the respiratory muscles is very small in the healthy resting subject. Under these circumstances the oxygen consumption of the respiratory muscles is only about 3 ml/min or less than 2 per cent of the metabolic rate. Furthermore, the efficiency of the respiratory muscles is only about 10 per cent. Thus 90 per cent of the work performed by the respiratory muscles is lost as heat generated within the muscles and only 10 per cent is available for moving gas against the frictional resistance of the airway and the tissues. The efficiency is further reduced in many forms of respiratory disease, certain deformities, pregnancy and when the minute volume is increased (*Figure 5.4*). When maximal ventilation is approached, the efficiency falls to such a low level that additional oxygen made available by further increases in ventilation will be entirely consumed by the respiratory muscles (Otis, 1954). This effectively limits the improvement in alveolar gas tensions which can be achieved by increasing the minute volume of spontaneous, but not artificial, ventilation. This 'ceiling' of ventilation is reached only at very high levels of ventilation in healthy patients. However, in severe diffuse obstructive respiratory disease, the 'ceiling' may be low enough to limit exercise tolerance.

Units of measurement of work

Work is performed when a force moves its point of application, and the work is equal to the product of force and distance moved. Similarly, work is performed when force is applied to the plunger of a syringe raising the pressure of gas contained therein. In this case the work is equal to the product of the mean pressure and the change in volume, or alternatively the product of the mean volume and the change in pressure. The units of work are identical whether the product is *force × distance* or *pressure × volume*. A multiplicity of units have been used for measuring work and are listed in Appendix A.

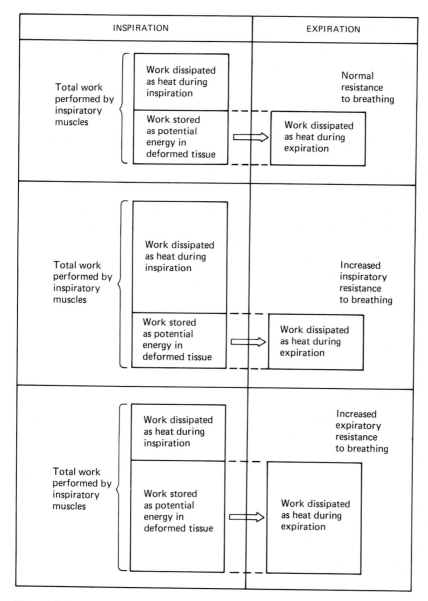

Figure 5.3 Source and dissipation of the work of breathing. The areas in each diagram correspond to the work of breathing. The total area on the left indicates the work done by the inspiratory muscles during inspiration.

Power is a measure of the rate at which work is being (or can be) performed. The term 'work of breathing', as it is normally used and when expressed in watts, is thus a misnomer since we are referring to the rate at which work is being performed and *power* is the correct term. 'Work of breathing' would be appropriate for a single event such as one breath, and joules would then be the appropriate units.

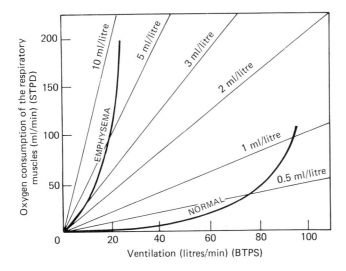

Figure 5.4 Oxygen consumption of the respiratory muscles plotted against minute volume of respiration. The isopleths indicate the oxygen cost of breathing in millilitres of oxygen consumed per litre of minute volume. The curve obtained from the normal subject shows the low oxygen cost of breathing up to a minute volume of 70 l/min. Thereafter the oxygen cost rises steeply. In the emphysematous patient, the oxygen cost of breathing is not only much higher at the resting minute volume, but it also rises steeply as ventilation is increased. At a minute volume of 20 l/min, the respiratory muscles are consuming 200 ml oxygen per minute, and a further increase of ventilation would consume more oxygen than it would make available to the rest of the body. (Reproduced after Campbell, Westlake and Cherniak (1957) by permission of the Editor of the Journal of Applied Physiology)

Dissipation of the work of breathing

The work of breathing overcomes two main sources of impedance. The first is the elastic recoil of the lungs and chest wall (Chapter 2) and the second is the frictional resistance to gas flow afforded by the air passages (Chapter 3). Further but minor sources of impedance are the frictional resistance of tissue deformation, and the inertance of tissue and gases which must be overcome as the direction of flow is reversed at the beginning and end of inspiration.

Work against elastic recoil. When a perfectly elastic body is deformed, none of the work is dissipated as heat and all work is stored as potential energy. No body is perfectly elastic but a satisfactory conversion to potential energy is obtained in such devices as the clockwork motor.

In the case of respiration, it is easiest to consider passive inflation of the lung. *Figure 5.5a* shows a section of the pressure/volume diagram taken from *Figure 2.8*. As the lungs are inflated, the relevant section of the alveolar pressure/volume curve forms the hypotenuse of triangle whose area represents the work done against elastic resistance. The area of the triangle (half the base times the height) will thus equal either half the tidal volume times the pressure change or the mean pressure times the volume change. The products have the units of work or energy (joules) and represent the potential energy available for expiration. In *Figure 5.5b*, the pressure/volume curve is flatter, indicating stiffer or less compliant lungs. For the

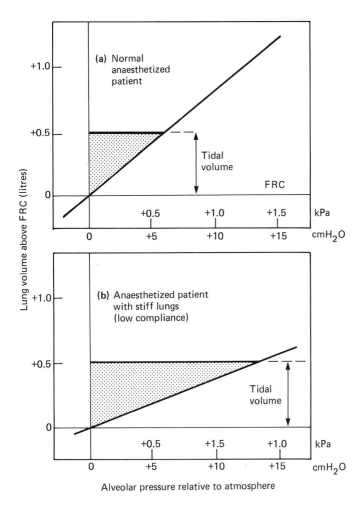

Figure 5.5 Work of breathing against elastic resistance during passive inflation. Pressure/volume plots of the lungs of anaesthetized patients (see Figure 2.8). The length of the pressure/volume curve covered during inspiration forms the hypotenuse of a right-angled triangle whose area equals the work performed against elastic resistance. Note the area is greater when the pressure/volume curve is flatter (indicating stiffer or less compliant lungs).

same tidal volume, the area of the triangle is increased. This indicates the greater amount of work performed against elastic resistance and the greater potential energy available for expiration.

Work against resistance to gas flow. Figure 5.5 describes conditions under which air flow resistance is ignored by measuring alveolar pressure. Additional pressure is required to overcome the resistance to breathing afforded by the respiratory tract. This is reflected in the mouth pressure which, during inspiration, is above the alveolar pressure by the driving pressure required to overcome airway resistance. When mouth pressure is plotted as in *Figure 5.6*, the inspiratory curve is bowed to

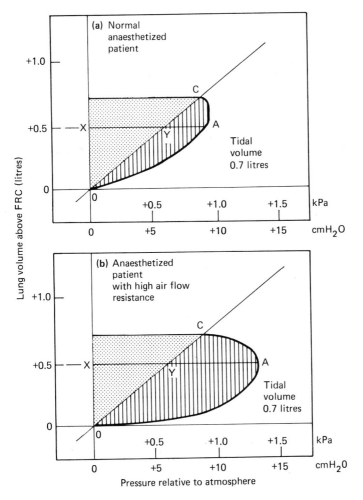

Figure 5.6 Work of breathing against air flow resistance during passive inflation. The sloping line (OYC) is the alveolar pressure/volume curve. The curve (OAC) is the mouth pressure/volume curve during inflation of the lungs. The area shaded with vertical stripes indicates the work of inspiration performed against air flow resistance. This work is increased in the patient with high resistance (b). At the point when 500 ml gas has entered the patient, XY represents the pressure distending the lungs, while YA represents the pressure overcoming air flow resistance. XA is the inflation pressure at that moment. The stippled areas represent work done against elastic resistance (see Figure 5.5).

the right and the area shaded with vertical lines to the right of the pressure volume curve indicates the work performed in overcoming airway resistance. *Figure 5.6b* represents a patient with increased airway resistance. The diagram clearly shows the partitioning of inflation pressure and work of breathing between the component required to overcome elastance and the component required to overcome airway resistance.

The expiratory curve, not shown in *Figure 5.6*, is bowed to the left as the mouth-to-alveolar pressure gradient is reversed during expiration.

The minimal work of breathing

For a constant minute volume, the work performed against elastic resistance is increased when breathing is slow and deep. Conversely, the work performed against air flow resistance is increased when breathing is rapid and shallow. If the two components are summated and the total work is plotted against respiratory frequency, it will be found that there is an optimal frequency at which the total work of breathing is minimal (*Figure 5.7*). If there is increased elastic resistance (as in patients with pulmonary fibrosis), the optimal frequency is increased while in the presence of increased air flow resistance the optimal frequency is decreased.

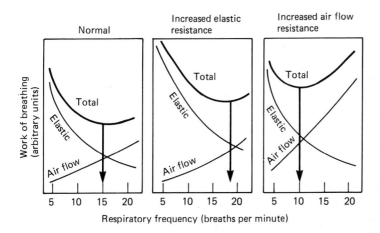

Figure 5.7 The diagrams show the work done against elastic and air flow resistance separately and summated to indicate the total work of breathing at different respiratory frequencies. The total work of breathing has a minimum value at about 15 breaths per minute under normal circumstances. For the same minute volume, minimum work is performed at higher frequencies with stiff (less compliant) lungs and at lower frequencies when the air flow resistance is increased.

Man and animals tend to select a respiratory frequency which is close to that which minimizes respiratory work (McIlroy et al., 1956). This applies to different species, to different age groups in the same species and to pathological conditions.

Work of breathing through apparatus

In many situations subjects and patients are required to breathe through external breathing apparatus which offers appreciable resistance to air flow. We have already considered the problems of quantifying the 'resistance' of such apparatus (page 69). It is, however, possible to quantify the work of breathing through external apparatus by measurement of the area of a loop of which one axis is the volume passing through the apparatus and the other axis is the driving pressure required to pass the gas through the apparatus. This is simpler than quantifying work against resistance in the lungs as the problem of compliance does not arise unless there is an elastic component in the apparatus.

The minute volume of pulmonary ventilation

It is the function of the respiratory system to ensure the normality of oxygen and carbon dioxide levels in the arterial blood. This requires that the minute volume of pulmonary ventilation is adequate to maintain arterial P_{O_2} and P_{CO_2} within the normal limits. P_{O_2} and P_{CO_2} also depend upon other factors such as the metabolic rate, the composition of the inspired gas and the gas exchange function of the lung. These factors are considered elsewhere in this book and the present section is concerned solely with pulmonary ventilation. The normal value for P_{CO_2} is considered on page 225 and for P_{O_2} on page 270.

Minute volume and alveolar ventilation

Calculations of the adequacy of minute volume and the effect of changes in the minute volume all depend upon the corresponding alveolar ventilation. Minute volume equals the product of tidal volume and respiratory frequency while alveolar ventilation equals the product of (tidal volume less dead space) and respiratory frequency. The subject of dead space is considered in detail on pages 156 et seq. but in the healthy subject approximates to one-third of tidal volume over quite a wide range of tidal volume. Thus the alveolar ventilation normally approximates to two-thirds of the minute volume.

Effect of alveolar ventilation on alveolar gas tensions

As alveolar ventilation increases, the composition of the alveolar gas tends to approach that of the inspired gas. The difference between inspired and alveolar gas concentrations is equal to the ratio of the output (or uptake) of the gas to the alveolar ventilation. The following is a universal alveolar air equation:

$$\begin{array}{c}\text{alveolar} \\ \text{concentration} \\ \text{of gas X}\end{array} = \begin{array}{c}\text{inspired} \\ \text{concentration} \\ \text{of gas X}\end{array} + \text{ (or } -\text{) } \frac{\text{output (or uptake) of gas X}}{\text{alveolar ventilation}}$$

Note:

1. Concentrations are here expressed as fractions and must be multiplied by 100 to give the more familiar percentages.
2. The equation does not correct for any difference between inspired and expired minute volumes. Corrections for this factor are considered on page 182.
3. The sign on the right-hand side is + for output of a gas (e.g. carbon dioxide) and − for uptake (e.g. oxygen).
4. The tension or partial pressure of gas X may be obtained by multiplying the fractional concentration by the dry barometric pressure (total barometric pressure less saturated water vapour pressure at body temperature).
5. Values for gas exchange and alveolar ventilation must both be expressed under the same conditions of temperature, pressure and humidity.

In the case of carbon dioxide, the normal value for alveolar concentration derived from this equation would be:

$$0 + 200/3600 = 0.56 \text{ or } 5.6\%$$

For oxygen the corresponding value would be:

$$0.21 - 250/3600 = 0.14 \text{ or } 14\%$$

0 is the inspired concentration of carbon dioxide, 200 is the carbon dioxide output (ml), 250 is the oxygen consumption (ml), 3600 is the alveolar ventilation (ml)and 0.21 is the inspired oxygen concentration (gas volumes being expressed under conditions of body temperature and pressure saturated).

The universal alveolar air equation indicates that the relationship between alveolar concentration and alveolar ventilation is non-linear. In fact, it is a rectangular hyperbola, and examples for carbon dioxide and oxygen are shown in *Figure 5.8.*

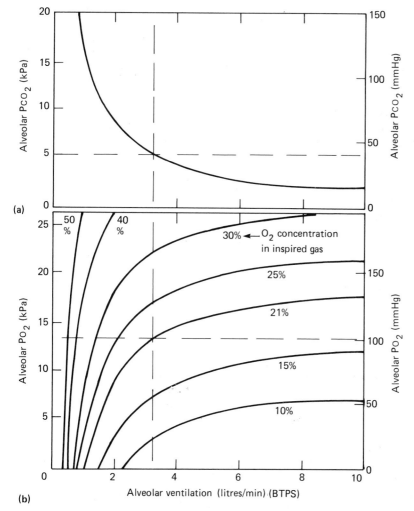

Figure 5.8 Alveolar gas tensions produced by different levels of alveolar ventilation. (a) The hyperbolic relationship between alveolar P_{CO_2} and alveolar ventilation. (b) The relationship between alveolar P_{O_2} and alveolar ventilation for different levels of oxygen concentration in the inspired gas. The broken vertical line indicates an alveolar ventilation of 3.2 l/min. Dry barometric pressure, 95 kPa = 713 mmHg; carbon dioxide output, 150 ml/min (STPD) = 180 ml/min (BTPS); oxygen uptake, 190 ml/min (STPD) = 225 ml/min (BTPS). No allowance has been made for the difference between inspired and expired minute volumes.

The curves have great practical and clinical relevance, making clear many aspects of the effect of changes in ventilation. Rectangular hyperbolas relating alveolar gas concentrations to alveolar ventilation all obey the following general rules:

1. The vertical asymptote is zero alveolar ventilation.
2. The horizontal asymptote is the ambient concentration of the gas under consideration (i.e. effectively zero for carbon dioxide and approximately 21 kPa or % for oxygen while breathing air).
3. The curve is concave upwards for gases being eliminated from the body and concave downwards for gas being taken up into the body.
4. The curves move away from the intersection of the asymptotes as the volume of the gas being exchanged increases.

Figure 5.8a shows a curve for carbon dioxide in a patient with a metabolic rate about 15 per cent below basal. Normal alveolar P_{CO_2} is attained with an alveolar ventilation of slightly more than 3 l/min. Increases in ventilation cause a relatively small reduction in P_{CO_2} while reductions in ventilation cause a progressively greater change as ventilation is reduced. The curve is asymptotic to zero P_{CO_2} but would be displaced bodily upwards if the patient were inhaling a carbon dioxide gas mixture. An increased metabolic rate would move the curve upwards and to the right without changing the asymptotes.

Figure 5.8b shows a family of curves for a patient breathing gas mixtures containing different concentrations of oxygen. Since oxygen is being taken up into the body the curves are concave downwards. All have a vertical asymptote of zero alveolar ventilation; however, each has its own horizontal asymptote corresponding to the inspired oxygen concentrations. A normal alveolar P_{O_2} is obtained with an alveolar ventilation of slightly more than 3 l/min while breathing 21% oxygen, but only 2 l/min when breathing 25%. This has great relevance to oxygen therapy in ventilatory failure and is discussed further on page 388. Note in particular that an alveolar ventilation of only 0.5 l/min will give a near normal alveolar P_{O_2} when the patient is breathing 50% oxygen but the P_{CO_2} will be well in excess of 20 kPa (150 mmHg). For clarity, the illustration does not show the effect of changes in metabolic rate. However, the general rules apply and an increase in metabolic rate would move each curve downwards and to the right without changing the asymptotes.

Measurement of ventilation

The first part of this section is concerned with the measurement of actual ventilation of the subject, while the second part deals with the maximal ventilation which he is able to achieve and which provides a measure of his ventilatory capacity.

Volume is the integral of gas flow rate and may be measured either directly or, alternatively, by the integration of instantaneous gas flow rate (*Figure 5.9*). Integration of a flow trace may be undertaken by estimation of the area under the flow curve or, more conveniently, by electrical integration of a flow signal. Conversely, flow rate may be derived as the slope of a trace of volume against time (e.g. a spirometer trace) or again, more conveniently, by electrical differentiation of a changing volume signal. It is important to distinguish between the instantaneous flow rate of gases during breathing and the minute volume of the subject which is of the order of one-quarter of the maximal flow rate (see *Figure 3.13*). This again

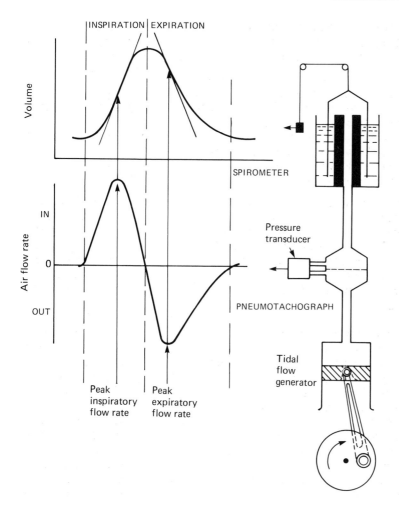

Figure 5.9 Relationship between volume and flow rate. The upper graph shows volume plotted against time; this type of tracing may be obtained with a spirometer. The lower graph shows instantaneous air flow rate plotted against time; this type of tracing may be obtained with a pneumotachograph. At any instant, the flow-rate trace indicates the slope of the volume trace, while the volume trace indicates the cumulative area under the flow-rate trace. Flow is the differential of volume; volume is the integral of flow rate. Differentiation of the spirometer trace gives a 'pneumotachogram'. Integration of the pneumotachogram gives a 'spirometer trace'.

is quite different from the peak flow rate which the patient is able to achieve (see below).

A final general point is to note that inspiratory and expiratory tidal volumes and minute volumes may be markedly different and the difference is important in calculations of gas exchange. The normal respiratory exchange ratio of about 0.8 means that inspiratory minute volume is about 50 ml larger than the expiratory minute volume in the resting subject. Much larger differences can arise during exercise and during uptake or wash-out of an inert gas such as nitrogen or, to a greater extent, nitrous oxide.

Direct measurement of respired volumes

Water-sealed spirometers. The reference method for the measurement of ventilation is the water-sealed spirometer (*Figure 5.9*), which may be calibrated by water displacement. The method provides negligible resistance to breathing and, by suitable design, may have a satisfactory frequency response up to very high respiratory frequencies (Bernstein and Mendel, 1951; Bernstein, D'Silva and Mendel, 1952). The technique is commonly used as a closed circuit but may be adapted to many different types of breathing systems (Nunn, 1956). Tissot spirometers have a capacity of about 200 litres and are used either as inspiratory gas reservoirs or for the collection of expired gas.

The box–bag spirometer (*Figure 5.10*) permits accurate measurement of inspiratory and expiratory tidal volumes without rebreathing (Donald and Christie, 1949). It provides a useful solution to a number of difficult problems of spirometery but suffers from the disadvantage of being very temperature sensitive and having a capacity which is sufficient for only a few breaths.

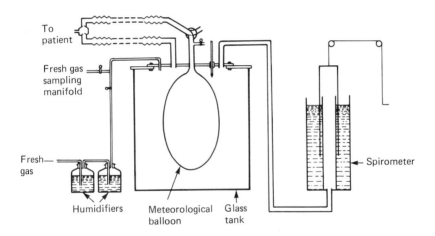

Figure 5.10 In the box–bag spirometer system, the patient inhales from the box and exhales into the bag. The tidal volume and the difference between the inspiratory and expiratory respiratory volumes are read directly from the spirometer. Inspiratory and expiratory gas may be sampled and analysis permits measurement of exchange of all gaseous components. The system may be reversed (i.e. inspiration from the bag) for studying the response to different inhaled gas mixtures. (Reproduced from Nunn and Pouliot (1962) by permission of the Editor of the British Journal of Anaesthesia*)*

The wet gas meter consists of a type of paddle wheel which is sealed with water. These instruments are rather cumbersome but are highly accurate for the measurement of a volume which is passed steadily through the meter. It is particularly suitable for the measurement of the expired volume collected in a Douglas bag.

Dry gas meters and spirometers. Dry spirometers, based on the wedge-shaped bellows, now approach the water-filled spirometer in accuracy. They can be used in much the same way as a traditional spirometer and are generally more convenient in use. Rotary gas meters measure the volume of gas which passes through the mechanism by means of two bellows which alternately drive a spindle by means of cranks. The principle is similar to the long-established design of meters used for measuring domestic gas consumption. They are not accurate for small volumes such as a single tidal volume but are very reliable for the measurement of larger volumes such as the volume exhaled over a few minutes. Errors in the use of dry gas meters have been exhaustively discussed by Cooper (1959).

Impellers and turbines. The best known of these instruments is the respirometer developed by Wright (1955). Although seemingly delicate in construction, these instruments appear to give good results even in the event of considerable mistreatment. The Wright respirometer automatically rectifies alternating gas flow and the dead space (22 ml) is sufficiently small for the patient to breathe to and fro through it. The essential mechanism is entirely mechanical with indication of volume on a dial but the output may be converted to an electrical signal to indicate either tidal volume or minute volume. The accuracy of the instrument was assessed by Nunn and Ezi-Ashi (1962). In general the respirometer tends to read low at low minute volumes and high at high minute volumes. Departure from normality is thus exaggerated and the instrument is essentially safe.

There are, in addition, a wide range of dry rotary meters, all somewhat larger than the Wright respirometer. Each has its own characteristics but there is a generic tendency to under-reading at low minute volumes.

Measurement of ventilatory volumes by integration of instantaneous gas flow rate

Technical advances in electronic circuitry have increased the attractions of measuring ventilatory volumes by integration of instantaneous flow rate. There are many methods of measurement of rapidly changing gas flow rates of which the original was pneumotachography. This employs measurement of the pressure gradient across a laminar resistance, which ensures that the pressure drop is directly proportional to flow rate (page 46). This is illustrated in *Figure 5.9* where the resistor is a wire mesh screen. It is necessary to take precautions to prevent errors due to different gas composition and temperature and to prevent condensation of moisture on the resistor. The pressure drop need not exceed a few millimetres of water and the volume can be very small. The pneumotachograph should not therefore interfere with respiration. Sources of error have been considered in detail by Smith (1964).

Alternative flow detectors include Venturi tubes which give a pressure signal proportional to the square of flow, Pitot tubes and the hot wire anemometer. The last device depends on the cooling of a very thin platinum wire heated to about 400°C. The hot wire anemometer is capable of considerable accuracy when run at high temperature and is little influenced by the temperature of the gas.

Measurement of ventilatory capacity

Measurement of ventilatory capcity is the most commonly performed test of respiratory function. The ratio of ventilatory capacity to actual ventilation is a measure of ventilatory reserve and of the comfort of breathing. In the normal subject the maximal breathing capacity is about 15–20 times the resting minute volume.

Maximal breathing capacity (MBC)

MBC is defined as the maximal minute volume of ventilation which the subject can maintain for 15 seconds. The test is exhausting to perform and is now seldom used. MBC cannot be sustained indefinitely but 75 per cent of MBC can be sustained with difficulty by young fit subjects for 15 minutes (Shephard, 1967). Dyspnoea ensues when ventilation reaches about a third of MBC. Thus there is dyspnoea at rest when MBC is reduced below about 30 l/min since resting minute volume is commonly increased to rather more than 10 l/min under such conditions (see *Figure 20.5*). The average fit young male adult should have an MBC of about 170 l/min but normal values depend upon body size, age and sex, the range being 47–253 l/min for men and 55–139 l/min for women (Cotes, 1975).

Forced expiration

A more practical test of ventilatory capacity is the forced expiratory volume (1 second) or $FEV_{1.0}$, which is the maximal volume exhaled in the first second starting from a maximal inspiration. It is far more convenient to perform than the MBC and less exhausting for the patient. It correlates well with the MBC, which is about 35 times the $FEV_{1.0}$.

Peak expiratory flow rate

Most convenient of all the indirect tests of ventilatory capacity is the peak expiratory flow rate. This can be measured with simple and inexpensive hand-held devices. This is most commonly done with the Wright peak flow meter, described in its original form by Wright and McKerrow (1959). Alternatively, the peak flow may be derived from a pneumotachogram but this is sensitive to very short transients and may give a spuriously high value. The Wright peak flow meter tends to give values about 5.7 times the MBC.

Interpretation of measurements of maximal expirations may be difficult. The tests are most commonly performed as a measure of airway obstruction and are extensively used in asthma and chronic obstructive airway disease. However, the results also depend on many other factors, including chest restriction, motivation and muscular power. The measurements may also be inhibited by pain. A more specific indication of airway resistance is the ratio of $FEV_{1.0}$ to vital capacity. This should exceed 75 per cent in the normal subject.

Use of bronchodilators

When there is a reduction in the ventilatory capacity measured by the techniques outlined above, it is helpful to administer a bronchodilator such as a beta-sympathomimetic agent. Any improvement in ventilatory capacity will then indicate the extent to which bronchoconstriction had been responsible. No change indicates that the reduction in ventilatory capacity was mainly caused by structural factors such as trapping or pulmonary fibrosis. No improvement is to be expected when reduced ventilatory capacity is due to non-pulmonary factors such as pain or muscle weakness.

Chapter 6

The pulmonary circulation

Fit autem comunicatio haec non per parierem cordis medium, vt vulgo creditur sed magno artificio a dextro cordis ventriculo, longo per pulmones ductu agitatur sanguis subtilis: a pulmonibus praeparatur, flavus efficitur . . . etc. (Michael Servetus, 1553). In a few words, interspersed in a theological writing, Michael Servetus was the first to suggest that venous blood did not pass through the middle wall of the heart, as was generally believed, but pursued a long course through the lungs to reach the right side of the heart.

The entire blood volume passes through the lungs during each circulation. This is an appropriate arrangement for gas exchange but is equally suitable for the filtering and metabolic functions of the lungs, which are considered in Chapter 11.

The flow of blood through the pulmonary circulation is approximately equal to the flow through the whole of the systemic circulation. It therefore varies from about 6 l/min under resting conditions to as much as 25 l/min in severe exercise. Although the flow rates are similar in the two systems, the pressures are greatly different, pulmonary arterial pressure being much less than that of the systemic circulation: consequently the pulmonary circulation has only limited ability to vary the distribution of blood flow within the lung fields. This is in marked contrast to the systemic circulation which is able to vary the distribution of blood flow within very wide limits in response to the changing requirements of the individual. We shall see that the pulmonary circulation, lacking much power of selective distribution, is very markedly affected by gravity, resulting in overperfusion of the dependent parts of the lung fields.

The distribution of the pulmonary blood flow has important consequences for gaseous exchange. Failure of perfusion of parts of the lung prevents exchange occurring with the gas which ventilates those parts, and it is convenient to consider the ventilation of unperfused regions as dead space ventilation (page 156). Localized failure of ventilation means that blood perfusing such parts cannot participate in gas exchange and thus constitutes venous admixture similar in effect to a right-to-left shunt.

Although blood flow is continuous while gas flow is tidal, it is helpful to represent both flows as continuous and to consider the lung as a black box with a gas inflow and outflow and a blood inflow and outflow (*Figure 6.1*). The object of this black box is to achieve equilibrium of oxygen and carbon dioxide tensions between the two outflow streams. However, the plumbing of neither side is perfect and in each case the effluent is contaminated with part of the corresponding inflow. The precise mechanism by which this takes place is often difficult to determine but it may be

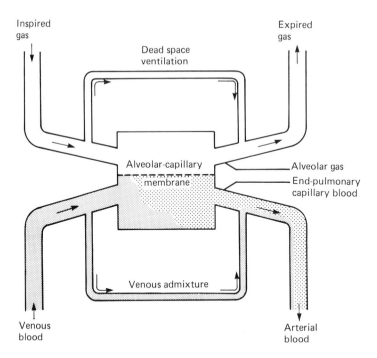

Figure 6.1 In this functional representation of gas exchange in the lungs, the flow of gas and blood is considered as a continuous process with movement from left to right. Under most circumstances, equilibrium is obtained between alveolar gas and end-pulmonary capillary blood, the gas tensions in the two phases being almost identical. However, alveolar gas is mixed with dead space gas to give expired gas. Meanwhile, end-pulmonary capillary blood is mixed with shunted venous blood to give arterial blood. Thus both expired gas and arterial blood have gas tensions which differ from those in alveolar gas and end-pulmonary capillary blood.

possible to obtain valuable guidance on the management of patients by considering the lung as though it functions in the manner shown in *Figure 6.1*. This illustration has been deliberately drawn without countercurrent flow. Such a system does not operate in mammals but, if it were present, it would be possible to bring the pulmonary ~~venous~~ PO_2 close to the PO_2 of the inspired gas.

ARTERIAL

Pulmonary blood volume

Haemodynamic considerations

As a first approximation the right heart pumps blood into the pulmonary circulation, while the left heart pumps away the blood which returns from the lungs. Therefore, provided that the output of the two sides is the same, the pulmonary blood volume will remain constant. However, very small differences in the outputs of the two sides will result in large changes in pulmonary blood volume if they are maintained for more than a few beats.

When we leave our first approximation and attempt to get nearer to the truth, we see that the relationship between the inflow and outflow of the pulmonary circulation is really rather complicated. *Figure 6.2* is a summary of some of the relevant anatomical features. The lungs receive a significant quantity of blood from the bronchial arteries which usually rise from the arch of the aorta. Blood from the bronchial circulation returns to the heart in two ways. From a plexus around the hilum, blood from the pleurohilar part of the bronchial circulation returns to the systemic veins via the azygos veins, and this fraction may thus be regarded as normal systemic flow neither arising from nor returning to the pulmonary circulation. However, another fraction of the bronchial circulation, distributed more peripherally in the lung, passes through postcapillary anastomoses to join the pulmonary veins, constituting an admixture of venous blood with the arterialized blood from the alveolar capillary networks (Marchand, Gilroy and Wilson, 1950).

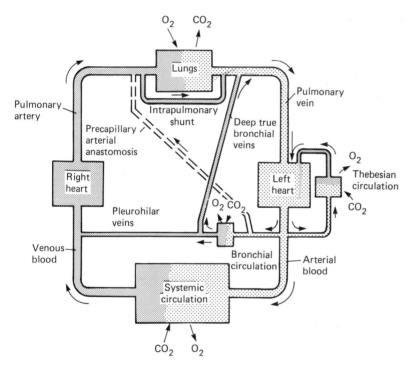

Figure 6.2 Schema of bronchopulmonary anastomoses and other forms of venous admixture in the normal subject. Part of the bronchial circulation returns venous blood to the systemic venous sytem (pleurohilar veins) while another part returns venous blood to the pulmonary veins and so constitutes venous admixture. Other forms of venous admixture are the thebesian circulation of the left heart and flow through atelectatic parts of the lungs. The existence of precapillary bronchopulmonary anastomoses in the normal subject is controversial. It will be clear from this diagram why the output of the left heart must be slightly greater than that of the right heart.

The paragraph above relates to the normal subject. The situation may be further complicated when blood flows through precapillary anastomoses from the bronchial arteries to the pulmonary arteries. The communications have been called 'sperr arteries' meaning muscular vessels which act as sluice gates. These anastomoses are thought to be present in the normal subject (Verloop, 1948; von Hayek, 1960), but they are of definite functional importance in cases of pulmonary oligaemia. This has been demonstrated after experimental ligation of a branch of the pulmonary artery in dogs (Cockett and Vass, 1951), but congenital pulmonary atresia is the most important natural cause of the condition. It should be noted that arterial bronchopulmonary anastomoses achieve the same purpose as a Blalock–Taussig operation.

The catalogue of abnormal communications between the pulmonary and systemic circulations can be continued almost indefinitely. It is not unusual for aberrant pulmonary veins to drain into the right atrium. Furthermore, flow may be reversed through normally occurring channels. Thus, in pulmonary venous hypertension due to mitral stenosis, pulmonary venous blood may traverse the bronchial venous system to gain access to the azygos system.

Factors influencing pulmonary blood volume

The quantity of blood within the pulmonary circulation is 10–20 per cent of total blood volume, between 0.5 and 1.0 litre. The volume fluctuates during the cardiac cycle since inflow exceeds outflow during systole. It is also likely that the cyclical pressure changes caused by respiration will influence pulmonary blood volume which decreases during a Valsalva manoeuvre, and during positive pressure breathing (Fenn et al., 1947). Conversely, pulmonary blood volume is increased during negative pressure breathing (Slome, 1965).

Posture. Pulmonary blood volume is directly influenced by posture (Harris and Heath, 1962). When a subject changes from the supine to the erect position the pulmonary blood volume falls by 27 per cent, a change which is of the same order as the decrease in cardiac output under the same circumstances. It is thought that both changes are due to pooling of blood in dependent parts of the systemic circulation.

Drugs. Since the systemic circulation has much greater vasomotor activity than the pulmonary circulation, it is to be expected that an overall increase in vascular tone will squeeze blood from the systemic into the pulmonary circulation. This may result from the administration of vasoconstrictor drugs, from release of endogenous catecholamines or by passive compression of the body in a G-suit. Conversely, it seems likely that pulmonary blood volume would be diminished when systemic tone is diminished, as for example by sympathetic ganglion blockade. Large decreases in pulmonary blood volume have been reported during spinal anaesthesia, but increases sometimes occurred when the patient was in the Trendelenburg position (Johnson, 1951). In general it may be said that vasoactive drugs produce a complementary relationship between pulmonary and systemic blood volumes.

Left heart failure. Pulmonary venous hypertension (due, for example, to mitral stenosis) would be expected to result in an increased pulmonary blood volume. There has, however, been difficulty in the experimental demonstration of any significant change.

The extent of the 'pulmonary blood volume'

Methods of measurement are outlined at the end of this chapter, where it will be seen that the pulmonary blood volume as measured is really the central blood volume which lies between the two anatomical sites chosen for injection and sampling of dye. This usually includes the chambers of the left heart and also certain parts of the systemic vascular system depending upon the placement of the catheters used in the measurement technique. Pulmonary capillary volume may be calculated from measurements of diffusing capacity (page 197), and this technique yields values of the order of 80 ml.

In view of the difficulties in definition and measurement, it is perhaps fortunate that pulmonary blood volume is of limited interest from the clinical standpoint, and can often be estimated with sufficient accuracy from the density of the vascular markings seen in a chest radiograph. Considerably greater importance attaches to pulmonary vascular pressures and flow, which are considered in the next two sections of this chapter.

Pulmonary vascular pressures

Pulmonary arterial pressure is only about one-sixth of systemic arterial pressure, although the capillary and venous pressures are not greatly different for the two circulations (*Figure 6.3*). There is thus only a small pressure drop along the pulmonary arterioles and consequently relatively little possibility for active regulation of the distribution of the pulmonary circulation. There is also little damping of the arterial pressure wave, so the pulmonary capillary blood flow is markedly pulsatile.

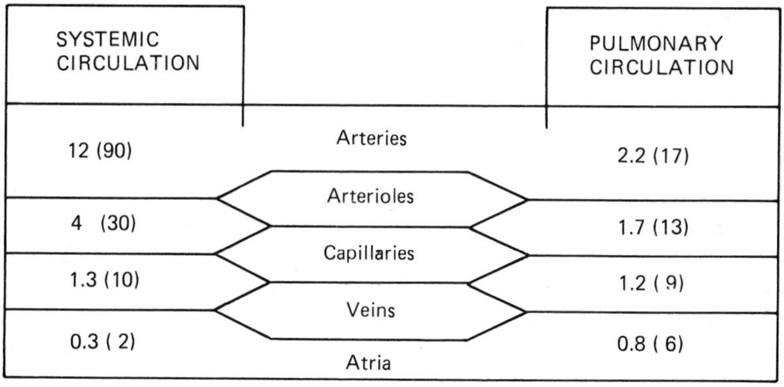

SYSTEMIC CIRCULATION		PULMONARY CIRCULATION
12 (90)	Arteries	2.2 (17)
4 (30)	Arterioles	1.7 (13)
1.3 (10)	Capillaries	1.2 (9)
0.3 (2)	Veins	0.8 (6)
	Atria	

Figure 6.3 Comparison of typical mean pressure gradients along the systemic and pulmonary circulations. (Mean pressures relative to atmosphere in kPa, with mmHg in parentheses)

Consideration of pulmonary vascular pressures carries a special difficulty in the selection of the reference pressure. Systemic pressures are customarily measured with reference to ambient atmospheric pressure. Thus a systolic pressure of 16 kPa (120 mmHg) implies a presure of 16 kPa above atmospheric (i.e. an absolute pressure of 16 + 101 = 117 kPa or 120 + 760 = 880 mmHg). This approach is not always appropriate when considering the pulmonary circulation because it does not indicate the important transmural pressure gradients between the inside of the pulmonary vasculature and the extravascular space. Neither does it tell us anything about the pressure gradients which cause the blood to flow onwards against the pulmonary vascular resistance into the left atrium. We therefore require to distinguish between pressures within the pulmonary circulation expressed in the three different forms listed below. Measurement techniques may be adapted to indicate these pressures directly (*Figure 6.4*).

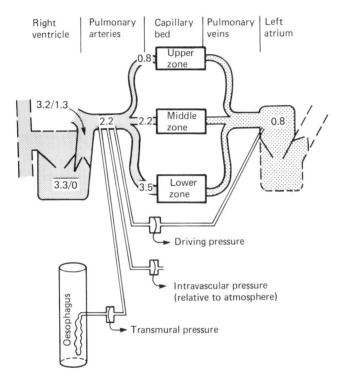

Figure 6.4 Normal values for pressures in the pulmonary circulation relative to atmosphere (kPa). Systolic and diastolic pressures are shown for the right ventricle and pulmonary trunk. Note the effect of gravity on pressures at different levels in the lung fields. Three differential manometers are shown connected to indicate driving pressure, intravascular pressure and transmural pressure.

Intravascular pressure is the pressure at any point in the circulation relative to atmosphere. This is the customary way of expressing pressures in the systemic circulation.

Transmural pressure is the difference in pressure between the inside of a vessel and the tissue surrounding the vessel. In the case of the larger pulmonary vessels, the outside pressure is the intrathoracic pressure (commonly measured as the oesophageal pressure as in *Figure 6.4*). In the case of the capillaries, the outside pressure is closer to alveolar pressure, but its precise value is difficult to determine since the relevant extravascular space is the interstitial space between the alveolar membrane and the capillary membrane (see *Figures 1.7* and *1.8*). The pressure in this space is probably intermediate between alveolar and intrathoracic.

The capillary transmural pressure gradient would drive fluid out of the circulation were it not prevented by the osmotic pressure of the plasma proteins, normally about 3.3 kPa (25 mmHg). Should this pressure be exceeded by the transmural pressure, pulmonary oedema results (see page 433).

Driving pressure is the difference in pressure between one point in the circulation and another point downstream. The driving pressure of the pulmonary circulation as a whole is the pressure difference between pulmonary artery and left atrium. This is the pressure which overcomes the flow resistance and should be used for determination of vascular resistance.

These differences are far from being solely academic. The capillary transmural pressure gradients may be markedly influenced by the intra-alveolar pressure, which may be raised by positive pressure respiration or reduced by the use of a subatmospheric pressure phase during expiration. However, the intracapillary pressure is directly influenced by changes in alveolar pressure (page 124) and account must therefore be taken of the induced change in intravascular pressure.

The difference between pulmonary arterial intravascular pressure (relative to atmosphere) and the pulmonary driving pressure is of importance in distinguishing between different causes of pulmonary hypertension. If the primary lesion is a raised left atrial pressure, the pulmonary arterial intravascular pressure will be raised but the driving pressure will not be increased unless there is a secondary rise in pulmonary vascular resistance. Left atrial pressure is measured by one of four possible techniques.

1. Wedge pressures are obtained by advancing the cardiac catheter into the pulmonary artery until it impacts. The Swan–Ganz catheter is now widely used for this purpose.
2. The left atrium may be punctured by a needle at bronchoscopy.
3. The atrial septum may be pierced from a catheter in the right atrium.
4. A catheter may be passed retrogradely from a peripheral systemic artery.

Typical normal values within the pulmonary circulation are shown in *Figure 6.4*. The effect of gravity on the pulmonary vascular pressure may be seen, and it will be clear why pulmonary oedema is most likely to occur in the lower zones of the lungs where the intravascular pressures and the transmural pressure gradients are highest.

Factors influencing pulmonary vascular pressures

Many very important factors which influence pulmonary vascular resistance have a direct effect on pulmonary vascular pressures. These are discussed below under the heading 'Pulmonary vascular resistance' (pages 125 et seq.) and will not be considered here. However, it is convenient at this point to mention cardiac output, changes in alveolar pressure, posture and disease.

Cardiac output. The pulmonary circulation can adapt to large changes in cardiac output with only small increases in pulmonary arterial pressure. This is achieved partly by recruitment of vessels and partly by passive dilatation. Thus pulmonary vascular resistance decreases as flow increases. This may not be the case if the pulmonary vascular bed is diminished by disease or surgery.

Changes of intra-alveolar pressure up to about 1.1 kPa (8 mmHg) normally cause an equal change in pulmonary arterial pressure (Lenfant and Howell, 1960). There is a rise in pressure during a Valsalva manoeuvre, and cyclical changes occur during spontaneous respiration with pressures higher during expiration and lower during inspiration. Since small rises in alveolar pressure cause an equal rise in pulmonary arterial intravascular pressure, there should be no reduction in capillary transmural pressure gradient unless the capillary pressure fails to rise as much as the arterial pressure. With larger changes in alveolar pressure it is known that the rise in pulmonary arterial pressure is less than the rise in alveolar pressure, and the disparity may be greater in patients with circulatory disorders. In haemodynamic pulmonary oedema, the intravascular pulmonary capillary pressure is considerably higher than the alveolar pressure. Elevation of the mean alveolar pressure (by IPP ventilation with or without PEEP) will not necessarily raise the capillary pressure under these conditions, and may therefore reduce the transmural pressure gradient.

Posture. It is difficult to study the effect of change of posture on pulmonary blood pressure, since the actual levels of pressure are so low that they are markedly influenced by movement of the reference level. However, it seems likely that the upright position is associated with a lower pulmonary arterial pressure in patients with pulmonary hypertension (Donald et al., 1953). Wedge pressures are also reduced. Intrathoracic pressure is also lower in the upright position, so it is unlikely that capillary transmural pressure is greatly affected.

Disease. Many forms of pulmonary and cardiac disease are associated with a rise in pulmonary vascular pressures. Mitral stenosis and incompetence are the principal conditions leading to an elevation of pressure in the left atrium. The maintenance of the pulmonary driving pressure requires a corresponding increase of the pulmonary arterial pressure, and there must therefore be a rise of pulmonary capillary pressure as well. In many cases of mitral stenosis, there is a secondary increase in pulmonary vascular resistance which results in further elevation of the pulmonary arterial pressure. The cause of this change is unknown. The work of the right ventricle is increased and, in severe cases, increased vascular resistance limits the benefit accruing from mitral valvotomy since the mitral valve is no longer the only site of increased resistance to the circulation. Pulmonary vascular resistance rises in many forms of chronic lung disease (cor pulmonale) and also in cases of pulmonary embolus. In a small number of patients the change appears to be primary and analogous to systemic hypertension.

Pulmonary hypertension may result from an increased pulmonary blood flow. However, following pneumonectomy, the remaining lung, if healthy, appears to be able to take the entire resting pulmonary blood flow without rise in pulmonary arterial pressure. The most important pathological cause of increased flow is left-to-right shunting through a patent ductus arteriosus or through atrial or ventricular septal defects. Under these circumstances the pulmonary circulation is greater than the systemic circulation and may be sufficient to result in pulmonary hypertension, even with normal vascular resistance. However, secondary changes commonly result in an increase in vascular resistance, causing a further rise in pulmonary arterial pressure.

The very important effect of chronic hypoxia on pulmonary arterial pressure is considered below under 'Hypoxia'.

Pulmonary hypotension results from pulmonary atresia and, as we have seen, this induces an increased flow through precapillary anastomoses from the bronchial circulation, collateral flow sometimes being as great as 1 l/min.

Pulmonary blood flow

Total pulmonary blood flow is approximately equal to cardiac output and is a topic which belongs to the field of circulation rather than respiration. We shall not therefore consider pulmonary blood flow in any more detail than is necessary for an understanding of the changes in pulmonary vascular pressure and resistance. Pulmonary gas exchange is, however, greatly influenced by the distribution of pulmonary blood flow, and this is considered in Chapter 7.

Methods for the measurement of pulmonary blood flow are outlined at the end of this chapter, but at this stage it should be pointed out that most methods of mesurement of cardiac output (Fick, dye and thermal dilution) measure the total pulmonary blood flow, together with the venous admixture (see *Figure 6.1*). On the other hand, the body plethysmograph measures only the pulmonary capillary blood flow. In this method, the alveoli are filled with nitrous oxide at a concentration of about 15%, and the amount of nitrous oxide taken up by the blood is measured by whole body plethysmography. If the mean alveolar P_{N_2O} and the solubility of nitrous oxide in blood are known, it is possible to calculate the pulmonary blood flow on the assumption that the alveolar P_{N_2O} equals the arterial P_{N_2O} and the mixed venous P_{N_2O} is zero. The method may be used to measure the instantaneous capillary blood flow, which is found to be pulsatile.

Pulmonary vascular resistance

Vascular resistance is an expression of the relationship between driving pressure and flow, as in the case of resistance to gas flow (see *Figure 3.1*). There are, however, important differences. When gases flow through rigid tubes the flow is laminar, or turbulent, or a mixture of the two. In the first case pressure increases in direct proportion to flow rate and the resistance remains constant (Poiseuille's law). In the second case pressure increases according to the square of the flow rate, and the resistance increases with flow. When the type of flow is mixed, the pressure rises in proportion to the flow rate raised to a power between one and two.

The circumstances differ in the case of blood since the tubes through which the blood flows are not rigid but tend to expand as flow is increased, particularly in the pulmonary circulation. Consequently the resistance tends to fall as flow increases and the plot of pressure against flow rate may be neither linear (see *Figure 3.2*) nor curved with the concavity upwards (see *Figure 3.3*) but curved with the concavity downwards. As an added complication, blood is a non-newtonian fluid (due to the presence of the corpuscles) and its viscosity varies with the shear rate and therefore its linear velocity through tubes. The situation is thus two degrees more complicated than in the case of gas flow, although the practical importance of these points should not be exaggerated. In fact, regardless of these considerations, there is a widespread convention that vascular resistance should be expressed as though the vessels were rigid and Poiseuille's law was obeyed. Resistance is usually expressed in the form directly analogous to electrical resistance which is used for laminar gas flow (see *Figure 3.1*).

$$\text{resistance} = \frac{\text{driving pressure}}{\text{blood flow rate}}$$

In the case of pulmonary circulation, the driving pressure is the difference in mean pressures between pulmonary artery and left atrium, the latter usually measured as the 'wedge pressure'. Flow rate is usually taken as cardiac output.

Vascular resistance is expressed in units derived from those which are used for expression of pressure and flow rate. The appropriate SI units will probably be kilopascal litre^{-1} minute. Using conventional units, vascular resistance may be expressed in units of mmHg litre^{-1} minute. In absolute CGS units, vascular resistance is usually expressed in units of dynes/square centimetre per cubic centimetre/second (dyn sec cm^{-5}). Normal values for the pulmonary circulation in the various units are as follows:

	Driving pressure	Pulmonary blood flow	Pulmonary vascular resistance
SI units	1.2 kPa	5 l/min	0.24 kPa l^{-1} min
Conventional units	9 mmHg	5 l/min	1.8 mmHg l^{-1} min
Absolute CGS units	12 000 dyn/cm^2	83 cm^3/sec	144 dyn sec cm^{-5}

The measurement of pulmonary vascular resistance is important, not only in the diagnosis of the primary cause of pulmonary hypertension but also for the detection of increased pulmonary vascular resistance which often develops in patients in whom the primary cause of pulmonary hypertension is raised left atrial pressure.

Localization of the pulmonary vascular resistance

By far the greatest part of the systemic resistance is within the arterioles, along which the pressure falls from a mean value of about 12 kPa (90 mmHg) down to about 4 kPa (30 mmHg) (see *Figure 6.3*). This pressure drop largely obliterates the pulse pressure wave, and the capillary flow is not pulsatile to any great extent. In the pulmonary circulation, the pressure drop along the arterioles is very much smaller than in the systemic circulation and, as an approximation, the pulmonary vascular resistance is equally divided between arteries, capillaries and veins. If the whole of the pulmonary microcirculation (i.e. vessels without muscular walls—page 20) is considered, then well over half of the total resistance lies in these vessels. Thus in the pulmonary circulation, vessels without the power of active vasoconstriction play a major role in governing total vascular resistance and the distribution of the pulmonary blood flow.

Autonomic control

The pulmonary circulation has both sympathetic and, to a less extent, parasympathetic control. There are both alpha and beta adrenergic endings, the former vasoconstrictor and the latter vasodilator, both acting on the smooth muscle of arteries and arterioles of diameter greater than 30 µm (Fishman, 1985). Noradrenaline is vasoconstrictor and isoprenaline vasodilator. The influence of the sympathetic system is not as strong as in the systemic circulation and appears to have little influence under resting conditions. It does, however, have an appreciable effect when there is general activation of the sympathetic system, as for example under conditions of flight or fight. Pulmonary vasoconstriction may be demonstrated when the stellate ganglion is stimulated, and also when the peripheral chemoreceptors are stimulated by hypoxia (see below).

The parasympathetic system causes pulmonary vasodilatation by release of acetylcholine but the role of this mechanism has not been established.

Effect of changes in oxygen and carbon dioxide tensions

Hypoxia has a vasoconstrictor effect on the pulmonary circulation which is the reverse of its effect on the systemic circulation. The effect is mediated primarily by the alveolar P_{O_2} but also by the pulmonary arterial P_{O_2} (*Figure 6.5*). The response to P_{O_2} is non-linear. This may be deduced from *Figure 6.5* by noting the pressure response for different values of the isobaric P_{O_2} (the broken line), and it will be

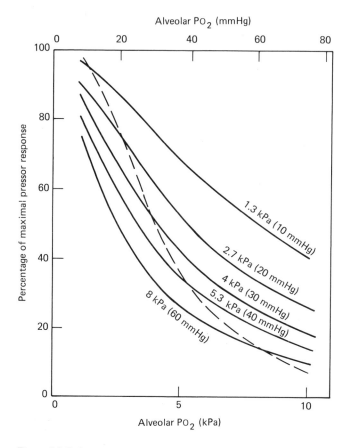

Figure 6.5 Pulmonary vasoconstriction (ordinate) as a function of alveolar P_{O_2} (abscissa) for different values of mixed venous P_{O_2} (indicated for each curve). The broken line shows the response when the alveolar and mixed venous P_{O_2} are identical. (Drawn from the data of Marshall and Marshall (1983))

seen that the general shape of the response curve resembles an oxyhaemoglobin dissociation curve with a P_{50} of about 4 kPa (30 mmHg).

Hypoxic pulmonary vasoconstriction is very important as a means of diverting the pulmonary blood flow away from regions in which the oxygen tension is low (Marshall et al., 1981). This is a major factor in the optimization of ventilation/ perfusion relationships and is discussed further in Chapter 7.

Hypoxic pulmonary vasoconstriction is also of major importance in the development of pulmonary hypertension and right heart failure (cor pulmonale) in patients with chronic respiratory disease. Furthermore, the sleep apnoea syndrome (page 306) results in recurrent bouts of arterial hypoxaemia which may be severe (see *Figure 13.3*) and pulmonary hypertension ensues. The long-term administration of oxygen to such patients, during the day and during sleep, retards the development of pulmonary hypertension, partially reverses established hypertension and improves survival (Abraham, Cole and Bishop, 1968; Abraham et al., 1969; Timms, Khaja and Williams, 1985; Flenley, 1985). Pulmonary hypertension is a feature of residence at high altitude and it has been suggested that high altitude pulmonary oedema may be caused by consequent stretching of the arteriolar endothelium with resultant increase in permeability to plasma (Chapter 14).

The pressor response to hypoxia appears to result from constriction of vessels of less than 1 mm diameter on the arterial side of the pulmonary capillaries. Constriction relates to the P_{O_2} in the vessel wall which is influenced by both alveolar and pulmonary arterial P_{O_2} (Marshall and Marshall, 1983). No hypoxic receptors have been identified and neither is there any evidence for release of a vasoconstrictor substance in response to hypoxia although histamine has been investigated for this possibility (Fishman, 1985). Some pulmonary vasoconstriction may result from hypoxic stimulation of the peripheral chemoreceptors by way of sympathetic efferent pathways (Daly and Daly, 1959) but this is manifestly less important than the local effect which is well known to operate in the isolated lung. Furthermore there is a unilateral increase in pulmonary vascular resistance when a gas mixture deficient in oxygen is breathed by one lung only. The similarity between the response curve and the oxyhaemoglobin dissociation curve suggests the possibility that a metalloporphyrin (e.g. a cytochrome) might act as a mediator, and Fishman (1980) has reviewed the evidence for this.

Hyperoxia has little effect upon pulmonary arterial pressure in the normal subject.

Hypercapnia has a slight pressor effect and reinforces hypoxic vasoconstriction, probably by causing acidosis. Hypoventilation of one lobe of a dog's lung reduces perfusion of that lobe but its ventilation/perfusion ratio is still reduced (Suggett et al., 1982).

Chemical mediators

Acetylcholine has been used extensively in studies of the pulmonary circulation. When introduced into the pulmonary artery, the rate of hydrolysis is so rapid that the drug is destroyed before it can act upon the systemic circulation. Acetylcholine results in a relaxation of vasomotor tone, causing the pulmonary vascular resistance and arterial pressure to fall by an amount which depends on the tone present before the administration of the drug. The response to acetylcholine may thus be used as an indicator of the degree of vasomotor tone which exists in the pulmonary circulation. Small falls of pressure occur in the normal subject but much greater falls occur in hypoxic subjects and those with pulmonary hypertension resulting from congenital heart disease, emphysema or mitral stenosis (Harris and Heath, 1962).

A number of references cited by those authors concur in the view that atropine does not affect pulmonary arterial pressure and is without vasomotor action of the pulmonary circulation. However, Daly, Ross and Behnke (1963) reported a fall in pressure following 2 mg of atropine (intravenously), and Nunn and Bergman (1964) suggested that this might be a cause of the increase in alveolar dead space which they found to follow the administration of atropine.

Adrenaline and dopamine, which act primarily upon the alpha receptors, result in an increase in pulmonary vascular resistance and arterial pressure. Isoprenaline and drugs which act primarily upon the beta receptors cause a fall of pressure, particularly when this is elevated. Ganglion-blocking agents generally cause a fall in pressure, and this has also been noted in the case of aminophylline.

Other pulmonary vasoconstrictors include 5-hydroxytryptamine (serotonin), thromboxane A_2, the prostaglandins $PGF_{2\alpha}$ and PGE_2. Histamine causes vasoconstriction by action at the H_1 receptors.

Other pulmonary vasodilators include bradykinin and the prostaglandins PGE_1 and PGI_2 (prostacyclin), the latter being released from capillary endothelium in response to sheer stress (Fishman, 1985). Histamine causes vasodilatation when acting at the H_2 receptors.

Almitrine is a drug which acts primarily to increase the drive of the peripheral chemoreceptors (page 84). However, it may improve arterial P_{O_2} without necessarily increasing pulmonary ventilation. Romaldini et al. (1983) have observed that it enhances hypoxic pulmonary vasoconstriction, and there is therefore the possibility that it improves the relative distribution of ventilation and perfusion, particularly in patients with diseased lungs.

Physical factors

Recruitment and distension in the pulmonary capillary bed. As the pulmonary blood flow increases from the resting level of about 5 l/min to exercise levels of the order of 20 l/min, there is a proportionately much smaller rise in pulmonary arterial pressure. Therefore, the vascular resistance is substantially reduced at the higher flow rate, implying an increase in the total cross-sectional area of the pulmonary vascular bed and particularly the capillaries. This is achieved mainly by recruitment of new capillaries with opening of new passages in the network lying in the alveolar septa (see *Plate 5*). Sections cut in lungs rapidly frozen while perfused with blood have shown that the number of open capillaries increase with rising pulmonary arterial pressure, particularly in the mid-zone of the lung (Glazier et al., 1969; Warrell et al., 1972). It seems likely that individual pulmonary capillaries show a spread of opening pressures, and the sequence of recruitment in the face of increasing pressure may be a purely physical phenomenon (West, 1974).

In addition to recruitment, it would be surprising if there were not an element of distension in the capillaries in response to increased transmural pressure gradient, since these vessels appear to be devoid of any vasomotor control. Sobin et al. (1972) have determined the distensibility of the capillary vessels and reported the diameter increasing from 5 to 10 µm as the transmural pressure increased from 0.5 to 2.5 kPa (5 to 25 cmH$_2$O). Distension plays the major role in zone 3 (see page 131) where most of the capillaries are already open (Glazier et al., 1969).

Effects of inflation of the lung. The effect of inflation of the lung on the pulmonary vascular resistance is complex. Confusion has arisen in the past because of failure to appreciate that pulmonary vascular resistance must be derived from driving pressure and not from pulmonary arterial or transmural pressure. This is very important since inflation of the lungs normally influences the pressure in the oesophagus, pulmonary artery and left atrium.

When pulmonary vascular resistance is correctly calculated from the driving pressure, there is reasonable agreement that, in the open-chested or isolated preparation, the pulmonary vascular resistance is minimal at an inflation pressure of the order of 0.5-1 kPa (5–10 cmH$_2$O). Change in inflation pressure may have very little effect upon resistance but the usual response is for the resistance to increase.

Although it is possible to determine the gross effect of inflation of the lungs upon pulmonary vascular resistance, it is less easy to discover the mechanism of this effect. It seems likely that inflation of the lungs increases the calibre and the volume of the larger blood vessels. This is achieved by the tethering effect of surrounding lung tissue which is sufficient to develop substantial subatmospheric pressures in the large vessels during expansion of the isolated non-perfused lung (Howell et al., 1961). However, opposite changes occur in the smaller vessels which are collapsed as the lung is expanded by inflation.

The effect of lung collapse. The effect of lung collapse on pulmonary blood flow is important because there is a clear physiological advantage in minimizing the perfusion of parts of the lung without ventilation. A most important series of studies by Barer and her colleagues (1969) clearly showed that it was the Po$_2$ within the collapsed lung which was important and not the volume or the inflation pressure. Perfusion decreased only when the alveolar Po$_2$ was reduced and, in total collapse, flow was controlled by the pulmonary arterial Po$_2$. Thus, perfusion of a collapsed lobe with systemic arterial blood restored normal blood flow. The increased vascular resistance in the collapsed lobe could also be reversed with vasodilator drugs, and the authors concluded that there was no evidence for any mechanical cause of increased vascular resistance in the collapsed lobe, as has been suggested in the past. However, flow was not reduced to zero and factors such as general anaesthetics impair hypoxic vasoconstriction (page 376). Therefore it should not be assumed that there will be no flow through the collapsed lung during one-lung anaesthesia (page 377). In long-standing collapse, the circulation is further reduced by structural changes in the vessels.

The vascular weir. The interplay of alveolar pressure, flow rate and vascular resistance is best considered by dividing the lung field into three zones (West, Dollery and Naimark, 1964; West and Dollery, 1965). In the upper zone (zone 1 of *Figure 6.6*) the pressure within the arterial end of the collapsible vessels is less than the alveolar pressure, and therefore insufficient to open the vessels which remain collapsed. The behaviour of these vessels is similar to that of a Starling resistor (see *Figure 3.5*). Provided the pressure outside the tube exceeds the pressure inside, there can be no flow regardless of the venous pressure, which is thus irrelevant. The situation is analogous to a weir in which the upstream water level is below the top of the weir and this is the condition in the uppermost parts of the lungs of the human subject in the upright position.

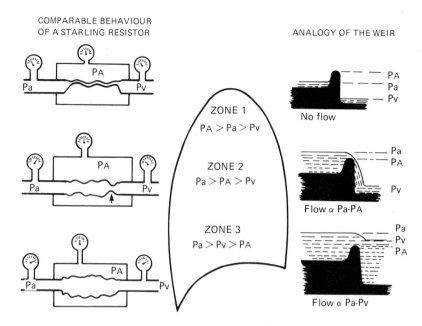

COMPARABLE BEHAVIOUR
OF A STARLING RESISTOR

ANALOGY OF THE WEIR

Figure 6.6 The effect of gravity upon pulmonary vascular resistance is shown by comparison with a Starling resistor (left) and with a weir (right). Pa, pressure in pulmonary artery; PA, pressure in alveoli; Pv, pressure in pulmonary vein (all pressures relative to atmosphere). This analogy does not illustrate zone 4 in which perfusion is reduced, apparently due to interstitial pressure acting on the larger vessels (Hughes et al., 1968). See text for full discussion.

In the mid-zone (zone 2 of *Figure 6.6*), the pressure at the arterial end of the collapsible vessels exceeds the alveolar pressure and, under these conditions, a collapsible vessel, behaving like a Starling resistor, permits flow in such a way that the flow rate depends upon the arterial/alveolar pressure difference. (Resistance in the Starling resistor is concentrated at the point marked with the arrows in *Figures 3.5* and *6.6*.) The larger the difference, the more widely the collapsible vessels will open and the lower will be the vascular resistance. Note that the venous pressure is still not a factor which affects flow or vascular resistance. This condition is still analogous to a weir with the upstream depth (head of pressure) corresponding to the arterial pressure, and the height of the weir corresponding to alveolar pressure. Clearly the flow of water over the weir depends solely on the difference in height between the top of the weir and the upstream water level. The depth of water below the weir (analogous to venous pressure) cannot influence the flow of water over the weir unless it rises above the height of the weir.

In the lower zone of the lungs (zone 3 of *Figure 6.6*), the pressure in the venous end of the capillaries is above the alveolar pressure, and under these conditions a collapsible vessel behaving like a Starling resistor will be held wide open and the flow rate will, as a first approximation, be governed by the arterial/venous pressure difference (the driving pressure) in the normal manner for the systemic circulation. However, as the intravascular pressure increases in relation to the alveolar pressure, the collapsible vessels will be further distended and their resistance will be correspondingly reduced. Returning to the analogy of the weir, the situation is now one in which the downstream water level has risen until the weir is completely submerged and offers little resistance to the flow of water, which is largely governed by the difference in the water level above and below the weir. However, as the levels rise further, the weir is progressively more and more submerged and what little resistance it offers to water flow is diminished still further. The concept of the weir is particularly helpful and was introduced by Permutt and Riley (1963) as the 'vascular waterfall'. Portrayal of a weir instead of a waterfall permits representation of zone 3 conditions.

To the three-zone model shown in *Figure 6.6*, Hughes et al. (1968) added a fourth zone of reduced blood flow in the most dependent parts of the lung. This reduction in blood flow appears to be due to compression of the larger blood vessels by increased interstitial pressure. This effect is more pronounced at reduced lung volumes. It is not shown in the weir analogy.

So far we have not mentioned the critical closing pressure of the pulmonary vessels (Burton, 1951). Current views suggest that the vessels of the lungs collapse at a pressure which is very close indeed to the alveolar pressure; that is to say, their critical closing pressure is extremely low (West and Dollery, 1965). The observations of these authors (and those reported by West, Dollery and Naimark in 1964) suggest that pulmonary blood flow ceases in any region where the alveolar pressure is in excess of the pressure at the arterial end of the collapsible vessels but that it recommences as soon as the vascular pressure exceeds the alveolar pressure. Simple hydrostatic considerations thus seem to define the amount of lung which is not perfused.

If the lungs are passively inflated by positive pressure, the pulmonary capillaries would clearly collapse if the pulmonary vascular pressures were to remain unchanged. In fact, the pulmonary vascular pressures normally rise by an amount almost exactly equal to the change in alveolar pressure up to inflation pressures of about 1.1 kPa (8 mmHg) (Lenfant and Howell, 1960). Beyond this the rise in intravascular pressure is less than the rise in alveolar pressure and the cut-off by the mechanism of the Starling resistor operates over a larger area of the lung field. This has been demonstrated as an increase in physiological dead space during positive pressure breathing (Bitter and Rahn, 1965; Folkow and Pappenheimer, 1955) and by the application of positive end-expiratory pressure during artificial ventilation (Bindslev et al., 1981). One might therefore expect that the physiological dead space for anaesthetized patients would be greater during artificial ventilation than during spontaneous respiration; this is, however, not the case (Nunn and Hill, 1960).

Structural factors which influence pulmonary vascular resistance

Organic obstruction of pulmonary blood vessels is important in a wide variety of conditions. Obstruction from within the lumen may be caused by emboli (thrombus, fat or gas) or by thrombosis (e.g. the chicken fat thrombus formed when death is imminent). Obstruction arising within the vessel wall is probably the cause of eventual reduction of flow through collapsed areas, and medial hypertrophy causes an increase in vascular resistance in certain cases of pulmonary hypertension due to obstruction of the outflow tract (e.g. mitral stenosis). Kinking of vessels may cause partial obstruction during surgery. Obstruction arising from outside the vessel wall may be due to a variety of pathological conditions (tumour, abscess, etc.) or to surgical manipulations during thoracotomy. Finally, vessels may be destroyed in emphysema and certain inflammatory conditions, causing a reduction in the total pulmonary vascular bed and an increase in vascular resistance.

Principles of measurement of the pulmonary circulation

Detailed consideration of haemodynamic measurement techniques must lie outside the scope of this book. The following section presents only the broad principles of measurement such as may be required for an understanding of respiratory physiology.

Pulmonary blood volume

Available methods are based on the technique used for measurement of cardiac output by dye dilution (see page 137). In essence, the dye is injected into a central vein and its concentration is recorded in samples aspirated from some point in the systemic arterial tree. Cardiac output is determined by the method described below, and then the interval is measured between the time of the injection of the dye and the mean arrival time of the dye at the sampling point. Cardiac output is multiplied by this time interval to indicate the amount of blood lying between injection and sampling sites. Assumed values for the extrapulmonary blood are then subtracted to indicate the intrapulmonary blood volume.

It is not at all easy to obtain satisfactory results with this method. The 'mean arrival time of the dye' is difficult to determine and the correction for the extra-pulmonary blood volume can be little more than an inspired guess but may be improved by injection into the pulmonary artery with sampling from the left ventricle. It may therefore be better to omit the correction and use the term 'central blood volume' which implies an appropriate lack of definition.

Pulmonary capillary blood volume may be measured as a byproduct of the measurement of pulmonary diffusing capacity, and the method is discussed in Chapter 8.

Pulmonary vascular pressures

Pressure measurements within the pulmonary circulation are almost always made with electronic differential pressure transducers. These invariably have a diaphragm which is deformed by a pressure difference across it. The movement of the diaphragm may be transduced to an electrical signal in a variety of ways. Its movement may influence special resistors of which the resistance is a function of their length (strain gauge). The diaphragm may form one plate of a capacitor of which the other plate is fixed. As the diaphragm is moved, the distance between the plates changes and this alters the capacitance of the device (capacitance manometer). Finally, the diaphragm may be linked to the core of a coil whose inductance is thus altered by movements of the diaphragm (inductance manometer). It is relatively simple for changes in resistance, capacitance or inductance to be detected, amplified and displayed as indicative of the pressures across the diaphragm of the transducer.

The space on the reference side of the diaphragm is in communication with atmosphere, oesophageal balloon or left atrial blood, as the case may be (see *Figure*

6.4). The other side of the diaphragm is filled with a liquid (usually heparinized saline) which is in direct communication with the blood of which the pressure is being measured.

If the system is to have the ability to respond to rapid changes of pressure, damping must be reduced to a minimum. This requires the total exclusion of bubbles of air from the manometer and connecting tubing, and the intravascular cannula must be unobstructed. Damping does not influence the measurement of mean pressure but reduces the apparent systolic pressure and increases the apparent diastolic pressure. The basic principles of pressure transducers and sources of error in their use have been reviewed by Gersh (1980).

These methods do not measure absolute pressure and can be used only for comparison with a primary standard (such as a column of mercury of known height). Electrical signals are often used as secondary standards, but must be checked at intervals against primary standards.

Electrical manometry yields a plot of instantaneous pressure against time (*Figure 6.7a*). From this it is often necessary to calculate the mean pressure. This is not simply the arithmetic mean of systolic and diastolic pressure, since the duration of diastole is greater than that of systole and therefore the effective or integrated mean

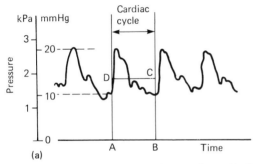

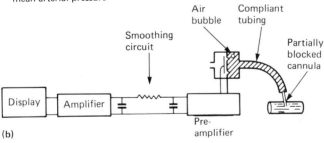

Figure 6.7 Determination of mean pulmonary arterial pressure. (a) An actual trace of instantaneous intravascular pulmonary arterial pressure during four cardiac cycles. For the second cycle, a rectangle has been constructed (ABCD) which has an area equal to that under the curve over the same time interval. The height of the rectangle (AD) indicates the effective integrated mean pressure. It will be seen to be approximately equal to diastolic pressure plus one-third of pulse pressure. (b) Factors which tend to damp the recording of instantaneous pressure (i.e. lower the indicated systolic pressure and raise the indicated diastolic pressure) tending towards an indication of the integrated mean pressure. Some of these factors are accidental (e.g. air bubble or blocked cannula) but others (e.g. smoothing circuit) may be employed deliberately to avoid the tedious method of calculation of mean pressure shown in (a).

must be weighted in favour of the diastolic pressure. Mean pressure is often taken to be one-third of the way from diastolic to systolic pressure (i.e. diastolic plus one-third of pulse pressure), but it is more correctly derived from assessing the area under the instantaneous pressure curve. A rectangle is constructed with length equal to the duration of one cardiac cycle and area equal to the area under the pressure curve over the same time interval. The height of the rectangle indicates the mean pressure.

More simply, the mean pressure may be determined by damping the measurement (or display) of the instantaneous pressure. This may be done on the actual measurement system (e.g. by allowing the intravascular cannula to become partly occluded) or by electrical means. These methods are illustrated in *Figure 6.7*. It should be noted that it is generally easier to measure mean pressure than instantaneous pressure. Exactly similar considerations apply to the determination of mean intrathoracic pressure. In the case of the intrathoracic pressure, the relevant cycle is, of course, that of respiration and not the heart beat.

Pulmonary blood flow

The total flow of blood through the pulmonary circulation may be measured by four groups of methods, each of which contains many variants (Kelman, 1971).

The Fick principle states that the amount of oxygen picked up from the respired gases equals the amount added to the blood which flows through the lungs. Alternatively, the amount of carbon dioxide exhaled equals the amount lost by the blood which flows through the lungs. In the case of oxygen it is evident that the oxygen uptake of the subject must equal the product of pulmonary blood flow and arteriovenous oxygen content difference. This is conveniently expressed in Pappenheimer symbols (see Appendix D):

$$\dot{V}_{O_2} = \dot{Q} \, (Ca_{O_2} - C\bar{v}_{O_2})$$

therefore:

$$\dot{Q} = \frac{\dot{V}_{O_2}}{Ca_{O_2} - C\bar{v}_{O_2}}$$

All the quantities on the right-hand side can be measured, although determination of the oxygen content of the mixed venous blood requires catheterization of the right ventricle or, preferably, the pulmonary artery.

Interpretation of the result is less easy. The calculated value includes the intrapulmonary arteriovenous shunt, but the situation is complicated beyond the possibility of easy solution if there is appreciable extrapulmonary admixture of venous blood (see *Figure 6.2*).

Indirect methods avoid right heart catheterization by calculating the composition of mixed venous blood by measurement of changes in composition of rebreathed gas. This is practicable only in the case of carbon dioxide, and determination of mixed venous P_{CO_2} is described in Chapter 9. Unfortunately, the derivation of mixed venous carbon dioxide content is not sufficiently accurate for the method to be a satisfactory alternative to the direct Fick method.

One important source of error is of particular concern to the anaesthetist. Between the pulmonary capillaries and the apparatus for measurement of oxygen consumption is a large volume of gas, comprising the subject's lungs, air passages, mouthpiece, valve box, etc. The method requires that the amount of oxygen in this volume remain constant throughout the period of measurement (1–5 minutes). Clearly both the volume of the space and the composition of its content must not be allowed to vary, and this can usually be achieved when the subject is breathing air. If the concentration of oxygen is allowed to alter during the period of measurement, a considerable error may be introduced. Thus if a patient breathing nitrous oxide and oxygen is connected to a closed-circuit spirometer containing oxygen for the measurement of oxygen uptake, nitrous oxide will pass from the patient to the spirometer and change both the total gas volume and its composition. This difficulty may be overcome, but only by quite elaborate methodology (Nunn and Pouliot, 1962). Measurement of oxygen consumption is discussed at the end of Chapter 10.

Methods based on uptake of inert tracer gases. A modified Fick method of measurement of cardiac output may be employed with fairly soluble inert gases such as acetylene (Grollman, 1929). With this technique, a single breath of a dilute acetylene mixture is taken and held. It is then exhaled and the alveolar (or, more correctly, end-expiratory) concentration of acetylene determined. Analysis of volume and composition of expired gas permits measurement of acetylene uptake. Since the duration of the procedure does not permit recirculation, it may be assumed that the mixed venous concentration of acetylene is zero. The Fick equation then simplifies to the following:

acetylene uptake = cardiac output × arterial acetylene concentration

The arterial acetylene concentration is derived from the assumption that the arterial acetylene tension equals the alveolar acetylene tension which is directly measured on the expired gas. Content is derived from tension using an assumed value for the solubility coefficient of acetylene in blood. This method entirely avoids sampling of blood and does not therefore require cannulation of vessels, a feature which appeals to the subjects.

This technique fell into disuse for a variety of reasons principally concerned with technical difficulties in making the various measurements. However, the concept came back into use following the introduction of the body plethysmograph, which has already been mentioned in connection with the measurement of lung volume and airway resistance. Its use in the determination of cardiac output is for the measurement of the uptake of the tracer gas (usually nitrous oxide at the present time). The subject inhales a mixture of about 15% nitrous oxide, and holds his breath with his mouth open. Nitrous oxide uptake is measured directly from the fall of the pressure within the box, and the arterial nitrous oxide content is derived from the alveolar nitrous oxide tension and its solubility coefficient in blood (Lee and DuBois, 1955).

All the methods based on the uptake of inert tracer gases have the following characteristics in common.

1. They measure pulmonary capillary blood flow, excluding any flow through shunts. This is in contrast to the Fick and dye methods.
2. The assumption that the tension of the tracer gas is the same in end-expiratory gas and arterial blood is invalid in the presence of disorders of blood and gas distribution within the lungs.

3. Some of the tracer gas dissolves in the tissues lining the respiratory tract and is carried away by blood perfusing these tissues. The indicated blood flow is therefore greater than the actual pulmonary capillary blood flow which is usually less than the total cardiac output.

When the body plethysmograph is used to measure the tracer gas uptake, it is possible to detect pulsatile uptake synchronous with systole. This is taken as evidence that pulmonary capillary blood flow is pulsatile.

Dye or thermal dilution. Currently the most popular technique for measurement of cardiac output is by dye dilution. Measurement can be repeated at least 20 times at 3-minute intervals with dye and indefinitely with a thermal indicator.

An indicator substance is introduced as a bolus into a large vein and its concentration is measured continuously at a sampling site in the systemic arterial tree. *Figure 6.8a* shows the method as it is applied to continuous non-circulating flow as, for example, of fluids through a pipeline. In the top right-hand corner is shown the sudden injection of the bolus of dye. It is carried downstream past a sampling point where some of the fluid in the pipe is drawn through a device which performs a continuous analysis of the concentration of the dye in the fluid. The concentration is displayed on the Y axis of the graph against time on the X axis. The dye is injected at time t_1 and is first detected at the sampling point at time t_2. The uppermost curve shows the form of a typical curve. There is a rapid rise to maximum concentration followed by a decay which is an exponential wash-out in form (see Appendix F), reaching insignificant levels at time t_3. The second graph shows the concentration (Y axis) on a logarithmic scale. Under these circumstances the exponential part of the decay curve becoms a straight line (see *Figure F.2*). If we consider only the part of the graph between times t_2 and t_3, the mean concentration of dye equals the amount of dye injected, divided by the volume of fluid flowing past the sampling point during the interval $t_2 - t_3$. The denominator is the product of the fluid flow rate and the time interval $t_2 - t_3$. The equation may now be rearranged to indicate the flow rate of the fluid as the following expression:

$$\frac{\text{amount of dye injected}}{\text{mean concentration of dye} \times \text{time interval } t_2 - t_3}$$

The denominator will be indicated by the area under the curve, and the flow rate may thus be readily calculated provided that the calibration of the dye analyser has been established.

Figure 6.8b shows the more complicated situation when fluid is flowing round a circuit. Under these conditions, the front of the dye-laden fluid may lap its own tail so that a recirculation peak appears on the graph before the primary peak has decayed to insignificant levels. This commonly occurs when cardiac output is determined in man, and steps must be taken to reconstruct the tail of the primary curve as it would have been had recirculation not taken place. To do this we make use of the fact that the exponential wash-out phase has usually been entered before the recirculation peak appears. This is clearly shown in the lowermost of the four graphs. On the logarithmic plot, the wash-out curve appears as a straight line until it is deflected upwards by recirculation. Having detected the point at which recirculation appears, the initial straight part of the descending curve is extrapolated as shown by the broken line in the lowest graph of *Figure 6.8*. This is then replotted on a linear scale (penultimate graph) and the area of the reconstructed primary

(a) NON-CIRCULATING FLOW

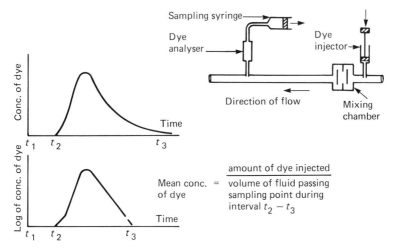

(b) CIRCULATING FLOW

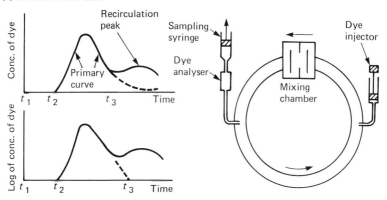

Figure 6.8 Measurement of flow by dye dilution. (a) The measurement of continuous non-circulating flow rate of fluid in a pipeline. The bolus of dye is injected upstream and its concentration is continuously monitored downstream. The relationship of the relevant quantities is shown in the equation. Mean concentration of dye is determined from the area under the curve as shown in Figure 6.7. (b) The more complicated situation when recirculation occurs and the front of the circulating dye laps its own tail, giving a recirculation peak. Reconstruction of the primary curve is based on extrapolation of the primary curve before recirculation occurs. This is facilitated by the fact that the down curve is exponential and therefore a straight line on a logarithmic plot

curve determined. This laborious procedure used to be undertaken manually. Nowadays it is almost invariably undertaken by a dedicated computer which is an integral part of the apparatus for measuring cardiac output.

Many different indicators have been used for the dye dilution technique, but currently the most satisfactory appears to be 'coolth'. A bolus of cold saline is injected and the dip in temperature is recorded downstream with the temperature record corresponding to the dye curve. No blood sampling is required and temperature is measured directly with a thermometer mounted on the catheter. The 'coolth' is dispersed in the systemic circulation and therefore there is no recirculation peak to complicate the calculation. The thermal method is particularly suitable for repeated measurements.

Direct measurements of intravascular flow rate. The instantaneous flow through a blood vessel may be measured with an electromagnetic flow meter probe in the form of a cuff attached directly to the blood vessel. The method is clearly of limited application to man but it has had important application in animal studies. These transducers may be used, for example, for comparisons of left and right pulmonary artery blood flows, which would be very difficult to make by any other means. The *velocity* of blood flow in a vessel may be measured by the Doppler shift using ultrasound. This can be translated into flow rate only if the diameter of the vessel is known. Practical difficulties arise in being sure that the signal arises solely from the vessel under consideration. Furthermore, it is erroneous to assume that the velocity profile is constant across the diameter of the vessel.

Chapter 7

Distribution of pulmonary ventilation and perfusion

Chapter 5 has considered pulmonary ventilation and Chapter 6 the pulmonary circulation. The present chapter is concerned with their distribution, particularly in relation to each other. The plan of the chapter is first to consider the spatial and temporal distribution of ventilation. The same consideration is then given to the pulmonary circulation. Following this, distribution of ventilation and perfusion are considered in relation to one another. Finally the concepts of dead space and shunt are presented.

Distribution of ventilation

The distribution of the inspired gas may be considered in a number of contexts. Firstly, it may be considered purely as spatial distribution in relation to anatomical structures. Secondly, the distribution of inspired gas may be considered in terms of the rate at which different alveoli fill and empty. Finally, it may be considered in relation to the distribution of pulmonary blood flow, differentiating between the ventilation of unperfused alveoli at one extreme and the failure of ventilation of perfused alveoli at the other extreme.

It frequently happens that these distinctions are not clearly made, and confusion may result from a failure to appreciate the precise meaning of the phrase 'distribution of inspired gas' in a particular situation.

Spatial and anatomical distribution of inspired gas

The spatial distribution of inspired gas can be considered either in relation to the anatomy of the lungs or in terms of zones which relate to the anatomy of the trunk rather than the lungs themselves.

Distribution between the two lungs is influenced by posture and by the manner of ventilation. In the normal conscious subject, the right lung enjoys a ventilation slightly greater than the left lung in both the upright and the supine position (*Table 7.1*). The studies of Svanberg (1957) showed that, in the lateral position, the lower lung is always better ventilated regardless of the side on which the subject is lying although there still remains a bias in favour of the right side (*Table 7.1*). It appears surprising at first sight that the lower lung should be better ventilated than the upper since the volume of the lower lung is less, and it is especially liable to collapse.

Table 7.1 Distribution of resting lung volume (FRC) and ventilation between the two lungs in man
(The first figure is the unilateral FRC (litres) and the second the percentage partition of ventilation)

	Supine		Right lateral (left side up)		Left lateral (right side up)	
	Right lung	Left lung	Right lung	Left lung	Right lung	Left lung
Conscious man	1.69	1.39	1.68	2.07	2.19	1.38
(Svanberg, 1957)	53%	47%	61%	39%	47%	53%
Anaesthetized man—	1.18	0.91	1.03	1.32	1.71	0.79
spontaneous breathing	52%	48%	45%	55%	56%	44%
(Rehder and Sessler, 1973)						
Anaesthetized man—						
artificial ventilation	1.36	1.16	1.33	2.21	2.29	1.12
(Rehder et al., 1972)	52%	48%	44%	56%	60%	40%
Anaesthetized man—thoracotomy	—	—	—	—	—	—
(Nunn, 1961a)	—	—	—	—	83%	17%

Each study refers to separate subjects or patients.

However, the diminished volume of the dependent lung is associated with the lower diaphragm lying higher in the chest and so being more sharply curved. It will therefore be able to contract more effectively during inspiration (see *Figure 5.2*). Fortunately, the preferential ventilation of the lower lung accords with increased perfusion of the same lung, so the ventilation/perfusion ratios of the two lungs are not greatly altered on assuming the lateral position. Rehder's group from the Mayo Clinic have reported that the preferential ventilation of the lower lung in the lateral position does not occur in anaesthetized or artificially ventilated man (*Table 7.1*).

Gross differences in ventilation between the two lungs may be assessed by inspection and auscultation of the chest. Additional information may be obtained by chest radiography and screening. Bronchospirometry is the definitive technique to differentiate the ventilation of the two lungs.

Spatial distribution in relation to the external anatomy of the trunk may be determined by a variety of techniques. The simplest approach is to distinguish between expansion of rib cage and abdomen. This can be done by magnetometers which measure anteroposterior or lateral diameters, tape and strain gauges which measure circumference or, best of all, by impedance plethysmography which measures the cross-sectional area and so relates most closely to volume changes (Milledge and Stott, 1977).

Optical contouring can provide a full quantification of the geometric change in shape of the trunk during breathing. Striped bands of light are projected from the sides of the torso which is then photographed from front and back (Peacock et al., 1984). The most complete information is provided by computerized tomography which can also indicate the position of the diaphragm. However, application is usually restricted to patients in the horizontal position and also the number of sections is limited by total radiation dosage. Techniques for geometric estimation of lung and chest wall function have been reviewed by Denison (1984).

Distribution to horizontal slices of lung was first studied by West (1962) using a radioactive isotope of oxygen. He found the slices to have different degrees of ventilation with a threefold increase in ventilation at the bottom compared with the top of the lung (*Figure 7.1*). The original studies were carried out with slow vital capacity inspirations starting from residual volume, but circumstances are different during normal tidal ventilation. Firstly, there is the end-expiratory lung volume and the range of lung volume over which the patient breathes. Slow inspirations from FRC to total lung capacity show the same preferential ventilation of the bases but the degree of inequality is reduced and Hughes et al. (1972) reported a mean ratio of 1.5:1 for basal ventilation compared with apical (*Figure 7.1*). The second factor

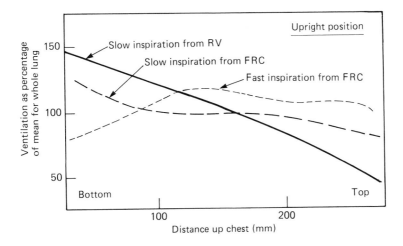

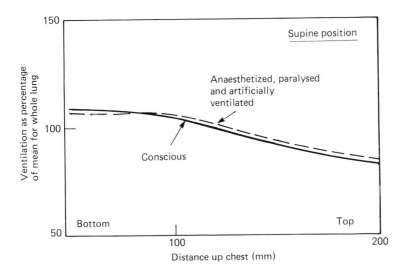

Figure 7.1 Relative distribution of ventilation in horizontal strata of the lungs. Data for the upright position from West (1962), and Hughes et al. (1972). Data for the supine position from Hulands et al. (1970), comprising inspirations of 1 litre from FRC with normal inspiratory flow rate.

is the rate of inspiration, since regional airway resistance then becomes relatively more important than regional compliance which governs distribution of ventilation during a very slow inspiration. Hughes et al. (1972) showed that fast inspirations from FRC did in fact reverse the distribution of ventilation with preferential ventilation of the upper parts of the lungs. Since this is contrary to the distribution of pulmonary blood flow, gas exchange would be impaired.

Bake et al. (1974) also studied the effect of inspiratory gas flow rate on distribution of ventilation and found that the preferential ventilation of the dependent parts of the lung was present only at flow rates below 1.5 l/s, starting from FRC. At higher flow rates, distribution was approximately uniform. Normal inspiratory flow rate is much less than 1.5 l/s (see *Figure 3.13*).

Posture affects distribution since *inter alia* the vertical height of the lung is reduced by about 30 per cent in the supine position. The gravitational force generating maldistribution is thus reduced. Hulands et al. (1970) investigated normal tidal breathing in the supine position and found slight preferential ventilation of the posterior slices of the lungs compared with the anterior slices (*Figure 7.1*). The inequality was not greatly different from that found in the upright position. Huland's group also found no major changes during anaesthesia with paralysis and artificial ventilation. The effect of gravitation on ventilation is of minor importance in comparison to its effect on perfusion, which will be considered below.

Distribution to zones of the lung can be conveniently studied with the gamma camera following inhalation of a suitable radioactive gas which is not too soluble in blood. Xenon-133 is suitable for this purpose and the technique has become a routine clinical investigation. The technique defines zones of the lung which can be related to anatomical subdivisions by comparing anteroposterior and lateral scans. The technique is useful for defining pathological causes of failure of regional ventilation and can be related to scans which indicate perfusion.

Distribution of inspired gas in relation to the rate of alveolar filling

The rate of inflation of the lung as a whole is a function of inflation pressure, compliance and airway resistance (page 398). The product of the compliance and resistance equals the time constant which is:

1. The time required for inflation to 63 per cent of the final volume attained if inflation is prolonged indefinitely.
   or
2. The time which would be required for inflation of the lungs if the initial gas flow rate were maintained throughout inflation (see Appendix F, *Figure F.3*).

These considerations apply equally to large and small areas of the lungs; *Figure 2.6* shows fast and slow alveoli, the former with a short time constant and the latter with a long time constant. We may now consider ventilation of the lungs when different zones have different time constants. *Figure 7.2* shows a range of different *functional units* of the lung with different time constants. Pairs of units are compared in each of the five parts of the diagram.

The considerations are fundamentally similar for spontaneous respiration and for artificial ventilation with a constant or sine-wave flow generator (see *Figures 21.4*

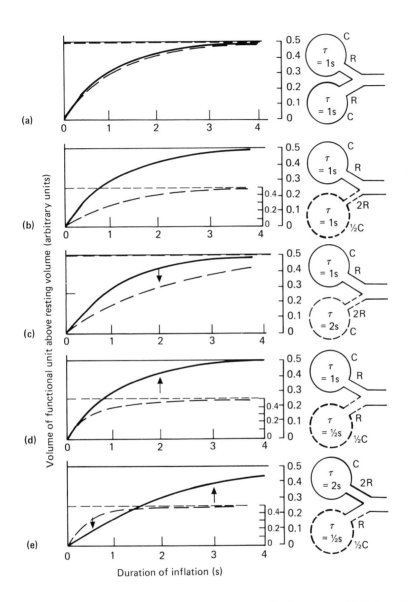

Figure 7.2 The effect of mechanical characteristics on the time course of inflation of different functional units of the lung when exposed to a sustained constant inflation pressure. The Y co-ordinate is volume change, but a scale showing intra-alveolar pressure is shown on the right. The continuous curve relates to the upper unit and the broken curve to the lower unit, in each case. Separate pressure scales are necessary when the compliances are different. Arrows show the direction of gas redistribution if inflow is checked by closure of the upper airway at the times indicated. See text for explanation of the changes.

and *21.5*). However, consideration of the special case of passive inflation of the lungs by development of a constant mouth pressure (see *Figure 21.1*) simplifies the presentation.

Figure 7.2a shows two functional units of equal compliance and resistance. If the mouth pressure is increased to a constant level, there will be an increase in volume of each unit, which is equal to the mouth pressure multiplied by the compliance of the unit. The time course of inflation will follow the wash-in type of exponential function (Appendix F) and the time constant will be equal to the product of compliance and resistance of each unit. The time courses will thus be identical, and if the inspiratory phase is terminated at any instant, the pressure in each unit will be identical and no redistribution of gas will occur between the two units.

Figure 7.2b shows two functional units, one of which has half the compliance but twice the resistance of the other. The time constants of the two will thus be equal. If a constant inflation pressure is maintained, the one with the lower compliance will increase in volume by half the volume change of the other. Nevertheless, the pressure build-up within each unit will be identical. Thus, as in the previous example, the relative distribution of gas between the two functional units will be independent of the rate or duration of inflation. If the inspiratory phase is terminated at any point, the pressure in each unit will be identical and no redistribution will occur between the different units.

In *Figure 7.2c*, the compliances of the two units are identical but the resistance of one is twice that of the other. Therefore, its time constant is double that of its fellow and it will fill more slowly, although the volume increase in both units will be the same if inflation is prolonged indefinitely. Relative distribution between the units is thus dependent upon the rate and duration of inflation. If inspiration is checked by closure of the upper airway after 2 seconds (for example), the pressure will be higher in the unit with the lower resistance. Gas will then be redistributed from one unit to the other as shown by the arrow in the diagram.

Figure 7.2d shows a pair of units with identical resistances but the compliance of one being half that of the other. Its time constant is thus half that of its fellow and it has a faster time course of inflation. However, since its compliance is half that of the other, the ultimate volume increase will only be half that of the other unit when the inflation is prolonged indefinitely. The relative distribution of gas between the two units is dependent upon the rate and duration of inflation. Pressure rises more rapidly in the unit with the lower compliance, and if inspiration is checked by closure of the upper airway at 2 seconds (for example), gas will be redistributed from one unit to the other as shown by the arrow.

An interesting and complex situation occurs when one unit has an increased resistance and another a reduced compliance (*Figure 7.2e*). This combination also features in the presentation of the concept of fast and slow alveoli in *Figure 2.6*. In the present example the time constant of one unit is four times that of the other, while the ultimate volume changes are determined by the compliance as in *Figure 7.2d*. When the inflation pressure is sustained, the unit with the lower resistance shows the greater volume change at first, but rapidly approaches its equilibrium volume. Thereafter the other unit undergoes the major volume changes, the inflation of the two units being out of phase with one another. Throughout inspiration, the pressure build-up in the unit with the shorter time constant is always greater and, if inspiration is checked by closure of the upper airway, gas will be redistributed from one unit to the other as shown by the arrows in *Figure 7.2e*.

These complex relationships may be summarized as follows. If the inflation pressure is sustained indefinitely, the volume change in different units of the lungs will depend solely upon their regional compliances. *If their time constants are equal*, the build-up of pressure in the different units will be identical at all times during inflation and therefore:

1. Distribution of inspired gas will be independent of the rate, duration or frequency of inspiration.
2. Dynamic compliance (so far as it is influenced by considerations discussed in relation to *Figure 2.6*) will not be affected by changes in frequency.
3. If inspiration is checked by closure of the upper airway, there will be no redistribution of gas within the lungs.

If, however, *the time constants of different units are different*, for whatever cause, it follows that:

1. Distribution of inspired gas will be dependent on the rate, duration and frequency of inspiration.
2. Dynamic compliance will be decreased as respiratory frequency is increased.
3. If inspiration is checked by closure of the upper airway, gas will be redistributed within the lungs.

In the healthy subject, the variations in time constants for different parts of the lung can be demonstrated by the effect on distribution of ventilation of fast and slow inspirations as described above. An increase in scatter of time constants in disease may be shown by an increase in the frequency dependence of compliance (page 28).

Spontaneous versus artificial ventilation

Intermittent positive pressure ventilation (IPPV) results in a spatial pattern of distribution which is determined by regional compliance and ventilation (*Figure 7.2*). It is still not clear how far similar considerations apply to spontaneous breathing. On the one hand there is the view that, during spontaneous breathing, the lungs simply expand passively in response to the reduction in intrapleural pressure created by the inspiratory muscles. In the other hand, it seems possible that the anatomical pattern of contraction of the inspiratory muscles may actually influence spatial distribution.

During anaesthesia, spontaneous respiration is predominantly abdominal, while there is a slight excess of rib cage movement during IPPV (see page 356). In the supine anaesthetized patient, the posterior part of the diaphragm moves more during spontaneous breathing, while the anterior part moves more during IPPV (see *Figure 19.6*). In spite of the major differences in these anatomical markers of the spatial distribution of inspired gas, indices of the efficiency of gas exchange (such as dead space and shunt) are not significantly different for the two types of breathing (pages 368 et seq.). Rather surprisingly, the two modes of ventilation cause no major difference in the distribution of inspired gas between the two lungs (see *Table 7.1*). It would thus seem that, however the spatial distribution of gas appears to be altered by IPPV, the functional effect is minimal.

Effect of maldistribution of inspired air on gas mixing

This subject is important for two reasons. Firstly, it constitutes one method of detecting certain types of maldistribution. Secondly, it has an adverse effect on most forms of inhalation therapy, including inhalational anaesthesia.

Various therapeutic manoeuvres require the replacement of the nitrogen in the alveolar gas with a different gas. Examples are the administration of 100% oxygen in severe shunting, the replacement of nitrogen with helium to diminish the resistance to breathing, and finally the replacement of alveolar nitrogen with anaesthetic gases. Replacement takes place, not only in the alveolar gas but also in all the tissues of the body and this is relatively more important in the case of the more soluble gases. Oxygen is a special case since it is consumed within the body and so can never come into equilibrium between the different tissues. The exchange of gases within the different body compartments is a complex story but we can confine discussion to exchange within the lungs at this stage.

If we ignore the exchange of a gas within the tissue compartments, the wash-in and wash-out of gases in the lungs may be considered as an exponential function (Appendix F). Thus if a patient inhales 100% oxygen, the alveolar nitrogen concentration falls according to a wash-out exponential function (*Figure F.2*). If, on the other hand, he inhales a helium mixture, the alveolar helium concentration rises according to a wash-in exponential function (*Figure F.3*) towards a plateau concentration equal to that in the inspired gas. In each case the time constant of change in the composition of the alveolar gas is the same and equals:

$$\frac{\text{functional volume of the lungs}}{\text{alveolar ventilation}}$$

If, for example, the lung volume is 3 litres and the alveolar ventilation is 6 l/min, the time constant will be 30 seconds. (This time constant should not be confused with the time constant of lung inflation and deflation which equals the product of compliance and resistance.)

This makes an important assumption—that every alveolus is ventilated in proportion to its volume. If this is not the case, there will be a whole family of time constants for different functional units of the lungs. Some units will therefore exchange rapidly and some slowly. The overall picture is that of delayed equilibrium, and after a finite interval (say 7 minutes) it is found that the mixed alveolar gas concentration has not changed as rapidly as would otherwise be expected. It may, furthermore, be shown that the wash-out curve is not that of a simple exponential, but shows two or more components, the areas with short time constants being dominant early and the areas with long time constants being dominant later.

If a patient breathes 100% oxygen, the alveolar nitrogen will normally be reduced to less than 2.5% after 7 minutes. This fall may be delayed by maldistribution. The fall of nitrogen concentration is the basis of the 'nitrogen wash-out test' but the rate of rise of oxygen concentration is often of direct interest to the anaesthetist and others who are concerned with patients with deranged lung function.

We have already considered the helium wash-in method of measurement of functional residual capacity (FRC) (page 45). The *rate* at which equilibrium is attained between spirometer and lungs is also a measure of the equality of distribution. Thus the measurement of FRC may be conveniently combined with a test of distribution.

Effect of maldistribution on the alveolar 'plateau'

If different functional units of the lung empty synchronously during expiration, the composition of the expired air will be approximately constant after the anatomical dead space has been flushed. This, however, does not occur when there is maldistribution with fast and slow units as shown in *Figure 2.6*. The slow units are slow both to fill and to empty, and thus are hypoventilated for their volume; therefore they are slow to respond to a change in the inspired gas composition. This forms the basis of an important test of maldistribution which, unlike the multi-breath nitrogen wash-out test (described above), will detect maldistribution only if there is sequential emptying of functional units of lung.

The single-breath nitrogen test is shown diagrammatically in *Figure 7.3*. The subject, who has been breathing air, takes a single deep breath of 100% oxygen sufficient to raise the alveolar oxygen concentration to about 50%. The patient then exhales deeply and the nitrogen concentration is measured at the patient's lips. (It would be just as satisfactory to monitor the oxygen concentration, but in the past it has been more convenient to measure nitrogen concentration.) We may now consider what is found under four different circumstances (*Figure 7.3a–d*):

1. *Figure 7.3a* shows two identical functional units. Following the inspiration of a single breath of oxygen, the nitrogen concentration in each unit is reduced to the same value and the exhaled nitrogen concentration must therefore remain constant throughout the latter part of expiration.
2. *Figure 7.3b* shows functional units of identical mechanical properties but which are subjected to unequal forces during inspiration. As a result, the nitrogen concentration is reduced by a greater amount in the better ventilated unit. If expiration is passive, the expirate will consist of the same proportion from each unit throughout expiration. Therefore the exhaled nitrogen concentration will be constant throughout the latter part of expiration, at a value intermediate between that of the two units.
3. *Figure 7.3c* shows two units of different mechanical properties but which nevertheless have the same time constant. (The unit on the right may be considered as having double the resistance and half the compliance of the unit on the left.) In these circumstances, ventilation will be preferentially distributed to the unit with the higher compliance and lower resistance (see *Figure 7.3b*). However, if expiration is passive, the expirate will again consist of the same proportion from each unit throughout expiration. Therefore the exhaled nitrogen concentration will remain constant throughout the latter part of expiration as in the previous example.
4. *Figure 7.3d* has two units with different time constants resulting from different mechanical properties, similar to the fast and slow alveoli in *Figure 2.6*. During inspiration of finite length, the faster unit will be preferentially ventilated, and its nitrogen concentration will therefore be lower. During expiration, the faster unit empties more rapidly at first while gas from the slower unit forms a proportionately greater part of the end-expiratory gas. Thus the proportion of gas from the two units changes during expiration and the nitrogen concentration rises progressively.

In the examples shown in *Figure 7.3b* and *c*, there is definite maldistribution of inspired gas, but this is not revealed by the single-breath nitrogen test. Only when the time constants of the units differ will the maldistribution be revealed by the test

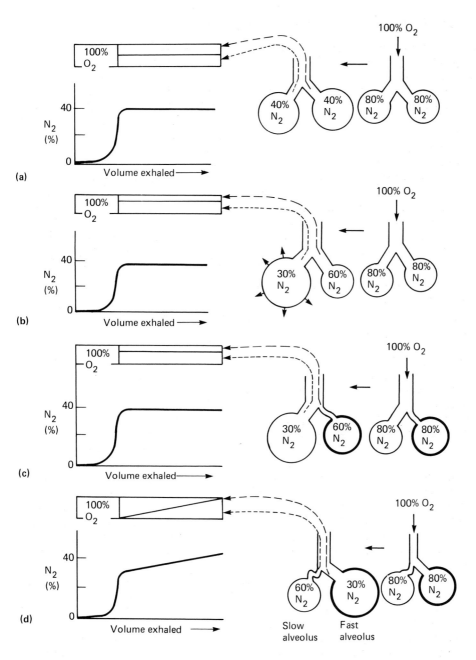

Figure 7.3 The single-breath nitrogen wash-out test in different types of maldistribution. Reading the diagram from right to left, the subject inhales a deep breath of 100% oxygen and then exhales into a nitrogen meter. (a) Normal subject with uniform distribution. (b) Maldistribution due to non-uniform pull of inspiratory muscles. (c) Maldistribution due to non-uniform mechanical factors in lung units but all having the same time constants. (d) Maldistribution due to non-uniform mechanical factors in lung units resulting in different time constants. Only this type of maldistribution alters the slope of the curve of the expired nitrogen.

(as in *Figure 7.3d*). This point is frequently glossed over by those who are chiefly concerned with maldistribution caused by lung disease. This is because maldistribution due to the commoner forms of lung disease is usually associated with different time constants and *sequential emptying*. Therefore, under these circumstances the single-breath nitrogen test is a valid method of detection of maldistribution of inspired gas. There are, however, other situations in which maldistribution is not associated with changes in time constants, and which could not therefore be demonstrated by the single-breath nitrogen test. Maldistribution of this type might result from the use of the lateral position, from intercostal paralysis or from artificial ventilation.

Before leaving the single-breath nitrogen test, two small points may be noted. Firstly, even with perfect distribution the exhaled nitrogen concentration rises slightly during the latter part of the exhalation. This is because oxygen is being consumed in greater volume than carbon dioxide is being produced. Therefore, the alveolar nitrogen concentration always rises slightly as expiration proceeds. (Normal alveolar gas contains 80–81 per cent nitrogen compared with 79 per cent in air.) The upper limit of normal is a rise of 1.5 per cent (more in older subjects) between the exhalation of 750 ml and 1250 ml after the inhalation of a large breath of oxygen. The second point is that fast alveoli must inhale more than their share of gas lying in the anatomical dead space. Thus the slow alveoli do have a marginal advantage in that their delayed filling results in the uptake of relatively more uncontaminated fresh gas.

Distribution of perfusion

Maldistribution of pulmonary blood flow is the commonest cause of impaired oxygenation of the arterial blood. The pulmonary blood flow is probably never distributed evenly to all parts of the lung field and the degree of non-uniformity is usually much greater than is the case for inspired gas. Uneven distribution may be present between the two lungs and between different lobes but always between successive horizontal slices of the lungs, except under conditions of zero gravity (Michels and West, 1978).

Maldistribution may also occur diffusely between tiny zones of lung which cannot be defined anatomically. The chief manifestation of this type of maldistribution is impairment of oxygenation of arterial blood, and the effect can be quantified in physiological terms although the disorder can seldom be explained in morphological terms.

Distribution between the two lungs

Use of a divided airway (such as a Carlen's tube) has permitted accurate estimation of the partition of the tidal volume between the two lungs. Unfortunately, no method of comparable simplicity exists to study the partition of the pulmonary blood flow in man. It might at first sight appear that a Carlen's tube would permit solution of the Fick equation for the two lungs separately. This, however, would require separate sampling of the blood leaving the two lungs, which could probably be contrived if it were not for the fact that each lung drains through two pulmonary veins. Representative sampling therefore requires blood to be sampled from each vein in proportion to its flow rate and this is not feasible. It is, however, possible to make a rough and ready estimate of the pulmonary venous oxygen content and this enables an approximate idea of unilateral flow to be obtained from the unilateral oxygen consumption, which is easily derived by using a Carlen's tube and a pair of bronchospirometers.

An alternative approach is to label the pulmonary circulation (with radioactive macroaggregates or ^{133}Xe dissolved in saline) and then to observe the activity in the two lung fields, either with suitably collimated counters or with a gamma camera. In animals, it is possible to implant electromagnetic flow probes around left and right branches of the pulmonary artery and so to obtain a continuous record of left and right lung blood flow.

Defares et al. (1960) studied supine subjects using an indirect method based on the Fick principle using CO_2 and obtained values for unilateral flow which agree closely with the distribution of ventilation observed in the supine position by Svanberg (1957) (see *Table 7.1*).

In the lateral position there is an increased perfusion of the dependent lung, as would be expected from considerations of the effect of gravity on the pulmonary circulation (page 151). In the dog, with its narrow chest, the effect is not large, and Rehder, Theye and Fowler (1961) reported only small increases in perfusion of the dependent lung when dogs were turned from the supine to the lateral position. Surprisingly, the effect was reversed when the thorax was opened.

In man the thorax is of the order of 30 cm in lateral diameter and so, in the lateral position, the column of blood in the pulmonary circulation exerts a hydrostatic pressure which is high in relation to the mean pulmonary arterial pressure. A fairly gross maldistribution is therefore to be expected with much of the upper lung comprising zone 2 and much of the lower lung comprising zone 3 (see *Figure 6.6*). Using the ^{133}Xe technique, Kaneko et al. (1966) showed uniform high perfusion of the dependent lung (apparently in zone 3) but with reduced perfusion of the upper lung which appeared to be mainly in zone 2. There was no evidence of the existence of a zone 1 (absent perfusion).

The increased perfusion of the lower lung is usually advantageous during thoracic surgery in the lateral position. Surgical intervention frequently limits or prevents ventilation of the exposed (upper) lung. Ventilation is thus deflected to the lower lung, which generally receives most of the pulmonary circulation. Gas exchange is impaired but the effects are mitigated by the gravitationally imposed distribution of the pulmonary circulation. Nevertheless, the high perfusion of the dependent lung, combined with its low relative lung volume (see *Figure 5.2*), causes the dependent lung to be at increased risk of absorption collapse (Potgieter, 1959).

Distribution in horizontal slices of the lung

In the previous chapter, it was shown how the pulmonary vascular resistance is mainly in the capillary bed and is governed by the relationship between alveolar, pulmonary arterial and pulmonary venous pressures. *Figure 6.6* presented the concept of the vascular weir with pulmonary vascular resistance decreasing and pulmonary blood flow increasing with distance down the lung, until zone 4 is entered where there is increased alveolar vascular resistance in larger vessels apparently due to increased interstitial pressure. This results in reduced perfusion of the most dependent part of the lung.

The first studies with radioactive gases took place at total lung capacity and showed flow increasing progressively down the lung in the upright position (West, 1963). However, it was later found that there was a significant reduction of flow in the most dependent parts of the lung (zone 4) which became progressively more important as lung volume was reduced from total lung capacity towards the residual volume (Hughes et al., 1968). *Figure 7.4* is redrawn from the work of Hughes' group and shows that pulmonary perfusion (per alveolus) is, in fact, reasonably uniform at the lung volumes relvant to normal tidal exchange. However, the dependent parts of the lung contain more but smaller alveoli than the apices at FRC and the perfusion *per unit lung volume* is still increased at the bases.

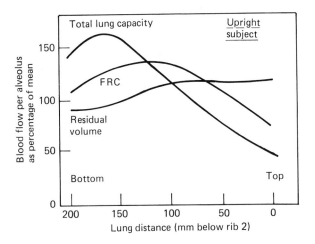

Figure 7.4 Pulmonary perfusion per alveolus as a percentage of that expected if all alveoli were equally perfused. At total lung capacity, perfusion increases down to 150 mm, below which perfusion is slightly decreased (zone 4). At FRC, zone 4 conditions apply below 100 mm, and at residual volume the perfusion gradient is actually reversed. It should be noted that perfusion has been calculated per alveolus. If shown as perfusion per unit lung volume, the non-uniformity at total lung capacity would be the same because alveoli are all the same size at total lung capacity. At FRC there are more but smaller alveoli at the bases and the non-uniformity would be greater. (Data are redrawn from Hughes et al. (1968))

In the *supine* position the differences in blood flow between apices and bases are replaced by differences between anterior and posterior aspects. Over the 20 cm height of the lung field in the average supine adult, the perfusion *per unit lung volume* increases progressively, with the most dependent parts receiving approximately double the perfusion of the uppermost parts at FRC (Kaneko et al., 1966; Hulands et al., 1970). However, as in the upright position, the dependent parts of the lungs contain more but smaller alveoli, and perfusion *per alveolus* is almost uniform down the lung (Kaneko et al., 1966). Zones 1 and 4 conditions were not observed in these studies.

Ventilation in relation to perfusion

Inspired gas distributed to regions which have no pulmonary capillary blood flow cannot take part in gas exchange and, conversely, pulmonary blood flow distributed to regions without ventilation cannot become oxygenated. This principle was appreciated by John Hunter who, in the eighteenth century, wrote:

> 'In animals where there is no circulation, there can be no lungs: for lungs are an apparatus for the air and blood to meet, and can only accord with motion of blood in vessels...As the lungs are to expose the blood to the air, they are so constructed as to answer this purpose exactly with the blood brought to them, and so disposed in them as to go hand in hand.'

It is convenient to consider the relationship between ventilation and perfusion in terms of the ventilation/perfusion ratio (abbreviated to $\dot{V}/\dot{Q}$. Each quantity is measured in litres per minute although ventilation is tidal and perfusion is continuous flow. Taking the lungs as a whole, typical resting values might be 4 l/min for alveolar ventilation and 5 l/min for pulmonary blood flow. Thus the overall ventilation/perfusion ratio would be 0.8 (which happens to be close to the respiratory exchange ratio but this is coincidental). If ventilation and perfusion of all alveoli were uniform then each alveolus would have an individual $\dot{V}/\dot{Q}$ ratio of 0.8.

In fact, ventilation and perfusion are not uniformly distributed but may range all the way from unventilated alveoli to unperfused alveoli with every gradation in between. Unventilated alveoli will have a $\dot{V}/\dot{Q}$ ratio of zero and the unperfused alveoli a $\dot{V}/\dot{Q}$ ratio of infinity. $\dot{V}/\dot{Q}$ ratios of other alveoli are ranged between these two extremes.

Alveoli with no ventilation ($\dot{V}/\dot{Q}$ ratio of zero) will have P_{O_2} and P_{CO_2} values which are the same as those of mixed venous blood since the trapped air in the unventilated alveoli will equilibrate with mixed venous blood. Alveoli with no perfusion ($\dot{V}/\dot{Q}$ ratio of infinity) will have P_{O_2} and P_{CO_2} values which are the same as those of the inspired gas since there is no gas exchange to alter the composition of the inspired gas which is drawn into these alveoli. Alveoli with intermediate values of $\dot{V}/\dot{Q}$ ratio will have P_{O_2} and P_{CO_2} values which are intermediate between those of mixed venous blood and inspired gas. *Figure 7.5* shows on a P_{O_2}/P_{CO_2} plot the line which joins all possible combinations of alveolar P_{O_2} and P_{CO_2} with an indication of the corresponding $\dot{V}/\dot{Q}$ ratios. The inhalation of higher than normal partial pressures of oxygen moves the inspired point of the curve to the right. The mixed venous point also moves to the right but only by a small amount for reasons which are explained on page 479. A new curve must be prepared for each combination of values for mixed venous blood and inspired gas (see appendix 2 of West, 1965). The curve can then be used to demonstrate the gas tensions in the horizontal strata of the lung according to their different $\dot{V}/\dot{Q}$ ratios (*Figure 7.5*).

It has been described above how collimated counters can be used with ^{133}Xe to measure ventilation and perfusion in horizontal strata of the lung. This technique can only discriminate rather thick slices of the lung and is unable to detect changes in small areas of lung within the slices. This limitation has been overcome by the multiple inert gas technique developed by West's group in San Diego. The methodology is outlined on page 181 but it is sufficient to say at this stage that it permits the plotting of the distribution of pulmonary ventilation and perfusion as a function of $\dot{V}/\dot{Q}$ ratios, expressed on a logarithmic scale.

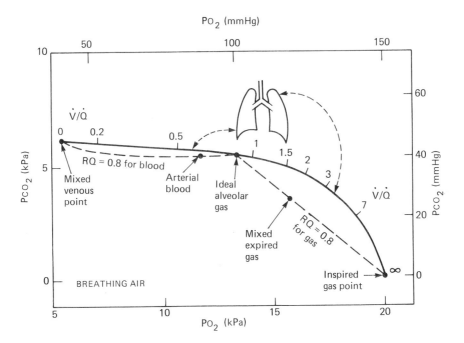

Figure 7.5 The heavy line indicates all possible values for P_{O_2} and P_{CO_2} of alveoli with ventilation/ perfusion ($\dot{V}/\dot{Q}$) ratios ranging from zero to infinity (subject breathing air). Values for normal alveoli are distributed as shown in accord with their vertical distance up the lung field. Mixed expired gas may be considered as a mixture of 'ideal' alveolar and inspired gas (dead space). Arterial blood may be considered as a mixture of blood with the same gas tensions as 'ideal' alveolar gas and mixed venous blood (the shunt).

Figure 7.6a shows a typical plot for a young healthy subject with both ventilation and perfusion largely confined to alveoli with $\dot{V}/\dot{Q}$ ratios in the range 0.3–3.0 (Wagner et al., 1974). There is no measurable distribution to areas of zero $\dot{V}/\dot{Q}$ ratio (i.e. shunt) but the method does not detect extrapulmonary shunt which must be present to a small extent (page 167). With advancing age, there is the appearance of a 'shelf' of distribution of blood flow to areas of low $\dot{V}/\dot{Q}$ ratio in the range 0.01–0.3 (*Figure 7.6b*). This probably represents gross underventilation of dependent areas of the lung due to airway closure when the functional residual capacity becomes less than the closing capacity (see *Figure 2.12*).

The spread of $\dot{V}/\dot{Q}$ ratios is also increased in a number of pathological conditions, including pulmonary oedema and pulmonary embolus (Wagner et al., 1975). Changes occurring during anaesthesia are described in Chapter 19, and the effects of breathing different concentrations of oxygen are described in Chapter 24.

Quantification of spread of $\dot{V}/\dot{Q}$ ratios as if it were due to dead space and shunt

The type of analysis illustrated in *Figures 7.5* and *7.6* is technically complex and unfortunately beyond the scope of all but a few centres in the world. A simpler and highly practical approach derived from the studies of Riley and his many colleagues

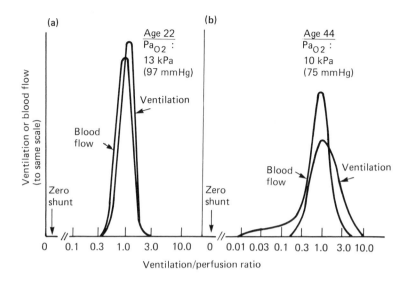

Figure 7.6 The distribution of ventilation and blood flow in relation to ventilation/perfusion ratios in two normal subjects. (a) A male aged 22 years with typical narrow spread and no measurable intrapulmonary shunt or alveolar dead space. This accords with the high arterial P_{O_2}, while breathing air. (b) The wider spread in a male aged 44 years. Note in particular the 'shelf' of blood flow distributed to alveoli with $\dot{V}/\dot{Q}$ ratios in the range 0.01–0.1. There is still no measurable intrapulmonary shunt or alveolar dead space. However, the appreciable distribution of blood flow to ~~underperfused~~ UNDERVENTILATED alveoli is sufficient to reduce the arterial P_{O_2} to 10 kPa (75 mmHg) while breathing air. (Redrawn from Wagner et al. (1974) by permission of the authors and the Editor of the Journal of Clinical Investigation

in Baltimore in the years 1945–1951. The essence of the 'Riley' approach is to consider the lung as if it were a three-compartment model comprising:

1. Ventilated but unperfused alveoli.
2. Perfused but unventilated alveoli.
3. Ideally perfused and ventilated alveoli.

The model is shown in *Figure 7.7*. The ventilated but unperfused alveoli comprise alveolar dead space (described below). The perfused but unventilated alveoli are here represented as a shunt. Gas exchange is confined to the 'ideal' alveolus. There is no suggestion that this is an accurate description of the actual state of affairs which is more accurately depicted by the type of plot shown in *Figure 7.6*. However, the parameters of the three-compartment model may be easily determined with equipment to be found in any department which is concerned with respiratory problems. Furthermore, the values obtained are of direct relevance to therapy. Thus an increased dead space can usually be offset by an increased minute volume, and arterial P_{O_2} can be restored to normal with shunts up to about 30 per cent by an appropriate increase in the inspired oxygen concentration (see *Figure 7.11* below).

Methods of calculation of dead space and shunt for the three-compartment model are deferred to the end of the chapter but no analytical techniques are required beyond measurement of blood and gas P_{CO_2} and P_{O_2}. It is then possible to determine what fraction of the inspired tidal volume does not participate in gas exchange and

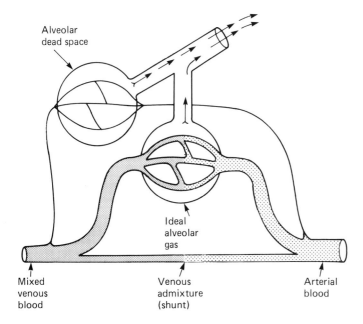

Figure 7.7 The assessment of the efficiency of gas exchange in the lungs considered as a three-compartment model. The lung is imagined to consist of three functional units comprising alveolar dead space, 'ideal' alveoli and venous admixture or shunt. Gas exchange occurs only in the 'ideal' alveoli. The measured alveolar dead space consists of true alveolar dead space together with a component caused by $\dot{V}/\dot{Q}$ scatter. The measured venous admixture consists of true venous admixture (shunt) together with a component caused by $\dot{V}/\dot{Q}$ scatter. Note that 'ideal' alveolar gas is exhaled contaminated with alveolar dead space gas (if present). Under such circumstances it is not possible to sample 'ideal' alveolar gas, the P_{CO_2} and P_{O_2} of which must therefore be derived indirectly.

what fraction of the cardiac output constitutes a shunt or venous admixture. However, the value for dead space will include a fraction representing ventilation of *relatively* underperfused alveoli and the value for shunt will include a fraction representing perfusion of *relatively* underventilated alveoli.

The concept of ideal alveolar gas is considered further elsewhere (page 182) but it will be clear from *Figure 7.7* that ideal alveolar gas cannot be sampled for analysis. The convention is that ideal alveolar P_{CO_2} is assumed to be equal to the arterial P_{CO_2}.

Dead space

It was realized in the last century that an appreciable part of each inspiration did not penetrate to those regions of the lungs in which gas exchange occurred and was therefore exhaled unchanged. This fraction of the tidal volume has long been known as the dead space, while the effective part of the minute volume of respiration is known as the alveolar ventilation. The relationship is as follows:

alveolar ventilation = respiratory frequency (tidal volume − dead space)

It is often useful to think of two ratios. The first is:

$$\frac{\text{dead space}}{\text{tidal volume}}$$

(often abbreviated to V_D/V_T and expressed as a percentage).

The second useful ratio is:

$$\frac{\text{alveolar ventilation}}{\text{minute volume}}$$

The first fraction is the wasted part of the breath, while the second is the utilized portion of the minute volume. The sum of the two fractions is unity and one may easily be calculated from the other.

Components of the dead space

The preceding section considers dead space as though it were a single homogeneous component of expired air. The situation is actually more complicated and *Figure 7.8* shows in diagrammatic form the various components of a single expirate. The

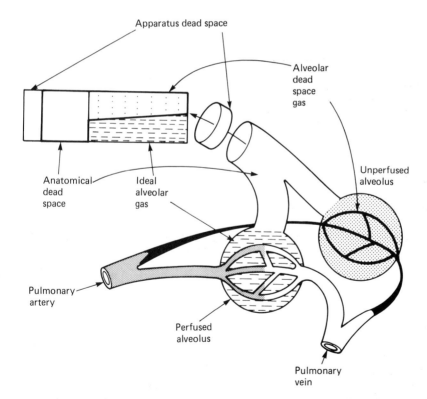

Figure 7.8 Components of expired gas. The rectangle is an idealized representation of a single expirate. The physiological dead space equals the sum of the anatomical and alveolar dead spaces and is outlined in the heavy black line. The alveolar dead space does not equal the volume of the unperfused spaces at alveolar level but only that part of their contents which is exhaled. This varies with the tidal volume.

first part to be exhaled will be from the *apparatus dead space* if the subject is employing any form of external breathing apparatus. The next component will be from the *anatomical dead space*, which is related to the volume of the conducting air passages. Thereafter gas is exhaled from the alveolar level and the diagram shows two representative alveoli, corresponding to the two ventilated compartments of the three-compartment lung model shown in *Figure 7.7*. One alveolus is perfused and, from this, 'ideal' alveolar gas is exhaled. The other alveolus is unperfused and so does not permit gas exchange. From this alveolus is exhaled gas approximating in composition to inspired gas. This component of the expirate is known as *alveolar dead space gas* which is important in many pathological conditions. The *physiological dead space* is the sum of the anatomical and alveolar dead spaces. It is defined as the whole of that part of the tidal volume which does not participate in gas exchange, as defined by the appropriate Bohr equation (see below).

In *Figure 7.8*, the final part of the expirate consists of a mixture of 'ideal' alveolar gas and alveolar dead space gas. A sample of this gas is called an *end-tidal* or, preferably, an *end-expiratory* sample. This corresponds to the alveolar sample defined by Haldane and Priestley (1905) as gas sampled at the end of a forced expiration. The composition of such a sample approximates to that of 'ideal' alveolar gas in a healthy resting subject. However, in many pathological states, an end-expiratory sample is contaminated by alveolar dead space gas and it is then necessary to distinguish between end-tidal gas and 'ideal' alveolar gas as shown in *Figure 7.7* and defined by Riley et al. (1946) (see page 182). For symbols, the small capital A relates to 'ideal' alveolar gas as in $P_{A_{CO_2}}$, while end-expiratory gas is distinguished by a small capital E, suffixed with a prime (e.g. PE'_{CO_2}). The term 'alveolar/arterial P_{O_2} difference' always refers to 'ideal' alveolar gas. Unqualified, the term 'alveolar' may mean either end-tidal or 'ideal' alveolar, depending on the context.

Figure 7.8 is only a model to simplify quantification. Alveoli do not fall into two watertight compartments, perfused and unperfused. There exists an infinite gradation between alveoli with zero blood flow and those with excessive blood flow. However, it is often helpful from the quantitative standpoint to consider alveoli *as though* they fell into the categories shown in the diagram, which represents the ventilatory aspects of the three-compartment lung model shown in *Figure 7.7*.

The Bohr equation

Bohr introduced his equation in 1891 when the dead space was considered simply as gas exhaled from the conducting airways (i.e. anatomical dead space). It may be simply derived as follows. During expiration all the CO_2 eliminated is contained in the alveolar gas. Therefore:

> The quantity of CO_2 eliminated in the alveolar gas
> = quantity of CO_2 eliminated in the mixed expired gas

that is to say:

> alveolar CO_2 concentration *multiplied by* alveolar ventilation
> = mixed-expired CO_2 concentration *multiplied by* minute volume

or, for a single breath:

> alv. CO_2 conc. × (tidal volume − dead space)
> = mixed-expired CO_2 conc. × tidal volume

There are four terms in this equation. There is no serious difficulty in measuring two of them, the tidal volume and the mixed-expired CO_2 concentration. This leaves the alveolar CO_2 concentration and the dead space. Therefore the alveolar CO_2 concentration may be derived if the dead space be known or, alternatively, the dead space may be derived if the alveolar CO_2 concentration be known. In the nineteenth century, it was not realized that alveolar gas could be sampled and therefore at that time it was customary to use the Bohr equation for calculation of the alveolar CO_2 concentration, substituting an assumed value for the dead space. After the historic discovery of the constancy of the alveolar gas (Haldane and Priestley, 1905), the position was reversed and the alveolar CO_2 concentration was measured directly and the Bohr equation used to calculate the dead space.

More recently the use of this equation has been expanded to measure various components of the dead space by varying the interpretation of the term 'alveolar'. So we must now return to the semantic problems surrounding the use of this word. In the paragraph above, the word 'alveolar' refers to that portion of the expirate which follows the anatomical dead space gas, and its composition would be similar to that of end-expiratory gas. The Bohr equation can only be employed to measure the anatomical dead space by using the end-expiratory CO_2 concentration if the alveolar CO_2 concentration remains reasonably constant during expiration.

If the 'ideal' alveolar CO_2 concentration is used, then the value for the dead space yielded by the calculation will be that of the physiological dead space comprising the sum of the anatomical and alveolar dead spaces (*Figure 7.8*). 'Ideal' alveolar gas cannot be sampled but Enghoff (1938) suggested that arterial P_{CO_2} should be substituted for alveolar P_{CO_2} in the Bohr equation. The value so derived is now, in effect, the definition of the physiological dead space:

$$V_D/V_T = (Pa_{CO_2} - P\bar{E}_{CO_2})/Pa_{CO_2}$$

This definition became widely accepted after the work of Riley and his colleagues (1946) who saw the arterial P_{CO_2} as an integration of the P_{CO_2} existing in different parts of the lung.

The use of the end-tidal P_{CO_2} in the Bohr equation needs further consideration. In exercise, in acute hyperventilation or if there is maldistribution of inspired gas with sequential emptying, the alveolar P_{CO_2} rises, often steeply, during expiration of the alveolar gas, and the end-tidal P_{CO_2} will not be appropriate for measuring the anatomical dead space by the Bohr equation. The end-tidal P_{CO_2} under these circumstances will depend on the duration and volume of expiration. It will not necessarily equal the arterial P_{CO_2} and so cannot be used to measure the physiological dead space, and the derived value would not, in fact, correspond to any of the compartments of the dead space shown in *Figure 7.8*. Fletcher (1984) has suggested that it be simply termed the Bohr dead space, which commits us to nothing beyond a tribute to Bohr's historic contribution.

The distinction between different meanings of the term 'alveolar gas' is fundamental for understanding dead space and is the clue to the controversy which existed for many years between Haldane and Krogh (reviewed by Bannister, Cunningham and Douglas, 1954). In the resting normal conscious healthy subject, the alveolar dead space is very small indeed. Therefore the anatomical and physiological dead spaces are, for practical purposes, identical and there is only a very small difference between the CO_2 concentration of the end-expiratory and the ideal alveolar gas, and their P_{CO_2} approximates closely to that of arterial blood. The distinctions arise only in special circumstances, particularly exercise, hyper-ventilation and respiratory disease.

Anatomical dead space

The gills of fishes are perfused by a stream of water which enters by the mouth and leaves by the gill slits. All of the water is available for gaseous exchange. Mammals, however, employ tidal ventilation which suffers from the disadvantage that a considerable part of the inspired gas comes to rest in the conducting air passages and is thus not available for gaseous exchange.

This imperfection was understood in the nineteenth century when the volume of the anatomical dead space was calculated from *post mortem* casts of the respiratory tract (Zuntz, 1882; Loewy, 1894). The value so obtained was used in the calculation of the composition of the alveolar gas according to the Bohr equation (1891). This was before the concept of alveolar dead space had arisen and at that time alveolar gas simply referred to that part of the expirate which followed the anatomical dead space gas.

The anatomical dead space is now generally defined as the volume of gas exhaled before the CO_2 concentration rises to its alveolar plateau, according to the technique of Fowler (1948) and outlined at the end of this chapter (see *Figure 7.14*). Fowler originally termed it the *physiological* dead space and Folkow and Pappenheimer (1955) suggested the term *series* dead space using an electrical analogy to distinguish it from alveolar dead space (parallel dead space). The boundary between anatomical dead space and alveolar gas is not clearly defined but is the zone where pre-dominantly convective gas transport gives way to transport which is predominately by diffusion.

The volume of the anatomical dead space, in spite of its name, is not constant and is influenced by many factors, some of which are of considerable clinical importance. Since many of these factors are not primarily anatomical, Fletcher (1984) has used yet another term—the airway dead space, but still with the Fowler definition.

Size of the subject must clearly influence the dimensions of the conducting air passages, and Radford (1955) drew attention to the fact that the volume of the air passages (in millilitres) approximates to the weight of the subject in pounds (1 pound = 0.45 kg).

Posture influences many lung volumes, including the anatomical dead space; Fowler (1950a) quoted the following mean values:

sitting	147 ml
semi-reclining	124 ml
supine	101 ml

Position of the neck and jaw has a pronounced effect on the anatomical dead space; studies by Nunn, Campbell and Peckett (1959) indicated the following mean values in three conscious subjects (not intubated):

neck extended, jaw protruded	143 ml
normal position	119 ml
neck flexed, chin depressed	73 ml

It is noteworthy that the first position is that which is used by resuscitators and anaesthetists to procure the least possible airway resistance. Unfortunately, it also results in the maximum dead space.

Age is usually accompanied by an increase in anatomical dead space but this may well be associated with an increased incidence of chronic bronchitis which usually results in an enlarged calibre of the major air passages (Fowler, 1950b).

Lung volume at the end of inspiration affects the anatomical dead space since the volume of the air passages is a function of the lung volume. The effect is not very large, being of the order of 20 ml additional anatomical dead space for each litre increase in lung volume (Shepard et al., 1957).

Tracheal intubation or tracheostomy will bypass the extrathoracic anatomical dead space. This was found to be 72 ml in six cadavers, while the intrathoracic anatomical dead space was found to be 66 ml in three intubated patients (Nunn, Campbell and Peckett, 1959). Intrathoracic anatomical dead space of 12 intubated anaesthetized patients had a mean value of 63 ml (Nunn and Hill, 1960). Between mask-breathing and intubated anaesthetized patients, a difference in total functional dead space of 82 ml was found by Kain, Panday and Nunn (1969). An undefined part of the difference would have been due to the additional apparatus dead space in the former state. Tracheal intubation or tracheostomy will bypass approximately half of the total anatomical dead space, although this advantage will clearly be lost if a corresponding volume of apparatus dead space is added to the circuit.

Pneumonectomy will result in a reduction of anatomical dead space if the excised lung was functional (Fowler and Blakemore, 1951).

Hypoventilation results in a marked reduction of the anatomical dead space as measured by Fowler's method. This effect limits the fall of alveolar ventilation resulting from small tidal volumes. It is important in the case of comatose or anaesthetized patients who are left to breathe for themselves when there is either heavy central depression of respiration or partial neuromuscular blockade of the respiratory muscles. Tidal volumes as small as 100 ml are not infrequently recorded. Tidal volumes of less than the supposed anatomical dead space are commonly used during high frequency ventilation, and this problem is discussed on page 407.

There are probably two factors which reduce the anatomical dead space during hypoventilation. Firstly, there is a tendency towards streamline or laminar flow of gas through the air passages. Inspired gas advances with a cone front and the tip of the cone penetrates the alveoli before all the gas in the conducting passages has been washed out (see *Figure 3.2*). This, in effect, reduces what we may call the 'functional anatomical dead space' below its value morphologically defined. The reduction of functional anatomical dead space at low tidal volumes was predicted by Rohrer in 1915 and, in the same year, Henderson, Chillingworth and Whitney demonstrated the axial flow of tobacco smoke through glass tubing. The second factor reducing dead space during hypoventilation is the mixing effect of the heart beat which tends to mix all gas lying below the carina. This effect is negligible at normal rates of ventilation, but becomes more marked during hypoventilation and during breath holding. Thus in one hypoventilating patient, Nunn and Hill (1960) found alveolar gas at the carina at the commencement of expiration. A similar effect occurs during breath holding when alveolar gas mixes with dead space gas as far up as the glottis.

In conscious subjects some inspired gas may be detected in the alveoli with tidal volumes as small as 60 ml (Briscoe, Forster and Comroe, 1954). In anaesthetized patients with tidal volumes less than 350 ml, Nunn and Hill (1960) found the 'functional' anatomical dead space to be about one-fifth of the tidal volume, a number of patients having values less than 25 ml at tidal volumes below 250 ml (see *Figure 19.12*)

Drugs acting on the bronchiolar musculature will affect the anatomical dead space, and an increase was noted after atropine by Higgins and Means (1915), Severinghaus and Stupfel (1955) and Nunn and Bergman (1964). Nunn and Bergman found a mean increase of 18 ml in six normal subjects, while Severinghaus and Stupfel reported an increase of 45 ml. The latter also reported significant increases with the ganglion-blocking agents hexamethonium and trimetaphan. Histamine caused a small decrease in anatomical dead space.

Hypothermia was reported to increase anatomical dead space in dogs (Severinghaus and Stupfel, 1955) but there seems to be little change in man (Nunn 1961a).

Alveolar dead space

Alveolar dead space may be defined as that part of the inspired gas which passes through the anatomical dead space to mix with gas at the alveolar level but which does not take part in gas exchange. The cause of the failure of gas exchange is lack of effective perfusion of the spaces to which the gas is distributed at the alveolar level. Parallel dead space (Folkow and Pappenheimer, 1955) is synonymous with alveolar dead space. The alveolar dead space is too small to be measured with confidence in healthy supine man but becomes appreciable in many conditions considered below.

Hydrostatic failure of alveolar perfusion. This cause of alveolar non-perfusion probably applies to the supraclavicular parts of the lungs of the normal subject in the upright position. However, if present, the effect is really too small to measure with available techniques.

Non-perfusion of alveoli will be markedly increased in pulmonary hypotension which occurs in many forms of low-output circulatory failure. The effect is particularly marked in severe haemorrhage which is associated with a large increase in physiological dead space, presumably due to failure of perfusion of a considerable proportion of the ventilated alveoli (Gerst, Rattenborg and Holaday, 1959; Freeman and Nunn, 1963).

Increased alveolar dead space is almost certainly the principal cause of the large increases in physiological dead space reported during anaesthesia with deliberate hypotension (Eckenhoff et al., 1963). The same study found that dead space was also influenced by head-up tilt and raised airway pressures, both of which factors would enhance the adverse effects of reduction of cardiac output (and presumably pulmonary arterial pressure) due to the hypotensive agents. These authors reported a number of patients with physiological dead space in excess of 75 per cent of the tidal volume.

Posture. In the supine position, the vertical height of the lungs and the hydrostatic head of pressure in the pulmonary artery are reduced from about 30 to 20 cm. It would therefore be reasonable to expect the alveolar dead space to be less in the supine than in the upright position. However, it is difficult to demonstrate the alveolar dead space at all in the upright position, and evidence of the effect of change of posture is not available.

In the lateral position, approximately two-thirds of the pulmonary blood flow is distributed to the dependent side. During spontaneous respiration the greater part of the ventilation is also distributed to the lower lung and there is probably little change in alveolar dead space. If, however, the patient is ventilated artificially in the lateral position, ventilation is distributed in favour of the upper lung (Rehder et al., 1972), particularly in the presence of an open pneumothorax (Nunn, 1961a). Under these conditions, it may be expected that much of the ventilation of the upper lung will constitute alevolar dead space. This problem is discussed further on page 377.

Embolism. Pulmonary embolism is considered separately in Chapter 25. Partial embolization of the pulmonary circulation results in the development of an alveolar dead space which may reach massive proportions.

Ventilation of non-vascular air space. The next form of alveolar dead space is the ventilation of an air space with no vasculature. This occurs in obstructive lung disease following widespread destruction of alveolar septa and the contained vessels. This is the principal cause of the very marked increase in physiological dead space reported in patients with chronic lung disease (Donald et al., 1952).

Constriction of precapillary pulmonary vessels. Alveolar dead space may be due to precapillary constriction of the pulmonary blood vessels. This cause is rather conjectural. Mechanisms and causes of pulmonary vasoconstriction are discussed in Chapter 6 but it is not yet clear under what circumstances this may result in the creation of an appreciable alveolar dead space.

Obstruction of the pulmonary circulation by external forces. There may be kinking, clamping or blocking of a pulmonary artery during thoracic surgery. This may be expected to result in an increase in dead space depending on the ventilation of the section of lung supplied by the obstructed vessel.

Physiological dead space

The physiological dead space is defined as that part of the tidal volume which does not participate in gaseous exchange. Nowadays it is universally defined by the Bohr mixing equation with substitution of arterial P_{CO_2} for alveolar P_{CO_2} thus:

$$\frac{\text{physiological}}{\text{dead space}} = \frac{\text{tidal}}{\text{volume}} \left(\frac{\text{arterial } P_{CO_2} - \text{mixed expired } P_{CO_2}}{\text{arterial } P_{CO_2} - \text{inspired } P_{CO_2}} \right)$$

It follows from this equation that the physiological dead space is the functionally ineffective part of the ventilation. Alveolar ventilation is therefore measured as:

respiratory frequency $\times$ (tidal volume $-$ physiological dead space) or, alternatively, as:

$$\left(1 - \frac{\text{physiological dead space}}{\text{tidal volume}}\right) \times \text{respiratory minute volume}$$

Thus if the physiological dead space is 30 per cent of the tidal volume ($V_D/V_T = $ 30 per cent), the alveolar ventilation will be 70 per cent of the respiratory minute volume. The use of the V_D/V_T ratio is useful since the ratio tends to remain fairly constant while the actual value for the physiological dead space may vary widely with changing tidal volumes. This approach is radically different from the assumption of a constant 'dead space' which is subtracted from the tidal volume, the difference then being multiplied by the respiratory frequency to indicate the alveolar ventilation.

The proportionality between dead space and tidal volume was first demonstrated by Enghoff in 1931. In a later publication (1938) he suggested that the dead space be measured by substitution of the arterial P_{CO_2} in Bohr's equation, thus introducing the modern concept of the physiological dead space, for which he used the term *volumen inefficax*. In practice, the concept of a relatively constant V_D/V_T ratio simplifies calculations of alveolar ventilation from minute volume.

Factors influencing the physiological dead space

This section summarizes information on the value of the total physiological dead space but reasons for the changes have been considered above in the sections on the anatomical and alveolar dead space.

Age. There is a tendency for V_D and also the V_D/V_T ratio to increase with age, with V_D increasing by slightly less than 1 ml per year (Harris et al., 1973). These authors found values for V_D in men of the order of 50 ml greater than in women but the former group had larger tidal volumes and there was a smaller sex difference in the V_D/V_T ratios (33.2–45.1 per cent for men; 29.4–39.4 per cent for women). All subjects were seated. The authors reviewed other studies of normal values for V_D/V_T ratios which tended to be slightly less than their own values, although there was general agreement that V_D/V_T increased with age.

Body size. It is evident that V_D, in common with other pulmonary volumes, will be larger in larger people. Harris' group recommended correlation with height, and reported that V_D increased by 17 ml for every 10 cm increase in height.

Posture. Craig et al. (1971) showed that the V_D/V_T ratio decreased from a mean value of 34 per cent in the upright position to 30 per cent in the supine position. The study was conducted in a group of 22 subjects, free of cardiovascular disease and aged from 21 to 78 years. The effect of posture was apparent in all subgroups, broken down according to age, smoking habits and closing volume.

Duration of inspiration and breath holding. It is well known that prolongation of inspiration reduces dead space by allowing gas mixing to take place between dead space and alveolar gas.

Smoking. Craig et al. (1971) showed a highly significant increase in the V_D/V_T ratio of smokers in whom the values were 37 per cent (upright) and 32 per cent (supine), compared with 29 per cent (upright) and 26 per cent (supine) for non-smokers. Smokers were evenly distributed among their age groups.

Pulmonary disease. The previous part of this chapter has considered the enlargement of the alveolar dead space which occurs when parts of the lung are deprived of circulation. Very large increases in V_D/V_T occur in pulmonary embolus and, to a lesser extent, in pulmonary hypoperfusion and emphysema. Patients with emphysema suffer a further increase in the V_D/V_T ratio following induction of anaesthesia (Pietak et al., 1975).

Anaesthesia. Many studies have now shown that the V_D/V_T ratio of a healthy, anaesthetized intubated patient is of the order of 30–35 per cent whether breathing spontaneously or ventilated artificially (see Chapter 19).

Artificial ventilation. Artificial ventilation itself seems to have little effect upon the V_D/V_T ratio compared with the value obtained during anaesthesia with spontaneous breathing. However, it seems likely that prolonged use of positive end-expiratory pressure causes an increase in the dead space (pages 414 and 416).

Effect of apparatus. When a subject or patient is connected to breathing apparatus, there will usually be apparatus dead space which is in series with the anatomical dead space and has a similar effect. When using cited values of the V_D/V_T ratio, for calculation of the effective part of the tidal volume, it is important to be quite clear whether the author made allowance for apparatus dead space.

Effects of an increased physiological dead space

Regardless of whether an increase in physiological dead space is due to the anatomical or the alveolar components, alveolar ventilation is reduced, unless there is a compensatory increase in minute volume.

Reduction of alveolar ventilation due to an increase in physiological dead space produces changes in the 'ideal' alveolar gas tensions which are identical to those produced when alveolar ventilation is decreased by reduction in respiratory minute volume (see *Figure 5.8*). The directions of changes in Po_2 and Pco_2 for different inspired oxygen concentrations are shown in *Figure 7.9*.

It is almost always possible to counteract the effects of an increase in physiological dead space by a corresponding increase in the respiratory minute volume. If, for example, the minute volume is 10 l/min and the V_D/V_T ratio 30 per cent, the alveolar ventilation will be 7 l/min. If the patient were then subjected to pulmonary embolism resulting in an increase of the V_D/V_T ratio to 50 per cent, the minute volume would need to be increased to 14 l/min to maintain an alveolar ventilation of 7 l/min. Should the V_D/V_T increase to 80 per cent, the minute volume would need to be increased to 35 l/min and so on.

Apparatus dead space and rebreathing

Thus far, we have considered apparatus dead space as though it were always a simple extension of the patient's anatomical dead space and could be treated as such during measurement. This approach is perfectly valid provided that we are considering only endotracheal tubes, mouthpieces and such equipment. A facemask,

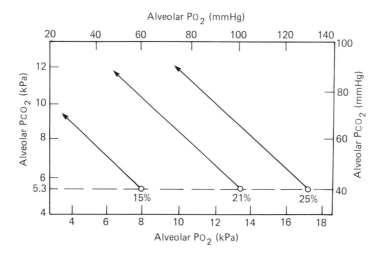

Figure 7.9 Pathways of changes in alveolar gas tensions during alveolar hypoventilation. The information may be derived from Figure 5.8. *Alveolar hypoventilation may result either from reduction of minute volume or from increase in any component of the dead space. The resultant effect upon both PO_2 and PCO_2 is similar, although the alveolar PO_2 is also influenced directly by the inspired oxygen concentration, which is indicated at the foot of the three lines in the diagram.*

however, presents a more difficult problem since the whole of the gas space under the mask may not be washed out by the tidal volume. The functional volume may then be less than the geometric volume as determined by filling it with water. Measurement of the functional apparatus dead space may, however, be made by means of modification of the technique of Fowler (1948) (page 177). In this case, the gas sampling point must lie at the junction between the apparatus dead space and the anatomical dead space; with carbon dioxide being used as the tracer gas, the measurement is made during inspiration. In effect, one measures the volume which must be inhaled through the apparatus dead space before uncontaminated inspired air is reached. Functional apparatus dead space may also be determined by measuring physiological dead space with and without added apparatus dead space and noting the difference.

Concepts of apparatus dead space and rebreathing have been explored in some detail by Nunn and Newman (1964). The authors found the problem far more complicated than might appear at first sight. The principal points which they made are as follows:

1. A variety of gas circuits are in common use, particularly by anaesthetists, and these circuits impose many different patterns of rebreathing.
2. The gas rebreathed may be end-expiratory gas (as with a simple facemask), mixed expired gas (as in circuit C, described by Mapleson, 1954), or even expired dead space gas (as in circuit A, described by Mapleson, 1954).
3. Contamination of inspired gas may occur early in inspiration, for example, with the use of simple mouthpieces. However, in other circuits (such as Ayre's T-piece) contamination may occur late in inspiration. This gas may come to rest in the patient's anatomical dead space and therefore take no part in gas exchange although it has been inhaled into the patient's respiratory tract.

4. If gas exhaled from the patient's anatomical dead space is stored and then re-inhaled (as with circuit A mentioned above), this will not influence gas exchange although, considered in terms of gas volumes, rebreathing has occurred.

5. The effective 'mean inspired gas composition' has two alternative meanings. The first refers to the mean composition of the gas which enters the patient's respiratory tract. The second is restricted to the gas which enters functioning alveoli and is the only part which can influence gas exchange.

6. 'Mean inspired gas composition' is difficult to measure in the presence of rebreathing. It cannot be derived from a plot of instantaneous gas composition against time, since the required value is the concentration integrated with respect to volume and not to time. An inspiratory gas sampler which will indicate the effective mean inspired gas composition in the presence of changes in inspired gas composition must sample not necessarily at a steady rate, but at a rate which is proportional to the instantaneous inspiratory gas flow rate. Such a device is practicable and was developed by Bookallil and Smith (1964).

The concept of venous admixture

Nomenclature of venous admixture

Venous admixture refers to the degree of admixture of mixed venous blood with pulmonary end-capillary blood which would be required to produce the observed difference between the arterial and the pulmonary end-capillary P_{O_2}. Pulmonary end-capillary P_{O_2} is usually taken as equal to ideal alveolar P_{O_2}, and the calculation is shown in *Figure 7.10*. Note that the venous admixture is not the *actual* amount of venous blood which mingles with the arterial blood but the *calculated* amount which would be required to produce the observed value for the arterial P_{O_2}. The difference is due to the contribution to the arterial blood of blood from alveoli having a ventilation/perfusion ratio of more than zero but less than the normal value, this problem being discussed in greater detail below. The strict quantitative basis of the calculation is also destroyed by the admixture of bronchial and thebesian venous blood of unknown oxygen content. *Venous admixture* is thus a convenient index but does not define the anatomical pathway of shunt. It is often termed simply as 'shunt'.

Anatomical shunt refers to the amount of venous blood which mingles with the pulmonary end-capillary blood on the arterial side of the circulation. The term embraces bronchial and thebesian venous blood flow and also admixture of mixed venous blood caused by atelectasis, bronchial obstruction, congenital heart disease with right-to-left shunting, etc. Clearly different components may have different oxygen contents which will not necessarily equal the mixed venous oxygen content. Anatomical shunt excludes blood draining any alveoli with a $\dot{V}/\dot{Q}$ ratio of more than zero.

Pathological shunt is sometimes used to describe the forms of anatomical shunt which do not occur in the normal subject.

Physiological shunt. This term is, unfortunately, used in two senses. In the first sense it is used to describe the degree of venous admixture which occurs in a normal

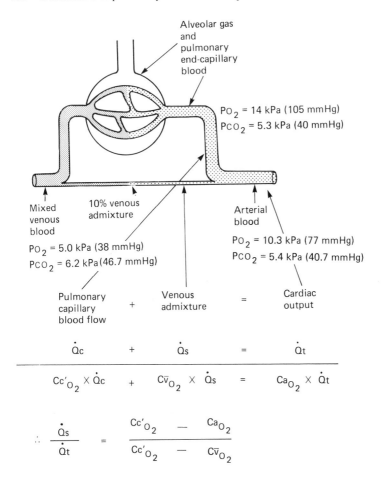

Figure 7.10 A schematic representation of venous admixture. It makes the simplifying assumption that all the arterial blood has come either from alveoli with normal $\dot{V}/\dot{Q}$ ratio or from a shunt. This is never true but it forms a convenient method of quantifying venous admixture and can be used as a basis for oxygen therapy. The shunt equation is similar to the Bohr equation and is based on the axiomatic relationship that the total amount of oxygen in 1 minute's flow of arterial blood equals the sum of the amount of oxygen in 1 minute's flow through the pulmonary capillaries and the amount of oxygen in 1 minute's flow through the shunt. Amount of oxygen in 1 minute's flow of blood equals the product of the blood flow rate and the concentration of oxygen in the blood. $\dot{Q}t$, total cardiac output; $\dot{Q}c$, pulmonary capillary blood flow; $\dot{Q}s$, flow of blood through shunt; Ca_{O_2}, concentration of oxygen in arterial blood; Cc'_{O_2}, concentration of oxygen in pulmonary end-capillary blood; $C\bar{v}_{O_2}$, concentration of oxygen in mixed venous blood.

healthy subject. Differences between the actual measured venous admixture and the normal value for the 'physiological shunt' thus indicate the amount of venous admixture which results from the disease process. In its alternative sense, physiological shunt is synonymous with venous admixture as derived from the mixing equation (*Figure 7.10*). It is probably best to avoid the term 'physiological shunt'.

Effects of venous admixture

Qualitatively, it will be clear that venous admixture reduces the overall efficiency of gas exchange and results in arterial blood gas tensions which are closer to those of mixed venous blood than would otherwise be the case. Quantitatively, the effect is simple provided that we consider the *contents* of gases in blood. Considering a simple anatomical shunt such as that shown in *Figure 7.10* we may take as an example:

Pulmonary end-capillary oxygen content	20 ml/100 ml
Mixed venous blood oxygen content	10 ml/100 ml

It will be clear that a 50 per cent venous admixture will result in an arterial oxygen content of 15 ml/100 ml, a 25 per cent venous admixture will result in an arterial oxygen content of 17.5 ml/100 ml, and so on. The calculation is based on the conservation of mass:

the amount of oxygen flowing in the arterial system	=	the amount of oxygen leaving the pulmonary capillaries	+	the amount of oxygen flowing through the venous admixture

For each term in this equation the amount of oxygen flowing may be expressed as the product of the blood flow rate and the oxygen content of blood flowing in the vessel. Thus, in the case of the pulmonary capillary blood flow, this equals $\dot{Q}c \times Cc'_{O_2}$ and so on (the symbols are explained in *Figure 7.10* and Appendix D). *Figure 7.10* shows how the equation may be cleared and solved for the ratio of the venous admixture to the cardiac output. The final equation has a form similar to that of the Bohr equation for the physiological dead space (page 159).

To calculate the venous admixture, one must first determine the gas contents of the arterial, pulmonary end-capillary and mixed venous blood. In practice these are usually measured or calculated as oxygen tensions, and content is then derived from the oxygen dissociation curve and the oxygen capacity of the blood, allowance being made for dissolved oxygen. Conversely, if we know the degree of venous admixture, the effect on arterial blood gas *contents* may be easily calculated. If, however, we require to know the effect on arterial blood P_{O_2}, we must undertake the tiresome calculation of tension from content using the oxygen dissociation curve and the oxygen capacity of the blood.

The shape of the oxygen dissociation curve looms very large in any consideration of venous admixture. If a normal subject has a pulmonary end-capillary P_{O_2} of 14 kPa (105 mmHg) (the normal value) and a venous admixture of 5 per cent of his cardiac output, the consequent reduction of his arterial oxygen content or saturation is too small to be measured easily (*Table 7.2*). However, due to the flatness of the oxygen dissociation curve in this range, there is a considerable fall in arterial P_{O_2} which may be detected without difficulty.

The effect of this degree of venous admixture on arterial CO_2 content is similar in magnitude to that of oxygen content. However, due to the relative steepness of the CO_2 dissociation curve in this range the effect on arterial P_{CO_2} is also very small and is far less than the change in arterial P_{O_2} (*Table 7.2*). Two conclusions may be drawn:

1. Arterial P_{O_2} is the most useful blood gas measurement for the detection of venous admixture.

Table 7.2 Effect of 5 per cent venous admixture on the difference between arterial and pulmonary end-capillary blood levels of carbon dioxide and oxygen

	Pulmonary end-capillary blood	Arterial blood
CO_2 content (ml/100 ml)	49.7	50.0
P_{CO_2} (kPa)	5.29	5.33
(mm Hg)	39.7	40.0
O_2 content (ml/100 ml)	19.9	19.6
O_2 saturation (%)	97.8	96.8
P_{O_2} (kPa)	14.0	12.0
(mm Hg)	105	90

It has been assumed that the arterial/venous oxygen content difference is 4.5 ml/100 ml and that the haemoglobin concentration is 14.9 g/dl. Typical changes in P_{O_2} and P_{CO_2} have been shown for a 10 per cent venous admixture in *Figure 7.10*.

2. Venous admixture reduces the arterial P_{O_2} markedly, but has relatively little effect on arterial P_{CO_2} or on the content of either CO_2 or O_2 unless the venous admixture is large.

Quite large degrees of venous admixture are needed to produce clinically recognizable reduction of arterial oxygen content, and elevations of P_{CO_2} are seldom seen. It is, in fact, more usual for venous admixture to *lower* the P_{CO_2} indirectly since the resultant lowering of the P_{O_2} commonly causes hyperventilation, which more than compensates for the slight elevation of P_{CO_2} which would otherwise result from the venous admixture (see *Figure 20.1*).

Since the effect of venous admixture on arterial P_{O_2} is so markedly influenced by the slope of the dissociation curve, it will clearly depend upon the section of the dissociation curve which is concerned in a particular situation. Thus if the pulmonary end-capillary P_{O_2} is high (above 40 kPa or 300 mmHg where the curve is flat), venous admixture causes a very marked fall in arterial P_{O_2} (approximately 2.3 kPa or 17 mmHg) for 1 per cent venous admixture). If, however, the pulmonary end-capillary P_{O_2} is low (below 9.3 kPa or 70 mmHg) where the curve is steep, venous admixture has relatively little effect on arterial P_{O_2} (see *Figure 10.8*). It would probably be wrong to consider this from the teleological standpoint, but it is nevertheless convenient to remember that a given degree of venous admixture causes a greater fall of P_{O_2} in the better oxygenated patients and a smaller fall in the less well oxygenated patients.

The iso-shunt diagram

If we consider arterial P_{CO_2}, haemoglobin and arterial/mixed venous oxygen content difference to be constant, the arterial P_{O_2} is determined mainly by the inspired oxygen concentration and venous admixture considered in the context of the three-compartment model (*Figure 7.7*). The relationship between inspired oxygen concentration and arterial P_{O_2} is a matter for constant attention in such situations as intensive therapy, and it has been found a matter of practical convenience to prepare a graph of the relationship at different levels of venous admixture (Benatar,

Hewlett and Nunn, 1973). The arterial/mixed venous oxygen content difference is often unknown in the clinical situation and therefore the diagram has been prepared for an assumed content difference of 5 ml oxygen/100 ml of blood. Iso-shunt bands have then been drawn on a plot of arterial P_{O_2} against inspired oxygen concentration (*Figure 7.11*). The bands are sufficiently wide to encompass all values of P_{CO_2} between 3.3 and 5.3 kPa (25–40 mmHg) and haemoglobin levels between 10 and 14 g/dl. Normal barometric pressure is assumed. Since calculation of the venous

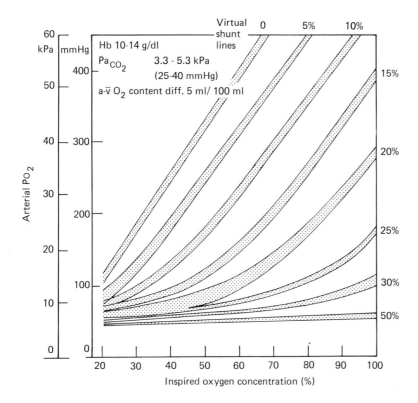

Figure 7.11 Iso-shunt diagram. On co-ordinates of inspired oxygen concentration (abscissa) and arterial P_{O_2} (ordinate), iso-shunt bands have been drawn to include all values of Hb, P_{CO_2} and a-v̄ oxygen content difference shown above. (Redrawn from Benatar, Hewlett and Nunn (1973) by permission of the Editor of the British Journal of Anaesthesia*)*

admixture requires knowledge of the actual arterial/mixed venous oxygen content difference, the iso-shunt lines in *Figure 7.11* refer to the 'virtual shunt' which is defined as the calculated shunt on the basis of an assumed value of the arterial/mixed venous oxygen content difference of 5 ml/100 ml.

In practice, the iso-shunt diagram is useful for adjusting the inspired oxygen concentration to obtain a required level of arterial P_{O_2}. For example, if a patient is found to have an arterial P_{O_2} of 30 kPa (225 mmHg) while breathing 90% oxygen, he has a virtual shunt of 20 per cent and, if it is required to attain an arterial P_{O_2} of 10 kPa (75 mmHg), this should be achieved by reducing the inspired oxygen concentration to 45%. The new value for arterial Po_2 should then be checked by direct measurement. Resolution of conditions such as pulmonary oedema, infection or collapse is shown by a reduction of the virtual shunt which may therefore be used as an indication of progress.

Finger clubbing

It is believed that finger clubbing (hypertrophic pulmonary osteoarthropathy in its most advanced stage) is due to shunting rather than hypoxaemia since it is absent in certain forms of hypoxaemia without shunting such as residence at high altitude. The association with shunting is strong (Pain, 1964) and it has also been suggested that bronchopulmonary anastomoses may be responsible for the transfer of a substance to the systemic circulation which is normally detoxified in the lung (Weatherall, Ledingham and Warrell, 1983). These authors suggest a role for reduced ferritin but it is not immediately obvious how this could be so.

Forms of venous admixture

Venae cordis minimae (thebesian veins). Some small veins of the left heart drain directly into the chambers of the left heart and so mingle with the arterial blood. The oxygen content of this blood is probably very low, and therefore the flow (believed to be about 0.3 per cent of cardiac output; Ravin, Epstein and Malm, 1965) causes an appreciable fall in the mixed arterial oxygen tension. It was thought by Cole and Bishop (1963) that the venae cordis minimae constitute the major part of the venous admixture in healthy man.

Bronchial veins. Figure 6.2 shows that a part of the venous drainage of the bronchial circulation passes by way of the deep true bronchial veins to reach the pulmonary veins. It is uncertain how large this component is in the healthy subject but is probably less than 1 per cent of cardiac output. In bronchial disease and coarctation of the aorta, the flow through this channel may be greatly increased, and in bronchiectasis and emphysema may be as large as 10 per cent of cardiac output. Under these circumstances it becomes a major cause of arterial desaturation.

Congenital heart disease. Right-to-left shunting in congenital heart disease is the cause of the worst examples of venous admixture. In patients with pulmonary atresia, right-to-left shunting is often present at all times. When there are abnormal communications between right and left hearts without pulmonary atresia, shunting will normally be from left to right unless the pulmonary arterial pressure is raised above that of the systemic circulation. In that event the shunt is reversed and venous admixture occurs. Although there is usually a progressive tendency to reversal as a result of hypertrophic changes in the pulmonary arterioles, sudden reversal may occur as a result of increases in alveolar pressure. This may occur during anaesthesia, for example during artificial ventilation, or straining during induction of anaesthesia.

Pulmonary infection. In the days when lobar pneumonia was common, it was a familiar sight to see a patient hyperventilating but deeply cyanosed. The hypoxaemia was due to a large shunt through the lobe which was affected by the pneumonic process. It seems likely that the infection increased the blood flow through the affected lobe above its normal value.

Although lobar pneumonia is now rare, bronchopneumonia is still relatively common, particularly in the elderly, and also, on occasion, after operation and in patients undergoing prolonged artificial ventilation. Under these conditions, pulmonary infection is a common cause of venous admixture and the alveolar/arterial P_{O_2} difference is a useful aid to diagnosis and assessment of progress.

Pulmonary oedema. Pulmonary oedema is considered in detail in Chapter 23. Once alveolar flooding has occurred, perfusion through the affected alveoli constitutes venous admixture and the alveolar/arterial P_{O_2} difference increases. When froth enters the bronchial tree there is failure of ventilation of whole regions of the lungs and venous admixture reaches high levels, resulting in gross hypoxaemia.

Pulmonary collapse is considered separately in Chapter 24.

Pulmonary neoplasm. Any pulmonary neoplasm is likely to cause a shunt as its venous drainage mingles with the pulmonary venous blood. With bronchial or secondary carcinoma, the flow through the neoplasm may be high, resulting in appreciable arterial hypoxaemia. Pulmonary haemangioma is rare but may first present as an unexplained venous admixture.

Pulmonary arteriovenous shunts. The existence of potential channels has been demonstrated by von Hayek (1960). The channels are 'sperr' arteries, structurally similar to those linking the pulmonary and bronchial arteries (pages 21 and 119), and forming a T-network allowing blood to flow from bronchial artery to pulmonary artery, or from pulmonary artery to bronchial veins (and thence to pulmonary veins) according to the relaxation of these muscular vessels. There is also the possibility of direct shunting through the giant capillaries below the pleura.

Although these possibilities exist, very little is known of the role of these vessels in the regulation of the pulmonary circulation (Krahl, 1964). The functional significance of these potential shunts remains in doubt, but flow through them must be negligible in the healthy conscious subject.

Effect of cardiac output on shunt

Cardiac output has an important bearing on shunt and this must be considered from three standpoints. Firstly, a reduction of cardiac output causes a decrease in mixed venous oxygen content with the result that a given shunt causes a greater reduction in arterial P_{O_2} *provided the shunt fraction is unaltered*, a relationship which is illustrated in *Figure 10.9*. Secondly, it has been observed that, in a very wide range of pathological and physiological circumstances, a reduction in cardiac output causes an approximately proportional reduction in the shunt fraction (Lynch, Mhyre and Dantzker, 1979; Dantzker, Lynch and Weg, 1980), the only apparent exception being a shunt through regional pulmonary atelectasis (Cheney and Colley, 1980). It is remarkable that these two effects tend to have approximately equal and opposite effects on arterial P_{O_2}. Thus with a decreased cardiac output there is usually a reduced shunt of a more desaturated mixed venous blood with the result that the arterial P_{O_2} is scarcely changed. Marshall and Marshall (1985) advance convincing reasons for believing that the reduction in shunt is due to pulmonary vasconstriction in consequence of the reduction in P_{O_2} of the mixed venous blood flowing through the shunt. The magnitude of the flow diversion is inversely related to the size of the hypoxic segment (Marshall et al. 1981). The third consideration concerns the oxygen flux. Even though a reduced cardiac output may have little effect on arterial oxygen content, it must have a direct effect on the oxygen flux which is the product of cardiac output and arterial oxygen content (page 256).

Scatter of V̇/Q̇ ratios considered as a shunt

Parts of the lung with a very low V̇/Q̇ ratio are often considered as though they constitute a shunt. This is partly because the arterial blood gases present a common picture which cannot easily be distinguished, partly because quantification of scatter of V̇/Q̇ ratios is difficult and partly because it is a convenient approach in the clinical situation.

Quantification of the effect on gas tensions of an increased scatter of V̇/Q̇ ratios is a tedious calculation but an example may help to clarify the general principles. *Figure 7.12* represents an imaginary subject in whom we may consider the functioning alveoli as falling into three groups (which might perhaps correspond to three horizontal strata), each group having its own V̇/Q̇ ratio. The Figure also shows the percentage contribution that each group makes to the mixed alveolar gas and the pulmonary end-capillary blood. The PO_2 of the alveolar gas in each group has been calculated from the V̇/Q̇ ratio and it is assumed that the pulmonary end-capillary PO_2 equals the alveolar PO_2 in each group. The pulmonary end-capillary oxygen saturation of each group has then been determined from the oxygen dissociation curve. Saturation can easily be converted into oxygen content, and the content of the mixed arterial blood has been determined making allowance for the different volume contributions of blood from the three zones. Arterial PO_2 was derived from the arterial saturation, using the dissociation curve. Mixed alveolar PO_2 was determined by a similar procedure but without the necessity of using the dissociation curve (since PO_2 of a gas is directly proportional to the oxygen content provided that the barometric pressure remains constant).

It will be seen that the saturation of the mixed arterial blood (97.4%) is less than the arithmetic mean of the saturations from the three groups (97.7%). This is partly due to the curvature of the oxygen dissociation curve (see below) but also because the group of alveoli with the lowest saturation makes the largest contribution to the arterial blood. As a result of these two effects the arterial PO_2 is always less than the alveolar PO_2, and in this example there is an alveolar/arterial PO_2 difference of 0.7 kPa (5 mmHg). In contrast, the scatter of PCO_2 between the three groups of alveoli is small and alveolar/arterial PCO_2 difference is only 0.1 kPa (0.75 mmHg). This is mainly because the mixed venous/arterial PCO_2 difference is small.

It is only possible to measure the scatter of V̇/Q̇ ratios of different parts of the lung by the use of sophisticated techniques which are not generally available. In the clinical field, it is usual to rely on measurements of blood and gas PO_2 and PCO_2 using routine equipment. However, sometimes the gamma camera may be used to indicate the V̇/Q̇ ratio of identifiable anatomical areas.

Effect of mean alveolar PO_2. Overventilated alveoli fail to compensate for underventilated alveoli in the maintenance of the arterial oxygen level. There are two reasons for this. The first is shown in *Figure 7.12* and arises from the fact that the relatively underventilated alveoli usually contribute more blood than the relatively overventilated alveoli to the mixed arterial blood. The second reason is that, due to the shape of the oxygen dissociation curve, the overventilated alveoli cannot

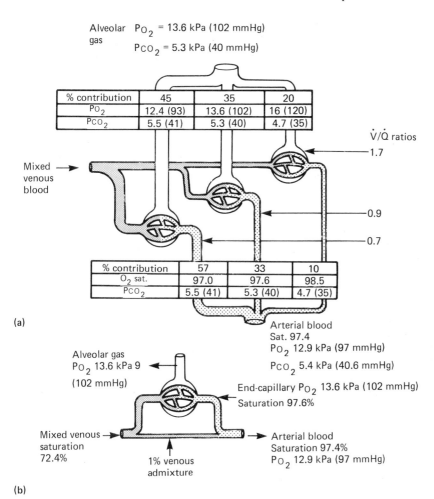

Figure 7.12 Alveolar/arterial Po_2 difference caused by scatter of $\dot{V}/\dot{Q}$ ratios and its representation by an equivalent degree of venous admixture. (a) Scatter of $\dot{V}/\dot{Q}$ ratios corresponding roughly to the three zones of the lung in the normal upright subject. Mixed alveolar gas Po_2 is calculated with allowance for the volume contribution of gas from the three zones. Arterial saturation is similarly determined and the Po_2 derived. There is an alveolar/arterial Po_2 difference of 0.7 kPa (5 mmHg). (b) An entirely imaginary situation which would account for the difference. This is a useful method of quantifying the functional effect of scatter of $\dot{V}/\dot{Q}$ ratios but should be carefully distinguished from the actual situation.

return blood with a saturation of much more than 98.5% saturation (when breathing air), and so cannot offset the contribution of desaturated blood from the under-ventilated alveoli. Asmussen and Nielsen (1960) have pointed out that this effect will be more pronounced if the mean alveolar Po_2 is reduced to the tension corresponding to the bend of the dissociation curve. This is a Po_2 of about 6.7 kPa (50 mmHg), which is encountered only in fairly severe underventilation or during the inhalation of oxygen mixtures of less than 20%. However, the effect is still appreciable at higher levels of alveolar Po_2. In the example shown in *Figure 7.13*,

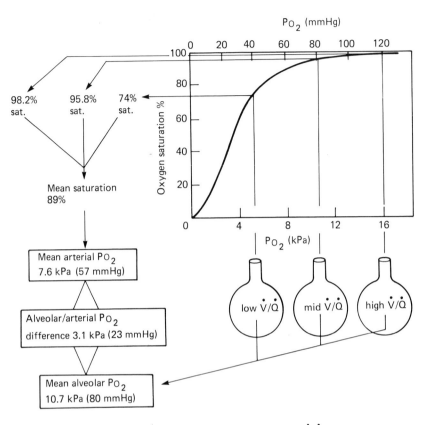

Figure 7.13 Alveolar/arterial Po_2 difference caused by scatter of $\dot{V}/\dot{Q}$ ratios resulting in oxygen tensions around the bend of the oxygen dissociation curve. The diagram shows the effect of three groups of alveoli with Po_2 values of 5.3, 10.7 and 16.0 kPa (40, 80 and 120 mmHg). Ignoring the effect of the different volumes of gas and blood contributed by the three groups, the mean alveolar Po_2 is 10.7 kPa. However, due to the bend of the dissociation curve, the saturations of the blood leaving the three groups are not proportional to their Po_2. The mean arterial saturation is, in fact, 89% and the Po_2 therefore is 7.6 kPa. The alveolar/arterial Po_2 difference is thus 3.1 kPa. The actual difference would be somewhat greater since gas with a high Po_2 would make a relatively greater contribution to the alveolar gas, and blood with a low Po_2 would make a relatively greater contribution to the arterial blood. In this example a calculated venous admixture of 27 per cent would be required to account for the scatter of $\dot{V}/\dot{Q}$ ratios in terms of the measured alveolar/arterial Po_2 difference, at an alveolar Po_2 of 10.7 kPa.

where the mean alveolar Po_2 is 10.7 kPa (80 mmHg), there is an equivalent shunt of 27 per cent.

It follows from the latter consideration that the degree of calculated shunt which is equivalent in effect to a fixed degree of scatter of $\dot{V}/\dot{Q}$ ratio will depend upon the actual level of the alveolar Po_2. At high levels of alveolar Po_2 the effect of $\dot{V}/\dot{Q}$ scatter will be small since blood from all alveoli will be close to 100% saturation, even if the $\dot{V}/\dot{Q}$ ratios vary widely. When the alveolar Po_2 is less than normal, scatter of $\dot{V}/\dot{Q}$ ratios may result in a very large equivalent shunt, the effect being maximal at an alveolar Po_2 of 6.7 kPa (50 mmHg).

Principles of assessment of distribution of ventilation and pulmonary blood flow

Distribution of inspired gas

Since the methodology is essential to an understanding of basic principles, the techniques have been outlined in the text above and will not be repeated here.

Measurement of anatomical dead space

The anatomical dead space can be measured only by solution of the Bohr equation using the CO_2 concentration of the end-expiratory gas if the alveolar CO_2 plateau is almost flat (see page 200). Therefore it is now universal practice to use a method based on the technique described by Fowler (1948) which is a development of the concept of Aitken and Clarke-Kennedy (1928). The CO_2 concentration at the lips is measured continuously with a rapid gas analyser, and then displayed against the volume actually expired. A typical normal plot is shown in *Figure 7.14*. The 'alveolar plateau' of CO_2 concentration is not flat but slopes gently. Anatomical dead space is derived by the graphical solution shown in the Figure.

The technique as introduced by Fowler (1948) used a rapid nitrogen analyser to follow a single expiration after the inspiration of a single breath of 100% oxygen. After 1950, infrared carbon dioxide analysers came into use and have now replaced the nitrogen analyser for this purpose. The same value for the anatomical dead space is obtained with both nitrogen and carbon dioxide as the tracer gas.

Measurement of physiological dead space

The measurement of physiological dead space is quite simple. Arterial blood and expired air are collected simultaneously over a period of two or three minutes (*Figure 7.15*). After collection, the P_{CO_2} of blood and gas are determined, the CO_2-sensitive electrode being suitable for both samples. Provided that the inspired gas is free from carbon dioxide, physiological dead space is indicated by the following form of the Bohr equation:

physiological dead space

$$= \text{tidal volume} \left(\frac{\text{arterial } P_{CO_2} - \text{mixed-expired gas } P_{CO_2}}{\text{arterial } P_{CO_2}} \right) - \text{apparatus dead space}$$

Apparatus dead space includes such items as the facemask and unidirectional valve box. It is usually measured by water displacement and is often found to be surprisingly large. Tidal volume may be determined by a variety of techniques; the Wright respirometer is the most convenient and may easily be incorporated in the gas-collection apparatus.

The result is often most conveniently expressed as the ratio of the physiological dead space to the tidal volume. Scatter of ventilation/perfusion ratios (page 154) undoubtedly contributes to the measured physiological dead space from which it cannot be distinguished by this method.

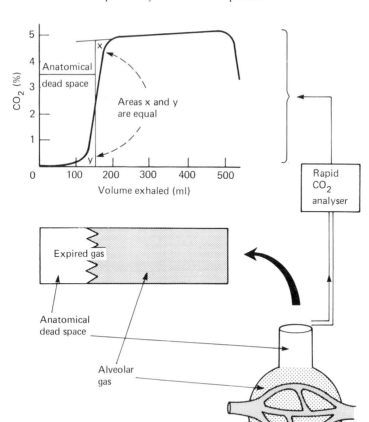

Figure 7.14 Measurement of the anatomical dead space using carbon dioxide as the tracer gas. If the gas passing the patient's lips is continuously analysed for carbon dioxide concentration, there is a sudden rise to the alveolar plateau level, after the expiration of gas from the anatomical dead space (conducting air passages). If the instantaneous CO_2 concentration is plotted against the volume exhaled (allowing for delay in the CO_2 analyser), a graph similar to that shown is obtained. A vertical line is constructed so that the two areas x and y are equal. This line will indicate the volume of the anatomical dead space.

Measurement of alveolar dead space

The alveolar dead space is measured as the difference between the physiological and anatomical dead space, determined separately but at the same time. When only the physiological dead space is measured, it is often possible to attribute a large increase in physiological dead space to an increase in the alveolar component, since there are few circumstances in which the anatomical dead space is greatly enlarged.

The arterial/end-expiratory $P\text{CO}_2$ *difference* is a convenient and relatively simple method of assessing the magnitude of the alveolar dead space. In *Figure 7.8* expired gas is shown as consisting of four components. The final portion of an expirate

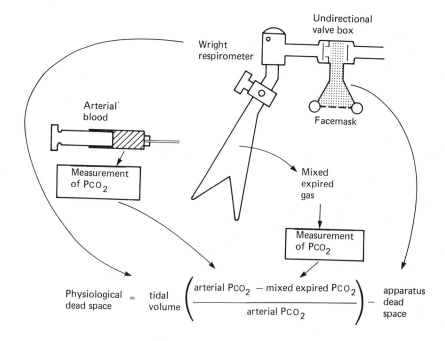

Figure 7.15 Clinical measurement of physiological dead space. Arterial blood and mixed expired gas are collected simultaneously over a period of 2–3 minutes. Values for Pco_2 are then substituted in the Bohr equation. Tidal volume is conveniently determined with a Wright respirometer and the apparatus dead space by water displacement.

consists of a mixture of 'ideal' alveolar gas and alveolar dead space gas. If the patient has an appreciable alveolar dead space, it follows that:

1. It is impossible to sample or analyse 'ideal' alveolar gas.
2. The Pco_2 of the end-expiratory gas will be less than that of 'ideal' alveolar gas since it is diluted with alveolar dead space gas which is practically free of CO_2.

If, for example, 'ideal' alveolar gas has a Pco_2 of 5.3 kPa (40 mmHg) and the end-expiratory Pco_2 is found to be 2.65 kPa (20 mmHg), it follows that the end-expiratory gas consists of equal parts of 'ideal' alveolar gas and alveolar dead space gas. Thus if the tidal volume is 500 ml and the anatomical dead space 100 ml, the components of the tidal volume would be as follows:

anatomical dead space	100 ml
alveolar dead space	200 ml
'ideal' alveolar gas	200 ml

The physiological dead space would be 100 + 200 = 300 ml and the V$_D$/V$_T$ ratio 60 per cent.

Changes in the end-expiratory Pco_2 provide a qualitative indication of the changes in the alveolar dead space. A pulmonary embolus (e.g. an air embolus during neurosurgery) when the minute volume is held constant will result in a sudden reduction in end-expiratory Pco_2, although a large reduction in cardiac output will have the same effect.

Measurement of unilateral pulmonary blood flow

Flow sensors, such as electromagnetic flow meters, may be applied to the pulmonary arteries but such methods are of limited scope in man. The measurement of unilateral pulmonary blood flow in man has been attempted by application of the Fick principle using oxygen as the indicator gas. Divided airway techniques such as the Carlen's catheter permit measurement of unilateral oxygen uptake and unilateral ventilation. The pulmonary arterial blood is common to both lungs and the only remaining problem is the measurement of the oxygen content of the blood draining each lung separately. This cannot be determined directly. Even if it were feasible to cannulate pulmonary veins, it would not be possible to sample proportionately from the two pulmonary veins which drain each lung. Their flow rate and oxygen content are both likely to be different, at least in the upright position. The usual approach is to measure the end-expiratory P_{O_2} and assume that the pulmonary venous P_{O_2} is less than this by a certain amount. Alternatively, the 'ideal' alveolar P_{O_2} may be calculated for each lung indirectly from its end-expiratory P_{CO_2}.

On a simpler plane, an approximate estimate of blood flow may be obtained from measurements of unilateral ventilation and oxygen uptake. Clearly, if the ventilation of the two lungs is similar and the oxygen uptake differs, it may be assumed that the blood flow rates differ by approximately the same extent. However, because ventilation and blood flow alter the pulmonary venous oxygen content, it is impossible to make a precise assessment of blood flow from the simple measurements made with the bronchospirometer.

A semi-quantitative estimate of the distribution of pulmonary blood flow between the two lungs may be made by injection of a suitable radioactive tracer into a vein and subsequently counting over the lung fields. A gamma radiation emitter is required and two different methods are employed. Firstly, a relatively insoluble gas such as ^{133}Xe may be dissolved in saline and injected into a systemic vein. The xenon is evolved in the lungs and may be counted in the alveolar gas. It is rapidly cleared by pulmonary ventilation and the method is therefore suitable only if counting can be completed during a breath hold. The second method is to inject labelled particles which have a diameter greater than about 50 μm and so lodge in the pulmonary circulation. They can then be counted at leisure without the limitation of breath-holding time. Different isotopes with different energy levels of radiation can be used at different times to study changes in the pulmonary circulation, and the lung fields are then counted for different energy levels. Counts may be obtained by stationary or moving scintillation counters and graphical representation of the circulation may be presented as a lung scan or by means of a gamma camera. The use of ^{133}Xe was first employed for studying the blood flow to horizontal slices of the lung and was introduced for this purpose by West (1962).

It is possible to deflect the pulmonary blood flow away from one lung, and so to study the ability of the other lung to take the whole of the pulmonary circulation. This may be achieved by inflation of a balloon on the end of a cardiac catheter within one branch of the pulmonary artery (Carlens, Hanson and Nordenström, 1951). It is also possible to combine this procedure with bronchial occlusion and so to reproduce the cardiorespiratory effects of pneumonectomy (Nemir et al., 1953).

Measurement of pulmonary lobar blood flow

By intubation, the right upper lobe bronchus may be isolated in man (Mattson and Carlens, 1955), and the oxygen consumption of this lobe may therefore be estimated.

It was found to be considerably less than proportionate to its ventilation and this indicated a low rate of perfusion.

End-expiratory gases sampled from different lobes at bronchoscopy will give some qualitative indication of blood flow, although precise calculation of flow is not possible. A simple estimate of ventilation/perfusion ratio may be obtained from the respiratory exchange ratio (Armitage and Taylor, 1956). A more complete assessment has been made by the simultaneous analysis of a number of gases exhaled from various bronchi, using a mass spectrometer at bronchoscopy (Hugh-Jones and West, 1960).

Measurement of ventilation and perfusion as a function of $\dot{V}/\dot{Q}$ ratio

The information of the type displayed in *Figure 7.6* is obtained by a technique developed by Wagner, Saltzman and West (1974). It employs a range of tracer gases ranging from very soluble (e.g. acetone) to very insoluble (e.g. sulphur hexafluoride). Saline is equilibrated with these gases and infused intravenously at a constant rate. After about 20 minutes a steady state is achieved and samples of arterial blood and mixed expired gas are collected. Levels of the tracer gases in the arterial blood are then measured by gas chromatography (Wagner, Naumann and Laravuso, 1974) and levels in the mixed venous blood are derived by use of the Fick principle. It is then possible to calculate the retention of each tracer in the blood passing through the lung and the elimination of each in the expired gas. Retention and elimination are related to the solubility coefficient of each tracer in blood and then, by numerical analysis, it is possible to compute a distribution curve for pulmonary blood flow and alveolar ventilation respectively in relation to the spectrum of $\dot{V}/\dot{Q}$ ratios. In practice, a number of finite values of $\dot{V}/\dot{Q}$ are employed. The range of $\dot{V}/\dot{Q}$ ratios between 0.005 and 100 is divided equally on a logarithmic scale into 48 compartments which, together with zero (shunt) and infinity (alveolar dead space), make 50 in all.

The technique is technically demanding and laborious. It has not become widely used, but results from a small number of laboratories have made major contributions to our understanding of gas exchange in a wide variety of circumstances.

Measurement of venous admixture or shunt

The classic method of calculation of venous admixture is by solution of the equation shown in *Figure 7.10*. When the alveolar P_{O_2} is less than about 27 kPa (200 mmHg), scatter of $\dot{V}/\dot{Q}$ ratios contributes appreciably to the total calculated venous admixture. This effect is maximal when the alveolar P_{O_2} is about 6.7 kPa (50 mmHg). When the subject breathes a high oxygen concentration, the calculated venous admixture contains only a small component due to scatter of $\dot{V}/\dot{Q}$ ratios (page 154). Nevertheless, the calculated quantity still does not indicate the precise value of shunted blood since some of the shunt consists of blood of which the oxygen content is unknown (i.e. from bronchial veins and venae cordis minimae). The calculated venous admixture is thus at best an index rather than a precise measurement of contamination of arterial blood with venous blood.

In the equation shown in *Figure 7.10*, some of the quantities on the right-hand side are amenable to direct measurement. The arterial and mixed venous oxygen contents may be derived by sampling and analysis. Arterial blood may be drawn from any convenient systemic artery, but the mixed venous blood must be withdrawn from the right ventricle or pulmonary artery. A Swan–Ganz catheter is suitable for this purpose. Blood in the right atrium is not perfectly mixed, and blood from inferior and superior venae cavae and coronary sinus forms separate streams. The major problem is, however, measurement of the pulmonary end-capillary P_{O_2}. This cannot be measured directly and is assumed equal to the alveolar P_{O_2}. If *Figure 7.7* is studied in conjunction with *Figure 7.10*, it will be seen that the 'alveolar' P_{O_2} required is the 'ideal' alveolar P_{O_2} and not the end-expiratory P_{O_2} which may be contaminated with alveolar dead space gas. Derivation of the 'ideal' alveolar P_{O_2} is considered in the next section.

The alveolar air equation. 'Ideal' alveolar gas cannot be sampled and its P_{O_2} must be derived by indirect means. Derivation of the 'ideal' alveolar P_{O_2} was first suggested by Benzinger (1937) and later by Rossier and Méan (1943). It was finally formulated with greater precision by Riley et al. (1946).

Derivation of the 'ideal' alveolar P_{O_2} is based on the following assumptions.

1. Quite large degrees of venous admixture or $\dot{V}/\dot{Q}$ scatter cause relatively little difference between P_{CO_2} of 'ideal' alveolar gas (or pulmonary end-capillary blood) and arterial blood (see *Table 7.2*). Therefore 'ideal' alveolar P_{CO_2} is approximately equal to arterial P_{CO_2}.
2. The respiratory exchange ratio of ideal alveolar gas (in relation to inspired gas) equals the respiratory exchange ratio of mixed expired gas (again in relation to inspired gas).

From these assumptions it is possible to derive an equation which indicates the 'ideal' alveolar P_{O_2} in terms of arterial P_{CO_2}, inspired gas P_{O_2}, respiratory exchange ratio or related quantities. As a very rough approximation, the oxygen and carbon dioxide in the alveolar gas replace the oxygen in the inspired gas. Therefore, very approximately:

$$\text{alveolar } P_{O_2} \doteq \text{ inspired } P_{O_2} - \text{arterial } P_{O_2}$$

This equation is not sufficiently accurate for use except in the special case when 100% oxygen is breathed. In other situations, three corrections are required to overcome errors due to the following factors: (1) usually, less carbon dioxide is produced than oxygen is consumed (respiratory exchange ratio); (2) the respiratory exchange ratio produces a secondary effect due to the fact that the expired volume does not equal the inspired volume; (3) the inspired and expired gas volumes may also differ because of inert gas exchange.

The simplest practicable form of the equation is that suggested by Benzinger (1937) and Rossier and Méan (1943). It makes correction for the principal effect of the respiratory exchange ratio (1), but not the small supplementary error due to the difference between the inspired and expired gas volumes which results from the respiratory exchange ratio (2):

$$\text{alveolar } P_{O_2} = \text{inspired } P_{O_2} - \text{arterial } P_{CO_2}/RQ$$

This form is suitable for rapid bedside calculations of alveolar P_{O_2}, when great accuracy is not required.

One stage more complicated is an equation which allows for differences in the volume of inspired and expired gas due to the respiratory exchange ratio, but still does not allow for differences due to the exchange of inert gases. This equation exists in various forms, all algebraically identical:

$$\text{alveolar } P_{O_2} = P_{I_{O_2}} - \frac{Pa_{CO_2}}{R}(1 - F_{I_{O_2}}(1 - R))$$

(derived from Riley et al., 1946)

This equation is suitable for use whenever the subject has been breathing the inspired gas mixture long enough for the inert gas to be in equilibrium. It is unsuitable for use when the inspired oxygen concentration has recently been changed, when the ambient pressure has recently been changed (e.g. during hyperbaric oxygen therapy) or when the inert gas concentration has recently been changed (e.g. soon after the start or finish of a period of inhaling nitrous oxide).

Perhaps the most satisfactory form of the alveolar air equation is that which was advanced by Filley, MacIntosh and Wright (1954). This equation makes no assumption that inert gases are in equilibrium and allows for the difference between inspired and expired gas from whatever cause. It also proves to be very simple in use and does not require the calculation of the respiratory exchange ratio:

$$\text{alveolar } P_{O_2} = P_{I_{O_2}} - Pa_{CO_2}\left(\frac{P_{I_{O_2}} - P\bar{E}_{O_2}}{P\bar{E}_{CO_2}}\right)$$

If the alveolar P_{O_2} is calculated separately according to the last two equations, the difference (if any) will be that due to inert gas exchange. This affords a method of study of such phenomena as the 'concentration' effect (page 248).

Distinction between shunt and the effect of $\dot{V}/\dot{Q}$ scatter

Shunt and scatter of $\dot{V}/\dot{Q}$ ratios will each produce an alveolar/arterial P_{O_2} difference from which a value for venous admixture may be calculated. It is, however, often impossible to say from the measurements whether the disorder is a true shunt or else an excessive scatter of $\dot{V}/\dot{Q}$ ratios. Three methods are available for distinction between the two conditions.

If the inspired oxygen concentration is altered, the effect on the arterial P_{O_2} will depend upon the nature of the disorder. If oxygenation is impaired by a shunt, the arterial P_{O_2} will increase as shown in the iso-shunt diagram (*Figure 7.11*). If, however, the disorder is due to scatter of $\dot{V}/\dot{Q}$ ratios, the arterial P_{O_2} will rise by more than or approximately the same amount as the inspired P_{O_2}.

Measurement of the alveolar/arterial P_{N_2} difference is a specific method for quantification of $\dot{V}/\dot{Q}$ scatter, since the P_{N_2} difference is entirely uninfluenced by true shunt. The method has not come into general use. Subjects must be in a state of complete nitrogen equilibrium which may be difficult to achieve in the clinical environment. Furthermore, the method is technically difficult, requiring the measurement of P_{N_2} to an accuracy which is not easily obtainable. The method was described by Rahn and Farhi (1964).

The multiple inert gas wash-out technique for analysis of distribution of blood flow in relation to $\dot{V}/\dot{Q}$ ratio is the best method of distinction between shunt and areas of low $\dot{V}/\dot{Q}$ ratio (see above).

Chapter 8

Diffusion and alveolar/capillary permeability

Fundamentals of the diffusion process

Diffusion of a gas is a process by which a net transfer of molecules takes place from a zone in which the gas exerts a high partial pressure to a zone in which it exerts a lower partial pressure. The mechanism of transfer is the random movement of molecules and the term excludes transfer by mass movement of gas in response to a total pressure difference (as occurs during expiration). The partial pressure (or tension) of a gas in a gas mixture is the pressure which it would exert if it occupied the space alone (equal to total pressure multiplied by fractional concentration). The tension of a gas in solution in a liquid is defined as being equal to the tension of the same gas in a gas mixture which is in equilibrium with the liquid.

Typical examples of diffusion are shown in *Figure 8.1*. In each case there is a net transfer of oxygen from one zone to another in response to a tension gradient. We may note certain points which are common to all three examples.

1. Total pressure differences play no significant part in gas transfer.
2. Gas transfer results from the random movement of the molecules and the rapidity with which equilibrium is attained is therefore dependent on temperature.
3. Gas molecules pass in each direction but at a rate proportional to the tension of the gas in the zone which they are leaving. The net transfer of the gas is the difference in the number of molecules passing in each direction, and it thus proportional to the difference in tension between the two zones.
4. In a static situation, such as the example in *Figure 8.1a*, the process of diffusion proceeds to equilibrium, when there will be no difference between the tension of the gas in the two zones. There will then be no net transfer of the gas, although molecules will continue to pass in both directions but at the same rate.

Conditions are not static for oxygen and carbon dioxide in the living body since oxygen is constantly being consumed while carbon dioxide is being produced. Therefore, static equilibrium cannot be attained as in the case of the open bottle of oxygen in *Figure 8.1a*. Instead, a dynamic equilibrium is attained with a cascade of oxygen tensions from 21 kPa (approx. 160 mmHg) in dry air, down to 1–3 kPa at the site of consumption in the mitochondria (see Chapter 10). The maintenance of these tension gradients is, in fact, a characteristic of life.

These considerations do not apply to gases and vapours which are not metabolized to a great extent, such as nitrogen, nitrous oxide and most volatile anaesthetic agents. In these cases, there is always a tendency towards a static equilibrium at

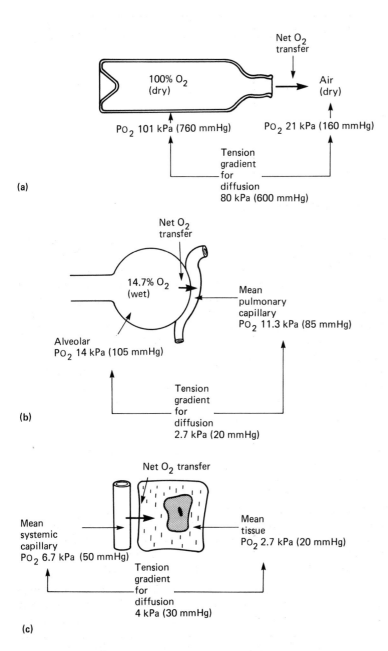

Figure 8.1 Three examples of diffusion of oxygen. In each case there is a net transfer of oxygen from left to right in accord with the tension gradient. (a) Oxygen passes from one gaseous phase to another. (b) Oxygen passes from a gaseous phase to a liquid phase. (c) Oxygen passes from one liquid phase to another.

which all tissue tensions become equal to the tension of the particular gas in the inspired air. This is attained in the case of nitrogen, and would also be attained with an inhalational anaesthetic agent if it were administered for a very long time.

Resistance to diffusion

In each of the examples shown in *Figure 8.1*, there is a finite resistance to the transfer of the gas molecules. In *Figure 8.1a*, the resistance is concentrated at the restriction in the neck of the bottle. Clearly, the narrower the neck, the slower will be the process of equilibration with the outside air. In *Figure 8.1b* the site of the resistance to diffusion is less circumscribed but includes the alveolar/capillary membrane, the diffusion path through the plasma, and the delay in combination of oxygen with the reduced haemoglobin in the erythrocyte. In *Figure 8.1c*, the resistance commences with the delay in the release of oxygen by haemoglobin, and includes all the interfaces between the erythrocyte cell membrane and the site of oxygen consumption in the cell (the mitochondria). There may then be an additional component in the rate at which oxygen enters into chemical combination.

There is a clear analogy between the diffusion of gases in response to a partial pressure gradient and the passage of an electrical current in response to a potential difference in an electrical circuit. Diffusing capacity is analogous to conductance (inverse of resistance):

$$\text{diffusing capacity} = \frac{\text{net rate of gas transfer}}{\text{partial pressure gradient}}$$

$$\text{conductance} = \frac{\text{current flow (amps)}}{\text{potential difference (volts)}}$$

It will be recalled that the unit of electrical conductance is the mho. The usual biological unit of diffusing capacity is ml/min/mmHg, or, in SI units, ml min^{-1} kPa^{-1}.

The size of gas molecules limits their ability to diffuse, and small molecules diffuse more easily than large molecules. Graham's law states that the rate of diffusion of a gas is inversely proportional to the square root of its density. This means that only large differences in density have any marked effect on the rate of diffusion within a gas phase. Thus, nitrous oxide has a density of 1.4 times that of oxygen, but the rate of gaseous diffusion of oxygen is only 1.2 times that of nitrous oxide.

When a gas is diffusing into or through an aqueous phase the solubility of the gas in water becomes an important factor, and the diffusing capacity under these circumstances is considered to be directly proportional to the solubility. Nitrous oxide would thus be expected to have about 20 times the diffusing capacity of oxygen in crossing a gas/water interface. High solubility does not confer an increased 'agility' of the gas in its negotiation of an aqueous barrier, but simply means that, for a given tension, more molecules of the gas are present in the liquid.

Apart from these factors, inherent in the gas, the resistance to diffusion is related directly to the length of the diffusion path and inversely to the area of interface which is available for diffusion. In the case of the lungs, for example, the diffusion path extends from the gas side of the alveolar membrane to some unspecified reference point within the erythrocyte. The area of interface probably corresponds to the total area of pulmonary capillary endothelium in contact with alveolar lining membrane. It is important to remember that the pulmonary diffusing capacity is as much a measure of the area of the interface as it is of the thickness of the tissues which comprise the diffusion path.

The diffusing capacity of oxygen in the lung is markedly influenced by the rate of combination of oxygen with reduced haemoglobin. Clearly, if this is slow, it will retard the whole process of oxygen transfer; similar considerations apply to release of carbon dioxide from chemical combination.

Tension and concentration gradients

In gas mixtures at the same total pressure, the tension of any component gas is directly proportional to its concentration. Therefore, when we consider a gas diffusing from one gas mixture to another, the tension gradient of the gas between the two mixtures will be directly proportional to the concentration gradient. This is not the case when a gas in solution in a liquid diffuses into a different liquid. When gases are in solution, the tension they exert is directly proportional to their concentration in the solvent but inversely to the solubility of the gas in the solvent. Thus, if water and oil have the same concentration of nitrous oxide dissolved in each, the tension of nitrous oxide in the oil will be only one-third of the tension in the water since the oil/water solubility ratio is about 3:1. If the two liquids are shaken up together, there will be a net transfer of nitrous oxide from the water to the oil until the tension in each phase is the same. At that time the concentration of nitrous oxide in the oil will be about three times the concentration in the water. Under all circumstances, the direction and rate of diffusion are governed by tension gradients and it is therefore more useful to consider tensions rather than concentrations in relation to movement of gases and vapours from one compartment of the body to another. The same units of pressure may be used in gas, aqueous and lipid phases.

Diffusion of oxygen within the lungs

It is now widely accepted that oxygen passes from the alveoli into the pulmonary capillary blood by a passive process of diffusion according to physical laws. For a long time this view was contested by a school of thought which believed that oxygen was actively secreted into the blood (Milledge, 1985b). A similar process was known to occur in the swim-bladders of certain fish, so the postulated mechanism was certainly feasible, but proof of secretion depended on the demonstration of an arterial Po_2 which was higher than the alveolar Po_2. In the earlier years of this century, a great controversy raged, with active secretion being upheld by Bohr and Haldane while the Kroghs and Barcroft took the opposite view. Much of the difficulty hinged on the analytical problems and on the sampling of representative alveolar gas, particularly under conditions of exercise. Finally the day was won by the diffusion school although it was for some time contended that secretion might play a part in adaptation to altitude.

There is now strong evidence for believing that diffusion equilibrium is very nearly achieved for oxygen during the normal pulmonary capillary transit time in the resting subject. Therefore, under these circumstances, the uptake of oxygen is limited by pulmonary blood flow and not by diffusing capacity. However, under conditions of exercise while breathing gas mixtures deficient in oxygen or at reduced barometric pressure, the diffusing capacity becomes important and may actually limit the oxygen uptake (page 318).

The diffusion path

The gas space within the alveolus. In the past there has been some doubt as to the degree of gas mixing which occurs within the alveolus. Some believed that gaseous diffusion would not be sufficiently rapid to maintain equality of gas composition between the core (freshly charged with inspired gas) and the periphery of the alveolus (where the oxygen concentration would be lowest, due to uptake by the pulmonary capillaries). 'Layering' of gas would clearly be a factor limiting the uptake of oxygen, and would impose a tension gradient between the centre of the alveolus and the alveolar/capillary membrane.

Georg et al. (1965) demonstrated unequal mixing of helium and the heavy gas, sulphur hexafluoride, within the alveolus. However, it seems unlikely that non-uniformity within a single alveolus is an important factor under normal conditions. At functional residual capacity, the diameter of the average human alveolus is of the order of 200 μm (Wiebel and Gomez, 1962), and it is likely that mixing is almost instantaneous over the very small distance from the centre to the periphery. Precise calculations are impossible on account of the complex geometry of the alveolus, but the overall efficiency of gas exchange within the lungs suggests that mixing must be complete within less than 10 ms (Forster, 1946b). Therefore, in practice it is usual to consider alveolar gas as uniformly mixed within a single alveolus.

The alveolar/capillary membrane. Electron microscopy has revealed details of the actual path between alveolar gas and pulmonary capillary blood, shown in *Figures 1.6–1.8.* Each alveolus is completely lined with epithelium which, with its basement membrane, is about 0.2 μm thick, except where its nuclei bulge into the alveolar lumen. Beyond the basement membrane is a tissue space which is very thin where it overlies the capillaries, particularly on the active side: elsewhere it is thicker and contains collagen, elastic fibres and lymphatics. The pulmonary capillaries are lined with endothelium, also with its own basement membrane, which is approximately the same thickness as the alveolar epithelium, except where it is expanded to enclose the endothelial nuclei. The total thickness of the active part of the alveolar/capillary membrane is thus about 0.5 μm. This arrangement is shown in *Figure 1.8.*

Pulmonary capillaries. Weibel (1962) suggested a mean diameter of 7 μm for the human pulmonary capillary. This is similar to the diameter of the erythrocyte, which is therefore forced into close proximity with the alveolar/capillary membrane. The pulmonary capillary network is seen by studying thick sections, which will occasionally reveal a face view of an alveolar septum. The space between the capillaries is normally less than the diameter of the capillaries themselves (see *Figures 1.6* and *1.10*).

Diffusion within the blood. Since the diameter of the erythrocytes is so close to that of the capillaries, the diffusion path through plasma may be very short indeed. Furthermore, since the diameter of the erythrocyte is about 14 times the thickness of the alveolar/capillary membranes, it is clear that the diffusion path within the erythrocyte is likely to be much longer than the path through the alveolar/capillary membrane, although the shape of the erythrocyte does tend to concentrate the cell mass at the periphery. Even so, the rim has a thickness of about 2.5 μm and the diffusion path within it is still large compared with the alveolar/capillary membrane. Once within the cell, diffusion of oxygen is aided by mass movement of the haemoglobin molecules caused by the deformation of the erythrocyte as it passes through the capillary bed. Other factors may be involved since oxygen diffuses through a layer of haemoglobin solution more rapidly than through a layer of water which might be expected to offer less resistance (Hemmingsen and Scholander, 1960).

Uptake of oxygen by haemoglobin. The greater part of the oxygen which is taken up in the lungs enters into chemical combination with haemoglobin. This chemical reaction takes a finite time and forms an appreciable part of the total resistance to the transfer of oxygen. Indeed, it now appears that the reaction of oxygen with haemoglobin is sufficiently slow to be the limiting factor in the rate of transfer of oxygen from the alveolar gas into chemical combination within the erythrocyte. This important discovery by Staub, Bishop and Forster (1961) resulted in an extensive reappraisal of the whole concept of diffusing capacity, since it followed that measurements of 'diffusing capacity' did not necessarily give an indication of the degree of permeability of the alveolar/capillary membrane. It will be seen below that methods exist for analysing the diffusing capacity of carbon monoxide into two components, one through the alveolar/capillary membrane and the other within the pulmonary blood. The latter component is determined by the pulmonary capillary volume and the rate of chemical combination of carbon monoxide with haemoglobin.

Quantification of the diffusing capacity for oxygen

The diffusing capacity of a gas is defined as the rate of its transfer, divided by the tension gradient across the interface. The rate of transfer of oxygen is simply the oxygen uptake, which may be easily measured. The tension gradient is from alveolar gas to pulmonary blood where the relevant tension is the mean pulmonary capillary P_{O_2}.

$$\text{oxygen diffusing capacity} = \frac{\text{oxygen uptake}}{\text{alveolar } P_{O_2} - \text{mean pulmonary capillary } P_{O_2}}$$

The alveolar P_{O_2} can be derived with some degree of accuracy (page 182) but there are serious problems in estimating the mean capillary P_{O_2}.

The mean pulmonary capillary P_{O_2}. It is clearly impossible to make a direct measurement of the mean P_{O_2} of the pulmonary capillary blood, and therefore attempts have been made to derive this quantity indirectly from the presumed changes of P_{O_2} which occur as blood passes through the pulmonary capillaries.

The earliest analysis of the problem was made by Bohr (1909). He made the assumption that, at any point along the pulmonary capillary, the rate of diffusion of oxygen was proportional to the P_{O_2} difference between the alveolar gas and the pulmonary capillary blood at that point. Using this approach, and assuming a value for the alveolar/end-pulmonary capillary P_{O_2} gradient, it seemed possible to construct a graph of capillary Po_2, plotted against the time the blood had been in the pulmonary capillary. The normal curve drawn on this basis is shown as the broken line in *Figure 8.2a*. Once the curve has been drawn, it is relatively easy to derive the effective or integrated mean pulmonary capillary Po_2, which then permits calculation of the oxygen diffusing capacity.

Unfortunately this approach, known as the Bohr integration procedure, was shown to be invalid when it was found that the fundamental assumption was untrue. The rate of transfer of oxygen is not proportional to the alveolar/capillary Po_2 gradient at any point along the capillary. It would no doubt be true if the transfer of oxygen were a purely physical process (as in the case of nitrous oxide, for example) but the rate of transfer is actually limited by the chemical combination of oxygen with haemoglobin, which is sufficiently slow to comprise the greater part of the total resistance to transfer of oxygen.

In vitro studies of the rate of combination of oxygen with haemoglobin have shown that this is not directly proportional to the Po_2 gradient, for two distinct reasons.

1. The combination of the fourth molecule of oxygen with the haemoglobin molecule ($Hb_4(O_2)_3 + O_2 \rightleftharpoons Hb_4(O_2)_4$) has a much higher velocity constant than that of the combination of the other three molecules (Staub, Bishop and Forster, 1961). This is discussed further on page 262.
2. As the capillary oxygen saturation rises, the number of molecules of reduced haemoglobin diminishes and the velocity of the forward reaction must therefore diminish by the law of mass action. This depends upon the haemoglobin dissociation curve and is therefore not a simple exponential function of the actual Po_2 of the blood.

When these two factors are combined it is found that the resistance to 'diffusion' due to chemical combination of oxygen within the erythrocyte is fairly constant up to a saturation of about 80% (Po_2 = 6 kPa or 45 mmHg). Thereafter, it falls very rapidly to become zero at full saturation (Staub, Bishop and Forster, 1962). These authors proceeded to elaborate the Bohr integration procedure to allow for changes in the rate of combinations of haemoglobin with oxygen. Assuming traditional values for the alveolar/end-capillary Po_2 difference, they obtained a curve lying to the left of the original Bohr curve shown in *Figure 8.2*. This indicated a mean pulmonary capillary Po_2 higher than had previously been believed, and therefore an oxyen diffusing capacity which was substantially higher than the accepted value. The situation is actually more complicated still, since quick-frozen sections prepared by Staub showed that the colour of haemoglobin begins to alter to the red colour of oxyhaemoglobin within the pulmonary arterioles before the blood has entered the pulmonary capillaries. Furthermore, pulmonary capillaries do not cross a single alveolus but may pass over three or more (see *Figures 1.6* and *1.10*).

Uncertainties about the pulmonary end-capillary Po_2. Both the classic and the modified Bohr integration procedures for calculation of mean capillary Po_2 depend critically on the precise value of the pulmonary end-capillary Po_2, and the constructed curve is considerably influenced by very small variations in the value which is assumed. It is therefore appropriate to consider the problems in derivation of this value which cannot be measured directly. In 1946, Riley et al. proposed the two-level method of resolution of the alveolar/arterial Po_2 gradient. This was undertaken with the subject breathing air and then 11% oxygen. At the alveolar

Po_2 of the first pair of observations, it was assumed that the component of the alveolar/arterial Po_2 difference due to resistance to diffusion would be small and the total difference would thus be largely due to venous admixture; under the conditions of the second pair of observations, it was assumed that the component of the difference due to venous admixture would become small while the difference due to resistance to diffusion would be appreciable. It was further assumed that both the diffusing capacity and the venous admixture would remain the same while breathing air and 11% oxygen. Typical normal values obtained by this approach were as follows.

	Breathing air	Breathing 11% oxygen
Venous admixture component	1.2 kPa (9 mmHg)	0.1 kPa (1 mmHg)
'Diffusion' component	0.1 kPa (1 mmHg)	1.2 kPa (9 mmHg)
Total alveolar/arterial Po_2 difference	1.3 kPa (10 mmHg)	1.3 kPa (10 mmHg)

Unfortunately, the two-level oxygen study made two assumptions which are now known to be incorrect. Firstly, the component of the alveolar/arterial Po_2 difference due to venous admixture does not fall to small values when the alveolar Po_2 is reduced, because a considerable part of it is now known to be due to regional scatter of ventilation/perfusion ratios (see *Figures 7.6* and *7.12*), and this component actually increases as the alveolar Po_2 falls (see *Figure 7.13*). The second fallacy is that the resistance to diffusion should be uninfluenced by the actual level of arterial Po_2. It has been explained above that the major part of the resistance to 'diffusion' is due to the rate of chemical combination of oxygen with haemoglobin, which is very markedly influenced by the actual level of Po_2.

We are thus at least two stages away from the possibility of measuring the alveolar/end-capillary Po_2 gradient. For this and the other reasons discussed above, we cannot determine the mean pulmonary capillary Po_2 and therefore cannot, in the present state of knowledge, measure the diffusing capacity of oxygen. Measurements reported in the earlier literature were based on false assumptions and cannot therefore be regarded as valid.

Forward integration. A new and entirely opposite approach was made by Staub in a most important paper in 1963. He started from what was known about the behaviour of oxygen in the pulmonary capillary, and, beginning at the pulmonary arterial end, calculated the Po_2 of the capillary blood progressively along the capillary until he was able to give an estimate of the remaining alveolar/capillary Po_2 gradient at the end of the capillary. This procedure of forward integration was thus the reverse of the classic approach which, starting from the alveolar/end-capillary Po_2 gradient, worked backwards to see what was happening along the capillary.

Staub's forward integrations gave important results. They suggested that alveolar/end-capillary Po_2 gradients were very much smaller than had previously been thought, although papers by Asmussen and Nielsen (1960) and Thews (1961) had anticipated much of Staub's conclusion. The results of Staub's calculations are summarized in *Table 8.1*.

Importance of the capillary transit time. It is convenient at this point to stress the importance of the capillary transit time as a factor determining both the pulmonary end-capillary Po_2 and the diffusing capacity. It will be seen from *Figure 8.2a* that,

Table 8.1 Values for the alveolar/end-capillary P_{O_2} gradient suggested by the forward integration procedure of Staub (1963a)

Conditions	Capillary Transit time(s)	Alveolar/end-capillary P_{O_2} gradient	
		kPa	mmHg
Resting subject $\dot{V}_{O_2}$ = 270 ml/min)			
Breathing air ($P_{A_{O_2}}$ = 13.3 kPa = 100 mmHg)	0.760	0.000 000 001	0.000 000 01
Breathing low oxygen ($P_{A_{O_2}}$ = 6.3 kPa = 47 mm Hg)	0.636	0.03	0.2
Moderate exercise $\dot{V}_{O_2}$ = 1500 ml/min)			
Breathing low oxygen ($P_{A_{O_2}}$ = 7.3 kPa = 55 mm Hg)	0.476	0.5	4.0
Heavy exercise $\dot{V}_{O_2}$ = 3000 ml/min)			
Breathing air ($P_{A_{O_2}}$ = 16 kPa = 120 mmHg)	0.496	<0.000 1	<0.001
Breathing low oxygen ($P_{A_{O_2}}$ = 7.9 kPa = 59 mm Hg)	0.304	2.1	16.0

Abbreviations: $\dot{V}_{O_2}$, oxygen consumption; $P_{A_{O_2}}$, alveolar P_{O_2}.

if the capillary transit time is reduced below 0.2 second, there will be an appreciable gradient between the alveolar and end-capillary P_{O_2}. Other things being equal, this will result in hypoxaemia. Since the diffusion gradient from alveolar gas to mean pulmonary capillary blood will be increased (and perhaps the oxygen consumption reduced), the oxygen diffusing capacity must be less than it would be with a normal capillary transit time.

The mean pulmonary capillary transit time equals the pulmonary capillary blood volume divided by the pulmonary blood flow (approximately equal to cardiac output). This gives a normal time of the order of 0.8 second with a subject at rest. However, there appears to be a wide range of values on either side of the mean, and times as short as 0.1 second have been suggested (McHardy, 1972). Blood from capillaries with the shortest time will yield desaturated blood and this will not be compensated by blood from capillaries with longer than average transit times, since capillary P_{O_2} probably reaches its maximum in about 0.3 second. Therefore a wide spread of transit times will increase the alveolar/arterial P_{O_2} gradient. This effect is rather similar to that of the spread of $\dot{V}/\dot{Q}$ ratios shown in *Figure 7.13* and it may be described as due to a spread of D/$\dot{Q}$ ratios. The concept of spread of D/$\dot{Q}$ ratios as a potential cause of hypoxaemia was proposed in two important papers by Piiper, Haab and Rahn (1961) and Piiper (1961). It also applies, of course, to reduced diffusing capacity due to causes other than diminished capillary transit time.

Possible causes of a reduction in oxygen 'diffusing capacity'

At this stage it is helpful to consider the possible causes of a reduction in the value of the oxygen diffusing capacity as defined by the equation on page 189.

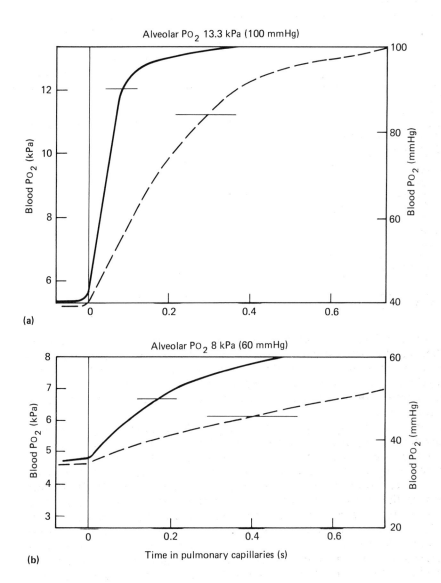

(a)

(b)

Figure 8.2 Each graph shows the rise in blood Po₂ as blood passes through the pulmonary capillaries. The horizontal line at the top of the graph indicates the alveolar Po₂ which the blood Po₂ is approaching. In (a) the patient is breathing air, while in (b) the patient is breathing about 14% oxygen. The broken curve shows the rise in Po₂ calculated according to the Bohr procedure on an assumed value for the alveolar/end-capillary Po₂ gradient. The continuous curve shows the values obtained by forward integration (Staub, 1963a). Horizontal bars indicate mean pulmonary capillary Po₂ calculated from each curve.

Decreased capillary transit time. In the section above, it has been explained how a reduction in capillary transit time may reduce the diffusing capacity. The mean transit time is reduced when the cardiac output is raised (as in anaemia or exercise), and the scatter of transit times may be increased in a number of diseases of the lungs.

The total area of the alveolar/capillary membrane may be reduced by any disease process or surgery which removes a substantial number of alveoli. In fact, occlusion of blood flow through one lung has little effect on the alveolar/arterial P_{O_2} difference in patients, even with pulmonary fibrosis (Staněk et al., 1967), but emphysema is thought to reduce the diffusing capacity mainly by destruction of alveolar septa.

A reduction in pulmonary capillary blood volume, sufficient to leave a substantial part of the lung unperfused, must reduce the diffusing capacity since the functioning interface is reduced in area.

Pulmonary congestion may reduce diffusing capacity by increasing the length of the diffusion pathway for oxygen within the pulmonary capillaries.

Severe maldistribution of ventilation relative to perfusion results in a physiological dysfunction which presents many of the features of a reduction in diffusing capacity. If, for example, most of the ventilation is distributed to the left lung and most of the pulmonary blood flow to the right lung, then the effective interface must be reduced. Minor degrees of maldistribution greatly complicate the interpretation of a reduced diffusing capacity, and a distinction between maldistribution and a true reduction of diffusing capacity cannot be made by simple means.

Alveolar/capillary block. At first sight, the most obvious cause of reduced diffusing capacity would seem to be an impediment at the alveolar/capillary membrane itself, which might either be thickened or else have its permeability to gas transfer reduced by some chemical abnormality. The term 'alveolar/capillary block' was introduced by Austrian et al. (1951) to describe a syndrome characterized by reduced lung volume, reasonably normal ventilatory capacity, hyperventilation and normal arterial P_{O_2} at rest, but with desaturation on exercise. A reduced diffusing capacity suggested an impermeability of the alveolar/capillary membrane, which was supported by the light microscopy appearance in such conditions as scleroderma, sarcoidosis, asbestosis, pulmonary fibrosis and pulmonary oedema. Evidence for such a condition at the magnification offered by electron microscopy has proved elusive. Elsewhere is described how interstitial pulmonary oedema tends to accumulate on the inactive side of the pulmonary capillary, leaving the active side relatively normal in appearance and thickness (page 16). This suggests that diffusion across the membrane should remain normal in spite of the presence of considerable pulmonary oedema. Something rather similar has been described for idiopathic interstitial pulmonary fibrosis (Hamman–Rich syndrome or fibrosing alveolitis). Electron microscopy showed that collagen was deposited on one side of the capillaries. Where capillaries were in contact with the alveolar membrane on the other (active) side of the capillary, the alveolar/capillary membrane was normal in appearance and thickness (Gracey, Divertie and Brown, 1968).

It will be seen that the oxygen-diffusing capacity may be influenced by many factors which are really nothing to do with diffusion *per se*. In fact, there is considerable doubt as to whether a true defect of diffusion (e.g. by a thickened alveolar/capillary membrane) is ever the limiting factor in transfer of oxygen from the inspired gas to the arterial blood. In view of these considerations, Cotes (1975) suggested that the term 'diffusing capacity' be abandoned and replaced by the term 'transfer factor' which implies that factors other than just diffusion may be involved. The symbol T may be used instead of D but the definition and methods of measurement remain the same. It is unfortunate that the term 'transfer factor' has an entirely different meaning in immunology.

The cause of hypoxaemia, previously thought to be due to alveolar/capillary block

The previous section suggests that a true impairment of diffusion is either never or seldom the limiting factor in the transfer of oxygen to the arterial blood. This must be reconciled with the fact that alveolar/capillary block is a well-recognized clinical entity, characterized by dyspnoea, hyperventilation (usually with reduced Po_2), cyanosis on exercise (if not at rest) and with radiological evidence of widespread involvement of the lungs by any of a wide variety of pathological processes. The syndrome is clearly distinguished from obstructive airway disease and the FEV/VC ratio is normal or only slightly reduced although the vital capacity itself may be substantially reduced. The syndrome of alveolar/capillary block may be due to a wide variety of diseases, including asbestosis, fibrosing alveolitis and alveolar cell carcinoma. Pulmonary fibrosis may have a known aetiology but otherwise is described as idiopathic interstitial fibrosis (fibrosing alveolitis or Hamman–Rich syndrome). Finally, interstitial pulmonary oedema presents a rather similar picture.

When doubts were cast on the validity of the classic concept of impaired diffusing capacity, Finley, Swenson and Comroe (1962) studied a group of patients previously diagnosed as having alveolar/capillary block and found that, in each case, the arterial hypoxaemia could be explained by disturbances of distribution without the need to invoke an alveolar/end-capillary Po_2 gradient.

A similar but more sophisticated study was carried out by Arndt, King and Briscoe (1970). They investigated 10 patients with the clinical syndrome of alveolar/capillary block. Arterial oxygenation was studied at different inspired oxygen concentrations and the results analysed in terms of a two-compartment lung model (see *Figure 2.6*). In 2 patients (alveolar cell carcinoma and idiopathic interstitial pulmonary fibrosis), hypoxaemia was present at rest while breathing air and could be explained by the existence of large shunts. In the next 4 patients (sarcoidosis, sarcoidosis with pulmonary fibrosis, desquamative interstitial pneumonia and eosinophilic granuloma), hypoxaemia could be explained in terms of the 'slow compartment' having a low V̇/Q̇ ratio (mean value 0.39) and yet sufficient perfusion (mean value 27 per cent of total pulmonary perfusion) to explain the hypoxaemia. This would correspond to a well-marked 'shelf' of the type shown for blood flow in *Figure 7.6a*. Arndt and his co-workers were then left with 4 patients (interstitial pulmonary oedema, sarcoidosis with pulmonary fibrosis and systemic sclerosis with pulmonary fibrosis) in whom there was no appreciable shunt and with identical V̇/Q̇ ratios in fast and slow alveolar compartments. Therefore, within the limits of their method of analysis, there were no demonstrable grounds for believing that maldistribution interfered with oxygenation of the arterial blood. In fact, this group had a mean arterial oxygen saturation of 96% when breathing air at rest, although this presumably fell during exercise. All 10 patients had severe reductions in their diffusing capacity (measured for carbon monoxide, see below), with gross reduction for the slow compartment. It would appear that this was the only remaining cause of desaturation on exercise in the last group of 4 patients.

Diffusion of carbon monoxide within the lungs

It has been explained above that the outstanding difficulty in the measurement of the oxygen diffusing capacity is derivation of the mean pulmonary capillary Po_2. Turning away from this intractable problem, it was reasonable to consider measuring the diffusing capacity of carbon monoxide as a substitute for oxygen, since the affinity of carbon monoxide for haemoglobin is so high that, for all practical purposes, the tension of the gas in the pulmonary capillary blood remains at zero throughout the usual procedures for measurement of the carbon monoxide diffusing capacity. The formula for calculation of this quantity then simplifies to the following:

$$\text{diffusing capacity for carbon monoxide} = \frac{\text{carbon monoxide uptake}}{\text{alveolar } P_{CO}}$$

(compare with equation for oxygen, page 189). The mean pulmonary capillary P_{CO} is deleted from the equation because it is effectively equal to zero. There are no insuperable difficulties in the measurement of either of the remaining quantities on the right-hand side of the equation, and the methods are outlined at the end of the chapter.

Measurement of the carbon monoxide diffusing capacity is firmly established as a valuable routine pulmonary function test which may show changes in a range of conditions in which other tests yield normal values. It does in fact provide an index which shows that something is wrong, and changes in the index provide a useful indication of progress of the disease. However, it is much more difficult to explain a reduced diffusing capacity for carbon monoxide in terms of the underlying physiology (see below).

The diffusion path for carbon monoxide

Diffusion of carbon monoxide within the alveolus, through the alveolar/capillary membrane and through the plasma is governed by the same factors which apply to oxygen and have been outlined above. The quantitative difference is due to the different vapour density and water solubility of the two gases. These factors indicate that the rate of diffusion of oxygen up to the point of entry into the erythrocyte is 1.23 times the corresponding rate for carbon monoxide.

Uptake of carbon monoxide by haemoglobin

At equilibrium the affinity of haemoglobin for carbon monoxide is about 250 times as great as for oxygen. Nevertheless, it does not follow that the rate of combination of carbon monoxide with haemoglobin is faster than the rate of combination of oxygen with haemoglobin; it is, in fact, rather slower (Forster, 1964a). The reaction is slower still when oxygen is displaced from oxyhaemoglobin according to the equation:

$$CO + HbO_2 \rightarrow O_2 + HbCO$$

Thus the reaction rate of carbon monoxide with haemoglobin is reduced when the oxygen saturation of the haemoglobin is high. The inhalation of different concentrations of oxygen thus causes changes in the reaction rate of carbon monoxide with the haemoglobin of a patient. Use has been made of this fact to study different components of the resistance to diffusion of carbon monoxide in man.

Quantification of the components of the resistance to difusion of carbon monoxide

When two resistances are arranged in series, the total resistance of the pair is equal to the sum of the two individual resistances. Diffusing capacity is analogous to conductance, which is the reciprocal of resistance. Therefore, when considering the diffusing capacity of a pair of structures in series, both of which offer resistance to diffusion, the reciprocal of the diffusing capacity of the total system equals the sum of the reciprocals of the diffusing capacities of the two components.

$$
\frac{1}{\text{total diffusing capacity for CO}} = \frac{1}{\substack{\text{diffusing capacity} \\ \text{of CO through the} \\ \text{alveolar/capillary} \\ \text{membrane}}} + \frac{1}{\substack{\text{'diffusing capacity'} \\ \text{of CO within the} \\ \text{erythrocyte}}}
$$

The second component on the right-hand side is not really a matter of diffusion, since the limiting factor to the passage of carbon monoxide within the erythrocyte is the rate of chemical combination with haemoglobin (exactly as in the case of oxygen). This 'diffusing capacity' within the erythrocyte is equal to the product of the pulmonary capillary blood volume (Vc) and the rate of reaction of carbon monoxide with haemoglobin (θco), a parameter which varies with the oxygen saturation of the haemoglobin. The equation may now be rewritten:

$$
\frac{1}{\text{total diffusing capacity for CO}} = \frac{1}{\substack{\text{diffusing capacity} \\ \text{of CO through the} \\ \text{alveolar/capillary} \\ \text{membrane}}} + \frac{1}{\substack{\text{pulmonary} \\ \text{capillary} \\ \text{blood} \\ \text{volume}} \times \substack{\text{reaction rate} \\ \text{of CO with} \\ \text{haemogloblin}}}
$$

The usual symbols for representation of this equation are as follows:

$$
\frac{1}{D_{L_{CO}}} = \frac{1}{D_{M_{CO}}} + \frac{1}{V_c \times \theta_{CO}}
$$

The term $D_{M_{CO}}$ equals 0.80 $D_{M_{O_2}}$ under similar conditions (*Table 8.2*).

The total diffusing capacity for carbon monoxide may be readily measured by the techniques outlined at the end of this chapter; θco may be determined, at different values of oxygen saturation, by *in vitro* studies. This leaves two unknowns—the diffusing capacity through the alveolar/capillary membrane and the pulmonary capillary blood volume. By repeating the measurement of total diffusing capacity at different values of θco (obtained by inhaling different concentrations of oxygen and so varying the oxygen saturation of the haemoglobin), it is possible

Table 8.2 The influence of physical properties on the diffusion of gases through a gas/liquid interface

Gas	Density relative to oxygen	Water solubility relative to oxygen	Diffusing capacity relative to oxygen
Oxygen	1.00	1.00	1.00
Carbon monoxide	0.88	0.75	0.80
Nitrogen	0.88	0.515	0.55
Carbon dioxide	1.37	24.0	20.5
Nitrous oxide	1.37	16.3	14.0
Helium	0.125	0.37	1.05
Ether	2.30	580	380
Halothane	5.07	27.3	12.1

to obtain two simultaneous equations with two unknowns. It is then possible to solve and derive values for the following.

1. Total diffusing capacity of carbon monoxide at different levels of oxygenation of the blood.
2. Diffusing capacity of the alveolar/capillary membrane (presumably independent of oxygenation).
3. Pulmonary capillary blood volume.
4. The 'diffusing capacity' of carbon monoxide within the erythrocyte at different values of oxygen saturation.

This elegant approach was introduced by Roughton and Forster (1957). Although the original data appeared to undergo an unreasonable amount of manipulation, confidence in the whole operation is engendered by the observed fact that the total diffusing capacity of carbon monoxide is undoubtedly reduced by the inhalation of high concentrations of oxygen. Furthermore, the change occurs very quickly and it would be unreasonable to expect that it was due to changes in the alveolar/capillary membrane. The technique yields normal values for pulmonary capillary blood volume within the range 60–110 ml. These appear astonishingly small, but morphometric studies by Weibel (1962) indicated a value of about 100 ml at a lung volume of 2.5 litres. This approximates to the functional residual capacity of the human lung in the supine position.

Normal values obtained by various methods of measurement of the carbon monoxide diffusing capacity were collected by Forster (1964b) as shown in *Table 8.3*.

Interpretation of the carbon monoxide diffusing capacity

Factors which may affect the oxygen diffusing capacity have been described above. Similar considerations apply to the carbon monoxide diffusing capacity and it will be clear that a low value does not necessarily imply a thickened impermeable alveolar/capillary membrane. It does, in fact, indicate that there is an impediment to gas transfer from inspired gas to arterial blood other than hypoventilation. In some cases, it will be clear that the reduced 'diffusing capacity' (or 'transfer factor') is due to a shunt or to well-perfused areas of low V̇/Q̇ ratio (see above). However, the present consensus of opinion is that there remain some patients in whom the main defect of oxygen transfer cannot be explained by maldistribution and in whom

Table 8.3 Values obtained by various methods of measurement of diffusing capacity (transfer factor) of carbon monoxide

Technique of measurement	Total diffusing capacity for CO		Membrane component of diffusing capacity		Pulmonary capillary blood volume
	$ml\ min^{-1}\ kPa^{-1}$	$ml/min/mm$ Hg	$ml\ min^{-1}\ kPa^{-1}$	$ml/min/mm$ Hg	(ml)
Steady state	113	15	195	26	73
Single breath	225	30	428	57	79
Rebreathing	203	27	300	40	110

(Data from Forster, 1964b)

it is probably reasonable to believe that it is due to a diffusion defect or perhaps to an abnormally wide scatter of diffusion/perfusion ratios. Even this does not mean that the patient has a thickened impermeable membrane. For reasons given above, the defect may be due to short capillary transit time or to excessive destruction of the alveolar/capillary membrane. The effective area of the membrane may also be reduced by pulmonary hypoperfusion.

In spite of these uncertainties, the carbon monoxide diffusing capacity remains a valuable diagnostic aid. It has the advantage of being sensitive. It may show changes long before these are reflected in altered blood gas values or other simple tests of pulmonary function. Apart from some measures of alveolar/capillary permeability (see below), it is, in fact, the most sensitive test of function which is generally available. The test also provides a most useful numerical index which may be observed during the course of a disease as a guide to deterioration or response to treatment, even if the physiological basis of the index is not precisely known. It is most useful in patients with the alveolar/capillary block syndrome (see above).

Certain non-pathological factors influence diffusing capacity, as follows.

Body size influences diffusing capacity directly. This is inevitable since alveolar/ capillary gas tension gradients are not greatly different in different species or in different-sized individuals while, of course, gas exchange volumes are related to body size.

Lung volume. Diffusing capacity is markedly increased when the lung volume is increased (Gurtner and Fowler, 1971).

Exercise results in an increase in diffusing capacity (Chapter 12) and it has been suggested that the increase proceeds to a plateau value which is known as the maximal diffusing capacity (Riley et al., 1954).

Age results in a diminution of both the diffusing capacity and the maximal diffusing capacity.

Posture. Diffusing capacity is substantially increased when the subject is supine rather than standing or sitting (Ogilvie et al., 1957). This change is explained in part by the increase in pulmonary blood volume, and the improvement in the uniformity of distribution of perfusion of the lungs.

Diffusion of carbon dioxide within the lungs

Carbon dioxide has a much higher water solubility than oxygen and, although its vapour density is greater, it may be calculated to penetrate an aqueous membrane about 20 times as rapidly as oxygen. Thus it was formerly believed that diffusion problems could not exist for carbon dioxide because the patient would have succumbed from hypoxia before hypercapnia could attain measurable proportions. All of this ignored the fact that chemical reactions of the respiratory gases were sufficiently slow to limit the rate of diffusion. Attention was therefore turned to the rate of release of carbon dioxide from its chemical combination in the pulmonary arterial blood.

The carriage of carbon dioxide in the blood is discussed in Chapter 9, but for the moment it is sufficient to say that the essential reactions in the release of all but dissolved carbon dioxide in the pulmonary capillaries are as follows:

1. Release of some carbon dioxide from carbamino carriage.
2. Conversion of bicarbonate ions to carbonic acid followed by dehydration to release molecular carbon dioxide.

The latter reaction involves the movement of bicarbonate ions across the erythrocyte membrane (Hamburger effect) but its rate is probably limited by the dehydration of carbonic acid. This reaction would be very slow indeed if it were not catalysed by carbonic anhydrase which is present in abundance in the erythrocyte. The important limiting role of the rate of this reaction was elegantly shown in a study by Cain and Otis (1961) of the effect of inhibition of carbonic anhydrase on carbon dioxide transport. This resulted in a large increase in the arterial/alveolar P_{CO_2} gradient, corresponding to a gross decrease in the apparent 'diffusing capacity' of carbon dioxide.

Equilibrium of carbon dioxide is probably very nearly complete within the normal pulmonary capillary transit time. However, even if it were not so, it would be of little significance since the mixed venous/alveolar P_{CO_2} difference is itself quite small (about 0.8 kPa or 6 mmHg). Therefore an end-gradient as large as 20 per cent of the initial difference would still be too small to be of any importance and, indeed, could hardly be measured by modern analytical methods.

Hypercapnia is, in fact, never caused by decreased 'diffusing capacity' except when carbonic anhydrase is inhibited by drugs such as acetazolamide (Diamox). Pathological hypercapnia may always be explained by other causes, usually an alveolar ventilation which is inadequate for the metabolic rate of the patient.

The assumption that there is no measurable difference between the P_{CO_2} of the alveolar gas and the pulmonary end-capillary blood is used when the alveolar P_{CO_2} is assumed equal to the arterial P_{CO_2}. The assumption is also made that there is no measurable difference beween end-capillary and arterial P_{CO_2}. We have seen in the previous chapter (page 170) that this is only partly true and a large shunt will cause an arterial/end-capillary P_{CO_2} gradient of up to 1 kPa.

Diffusion of 'inert' gases within the lungs

In the biological sense, inert gases are those which do not undergo chemical changes within the body. This definition includes nitrogen, helium and, for practical purposes, most of the anaesthetic gases and vapours. Diffusion of these gases is as important to the diver as it is to the anaesthetist, and is an essential consideration in the pharmacokinetics of the inhalational anaesthetic agents.

Since these substances are carried in the blood by purely physical means, their diffusing capacity consists only of the membrane component and there is no limitation due to chemical reaction as in the case of oxygen, carbon monoxide and carbon dioxide. Their diffusing capacities are therefore governed primarily by their water solubilities, and the diffusing capacities of the anaesthetic agents are all very much higher than for oxygen. Gases and vapours with high molecular weight, such as chloroform, halothane and methoxyflurane, have a high vapour density, but the effect of this is more than offset by their water solubility which is also very high and influences the diffusing capacity in direct proportion. Vapour density only affects diffusing capacity inversely according to its square root, so its influence is relatively unimportant. Physical properties influencing diffusing capacity are set out in *Table 8.2*.

Diffusion of gases in the tissues

In the case of oxygen there is a series of tension gradients from ambient air to the mitochondria of the cells, the site of oxygen consumption and the point at which the P_{O_2} is lowest (page 242). The series of tension gradients for carbon dioxide is in the reverse direction, with the highest values in the mitochondria and the lowest in ambient air.

During induction, anaesthetic gases and vapours diffuse outwards from the capillaries until the tissues reach tension-equilibrium with the incoming blood. During recovery, gases and vapours leave the tissues until zero tension is attained.

Oxygen

Oxygen leaves the systemic capillaries by the reverse of the process by which it entered the pulmonary capillaries. After leaving the tissue capillaries, oxygen passes to its site of utilization in the mitochondria by diffusion, although possibly aided by protoplasmic streaming.

Diffusion paths are much longer in tissues than in the parenchyma of the lung. In well-vascularized tissue, such as brain, each capillary serves a zone of radius about 20 μm, but the corresponding distance is about 200 μm in skeletal muscle and greater still in fat and cartilage.

It is impracticable to talk about mean tissue P_{O_2} since this varies from one organ to another and must also depend on perfusion in relation to metabolic activity. Furthermore, within an organ there must be some cells occupying more favourable sites towards the arterial ends of capillaries, while others must be content with accepting oxygen from the venous ends of the capillaries where the P_{O_2} is lower. This is well demonstrated in the liver where the centrilobular cells must exist at a lower P_{O_2} than their fellows at the periphery of the lobule. Even within a single cell, there is no uniformity of P_{O_2}. Not only are there 'low spots' around the mitochondria, but those mitochondria nearest to the capillaries presumably enjoy a higher P_{O_2} than those lying further away.

Figure 8.3 shows a model in which an area of tissue is perfused by three parallel capillaries. Vertical height indicates P_{O_2} which falls exponentially along the line of the capillaries, with troughs lying in between the capillaries. Five 'low spots'

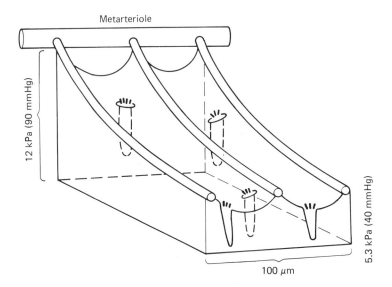

Figure 8.3 Diagrammatic representation of P_{O_2} within the tissues. The vertical axis represents the actual P_{O_2}; in the horizontal plane is represented the course of three parallel capillaries from the metarteriole to the point of entry into the venule (not shown). The P_{O_2} falls exponentially along the course of each capillary with a trough of P_{O_2} between the capillaries. The pits represent the low spots of P_{O_2} from about 12 kPa (90 mmHg) in the tissue close to the arterial end of the capillaries down to less than 1 kPa at the mitochondria near the venous end of the capillaries. This is the simplest of many possible models of tissue perfusion.

corresponding to mitochondria are shown. This diagram makes no pretence to histological accuracy but merely illustrates the difficulty of talking about the 'mean tissue P_{O_2}' which is not an entity like the arterial or mixed venous P_{O_2}.

There is uncertainty about the actual P_{O_2} within a mitochondrion. It is known that oxidative phosphorylation will continue down to a P_{O_2} of about 0.13 kPa (1 mmHg) (page 241), and some mitochondria may habitually operate at this level. Others, particularly those close to the arterial end of the capillaries, may have a much higher P_{O_2}.

Carbon dioxide

Little is known about the magnitude of carbon dioxide gradients between the mitochondria and the tissue capillaries. It is, however, thought that the tissue/venous P_{CO_2} gradient can be increased by two methods. The first is by inhibition of carbonic anhydrase which blocks the uptake of carbon dioxide by the blood. The second is by hyperoxygenation of the arterial blood caused by breathing 100% oxygen at high pressures. If the P_{O_2} of the arterial blood exceeds about 300 kPa (2250 mmHg), the dissolved oxygen will be sufficient for the usual tissue requirements. Therefore no significant amount of oxyhaemoglobin will be dissociated and reduced haemoglobin is not available for the carbamino carriage of carbon dioxide, for which it is more efficient than oxyhaemoglobin. This results in partial blocking of the uptake of carbon dioxide by the blood. This theory was advanced by Gessell (1923) as an explanation of the cause of oxygen convulsions.

However, it seems likely that the alternative method of carbon dioxide carriage as bicarbonate would be able to function quite adequately in the absence of the facilitated carbamino carriage. There are alternative explanations of oxygen convulsions (page 491).

Inert gases and anaesthetic agents

Inert gases will ultimately attain equilibrium in the tissues because, unlike oxygen, they are not constantly being consumed which must result in permanent tension gradients. The rate of attaining equilibrium with inert gases depends upon the perfusion of the tissue relative to its bulk and the solubility of the agent in the tissue. There is an important distinction between well-perfused and poorly perfused tissues. The former are those tissues in which all parts of the cells come into rapid equilibrium with the inert gas carried in the arterial blood, so that the tension of the gas in blood leaving the tissue may be considered equal to the mean tension of the gas in the tissue. Well-perfused tissues include brain, heart and liver. Poorly perfused tissues are those in which inert gases tend to diffuse slowly, forming tension gradients in the form of the cylinders and cones which were considered in the case of oxygen, above. Less well perfused tissues include fat, cartilage and, to a certain extent, resting muscle. The practical importance is that the tension of the gas in the venous blood draining the tissue does not give a representative value for the mean tissue tension, being higher during loading and lower during unloading of the agent. This greatly complicates measurement of exchange and also theoretical consideration of long-term changes in tissue levels. Appreciation of this problem has been of the greatest importance in establishing techniques for avoidance of the 'bends' after prolonged dives.

Alveolar/capillary permeability

The alveolar epithelium and the capillary endothelium have a very high permeability to water, most gases, alcohol and lipophilic substances such as the tracer antipyrene. However, for many hydrophilic substances of larger molecular diameter and for molecules carrying a charge, there is an effective barrier. Passage of these substances is mainly through the gaps between the cells and must be considered separately for epithelium and endothelium. It was explained in Chapter 1 (page 17) that the alveolar epithelial type I cells have very tight junctions, effectively limiting the molecular radius to about 0.6 nm. Endothelial junctions are much larger, with gaps of the order of 4–6 nm.

Passage of solutes across the alveolar/capillary membrane is usually quantified as in terms of the half-time of clearance or, alternatively, as the fractional clearance per minute, the one parameter being related to the reciprocal of the other. Clearance from the alveoli (i.e. across the epithelium) bears an approximate inverse relationship to the molecular weight (Effros and Mason, 1983). Urea (60 daltons) has a clearance of the order of 0.07/min, while for sucrose (342 daltons) the corresponding figure is 0.003/min and for albumin (64 000 daltons) is of the order of 0.0001/min. All of these clearances may be greatly increased if the alveolar epithelium is damaged, as in the permeability type of pulmonary oedema (page 435).

A useful tracer molecule is ^{99m}Tc DTPA (diethylene triamine penta-acetate) with a molecular weight of 492 daltons (Jones, Royston and Minty, 1983). After being aerosolized into the lungs, its concentration can be continuously measured over the lung fields *in vivo* by detection of its gamma emission. In the healthy non-smoker the clearance is very slow, about 0.01/min (half-time about 1 hour).The clearance is dramatically increased in many different types of pulmonary damage—including, for example, smoking, in which there is a threefold increase. It is, in fact, the very sensitivity of this test which limits its value.

Electrolytes such as sodium ions can cross the epithelial barrier fairly freely but the rate of passage is governed by concentration gradients. Thus, isotonic sodium solutions are cleared from the alveoli more quickly than hypertonic solutions (Efros and Mason, 1983).

In effect, the normal alveolar epithelium is almost totally impermeable to protein and small solutes, the half-time for turnover of albumin between plasma and the alveolar compartment being of the order of 36 hours (Staub, 1983).

The microvascular endothelium with its larger intercellular gaps, is far more permeable for all molecular sizes and there is normally an appreciable leak of protein. Thus the concentration of albumin in pulmonary lymph is about half the concentration in plasma and may increase to approximate the plasma concentration in conditions of damaged alveolar/capillary permeability (Staub, 1984). This problem is discussed further in relation to pulmonary oedema in Chapter 23 (pages 435 et seq.).

It should be noted that many lung diseases tend to decrease the carbon monoxide diffusing capacity, while the commonest pathological change in alveolar/capillary permeability is an increase.

Principles of methods of measurement of carbon monoxide diffusing capacity

All the methods are based on the general equation:

$$D_{CO} = \frac{\dot{V}_{CO}}{P_{A_{CO}} - P_{\bar{c}_{CO}}}$$

In each case it is usual to assume that the mean tension of carbon monoxide in the pulmonary capillary blood ($P_{\bar{c}_{CO}}$) is effectively zero. It is, therefore, only necessary to measure the carbon monoxide uptake ($\dot{V}_{CO}$), and the alveolar carbon monoxide tension ($P_{A_{CO}}$). The diffusing capacity indicated (D_{CO}) is the total diffusing capacity including that of the alveolar capillary membrane and the component due to the reaction of carbon monoxide with haemoglobin.

The steady state method

The subject breathes a gas mixture containing about 0.3% carbon monoxide for about a minute. After this time, expired gas is collected when the alveolar P_{CO} is steady but the mixed venous P_{CO} has not yet reached a level high enough to require consideration in the calculation.

The carbon monoxide uptake ($\dot{V}_{CO}$) is measured in exactly the same way as oxygen consumption by the open method (page 282): the amount of carbon monoxide expired ($\dot{V}E \times F\bar{E}_{CO}$) is subtracted from the amount of carbon monoxide inspired ($\dot{V}I \times F_{ICO}$). The alveolar P_{CO} is calculated from the form of the alveolar air equation derived by Filley, MacIntosh and Wright (1954):

$$P_{ACO} = P_{ICO} - P_{ACO_2} \left(\frac{F_{ICO} - F\bar{E}_{CO}}{F\bar{E}_{CO_2}} \right)$$

Rewritten for oxygen, this equation has proved of great value for the calculation of the alveolar P_{O_2} under the circumstances of general anaesthesia, and is discussed in Chapter 7 (page 183).

Measurement of inspiratory and expiratory carbon monoxide and expiratory carbon dioxide concentrations presents no serious difficulty, and infrared analysis has proved satisfactory. Alveolar P_{CO_2} may be determined by sampling arterial blood and assuming that the alveolar P_{CO_2} is equal to the arterial P_{CO_2}. This is not strictly true in the presence of maldistribution. As an alternative, some workers measure the end-expiratory P_{CO_2} but neither does this equal the arterial P_{CO_2} in the presence of maldistribution (page 232). Finally, it is possible to derive the alveolar P_{CO_2} from the mixed venous P_{CO_2} by the rebreathing technique, assuming a reasonable value for the mixed venous/alveolar P_{CO_2} difference (page 233).

The single-breath method

This method has a long history of progressive refinement. The patient is first required to exhale maximally. He then draws in a vital-capacity breath of a gas mixture containing about 0.3% carbon monoxide and about 10% helium. The breath is held for 10 seconds and a gas sample is then taken after the exhalation of the first 0.75 litre, which is sufficient to wash out the patient's dead space. The breath-holding time is sufficient to overcome maldistribution of the inspired gas.

It is assumed that no significant amount of helium has passed into the blood and, therefore, the ratio of the concentration of helium in the inspired gas to the concentration in the end-expiratory gas, multiplied by the volume of gas drawn into the alveoli during the maximal inspiration, will indicate the total alveolar volume during the period of breath holding. The alveolar P_{CO} at the commencement of breath holding is equal to the same ratio multiplied by the P_{CO} of the inspired gas mixture. The end-expiratory P_{CO} is measured directly.

From these data, together with the time of breath holding, it is possible to calculate the carbon monoxide uptake and the mean alveolar P_{CO}. A neat mathematical solution is available, and the interested reader is referred to Cotes (1975). Methodology has been discussed in detail by Bates, Macklem and Christie (1971).

The rebreathing method

Somewhat similar to the single-breath method is the rebreathing method by which a gas mixture containing about 0.3% carbon monoxide and 10% helium is rebreathed rapidly from a rubber bag. The bag and the patient's lungs are considered as a single system, with gas exchange occurring in very much the same way as during breath holding. The calculation proceeds in a similar way to that for the single-breath method.

Measurement of oxygen-diffusing capacity

For reasons which were developed in this chapter, it now appears that the measurement of oxygen-diffusing capacity is based on assumptions which can no longer be considered valid. Therefore, the method is not described here but, for historical purposes, reference may be made to Comroe et al. (1962).

Measurement of alveolar/capillary permeability

Reference has been made above to the use of ^{99m}Tc DPTA described by Jones, Royston and Minty (1983).

Chapter 9

Carbon dioxide

Carbon dioxide is the end-product of aerobic metabolism. It is produced in the cells and almost entirely in the mitochondria where the P_{CO_2} is highest. From its point of origin there are a series of tension gradients as carbon dioxide passes through the cytoplasm, and the extracellular fluid into the blood. In the lungs the P_{CO_2} of the blood entering the pulmonary capillaries is higher than the alveolar P_{CO_2}, and therefore carbon dioxide diffuses from the blood into the alveolar gas. Carbon dioxide finally passes into the expired air where it mixes with the ambient air.

Abnormal levels of carbon dioxide have important physiological effects throughout the body. There are many clinical situations in which the P_{CO_2} must be maintained at the optimal level.

Carriage of carbon dioxide in blood

In physical solution

Carbon dioxide belongs to the group of gases with moderate solubility in water. This group includes many of the anaesthetic gases, and the solubility of carbon dioxide is rather greater than that of nitrous oxide. According to Henry's law of solubility:

$$P_{CO_2} \times \text{solubility coefficient} = CO_2 \text{ concentration in solution} \quad \ldots (1)$$

The solubility coefficient of carbon dioxide (α) is expressed in units of mmol l^{-1} kPa^{-1} (or mmol/l/mmHg). The value depends on temperature, and values are listed in *Table 9.1*. The contribution of dissolved carbon dioxide to the total carriage of the gas in blood is shown in *Table 9.2*.

As carbonic acid

In solution, carbon dioxide hydrates to form carbonic acid:

$$CO_2 + H_2O \rightleftharpoons H_2CO_3 \quad \ldots (2)$$

The equilibrium of this reaction is far to the left under physiological conditions. Published work shows some disagreement on the value of the equilibrium constant, but it seems likely that less than 1 per cent of the molecules of carbon dioxide are in the hydrated form. It should be mentioned that there is a rather misleading

Table 9.1 Values for solubility of carbon dioxide in plasma and for pK' at different temperatures

Temperature (°C)	Solubility of CO_2 in plasma		pK'		
	$mmol\ l^{-1}\ kPa^{-1}$	$mmol/l/mmHg$	at pH 7.6	at pH 7.4	at pH 7.2
40	0.216	0.0288	6.07	6.08	6.09
39	0.221	0.0294	6.07	6.08	6.09
38	0.226	0.0301	6.08	6.09	6.10
37	0.231	0.0308	6.08	6.09	6.10
36	0.236	0.0315	6.09	6.10	6.11
35	0.242	0.0322	6.10	6.11	6.12
33	0.253	0.0337	6.10	6.11	6.12
30	0.272	0.0362	6.12	6.13	6.14
25	0.310	0.0413	6.15	6.16	6.17
20	0.359	0.0478	6.17	6.19	6.20
15	0.416	0.0554	6.20	6.21	6.23

(Values from Severinghaus, Stupfel and Bradley, 1956a, b)

Table 9.2 Normal values for carbon dioxide carriage in blood

	Arterial blood (Hb 95% sat.)	Mixed venous blood (Hb 70% sat.)	Arterial/venous difference
Whole blood			
pH	7.40	7.367	−0.033
P_{CO_2} (kPa)	5.3	6.1	+0.8
(mmHg)	40.0	46.0	+6.0
Total CO_2 (mmol/l)	21.5	23.3	+1.8
(ml/l)	48.0	52.0	+4.0
Plasma (mmol/l)			
Dissolved CO_2	1.2	1.4	+0.2
Carbonic acid	0.0017	0.0020	+0.0003
Bicarbonate ion	24.4	26.2	+1.8
Carbamino CO_2	Negligible	Negligible	Negligible
Total	25.6	27.6	+2.0
Erythrocyte fraction of 1 litre of blood			
Dissolved CO_2	0.44	0.51	+0.07
Bicarbonate ion	5.88	5.92	+0.04
Carbamino CO_2	1.10	1.70	+0.60
Plasma fraction of 1 litre of blood			
Dissolved CO_2	0.66	0.76	+0.10
Bicarbonate ion	13.42	14.41	+0.99
Total in 1 litre of blood (mmol/l)	21.50	23.30	+1.80

These values have not been drawn from a single publication but represent the mean of values reported in a large number of studies.

medical convention by which both forms of carbon dioxide in equation (2) are sometimes shown as carbonic acid. Thus the term H_2CO_3 may, in some situations, mean the total concentrations of dissolved CO_2 and H_2CO_3 and, to avoid confusion, it is preferable to use αP_{CO_2} as in equation (7) below. This does not apply to equations (4) and (5) below, where H_2CO_3 has its correct meaning.

It would be theoretically more correct to indicate the thermodynamic activities rather than concentrations, the two quantities being related as follows:

$$\frac{\text{activity}}{\text{concentration}} = \text{activity coefficient}$$

At infinite dilution the activity coefficient is unity, but in physiological concentrations it is significantly less than unity. In practice it is usual to work in concentrations, and values for the various equilibrium constants are adjusted accordingly, as indicated by a prime after the symbol thus—K'. This is one of the reasons why these 'constants' are not in fact constant but should be considered as parameters which vary slightly under physiological conditions.

The reaction of carbon dioxide with water (equation 2) is non-ionic and slow, requiring a period of minutes for equilibrium to be attained. This would be far too long for the time available for gas exchange in pulmonary and systemic capillaries were the reaction not speeded up enormously in both directions by the enzyme carbonic anhydrase which is present in erythrocytes but not in plasma. In addition to its role in the respiratory transport of carbon dioxide, this enzyme is concerned with the transfer and accumulation of hydrogen and bicarbonate ions in secretory organs including the kidney.

Carbonic anhydrase is a zinc-containing enzyme of low molecular weight, discovered by Meldrum and Roughton (1933). It is inhibited by a large number of unsubstituted sulphonamides (general formula $R-SO_2NH_2$). Sulphonilamide is an active inhibitor but the later antibacterial sulphonilamides are substituted ($R-SO_2NHR'$), and therefore inactive. Other active sulphonamides include the thiazide diuretics and various heterocyclic sulphonamides, of which acetazolamide is the most important. This drug produces complete inhibition at 5–20 mg/kg in all organs and has no other pharmacological effects of importance. Acetazolamide has been much used in the study of carbonic anhydrase and has revealed the surprising fact that it is not essential to life. With total inhibition, P_{CO_2} gradients between tissues and alveolar gas are increased. Pulmonary ventilation is increased and alveolar P_{CO_2} is decreased. The serious student is referred to the important review of carbonic anhydrase by Maren (1967).

As bicarbonate ion

The largest fraction of carbon dioxide in the blood is in the form of bicarbonate ion which is formed by ionization of carbonic acid:

$$H_2CO_3 \rightleftharpoons H^+ + HCO_3^- \rightleftharpoons 2H^+ + CO_3^{2-} \qquad \ldots (3)$$

first
dissociation
second
dissociation

The second dissociation occurs only at high pH (above 9) and is not a factor in the carriage of carbon dioxide by the blood. The first dissociation is, however, of the greatest importance within the physiological range. The pK'_1 is about 6.1 and carbonic acid is about 96 per cent dissociated under physiological conditions (Morris, 1968).

According to the law of mass action:

$$\frac{[H^+] \times [HCO_3^-]}{[H_2CO_3]} = K_1' \qquad \ldots (4)$$

where K'_1 is the equilibrium constant of the first dissociation. The subscript 1 indicates that it is the first dissociation, and the prime indicates that we are dealing with concentrations rather than the more correct activities.

Rearrangement of equation (4) gives the following:

$$[H^+] = K_1' \frac{[H_2CO_3]}{[HCO_3^-]} \qquad \ldots (5)$$

The left-hand side is the hydrogen ion concentration, and this equation is the non-logarithmic form of the Henderson–Hasselbalch equation (Henderson, 1909). The concentration of carbonic acid cannot be measured and the equation may be modified by replacing this term with the total concentration of dissolved CO_2 and H_2CO_3, most conveniently quantified as αP_{CO_2} as described above. The equation now takes the form:

$$[H^+] = K' \frac{\alpha P_{CO_2}}{[HCO_3^-]} \qquad \ldots (6)$$

The new constant K' is the *apparent* first dissociation constant of carbonic acid and includes a factor which allows for the substitution of total dissolved carbon dioxide concentration for carbonic acid.

The equation is now in a useful form and permits the direct relation of plasma hydrogen ion concentration, P_{CO_2} and bicarbonate concentration, all quantities which can be measured. The value of K' cannot be derived theoretically and is determined experimentally by simultaneous measurements of the three variables. Under normal physiological conditions, if $[H^+]$ is in nmol/l, P_{CO_2} in kPa, and HCO_3 in nmol/l, the value of the combined parameter $(\alpha K')$ is about 180. If P_{CO_2} is in mmHg, the value of the parameter is 24. This equation is very simple to use and was strongly recommended by Campbell (1962).

Those who prefer to use the pH scale may follow the approach of Hasselbalch (1916) and take logarithms of the reciprocal of each term in equation (6) with the following familiar result:

$$pH = pK' + \log \frac{[HCO_3^-]}{\alpha P_{CO_2}} = pK' + \log \frac{[CO_2] - \alpha P_{CO_2}}{\alpha P_{CO_2}} \qquad \ldots (7)$$

where pK' has an experimentally derived value of the order of 6.1, but variable with temperature and pH (see *Table 9.1*). '$[CO_2]$' refers to the total concentration of carbon dioxide in all forms (dissolved CO_2, H_2CO_3 and bicarbonate) as indicated by Van Slyke analysis.

It is sometimes useful to clear equation (7) for P_{CO_2}:

$$P_{CO_2} = \frac{[CO_2]}{\alpha\{\text{antilog (pH} - pK') + 1\}} \qquad \ldots (8)$$

It is important to remember that $[CO_2]$ refers to the carbon dioxide concentration in plasma and not in whole blood.

Carbamino carriage

Amino groups have the ability to combine directly with carbon dioxide thus:

$$\overset{\overset{\displaystyle H}{\displaystyle |}}{R-N-H} + CO_2 \rightleftharpoons \overset{\overset{\displaystyle H}{\displaystyle |}}{R-N}-\underset{\underset{\displaystyle O}{\displaystyle ||}}{C}-OH \rightleftharpoons \overset{\overset{\displaystyle H}{\displaystyle |}}{R-N}-\underset{\underset{\displaystyle O}{\displaystyle ||}}{C}-O^- + H^+$$

In a protein, the amino groups involved in the peptide linkages between amino acid residues cannot combine with carbon dioxide. Carbamino carriage is therefore restricted to the one terminal amino group in each protein and to the side chain amino groups in lysine and arginine. The terminal amino groups are the most effective at physiological pH, and one binding site per protein monomer is more than sufficient to account for the quantity of carbon dioxide carried as a carbamino compound.

Only very small quantities of carbon dioxide are carried in carbamino compounds with plasma protein. Almost all is carried by haemoglobin, and reduced haemoglobin is about 3.5 times as effective as oxyhaemoglobin (*Figure 9.1*). The actual P_{CO_2} has very little effect upon the quantity of carbon dioxide carried in this manner, throughout the physiological range of P_{CO_2} (Ferguson, 1936).

The Haldane effect. Although the amount of carbon dioxide carried in the blood in carbamino carriage is small (see *Table 9.2*), the *difference* between the amount carried in venous and arterial blood is about a third of the total arterial/venous difference. This accounts for the major part of the Haldane effect, which is the difference in the quantity of carbon dioxide carried, at constant P_{CO_2}, in oxygenated and reduced blood (*Figure 9.2*). The remainder of the effect is due to the increased buffering capacity of reduced haemoglobin, which is discussed below. It is interesting to recall that when the Haldane effect was described by Christiansen, Douglas and Haldane (1914) they believed that the whole effect was due to altered buffering capacity: carbamino carriage was not proved until much later (Ferguson and Roughton, 1934).

Formation of carbamino compounds does not require the dissolved carbon dioxide to be hydrated and so is independent of carbonic anhydrase. The reaction is very rapid and would be of particular importance in a patient who had received a carbonic anhydrase inhibitor. The arterial/venous difference in carbamino carriage is lost in certain regions of the body when a patient inhales 100% oxygen at a pressure of about 3 atmospheres absolute (ATA), since the oxygen dissolved in the

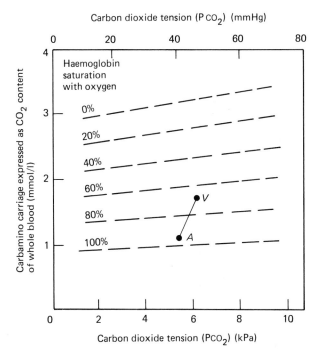

Figure 9.1 The broken lines on the graph indicate the carbamino carriage of carbon dioxide at different levels of saturation of haemoglobin with oxygen (15 g Hb/dl blood). It will be seen that this has a far greater influence on carbamino carriage than the actual P_{CO_2} (abscissa). A represents arterial blood (95% saturation and P_{CO_2} 5.3 kPa or 40 mmHg); V represents mixed venous blood (70% saturation and P_{CO_2} 6.1 kPa or 46 mmHg). Note that the arterial/venous difference in carbamino carriage is large in relation to the actual level of carbamino carriage, and accounts for about a third of the total arterial/venous blood CO_2 content difference (see Table 9.2). (These values have not been drawn from a single publication but present the mean of values reported from a number of studies.)

arterial blood is then sufficient for metabolic requirements and very little reduced haemoglobin appears in the venous blood.

Gessell (1923) suggested that the loss of the arterial/venous difference in carbamino carriage of carbon dioxide under these conditions resulted in tissue retention of carbon dioxide, and was a major factor in the cerebral toxic effects produced by high tensions of oxygen (page 491). It is, however, unlikely that this would cause a rise of tissue P_{CO_2} greater than 1 kPa (7.5 mmHg), and it is known that such a rise can be tolerated without any of the symptoms characteristic of oxygen toxicity. Furthermore, administration of carbonic anhydrase inhibitors does not produce a condition resembling oxygen toxicity.

Carbamino carriage has been reviewed by Roughton (1964) and Kilmartin and Rossi-Bernardi (1973).

Effect of buffering power of proteins on carbon dioxide carriage

Amino and carboxyl groups concerned in peptide linkages have no buffering power. Neither have most side chain groups (e.g. in lysine and glutamic acid) since their

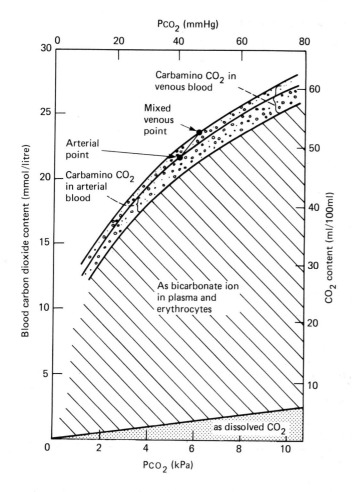

Figure 9.2 Components of the carbon dioxide dissociation curve for whole blood. Dissolved CO$_2$ and bicarbonate ion vary with P$_{CO_2}$ but are little affected by the state of oxygenation of the haemoglobin. (Increased basic properties of reduced haemoglobin causes slight increase in formation of bicarbonate ion.) Carbamino carriage of CO$_2$ is strongly influenced by the state of oxygenation of haemoglobin but hardly at all by P$_{CO_2}$. (These values have not been drawn from a single publication but represent the mean of values reported in a large number of studies.)

pK values are far removed from the physiological range of pH. In contrast is the imidazole group of the amino acid histidine which is almost the only effective buffer in the normal range of pH. Imidazole groups constitute the major part of the considerable buffering power of haemoglobin, each molecule of which contains 38 histidine residues. The buffering power of plasma proteins is less and is proportional to their histidine content.

$$\underset{\text{Basic form of histidine}}{
\begin{array}{c}
H \\
C \\
\diagup\diagdown \\
N \quad N^- \\
| \quad | \\
HC=C \\
| \\
CH_2 \\
| \\
NH_2-C-COOH \\
| \\
H
\end{array}}
\quad + H^+ \rightleftharpoons \quad
\underset{\text{Acidic form of histidine}}{
\begin{array}{c}
H \\
C \\
\diagup\diagdown \\
N \quad NH \\
| \quad | \\
HC=C \\
| \\
CH_2 \\
| \\
NH_2-C-COOH \\
| \\
H
\end{array}}$$

Basic form of histidine   *Acidic form of histidine*

The four haem groups of a molecule of haemoglobin are attached to the corresponding four amino acid chains by means of one of the histidine residues on each chain (page 259). The following is a section of a beta chain of human haemoglobin:

```
         haem   O₂
            \   /
             Fe
              |
—leucine—histidine—cysteine—aspartic acid—lysine—leucine—histidine—valine—
   91       92       93         94          95      96       97      98
```

The figures indicate the position of the amino acid residue in the chain. The histidine in position 92 is one to which a haem group is attached. The histidine in position 97 is not. Both have buffering properties but the dissociation constant of the imidazole groups of the four histidine residues to which the haem groups are attached is strongly influenced by the state of oxygenation of the haem. Reduction causes the corresponding imidazole group to become more basic. The converse is also true: in the acidic form of the imidazole group of the histidine, the strength of the oxygen bond is weakened. Each reaction is of great physiological interest and both effects were noticed many decades before their mechanisms were elucidated.

1. *The reduction of haemoglobin causes it to become more basic.* This results in increased carriage of carbon dioxide as bicarbonate, since hydrogen ions are removed, permitting increased dissociation of carbonic acid (first dissociation of equation 3). This accounts for part of the Haldane effect, the other and greater part being due to increased carbamino carriage (see above).
2. *Conversion to the basic form of histidine causes increased affinity of the corresponding haem group for oxygen.* This is, in part, the cause of the Bohr effect (page 263).

Total reduction of the haemoglobin in blood would raise the pH by about 0.03 pH units if the P_{CO_2} were held constant at 5.3 kPa (40 mmHg), and this would correspond roughly to the addition of 3 mmol of base to 1 litre of blood. The normal degree of desaturation in the course of the change from arterial to mixed venous blood is about 25 per cent, corresponding to a pH rise of about 0.007 if P_{CO_2} remains constant. In fact, P_{CO_2} rises by about 0.8 kPa (6 mmHg), which would cause a fall of pH of 0.040 units if the oxygen saturation were to remain the same. The combination of a rise of P_{CO_2} of 0.8 kPa and a fall of saturation of 25 per cent thus results in a fall of pH of 0.033 units (see *Table 9.2*).

Distribution of carbon dioxide within the blood

Table 9.2 shows the forms in which carbon dioxide is carried in normal arterial and mixed venous blood. Although the amount carried in solution is small, most of the carbon dioxide enters and leaves the blood as CO_2 itself (*Figure 9.3*). Within the plasma there is little combination of carbon dioxide, for three reasons. Firstly, there

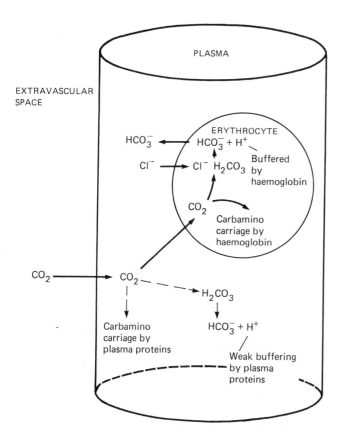

Figure 9.3 How carbon dioxide enters the blood in molecular form. Within the plasma, there is only negligible carbamino carriage due to the structure of the plasma proteins and a slow rate of hydration to carbonic acid due to the absence of carbonic anhydrase. The greater part of the carbon dioxide diffuses into the erythrocytes where conditions for carbamino carriage are much more favourable. In addition, hydration to carbonic acid occurs rapidly in the presence of carbonic anhydrase and subsequent ionization is promoted by the buffering capacity of haemoglobin for the hydrogen ions.

is no carbonic anhydrase in plasma and therefore carbonic acid is formed only very slowly. Secondly, there is little buffering power in plasma to promote the dissociation of carbonic acid. Thirdly, it is thought that the formation of carbamino compounds by plasma proteins is not great, and is presumably almost identical for arterial and venous blood.

Carbon dioxide can, however, diffuse freely into the erythrocyte, where two courses are open. Firstly, carbamino compounds may be formed with haemoglobin, not so much because the P_{CO_2} is raised but rather because the oxygen saturation is likely to be reduced at the same time as the P_{CO_2} is rising (see above). The second course is hydration and dissociation. Hydration is greatly facilitated by the presence of carbonic anhydrase in the erythrocyte, and dissociation is facilitated by the buffering power of the imidazole groups on the histidine residues of the haemoglobin, particularly reduced haemoglobin. In this way considerable quantities of bicarbonate ion are formed and these are able to diffuse into the plasma in exchange for chloride ions which diffuse in the opposite direction (Hamburger, 1918).

Dissociation curves of carbon dioxide

Figure 9.2 shows the classic form of the dissociation curve of carbon dioxide relating blood content to tension. Recently, there has been much greater interest in curves which relate any pair of the following: (1) plasma bicarbonate concentration; (2) P_{CO_2}; (3) pH. These three quantities are related by the Henderson–Hasselbalch equation and therefore the third variable can always be derived from the other two. For this reason the three possible plots may be used interchangeably and selection is largely a matter of custom or convenience. There is some doubt about the nomenclature of the plots. A plot of plasma $[CO_2]$ against P_{CO_2} is not really a dissociation curve, and a plot of plasma $[HCO_3^-]$ against pH (*Figure 9.4*) is not really a titration curve since in each case the relevant concentration is in plasma and not blood. The difference, however, is not very great, and the general shape of the curve is much the same when the ordinate is expressed as concentration in blood. With current analytical techniques a plot of P_{CO_2} (logarithmic) against pH has special attractions (*Figure 9.5*) and is best described as a CO_2 equilibration curve (Siggaard-Andersen, 1964).

It is important to appreciate that, if the P_{CO_2} of an entire patient is altered, the pH changes are not the same as those of a blood sample of which the P_{CO_2} is altered *in vitro*. This is because the blood of a patient is in continuity with the extracellular fluid (of very low buffering capacity) and also with intracellular fluid (of high buffering capacity). Bicarbonate ions pass rapidly and freely across the various interfaces, and experimental studies have shown the following changes to occur in the arterial blood of an intact subject when the P_{CO_2} is acutely changed.

1. The arterial pH reaches a steady state within minutes of establishment of the new level of P_{CO_2}.
2. The change in arterial pH is intermediate between the pH changes obtained *in vitro* with plasma and whole blood after the same change in P_{CO_2}. That is to say, the *in vivo* change in pH is greater than the *in vitro* change in the patient's blood when subjected to the same change in P_{CO_2}.

Numerous studies have been carried out in animals, and there is indication of some species differences (Shaw and Messer, 1932). Studies in conscious man show

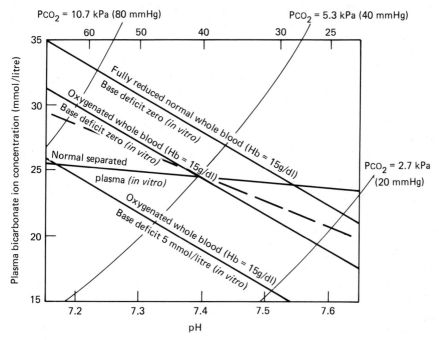

Figure 9.4 A number of CO_2 equilibration curves plotted on the co-ordinates $pH/[HCO_3^-]$. (Isobars are shown for P_{CO_2} 10.7, 5.3, 2.7 kPa = 80, 40 and 20 mmHg.) For most biological fluids, the plot is linear over the physiological range. $pH = 7.40$, $P_{CO_2} = 5.3$ kPa (40 mmHg) and $HCO_3^- = 24.4$ mmol/l is the accepted normal point through which all curves for normal oxygenated blood or plasma pass. The steepest curve passing through that point is the curve of normal oxygenated whole blood; the flattest is that of plasma, both curves being obtained in vitro. The broken curve describes blood of haemoglobin 10 g/dl equilibrated in vitro, or alternatively the arterial blood (Hb = 15 g/dl) equilibrated in vivo of a normal anaesthetized patient whose P_{CO_2} is acutely changed (Prys-Roberts, Kelman and Nunn, 1966). The uppermost curve is that of reduced but otherwise normal blood equilibrated in vitro. The lowermost curve is that of oxygenated blood with a metabolic acidosis (base deficit) of 5 mmol/l equilibrated in vitro.

in vivo changes close to the in vitro changes obtained in plasma (Cohen, Brackett and Schwartz, 1964). Prys-Roberts, Kelman and Nunn (1966) studied step changes of P_{CO_2} in anaesthetized patients and obtained in vivo dissociation curves of similar slope to those which would be obtained with the patient's blood in vitro if the haemoglobin concentration were reduced by a third (Figures 9.4 and 9.5).

This effect introduces a small potential error into the calculation of base excess in a patient whose P_{CO_2} is well outside the normal range. The error may be determined from Figures 9.4 and 9.5. The measured base excess will be about 2 mmol/l low (apparent metabolic acidosis) if blood is sampled when the P_{CO_2} is 10.7 kPa (80 mmHg), and the measured base excess will be about 2 mmol/l high (apparent metabolic alkalosis) if blood is sampled when the P_{CO_2} is 2.7 kPa (20 mmHg). Values of P_{CO_2} outside these limits are comparatively rare and a correction factor can easily be applied if necessary.

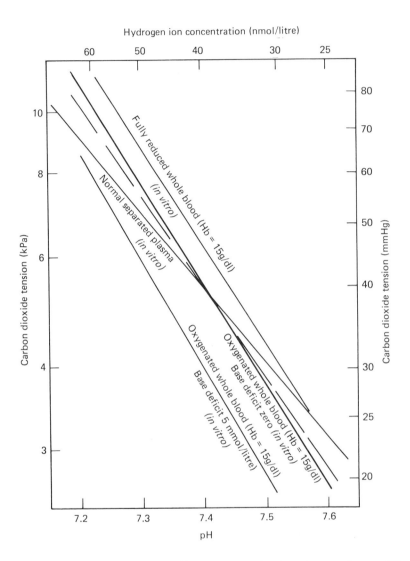

Figure 9.5 A number of CO₂ equilibration curves plotted on the co-ordinates pH/log Pco₂. For most biological fluids the plot is linear over the physiological range. pH = 7.40 and Pco₂ = 5.3 kPa (40 mmHg) is the accepted normal value through which all curves for normal oxygenated blood or plasma pass. The steepest curve passing through this point is that of normal oxygenated blood; the flattest is that of plasma, both curves being obtained in vitro. The broken curve describes blood of haemoglobin 10 g/dl, equilibrated in vitro, or alternatively the arterial blood, equilibrated in vivo (Hb = 15 g/dl), of a normal anaesthetized patient whose Pco₂ is acutely changed (Prys-Roberts, Kelman and Nunn, 1966). The uppermost curve is that of reduced but otherwise normal blood equilibrated in vitro. The lowermost curve is that of oxygenated blood with a metabolic acidosis (base deficit) of 5 mmol/l, equilibrated in vitro.

Transfer of carbon dioxide across cell membranes

It may readily be demonstrated in the laboratory that membranes made of most plastic materials (e.g. polytetrafluorethylene or Teflon) permit the free diffusion of carbon dioxide but will not permit the passage of hydrogen ions. This is, in fact, the principle of the CO_2-sensitive electrode (page 232).

Selectivity of a somewhat similar type exists across cell membranes in the living body. These membranes, particularly the blood/brain barrier, are relatively impervious to hydrogen ions but permit the rapid diffusion of carbon dioxide. Therefore, the intracellular hydrogen ion concentration is relatively uninfluenced by changes in extracellular pH but can be altered by perfusion with a solution containing dissolved carbon dioxide. The carbon dioxide passes through the membrane and, once inside the cell, is able to hydrate and ionize, thus producing hydrogen ions. This property is unique to carbon dioxide, which is the only substance, normally present in the blood, able to alter the intracellular pH in this manner.

The passage of carbon dioxide through the cell membrane to release hydrogen ions within the cell is reminiscent of the seige of Troy (Virgil, 19 BC). The city of Troy is analogous to the cell and its walls were impervious to Greek soldiers (hydrogen ions). However, the wooden horse (carbon dioxide) passed through the walls without difficulty and, once within the city (cell), was able to release the Greek soldiers (hydrogen ions).

This effect of carbon dioxide is of great physiological importance, and probably accounts for many of the effects of carbon dioxide. Chapter 4 describes how this mechanism underlies the effect of carbon dioxide on the central chemoreceptors (page 86).

Factors influencing the carbon dioxide tension in the steady state

In common with other catabolites, the level of carbon dioxide in the body fluids depends upon the balance between production and elimination. There is a continuous gradient of P_{CO_2} from the mitochondria (the site of production of carbon dioxide) through the cytoplasm, the venous blood, the alveolar gas and thence by way of expired air to dispersal in the ambient air. The P_{CO_2} in all cells is not identical, but is lowest in tissues with the lowest metabolic activity and the highest perfusion (e.g. skin) and highest in tissues with the highest metabolic activity for their perfusion (e.g. the myocardium). Therefore the P_{CO_2} of venous blood differs from one tissue to another, and the mixed venous P_{CO_2} is the integrated mean for the body as a whole.

In the pulmonary capillaries, carbon dioxide passes into the alveolar gas and this causes the alveolar P_{CO_2} to rise steadily during expiration. During inspiration, the inspired gas dilutes the alveolar gas and the P_{CO_2} falls by about 0.4 kPa. This imparts a sawtooth curve to the alveolar P_{CO_2} when it is plotted against time. The expiratory section of this curve may be determined from the carbon dioxide concentration determined at the mouth with a rapid analyser (*Figure 9.6*). The amplitude of the oscillations of alveolar P_{CO_2} is increased during exercise and this has implications in the control of breathing (page 83).

On the arterial side, the blood leaving the pulmonary capillary has a P_{CO_2} which is very close to that of the alveolar gas and, therefore, varies with *time* in the same

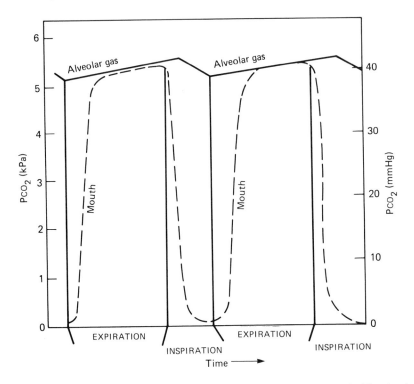

Figure 9.6 Changes in alveolar and mouth Pco₂ during the respiratory cycle. The alveolar Pco₂ is shown by a continuous curve, and the mouth Pco₂ (as determined by a rapid analyser) by the broken curve. The mouth Pco₂ falls at the commencement of inspiration but does not rise during expiration until the anatomical dead space gas is washed out. The alveolar Pco₂ rises during expiration and also during the early part of inspiration until fresh gas penetrates the alveoli after the anatomical dead space is washed out. The alveolar Pco₂ then falls until expiration commences. This imparts a sawtooth curve to the alveolar Po₂.

manner as the alveolar Pco_2. There is also a *regional* variation depending upon the ventilation/perfusion ratio of different parts of the lung. This exerts a marked effect upon regional Pco_2, which is inversely related to the ventilation/perfusion ratio (see *Figure 7.12*). The mixed arterial Pco_2 is the integrated mean of blood from different parts of the lung, and a sample drawn over several seconds will average out the cyclical variations resulting from breathing.

When discussing factors influencing the level of carbon dioxide, it is more convenient to consider tension than content. This is because carbon dioxide always moves in accord with tension gradients even if they are in the opposite direction to concentration gradients. Also, the concept of tension may be applied with equal significance to gas and liquid phases: content has a rather different connotation in the two phases. Furthermore, it seems likely that the effffects of carbon dioxide (e.g. upon respiration) are a function of tension rather than concept. Normal values for tension and content are shown in *Figure 9.7*.

Each factor which influences the Pco_2 has already been mentioned in this book and it only remains in this chapter to draw them together, illustrating their relationship to one another. The following section may therefore be used either as an introduction to the subject or as a summary.

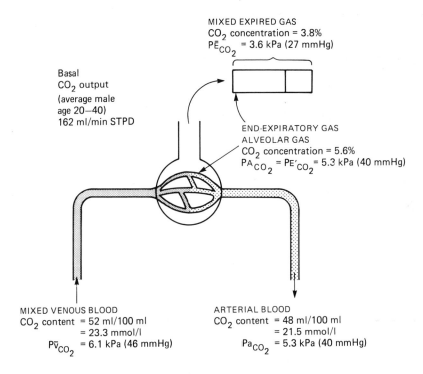

MIXED EXPIRED GAS
CO_2 concentration = 3.8%
$P\bar{E}_{CO_2}$ = 3.6 kPa (27 mmHg)

Basal
CO_2 output
(average male
age 20–40)
162 ml/min STPD

END-EXPIRATORY GAS
ALVEOLAR GAS
CO_2 concentration = 5.6%
PA_{CO_2} = PE'_{CO_2} = 5.3 kPa (40 mmHg)

MIXED VENOUS BLOOD
CO_2 content = 52 ml/100 ml
               = 23.3 mmol/l
$P\bar{v}_{CO_2}$ = 6.1 kPa (46 mmHg)

ARTERIAL BLOOD
CO_2 content = 48 ml/100 ml
               = 21.5 mmol/l
Pa_{CO_2} = 5.3 kPa (40 mmHg)

Figure 9.7 Normal values of CO_2 levels. These normal values are rounded off and ignore the small difference in P_{CO_2} between end-expiratory gas, alveolar gas and arterial blood. Actual values of P_{CO_2} depend mainly on alveolar ventilation but the differences depend upon maldistribution; the alveolar/end-expiratory P_{CO_2} difference depends on alveolar dead space and the very small arterial/alveolar P_{CO_2} difference on shunts. Scatter of $\dot{V}/\dot{Q}$ ratios makes a small contribution to both alveolar/end-expiratory and arterial/alveolar P_{CO_2} gradients. The arterial/mixed venous CO_2 content difference is directly proportional to CO_2 output and inversely proportional to cardiac output. Secondary symols: $\bar{E}$, mixed expired; E', end-expiratory'; A, alveolar; a, arterial; $\bar{v}$, mixed venous.

It is convenient first to summarize the factors influencing the alveolar P_{CO_2} and then to consider the factors which influence the relationship between the alveolar and the arterial P_{CO_2}.

The alveolar P_{CO_2} (PA_{CO_2}) (*Figure 9.8*)

Carbon dioxide is constantly being added to the alveolar gas from the pulmonary blood and removed from it by the alveolar ventilation. The concentration of carbon dioxide is equal to the ratio of the two, provided that carbon dioxide is not inhaled.

$$\text{alveolar } CO_2 \text{ concentration} = \frac{\text{carbon dioxide output}}{\text{alveolar ventilation}}$$

This axiomatic relationship is the basis of all the methods of predicting the P_{CO_2} and is, in fact, a form of the Bohr equation. Derivations from this equation have been presented in Chapter 5, and we may note the following equation which describes the principal factors influencing the alveolar P_{CO_2}:

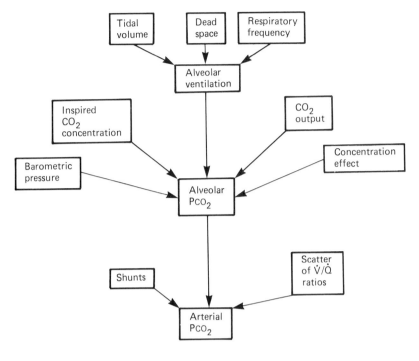

Figure 9.8 Summary of factors which influence P_{CO_2}; *the more important ones are indicated with the thicker arrows. In the steady state, the carbon dioxide output of an anaesthetized patient usually lies within the range 100–200 ml/min and the alveolar* P_{CO_2} *is largely governed by the alveolar ventilation, provided that the inspired* CO_2 *concentration is zero. The barometric pressure is the only limit to the elevation of* P_{CO_2} *which may be brought about by the inhalation of gas mixtures containing* CO_2. *See text for explanation of the concentration effect.*

$$\begin{array}{c} \text{alveolar} \\ P_{CO_2} \end{array} = \begin{array}{c} \text{dry} \\ \text{barometric} \\ \text{pressure} \end{array} \left(\begin{array}{c} \text{mean} \\ \text{inspired } CO_2 \\ \text{concentration} \end{array} + \frac{CO_2 \text{ output}}{\text{alveolar ventilation}} \right)$$

The equation is shown in graphical form in *Figure 9.9*. Prediction of P_{CO_2} from ventilation has been discussed on page 110.

The dry barometric pressure is not a factor of much importance in the determination of alveolar P_{CO_2}, and normal variations of barometric pressure at sea level are unlikely to influence the P_{CO_2} by more than 0.3 kPa (2 mmHg). At high altitude it is the hypoxic drive to ventilation which lowers the P_{CO_2} (page 312).

The mean inspired CO_2 concentration is a more difficult concept than it appears at first sight, and has been considered in relation to apparatus dead space on page 165. For the present we may note that the effect of inspired carbon dioxide on the alveolar P_{CO_2} is additive. If, for example, a patient breathes gas containing 4.2% carbon dioxide (P_{CO_2} = 4.0 kPa or 30 mmHg), the alveolar P_{CO_2} will be raised 4.0 kPa above the level it would be if there were no carbon dioxide in the

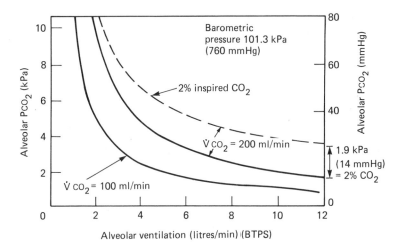

Figure 9.9 The effect of CO₂ output, alveolar ventilation and inspired CO₂ concentration on alveolar Pco₂. The lower continuous curve shows the relationship between ventilation and alveolar Pco₂ for a carbon dioxide output of 100 ml/min (STPD). The upper continuous curve shows the relationship when the carbon dioxide output is 200 ml/min (STPD). The broken curve represents the relationship when the carbon dioxide output is 200 ml/min and there is an inspired CO₂ concentration of 2%. Two per cent CO₂ is equivalent to about 1.9 kPa (14 mmHg) and each point on the broken curve is 1.9 kPa above the upper of the two continuous curves. The continuous curves are rectangular hyperbolas with identical asymptotes (zero alveolar Pco₂ and zero alveolar ventilation). The broken curve is also a rectangular hyperbola but the horizontal asymptote is Pco₂ 1.9 kPa (14 mmHg) which is the tension in the inspired gas.

inspired gas, provided other factors, including ventilation, remain the same. The barometric pressure is the only limit to the elevation of Pco_2 which may be obtained by the inhalation of carbon dioxide mixtures. Arterial tensions of over 27 kPa (200 mmHg) have been obtained by inhaling a few breaths of 30% carbon dioxide.

Carbon dioxide output is equal to carbon dioxide production in a steady state. However, during unsteady states, output may be quite different from production (Nunn and Matthews, 1959). For example, during acute hypoventilation, much of the carbon dioxide production is diverted into the body stores, so that the output may temporarily fall to very low figures until the alveolar carbon dioxide concentration has risen. Conversely, acute hyperventilation results in a transient increase in carbon dioxide output. A sudden fall in cardiac output decreases the carbon dioxide output until the carbon dioxide concentration in the mixed venous blood rises. The unsteady state is considered in more detail later (page 226).

Alveolar ventilation, for the present purposes, means the product of the respiratory frequency and the difference between the tidal volume and the physiological dead space (page 163). It can change over very wide limits and is the main factor influencing alveolar Pco_2. Changes in ventilation are considered elsewhere (page 110).

With gas circuits which result in rebreathing, it is possible for the fresh gas inflow rate to replace the alveolar ventilation in the relationship defined in the equation above. With the alveolar ventilation considerably in excess of the fresh gas inflow rate, the latter may then be used to control the level of the P_{CO_2} (Schofield and Williams, 1974).

The concentration effect. Apart from the factors shown in the equation above and in *Figure 9.9*, the alveolar P_{CO_2} is influenced by what is, for want of a better name, known as the concentration effect. This is caused by a sudden change in the net transfer of inert gases across the alveolar/capillary membrane which alters the concentration of carbon dioxide (and oxygen) in the alveolar gas. This occurs, for example, at the end of an anaesthetic when large quantities of nitrous oxide are passing from the body stores into the alveolar gas, and a much smaller quantity of nitrogen is returning to its accustomed place in the body. This leads to a dilution of the alveolar carbon dioxide. The fall in P_{CO_2} is usually quite small but may be sufficient to cause a transient reduction in ventilation when nitrous oxide is withdrawn at the end of an operation (see also page 248). The reverse effect occurs at the start of nitrous oxide inhalation.

The end-expiratory $P_{CO_2}(P_E'_{CO_2})$

In the normal, healthy, conscious subject, the end-expiratory gas consists almost entirely of alveolar gas. If, however, appreciable parts of the lung are ventilated but not perfused, they will contribute a significant quantity of CO_2-free gas from the alveolar dead space to the end-expiratory gas (see *Figure 7.8*). As a result, the end-expiratory P_{CO_2} (end-tidal or Haldane–Priestley sample) will have a lower P_{CO_2} than that of the alveoli which are perfused. Gas cannot be sampled selectively from the perfused alveoli but Chapter 7 explains how the arterial P_{CO_2} usually approximates closely to the mean value of the perfused alveoli in spite of scatter of ventilation/perfusion ratios. It is therefore possible to compare the arterial P_{CO_2} with the end-expiratory P_{CO_2} to demonstrate the existence of an appreciable proportion of unperfused alveoli. Studies during anaesthesia have, for example, shown an arterial/end-tidal P_{CO_2} gradient of about 0.7 kPa (5 mmHg) in patients without lung disease (Ramwell, 1958; Nunn and Hill, 1960).

The alveolar/arterial P_{CO_2} gradient

For reasons which have been discussed in Chapter 8, we may discount the possibility of any significant gradient between the P_{CO_2} of alveolar gas and that of pulmonary end-capillary blood. Arterial P_{CO_2} may, however, differ slightly from the mean alveolar P_{CO_2} as a result of shunting or scatter of ventilation/perfusion ratios. The magnitude of the gradient has been considered in Chapter 7 (page 168) where it was shown that a shunt of 10 per cent will cause an alveolar/arterial P_{CO_2} gradient of only about 0.1 kPa (0.7 mmHg). Since the normal degree of ventilation/ perfusion ratio scatter causes a gradient of the same order, neither can be considered to cause a significant gradient and, for practical purposes, there is an established convention by which the arterial and alveolar P_{CO_2} values are taken to be identical. It is only in exceptional patients that the gradient is likely to exceed 0.3 kPa (2 mmHg).

The arterial P_{CO_2}

Pooled results for the normal arterial P_{CO_2} reported by various authors show a mean of 5.1 kPa (38.3 mmHg) with 95 per cent limits (2 s.d.) of 1.0 kPa (7.5 mmHg). Five per cent of normal patients will lie outside these limits and it is therefore preferable to refer to this as the reference range rather than the normal range. There is no evidence that P_{CO_2} is influenced by age unless the patient goes into respiratory failure.

Causes of hypocapnia (respiratory alkalosis)

Hypocapnia can result only from an alveolar ventilation which is excessive in relation to carbon dioxide production. Low values of arterial P_{CO_2} are very commonly found, due to voluntary hyperventilation resulting from arterial puncture, and it is sometimes better to insert a cannula, returning for the sample when the patient has settled. Persistently low values may then be due to an excessive respiratory drive resulting from one of the following causes.

Hypoxaemia is a common cause of hypocapnia, occurring in congenital heart disease with right-to-left shunting, residence at high altitude, pulmonary collapse or consolidation and any other condition which reduces the arterial P_{O_2} below about 8 kPa (60 mmHg). Hypocapnia, secondary to hypoxaemia, counteracts the ventilatory response to the hypoxaemia.

Metabolic acidosis produces a compensatory hyperventilation (air hunger) which minimizes the fall in pH which would otherwise occur. This is a pronounced feature of diabetic ketosis and severe haemorrhagic shock. Arterial P_{CO_2} values below 3 kPa (22.5 mmHg) are not uncommon in severe metabolic acidosis.

Mechanical abnormalities of the lung may drive respiration through the vagus, resulting in moderate reduction of the P_{CO_2}. Thus conditions such as pulmonary fibrosis and asthma are usually associated with a low to normal P_{CO_2} until the patient passes into respiratory failure.

Hypotension may drive respiration directly but, in cases of haemorrhage, metabolic acidosis is usually a more important factor.

Hysteria, head injuries and various neurological disorders may result in hyperventilation.

The effects of hypocapnia are considered in Chapter 27.

Causes of hypercapnia (respiratory acidosis)

It is uncommon to encounter an arterial P_{CO_2} above the normal range in a healthy subject. Any value of more than 6.1 kPa (46 mmHg) should be considered abnormal. Values up to 6.7 kPa (50 mmHg) may be attained by breath holding but, by breathing mixtures of carbon dioxide in oxygen, the normal subject may easily attain a P_{CO_2} of 10 kPa (75 mmHg) without ill effect. Higher values, whether due to inhalation of carbon dioxide or to hypoventilation, result in confusion and loss of consciousness. *While breathing air*, it is not possible for a hypoventilating patient to have a P_{CO_2} in excess of about 13 kPa (100 mmHg) because, at that level of ventilation, the accompanying hypoxaemia will become critical (see *Figure 20.1*). P_{CO_2} values in excess of 13 kPa can occur only in patients breathing either oxygen-enriched gas mixtures or gas containing carbon dioxide: the condition can therefore be regarded as iatrogenic.

Hypoventilation

Pathological causes of hypoventilation leading to hypercapnia are considered in Chapter 20. In respiratory medicine, the commonest cause of hypercpania is chronic bronchitis. The type of patient known as the 'blue bloater' has reduced ventilatory capacity combined with reduced ventilatory response to carbon dioxide. It is an intractable, progressive condition which renders the patient a poor risk for anaesthesia and surgery (Milledge and Nunn, 1975). Fortunately, it is becoming far less common in Great Britain. In other respiratory diseases, including asthma and emphysema ('pink puffers') the ventilatory response to carbon dioxide is better preserved and a rise in P_{CO_2} is generally late and may be terminal.

Increased concentration of carbon dioxide in the inspired gas

Apart from hypoventilation, the only other cause of hypercapnia is an increased concentration of carbon dioxide in the inspired gas. This may be endogenous or exogenous, the former resulting from rebreathing while the latter is usually therapeutic or accidental. The only essential difference between the two is the rate at which the P_{CO_2} can increase. If all the carbon dioxide produced by metabolism is retained and distributed in the body stores, arterial P_{CO_2} rises by about 0.4–0.8 kPa/min (3–6 mmHg/min. This limits the rate of increase of P_{CO_2} during rebreathing. In contrast, the P_{CO_2} may rise extremely rapidly when exogenous carbon dioxide is inhaled (see page 227). The effects of hypercapnia are considered in Chapter 27.

Carbon dioxide stores and the unsteady state

The quantity of carbon dioxide and bicarbonate ion in the body is very large — about 120 litres, which is almost 100 times greater than the volume of oxygen (page 271). Therefore, when ventilation is altered out of accord with metabolic activity, carbon dioxide levels change only slowly. *Figure 9.10* shows a three-compartment hydraulic model in which depth of water represents P_{CO_2} and the volume in the various compartments corresponds to volume of carbon dioxide. The metabolic production of carbon dioxide is represented by the variable flow of water from the supply tank. The outflow corresponds to alveolar ventilation and the controller watching the P_{CO_2} represents the central chemoreceptors.

The rapid compartment represents circulating blood, brain, kidneys and other well perfused tissues. The medium compartment represents skeletal muscle (resting) and other tissues with a moderate blood flow. The slow compartment includes bone,

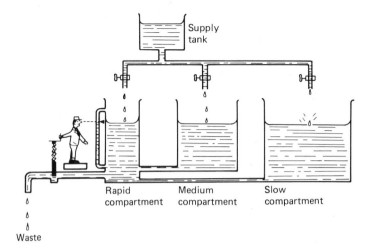

Figure 9.10 A hydrostatic analogy of the elimination of carbon dioxide. See text for full discussion.

fat and other tissues with a large capacity for carbon dioxide. Each compartment has its own time constant (see Appendix F), and the long time constants of the medium and slow compartments buffer changes in the rapid compartment.

Hyperventilation is represented by a wide opening of the outflow valve with subsequent exponential decline in the levels in all three compartments, the rapid compartment falling most quickly. During hypoventilation, the rise of the levels depends on the balance between inflow and outflow. In total apnoea, the change in P_{CO_2} is governed by the inflow and the capacity of the compartments—i.e. by the metabolic production of carbon dioxide and the capacity of the body stores.

It will be clear that the time course of the increase of P_{CO_2} following step decrease of ventilation is not the mirror image of the time course of decrease of P_{CO_2} when ventilation is increased. In fact, the rate of rise is much slower than the rate of fall, which is fortunate for patients in asphyxial situations. In the event of total respiratory arrest, the rate of rise of arterial P_{CO_2} is of the order of 0.4–0.8 kPa/min (3–6 mmHg/min), which is the resultant of the rate of production of carbon dioxide and the capacity of the body stores to accommodate the carbon dioxide which is produced. During actual hypoventilation, the rate of increase in P_{CO_2} will be less than this and *Figure 9.11* shows typical curves for P_{CO_2} increase and decrease following step changes in ventilation of anaesthetized patients. The time course of rise of P_{CO_2} after step reduction of ventilation is faster when the previous level of ventilation has been of short duration (Ivanov and Nunn, 1968).

In a later study, Ivanov and Nunn (1969) compared the rapidity with which P_{CO_2} could be elevated by three different techniques in a previously hyperventilated patient. As described above, reduction of minute volume was too slow a method to be used in an acute situation. Rebreathing with oxygen replenishment was the fastest practicable method without using exogenous carbon dioxide. However, even this did not compare with the rate of rise of P_{CO_2}, attainable by the use of exogenous carbon dioxide. The use of an inspired gas mixture containing 5% carbon dioxide elevated the P_{CO_2} by 2.3 kPa (17.3 mmHg) in 2 minutes, most of the change occurring in the first minute.

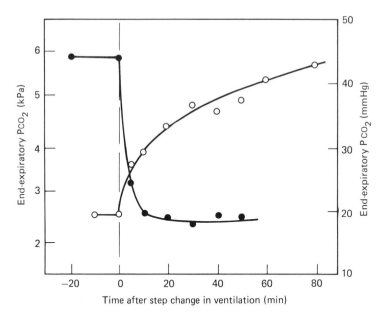

Figure 9.11 Time course of changes in end-expiratory P_{CO_2} *following step changes in ventilation. The solid circles indicate the changes in end-expiratory* P_{CO_2} *which followed a step change in ventilation from 3.3 to 14 l/min. The open circles show the change following a step change in ventilation from 14 to 3.3 l/min in the same patient. During the fall of* P_{CO_2}, *half the total change is completed in about 3 minutes. During the rise of* P_{CO_2}, *half-change takes approximately 16 minutes.*

Laparoscopy with carbon dioxide as the inflating gas seems at first sight to carry a hazard of exogenous carbon dioxide intoxication. However, a number of studies have now shown that the elevation of P_{CO_2} is minimal provided that pulmonary ventilation is properly maintained (Kelman et al., 1972). Surprisingly, the elevation of P_{CO_2} appears to be greater if nitrous oxide is used as the inflating gas.

It will be seen in Chapter 10 that, unlike the P_{CO_2}, the P_{O_2} changes very quickly after alterations in ventilation. Consequently, changes in ventilation are followed by temporary changes in the respiratory exchange ratio, although, if the ventilation is held constant, the respiratory exchange ratio must eventually return to the level determined by the metabolic process of the body. Carbon dioxide stores were reviewed by Farhi (1964).

Apnoeic mass-movement oxygenation (formerly known as **diffusion respiration**)

When a patient becomes apnoeic, the alveolar gas comes into equilibrium with the mixed venous blood, provided it continues to perfuse the lungs. Assuming normal initial values for the composition of the alveolar gas and mixed venous gas tensions, this would entail a rise of P_{CO_2} from 5.3 to 6.1 kPa (40 to 46 mmHg) and a fall of P_{O_2} from 14 to 5.3 kPa (105 to 40 mmHg). The *volume* of gas which would require to cross the alveolar/capillary membrane is directly proportional to the gas tension change. Ignoring changes in the composition of the mixed venous blood and assuming an average FRC, equilibration of alveolar gas with mixed venous blood would require the output of 21 ml of carbon dioxide and the uptake of 230 ml of oxygen at normal lung volume. The small quantity of carbon dioxide could be transferred within one circulation time while oxygen would take much longer. Thus, for practical purposes, carbon dioxide does reach equilibrium while oxygen is always *tending towards* equilibrium but never reaching it.

What actually happens to the arterial blood gases in apnoea depends upon the patency of the airway and the composition of the ambient gas if the airway is patent.

With airway occlusion the pattern of change is close to that described above. There is a rapid attainment of equilibrium between alveolar and mixed venous P_{CO_2}. The arterial, alveolar and mixed venous P_{CO_2} values remain close together and rise gradually at the rate of about 0.4–0.8 kPa/min (3–6 mmHg/min), with more than 90 per cent of the metabolically produced carbon dioxide passing into the body stores. Alveolar P_{O_2} falls rapidly towards the mixed venous P_{O_2} which itself falls continuously as the arterial P_{O_2} decreases. The lung volume falls by the difference between the oxygen uptake and the carbon dioxide output. Initially the rate would be $230 - 21 = 209$ ml/min. The change in alveolar P_{O_2} may be calculated, and gross hypoxia supervenes after about 90 seconds if apnoea follows air breathing and starts at the functional residual capacity.

With patent airway and air as ambient gas the oxygen is initially taken up and the carbon dioxide rises as described above. However, instead of the lung volume falling by the net gas exchange rate (initially 209 ml/min), this amount of ambient gas is drawn in by mass movement down the trachea. If the ambient gas is air, the oxygen in it will be removed but the nitrogen will accumulate and rise above its normal concentration until gross hypoxia supervenes after about 2 minutes. This is likely to occur when the accumulated nitrogen has reached 90% since the alveolar carbon dioxide concentration will then have reached about 8%. Carbon dioxide elimination cannot occur as there is mass-movement of gas down the trachea and this prevents the loss of carbon dioxide by diffusion. Measured at the mouth, there is oxygen uptake but no carbon dioxide output; the respiratory exchange ratio is thus zero.

With patent airway and oxygen as the ambient gas the situation is quite different. Oxygen is drawn in by mass-movement and replaces the oxygen which crosses the alveolar/capillary membrane. No nitrogen is added to the alveolar gas, and the alveolar P_{O_2} only falls as fast as the P_{CO_2} rises (about 0.4–0.8 kPa/min or 3–6 mmHg/min). Therefore the patient will not become seriously hypoxic for several minutes. If the patient has been breathing oxygen prior to the respiratory arrest, the starting alveolar P_{O_2} will be of the order of 88 kPa (660 mmHg) and therefore the patient can theoretically survive about 100 minutes of apnoea provided that his airway remains clear and he is connected to a supply of 100% oxygen. This does, in fact, happen and has been demonstrated in both animals and man (Draper and Whitehead, 1944; Enghoff, Holmdahl and Risholm, 1951; Holmdahl, 1956; Frumin, Epstein and Cohen, 1959).

The phenomenon has moved out of the laboratory into clinical anaesthesia (Holmdahl, 1953) and has been used as a practical anaesthetic technique, particularly for bronchoscopy without artificial ventilation (Barth, 1954; Payne, 1962). However, the technique causes total retention of carbon dioxide and the arterial

PCO_2 rises at a rate within the range 0.4–0.8 kPa/min (3–6 mmHg/min). Hypercapnia is thus an inevitable feature of the technique. Arterial PCO_2 values as high as 18.7 kPa (140 mmHg) have been reported by Payne (1962) after 11 minutes (with an initial PCO_2 of 11.1 kPa or 83 mmHg).

Therapeutic uses of carbon dioxide

The varied and powerful effects of increased PCO_2 suggest that the inhalation of carbon dioxide gas mixtures would have a clear place in therapy. In fact, this is not so and its therapeutic role is limited.

The main indication for the administration of carbon dioxide is to stimulate respiration. This is useful to expedite the uptake and elimination of inhalational anaesthetic agents, and carbon dioxide may be given to raise the arterial PCO_2 above the apnoeic threshold in order to encourage the resumption of spontaneous breathing after passive hyperventilation of an unconscious patient. Although carbon dioxide may be used to stimulate breathing in these situations, its use in the treatment of ventilatory failure is very limited. In many patients, the cause of the respiratory failure is a diminished or absent response to carbon dioxide and the administration of exogenous carbon dioxide to such patients would not only be ineffective but might also actually make things worse. Carbon dioxide is also likely to be ineffective or harmful if ventilation is limited by malfunction of the efferent motor pathway, the respiratory muscles or by raised airway resistance. Such patients will already have a raised PCO_2 and a flattened PCO_2/ventilation response curve.

Carbon monoxide poisoning remains one of the clearest indications for the administration of carbon dioxide gas mixtures. Not only will stimulation of respiration hasten the elimination of carbon monoxide, but also the venous and therefore the tissue PO_2 will be substantially increased by the shift of the dissociation curve of the remaining normal haemoglobin (page 265). Increasing PCO_2 will usually improve both cardiac output and regional perfusion of certain organs, particularly the brain. Raised intracranial pressure is a hazard of the latter effect.

If carbon dioxide is used clinically, careful attention must be paid to dosimetry. Maximal effectiveness as a respiratory stimulant requires control of the concentration of the inspired gas. Five per cent carbon dioxide in oxygen is generally available as Carbogen.

Outline of methods of measurement of carbon dioxide

Fractional concentration in gas mixtures

Chemical absorption remains the reference method of analysis. In medical circles the most accurate method usually employed is Lloyd's modification of the Haldane apparatus (Cormack, 1972). A simpler version of Haldane's apparatus, which is sufficiently accurate for clinical work, has been described by Campbell (1960a). The popularity of the Scholander apparatus has declined in Great Britain in recent years, but it may still be required for the analysis of samples of less than 1 ml (Scholander, 1947). All these methods are markedly influenced by the presence of nitrous oxide in gas samples, and modifications of technique are required (Nunn, 1958a; Glossop, 1963; Meade and Owen-Thomas, 1975).

Rapid analysis. For over 30 years, infrared absorption has been the most widely used method for rapid breath-to-breath analysis. Correction is required for the presence of other diatomic gases which introduce an error due to collision broadening (Cooper, 1957). This effect is best overcome by calibrating with a known concentration of carbon dioxide in a diluent gas mixture which is similar to the gas sample for analysis. Infrared analysers can be made to respond within less than a quarter of a second and will thus show the changes in carbon dioxide concentration during a single respiratory cycle. Cormack and Powell (1972) described refinements of technique which permit greater accuracy. The broken line in *Figure 9.6* shows a typical capnogram from which the following information may be derived.

1. The end-expiratory carbon dioxide concentration.
2. The inspiratory carbon dioxide concentration.
3. In conjunction with a record of the patient's tidal exchange, it is possible to see how much gas is exhaled before the carbon dioxide concentration at the lips rises to the alveolar plateau. This is the anatomical dead space.
4. The slope of the alveolar P_{CO_2} plateau indicates the rate of rise of the alveolar P_{CO_2} during the course of expiration. This is increased by maldistribution of inspired gas or by an increase in the mixed venous/arterial P_{CO_2} difference.

When the instantaneous expired carbon dioxide concentration is plotted against the expired volume (see *Figure 7.14*), it constitutes the single-breath expired carbon dioxide test. Not only may it be used to derive the anatomical dead space but also the slope of the plateau and its relationship to the arterial P_{CO_2} give useful information on other components of the dead space (page 224).

Within the last 10 years, mass spectrometry has at last become established as an acceptable alternative method for the rapid analysis of carbon dioxide. The cost is much greater than for infrared analysis but response times tend to be shorter and there is usually provision for analysis of up to four gases at the same time.

Blood carbon dioxide concentration

For more than half a century the concentration of carbon dioxide in blood or plasma has been measured by vacuum extraction followed by chemical absorption in the manometric apparatus of Van Slyke and Neill (1924). The microapparatus of Natelson (1951) is considerably easier to handle. An even simpler technique is dissociation of bicarbonate by adding a large volume of acid to blood followed by measurement of P_{CO_2} of the blood-plus-acid (Linden, Ledsome and Norman, 1965). P_{CO_2} of the mixture is conveniently measured by means of the P_{CO_2}-sensitive electrode (see below). By suitable calibration with solutions of known concentrations of sodium bicarbonate, the method is capable of satisfactory accuracy.

With the improved methods for direct measurement of pH and P_{CO_2}, there now seems to be less requirement for measurement of the carbon dioxide concentration of blood and plasma.

Blood P_{CO_2}

Four methods of measurement have been described and each in its time has enjoyed widespread popularity.

Bubble tonometry was the first practical method (Pflüger 1866). A tiny bubble of gas was equilibrated with blood at the patient's body temperature and then analysed quantitatively for carbon dioxide concentration of the bubble, which was assumed to have the same P_{CO_2} as the blood. The technique was progressively refined over 100 years, culminating in the 'Riley bubble method' (Riley, Campbell and Shepard, 1957). However, the technique always remained very difficult to master and disappeared from use after 1960.

The indirect method. For many years P_{CO_2} was derived from the form of the Henderson–Hasselbalch equation given earlier in this chapter (equation 8, page 211). It was a most laborious procedure requiring measurements of both pH and CO_2 content, and there was always uncertainty of the value which should be taken for pK'. Nevertheless, tolerable accuracy was attainable (Thornton and Nunn, 1960).

The interpolation technique. The death knell of the methods described above was sounded by the development of the interpolation method by Siggaard-Andersen and Astrup in Copenhagen. In their approach, P_{CO_2} of blood is measured by interpolating the actual pH in a plot of log P_{CO_2} against pH derived from aliquots of the same blood sample. The plot is linear (*Figures 9.5*, and *E.4* in Appendix E) and the whole operation became a practical proposition following the introduction of the microapparatus described by Siggaard-Andersen et al. (1960). A small error is introduced if the sample is desaturated. Minor refinements of technique and the level of accuracy were described by Kelman, Coleman and Nunn (1966). Accuracy is uninfluenced by the presence of anaesthetic gases. Between 1957 and 1960 the interpolation procedure was undertaken on separated plasma but this contained a conceptual source of error and the method was abandoned.

The P_{CO_2}-sensitive electrode. Finally, all the above methods have given way to the P_{CO_2}-sensitive electrode which, in its automated form, has removed the requirement for technical expertise. Analysis may now be satisfactorily performed by untrained staff on a do-it-yourself basis with results available within 5 minutes (Minty and Barrett, 1978).

P_{CO_2} of any gas or liquid may be determined directly by this technique (Severinghaus and Bradley, 1958; Severinghaus, 1965). The P_{CO_2} of a film of bicarbonate solution is allowed to come into equilibrium with the P_{CO_2} of a sample across a membrane permeable to carbon dioxide but not to hydrogen ions. The pH of the bicarbonate solution is constantly monitored by a glass electrode and the log of the P_{CO_2} is inversely proportional to the recorded pH. The accuracy obtainable is comparable to that of other techniques and is uninfluenced by the presence of anaesthetic gases.

The long and fascinating history of measurement of P_{CO_2} and acid–base has been recorded by Astrup and Severinghaus (1986) and Severinghaus and Astrup (1986).

Indirect measurement of arterial P_{CO_2}

Measurement of end-expiratory P_{CO_2} is of limited value due to the variable arterial/ end-expiratory P_{CO_2} gradient caused by lung disease or anaesthesia. However, the method is useful for recording changes. If a rapid carbon dioxide analyser is not available, end-expiratory samples may be collected (Rahn et al., 1946).

Measurement of mixed venous P_{CO_2} is of greater value than measurement of end-expiratory P_{CO_2} and it may be estimated indirectly with very simple apparatus, using the rebreathing technique of Campbell and Howell (1960). A modification of the technique for use in children was described by Sykes (1960). The collection of the gas sample which has been equilibrated with mixed venous blood is perfectly feasible in the unconscious patient, and the technique should be available in hospitals where there are no facilities for measurement of P_{CO_2} of blood samples.

It was originally recommended that 0.8 kPa (6 mmHg) should be subtracted from the mixed venous (rebreathing) P_{CO_2} to give the arterial P_{CO_2} since this is the normally accepted difference between mixed venous and arterial P_{CO_2}. However, many workers have found that the mixed venous P_{CO_2} measured by the rebreathing technique seems to give a higher value than would be expected. McEvoy, Jones and Campbell (1974) reconsidered the theoretical background of the method and drew attention to a number of factors which raise the rebreathing P_{CO_2}. Most important is the fact that the rebreathing method measures the P_{CO_2} of venous blood as it would be if fully oxygenated. The Haldane effect (see *Figure 9.2*) then raises the P_{CO_2} 0.5–1 kPa (3.8–7.5 mmHg) higher than the true mixed venous P_{CO_2}. Furthermore, the mixed venous/arterial P_{CO_2} gradient will be increased in hypercapnia (due to the curvature of the carbon dioxide dissociation curve), as well as with arterial hypoxaemia, reduced cardiac output and anaemia. An additional factor is the finite time required for the physicochemical equilibration of carbon dioxide in the blood, the rate-limiting step being equation (2) on page 207. The P_{CO_2} of arterial blood when sampled and analysed may be different from the value when the blood left the pulmonary capillary where it was in equilibrium with alveolar gas. In general, the observed mixed venous P_{CO_2} (as measured by the rebreathing technique) is likely to exceed the arterial P_{CO_2} by 1–2 kPa (7.5–15 mmHg) in the normal resting subject, and it certainly does so in the author. Since this difference rises with increasing P_{CO_2}, McEvoy and his co-workers suggested that the indirect arterial P_{CO_2} should be calculated as 0.8 times the mixed venous P_{CO_2} measured by the rebreathing technique. Denison et al. (1971) and Godfrey and Wolf (1972) described the use of the method in exercise.

Much of the above is now academic since, with modern techniques, it is generally easier to analyse a sample of arterial blood than to undertake the rebreathing procedure. Nevertheless, certain alternative sites for measurement of P_{CO_2} should be considered.

Transcutaneous P_{CO_2}. This is generally a satisfactory technique using a CO_2-sensitive electrode heated to about 44°C—which is, however, close to the temperature which burns the skin. Transcutaneous P_{CO_2} should be within about 0.5 kPa (3.8 mmHg) of the simultaneous arterial value, but it is necessary to apply a large correction factor for the difference in temperature between body and electrode (Severinghaus, 1981).

Measurement of P_{CO_2} *of venous blood draining skin* has been advanced as an alternative to arterial puncture. The results are quite acceptable for clinical purposes (Forster et al., 1972). However, it is surprisingly difficult to collect a good sample of blood anaerobically from the veins on the back of the hand. Cooper and Smith (1961) found that agreement between arterial and cutaneous venous P_{CO_2} was good in the majority of a series of anaesthetized patients, but considerable discrepancies appeared in a minority of patients, thought to have circulatory disturbances. Blood from veins draining muscles (e.g. the median cubital vein) has a P_{CO_2} much higher than the arterial level and is useless as an indication of the arterial P_{CO_2}.

Measurement of capillary P_{CO_2} on blood obtained from a skin prick suffers from the same uncertainties which surround cutaneous venous P_{CO_2}. However, the technique is clearly useful in neonates. It is perhaps important to remember that an error of 0.6 kPa (4.5 mmHg) is seldom of much consequence in the management of a patient.

Handling of blood samples

It is important that samples be preserved from contact with air or oil, to which they may lose carbon dioxide. Analysis should be undertaken quickly, as the P_{CO_2} of blood *in vitro* rises by about 0.013 kPa/min (0.1 mmHg/min) at 37°C. If analysis is not carried out at the patient's body temperature, a correction factor should be applied, as the P_{CO_2} of an anaerobic blood sample falls by about 4 per cent for each degree Celsius cooling. Nomograms for correction for both these errors were prepared by Kelman and Nunn (1966b) and are to be found in Appendix E (*Figures E.1* and *E.2*).

Chapter 10

Oxygen

The role of oxygen in the cell

Dissolved molecular oxygen (dioxygen) enters into many metabolic processes in the mammalian body (Fisher and Forman, 1985). Quantitatively much the most important is the cytochrome c oxidase system which is responsible for about 90 per cent of the total oxygen consumption of the body. However, cytochrome c oxidase is but one of more than 200 oxidases which may be classified as follows.

Electron transfer oxidases. As a group these oxidases involve the reduction of oxygen to superoxide anion, hydrogen peroxide or water, the last being the fully reduced state (see Chapter 29, *Figure 29.2*). The most familiar is cytochrome c oxidase. Located in the mitochondria, this is concerned in the production of the high energy phosphate bond in adenosine triphosphate (ATP) which is the main source of biological energy. This process is described in greater detail below under the heading 'Oxidative phosphorylation'. Another member of this group of oxidases is NADPH oxidase which is concerned in the generation of superoxide anion in phagocytes. This is discussed further in Chapter 29. Other electron transfer oxidases are responsible for the conversion of 5-hydroxytryptamine to 5-hydroxyindole-acetaldehyde and urate to allantoin.

Oxygen transferases (dioxygenases). This group of oxygenases incorporates oxygen into substrates without the formation of any reduced oxygen product. Familiar examples are cyclo-oxygenase and lipoxygenase which are concerned in the first stage of conversion of arachidonic acid into prostaglandins and leukotrienes (see Chapter 11, page 291). A dioxygenase is also concerned in the conversion of tryptophan to formylkynurenine.

Mixed function oxidases. These oxidases result in oxidation of both a substrate and a co-substrate, which is most commonly NADPH. Well known examples are the cytochrome P-450 hydroxylases, which play an important role in detoxification and are considered further on page 241. Mixed function oxidases are also concerned in the conversion of phenylalanine to tyrosine and of dopamine to noradrenaline, the co-substrate being NADPH for the former and ascorbate for the latter.

Oxidative phosphorylation

Most of the energy deployed in the mammalian body is derived from the oxidation of food fuels, of which the most important is glucose:

$$C_6H_{12}O_6 + 6O_2 = 6CO_2 + 6H_2O + energy$$

The equation accurately describes the combustion of glucose *in vitro*, but is only a crude, overall representation of the oxidation of glucose in the body. The direct reaction does not produce energy in a form in which it can be utilized for the various activities of the living body. The biological oxidation proceeds by a large number of stages, with phased production of energy. This energy is not all immediately released but is partly stored by means of the reaction of adenosine diphosphate (ADP) with inorganic phosphate ion to form adenosine triphosphate (ATP):

$$ADP + inorganic\ phosphate\ ion + energy \rightleftharpoons ATP$$

The third phosphate group in ATP is held by a high energy bond which releases its energy when ATP is split back into ADP and inorganic phosphate ion. ATP is thus recycled indefinitely, with ATP acting as a short-term store of energy available in a form which may be used directly for work such as muscle contraction, ion pumping, protein synthesis and secretion. ATP is commonly transported short distances between the sites of synthesis and utilization. For example, in voluntary muscles, it is formed in the mitochondria and used in the myofibrils.

There is no large store of ATP in the body and it must be synthesized continuously as it is being used. The ATP/ADP ratio is an indication of the level of energy which is currently carried in the ADP/ATP system, and the ratio is normally related to the state of oxidation of the cell. The ADP/ATP system is not the only short-term energy store in the body but it is the most important.

The uses of ATP in the body lie outside the scope of this book, but its production from ADP is highly relevant to this chapter since the most efficient methods of production of ATP require the consumption of oxygen. However, the anaerobic methods are of great biological importance and were universal in the early Pre-Cambrian era before the atmospheric Po_2 was sufficiently high for aerobic pathways of metabolism. Anaerobic metabolism is still the rule in certain organisms and in the mammalian body when energy requirements outstrip oxygen supply as, for example, during severe exercise and in hypoxia.

The aerobic pathway permits the release of far greater quantities of energy from the same amount of substrate and is therefore used whenever possible. In simplified form, the contrasting pathways can be shown as follows:

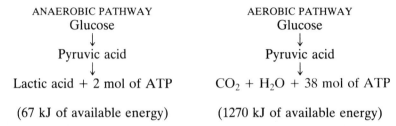

ANAEROBIC PATHWAY
Glucose
↓
Pyruvic acid
↓
Lactic acid + 2 mol of ATP

(67 kJ of available energy)

AEROBIC PATHWAY
Glucose
↓
Pyruvic acid
↓
CO₂ + H₂O + 38 mol of ATP

(1270 kJ of available energy)

In vitro combustion of glucose liberates 2820 kJ/mol as heat. Thus, under conditions of oxidative metabolism, 45 per cent of the total energy is made available for biological work and this compares favourably with most man-made machines.

Localization of oxidative phosphorylation in the cell. The oxygen consumption occurs in the mitochondria, where it combines with hydrogen to form water. The hydrogen has previously been removed from a variety of substrates by nicotinamide adenine dinucleotide (NAD), and then passed along a chain of hydrogen carriers to combine with oxygen at cytochrome a_3 which is the end of the chain. *Figure 10.1* shows the transport of hydrogen along the chain, which consists of structural entities just visible under the electron microscope and arranged in rows along the cristae of the mitochondria. Three molecules of ATP are formed at various stages of the chain during the transfer of two atoms of hydrogen. The process is not associated directly with the production of carbon dioxide, which is formed elsewhere in the

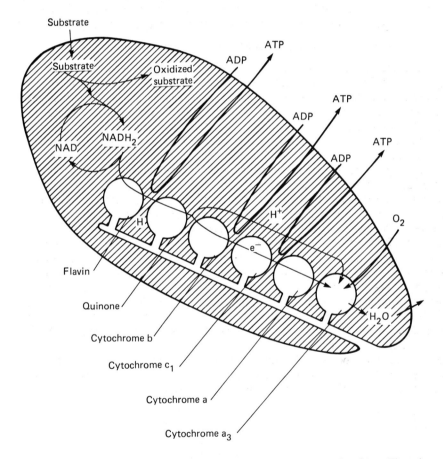

Figure 10.1 Diagrammatic representaton of oxidation within the mitochondrion. The substrate diffuses from the cytoplasm into the mitochondrion where hydrogen is removed under the influence of the appropriate dehydrogenase enzyme. The hydrogen is carried by intramitochondrial NAD to the first of the chain of hydrogen carriers which are attached to the cristae of the mitochondria. When the hydrogen reaches the cytochromes, ionization occurs; the proton passes into the lumen of the mitochondrion while the electron is passed along the cytochromes where it converts ferric iron to the ferrous form. The final stage is at cytochrome a_3 where the proton and the electron combine with oxygen to form water. Three molecules of ADP are converted to ATP at the stages shown in the diagram. ADP and ATP can cross the mitochondrial membrane freely while there are separate pools of intra- and extramitochondrial NAD which cannot interchange.

metabolic pathways. Oxidative phosphorylation can take place only when the Po_2 within the mitochondrion is above a critical level, thought to be of the order of 0.1 kPa. When the Po_2 falls below this level, metabolism reverts to anaerobic pathways. The reduction of oxygen to water by cytochrome a_3 is inhibited by cyanide.

The role of oxidative phosphorylation in the aerobic degradation of glucose is illustrated in *Figure 10.2*. One molecule of glucose is converted into two molecules

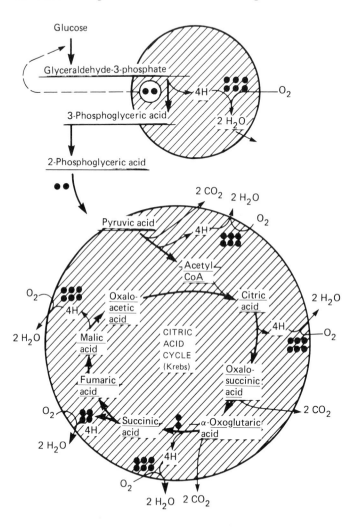

Figure 10.2 Successive stages in the principal oxidative metabolic pathway of glucose by the citric acid cycle. Many stages have been omitted for clarity. The two shaded circles represent mitochondria and indicate the reactions which can only take place within them. The names of substances which cross the membranes show those which are capable of diffusion into and out of the mitochondria. Underlining indicates that two molecules are formed from one of glucose. Black dots show where ATP is formed (the first two to be produced are offset by two which are required for the conversion of glucose to glyceraldehyde-3-phosphate). Note the dissociation between O_2 consumption and CO_2 production. The conversion of glyceraldehyde-3-phosphate to 3-phosphoglyceric acid can also take place in the cytoplasm as shown in Figure 10.3 but, in that case, it is not possible for the liberated hydrogen to be oxidized to water, since the $NADH_2$ cannot diffuse into the mitochondria.

of glyceraldehyde-3-phosphate in the cytoplasm of the cell. The latter then diffuses into the mitochondria where it is converted into 3-phosphoglyceric acid when hydrogen is removed by NAD and oxidized after transport along the chain shown in *Figure 10.1*. The next reactions can take place in the cytoplasm down to the point where pyruvic acid is formed. The oxidation of pyruvic acid, however, can take place only in the mitochondria where hydrogen is removed and oxidized at successive stages of the familiar citric acid cycle. It will be seen that the production of carbon dioxide also occurs within the mitochondria but that it is not directly associated with oxygen consumption. The scheme shown in *Figure 10.2* also accounts for the consumption of oxygen in the metabolism of fat. After hydrolysis, glycerol is converted into pyruvic acid while the fatty acids shed a series of 2-carbon molecules in the form of acetyl CoA. Pyruvic acid and acetyl CoA enter the citric acid cycle and are then degraded in the same manner as though they had been derived from glucose. Amino acids are dealt with in similar manner after deamination.

Figure 10.3 illustrates the anaerobic metabolism of glucose, a pathway which is followed either when there is a shortage of oxygen or, in the case of erythrocytes, when there is an absence of the respiratory enzymes located in the mitochondria. Two molecules of ATP are consumed in the priming stages prior to the formation of fructose-1,6-diphosphate, 6-phosphofructokinase being the rate-limiting enzyme. These ATP molecules are regenerated in the conversion of two molecules of 1,3-diphosphoglyceric acid to two of 3-phosphoglyceric acid, but there is generation of a further two molecules of ATP (from one molecule of glucose) at the conversion of phosphoenolpyruvic acid to pyruvic acid. The conversion of glyceraldehyde-3-phosphate to 3-phosphoglyceric acid can take place in the cytoplasm with hydrogen released as in the aerobic pathway but, in this case, to extramitochondrial NAD. This hydrogen cannot be oxidized but it is taken up lower down the pathway by the reduction of pyruvic acid to lactic acid.

This series of changes is associated with the net formation of only two molecules of ATP from one of glucose, in contrast to the 38 produced in the course of aerobic metabolism.

$$\text{Glucose} + 2\text{Pi} + 2\text{ADP} \rightarrow 2\text{Lactic acid} + 2\text{ATP} + 2\text{H}_2\text{O}$$
$$(\text{Pi} = \text{inorganic phosphate})$$

However, considerable chemical energy remains in the lactic acid which, in the presence of oxygen, can be reconverted to pyruvic acid and then oxidized in the citric acid cycle, producing the balance of 36 molecules of ATP. Alternatively, lactic acid may be converted into liver glycogen to await more favourable conditions for oxidation.

All the acids shown in *Figure 10.3* are highly ionized in the body, and the anaerobic pathway may result in severe acidosis. It is now clear that 6-phosphofructokinase is inhibited by lactacidosis and this limits the generation of ATP. Fructose-1,6-diphosphate bypasses both the rate-limiting stage of 6-phosphofructokinase and also the requirement for two molecules of ATP for priming. It therefore gives twice the yield of ATP compared with glucose and is not subject to rate limitation from acidosis. Its clinical role is considered in Chapter 28.

Significance of oxidative phosphorylation. The production of a high yield of ATP requires oxygen. The alternative anaerobic pathways must either consume very much larger quantities of glucose or, alternatively, yield less ATP. In high-energy-consuming organs such as brain, kidney and liver it is not, in fact, possible to

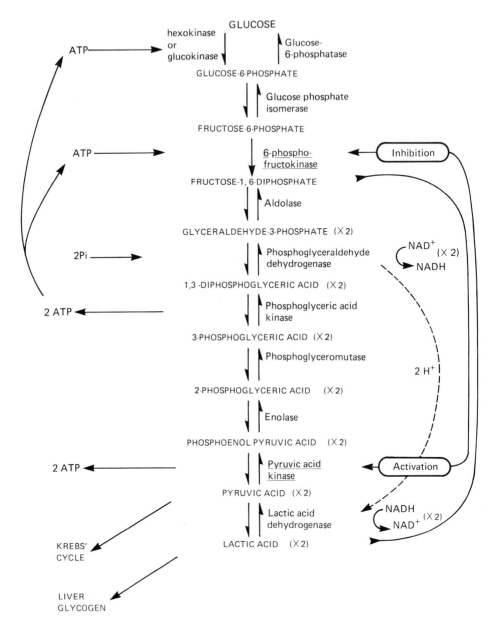

Figure 10.3 The Embden–Meyerhof pathway for anaerobic metabolism of glucose. From glyceraldehyde-3-phosphate downwards, two molecules of each intermediate are formed from one of glucose. Note the consumption of two molecules of ATP in the first three steps. These must be set against the total production of four molecules of ATP, leaving a net gain of two molecules of ATP from the consumption of one molecule of glucose. The hydrogen ions produced at the fifth step are used in the reduction of pyruvic acid to lactic acid. All the acids are largely ionized at tissue pH.

transfer the increased quantities of glucose and therefore these organs suffer ATP depletion under hypoxic conditions. In contrast, voluntary muscle is able to function satisfactorily on anaerobic metabolism during short periods of time and this is normal in the diving mammals.

Anaerobic metabolism carries not only the penalty of ATP depletion but also the serious disadvantage of production of two moles of lactic acid from one of glucose (*Figure 10.3*). At normal intracellular pH, the lactic acid so formed is almost entirely ionized. In most organs both hydrogen and lactate ions escape into the circulation, producing 'lactacidosis'. However, the situation in the brain is quite different. The blood–brain barrier is relatively impermeable to charged ions and both hydrogen and lactate ions are largely retained within the neurone, lowering the intracellular pH. The biochemical and physiological consequences of hypoxia are discussed in Chapter 28.

The critical oxygen tension for aerobic metabolism. When the mitochondrial Po_2 is reduced, oxidative phosphorylation continues normally down to a level of about 0.3 kPa (2 mmHg). Below this level, oxygen consumption falls and the various members of the electron transport chain revert to the reduced state. $NADH/NAD^+$ and lactate/pyruvate ratios rise and the ATP/ADP ratio falls. The critical oxygen tension varies between different organs and different species but, as an approximation, a mitochondrial Po_2 of about 0.13 kPa (1 mmHg) may be taken as the level below which there is serious impairment of oxidative phosphorylation and a switch to anaerobic metabolism. This level is, of course, far below the critical arterial Po_2 because there normally exists a large gradient of Po_2 between arterial blood and the site of utilization of oxygen in the mitochondria. This gradient is discussed as the oxygen cascade, below.

The critical Po_2 for oxidative phosphorylation is also known as the Pasteur point and has applications beyond the pathophysiology of hypoxia in man. In particular, it has a powerful bearing on putrefaction, many forms of which are the results of anaerobic metabolism resulting from a fall of Po_2 below the Pasteur point in, for example, polluted rivers.

Cytochrome P-450

The cytochrome P-450 enzymes are the terminal oxidases for many mixed function oxidase systems, the typical overall reaction being:

$$RH + NADPH + H^+ + O_2 \rightarrow ROH + NADP^+ + H_2O$$

Cytochrome P-450 enzymes are at the end of an electron transport chain in a position analogous to cytochrome a_3 (see *Figure 10.1*) but there are very important differences. Firstly, these enzymes are bound to the membrane of the smooth endoplasmic reticulum (microsomes in homogenized and centrifuged preparations). Secondly, they are not concerned with synthesis of ATP but with hydroxylation of a wide range of substrates, including many drugs. They are thus very important not only in detoxification but also in the formation of biotransformation products which may be more toxic than the original drug. These functions are largely carried out in the liver but also in other tissues, including the lung. It is generally possible to demonstrate that the substrate for hydroxylation is bound to cytochrome P-450 *in vitro* with characteristic changes of its spectral properties.

The cytochrome P-450 enzymes derive their name from the difference spectrum between preparations treated with nitrogen and carbon monoxide. The difference spectrum shows a strong band at a wavelength of 450 nm. It is likely that a number of mixed function oxidases share this property, and they are known collectively as cytochrome P-450.

The hepatic smooth endoplasmic reticulum hypertrophies as a result of *in vivo* treatment with enzyme inducers such as phenobarbitone. There is also an increased level of cytochrome P-450 with enhanced activity towards a wide variety of substrates. Induction with 3-methylcholanthrene causes synthesis of different structural form of cytochrome with the peak of the difference spectrum at 448 nm (cytochrome P-448).

The likely scheme of action of cytochrome P-450 is shown in *Figure 10.4*. Biotransformation by the P-450 system does not only detoxify compounds but may also actually convert an inert molecule into a toxic moiety. A classic example is the anaesthetic fluroxene. Enzyme induction with phenobarbitone increases conversion to trifluoroethanol and thereby the toxicity of fluroxene in animals but not man (Cascorbi and Singh-Amaranath, 1972).

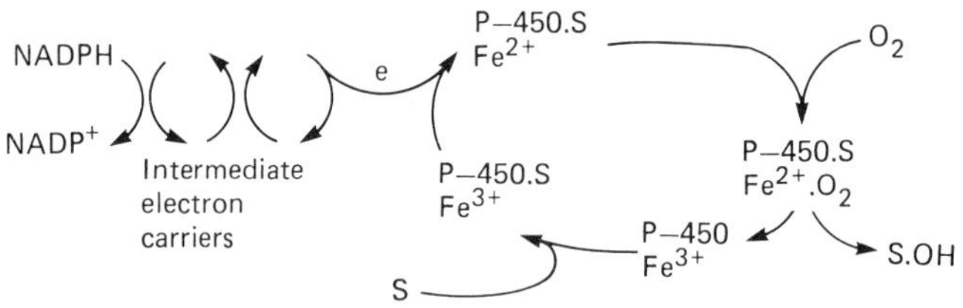

Figure 10.4 The likely scheme of action of cytochrome P-450. S indicates the substrate: both C- and N-oxygenations can occur.

Cytochromes have a range of different P_{50} values and it has been suggested that herein lie the mechanisms for P_{O_2} sensors in the carotid body (page 84) and the pulmonary circulation (page 128).

The oxygen cascade

The P_{O_2} of dry air at sea level is 21.2 kPa (159 mmHg). Oxygen moves down a partial pressure gradient from air, through the respiratory tract, the alveolar gas, the arterial blood, the systemic capillaries and the cell, and finally reaches its lowest level within the mitochondria where it is consumed (*Figure 10.5*). At this point, the P_{O_2} is probably within the range 0.5–3 kPa (3.8–22.5 mmHg) varying from one tissue to another, from one cell to another, and from one part of a cell to another.

The steps by which the P_{O_2} decreases from air to the mitochondria are known as the oxygen cascade and are of great practical importance. Any one step in the cascade may be increased under pathological circumstances and this may result in hypoxia. The steps will now be considered *seriatim*.

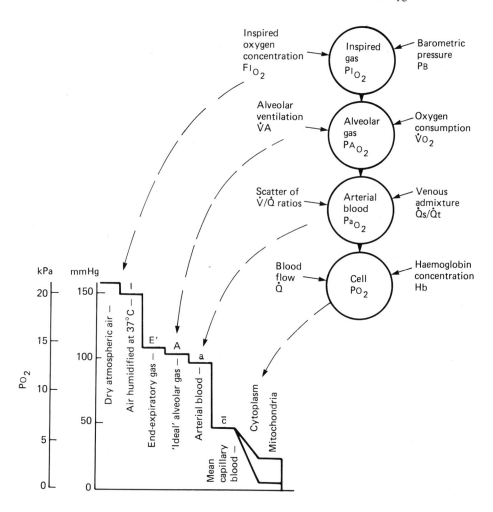

Figure 10.5 On the left is shown the oxygen cascade with Po_2 falling from the level in the ambient air down to the level in mitochondria, which is the site of utilization. On the right is shown a summary of the factors influencing oxygenation at different levels in the cascade.

Dilution of inspired oxygen by water vapour

Analysis with the Haldane apparatus indicates the true fractional concentration of oxygen in a dry gas mixture. If the gas sample is humidified, the added water vapour is ignored and the indicated fractional concentration of oxygen is still that of the dry part of the gas mixture. Thus the normal value for atmospheric oxygen (20.94% or 0.2094 fractional concentration) indicates the concentration of oxygen in the dry gas phase regardless of whether the gas is humidified or not. However, humidification such as occurs when dry air is inhaled through the upper respiratory tract, dilutes air with water vapour and so reduces the Po_2. The process is similar to the reduction in Po_2 which occurs when ether vapour is added to air (Scott, 1847).

When dry gas kept at normal barometric pressure is humidified with water vaporized at 37°C, 100 volumes of the dry gas take up about 6 volumes of water vapour, giving a total gas volume of 106 units but containing the same number of molecules of oxygen. The Po_2 is thus reduced by the fraction 6/106. It follows from Boyle's law that Po_2 after humidification is indicated by the following expression:

$$\begin{array}{c}\text{fractional concentration of oxygen} \\ \text{in the dry gas phase} \\ \text{(Haldane value)}\end{array} \times \left(\begin{array}{cc}\text{barometric} & \text{saturated water} \\ \text{pressure} & - & \text{vapour pressure}\end{array}\right)$$

(the quantity in parentheses is known as the dry barometric pressure).

Therefore the effective Po_2 of inspired air at a body temperature of 37°C is:

$$0.2094 \times (101.3 - 6.3) = 0.2094 \times 95$$

$$= 19.9 \text{ kPa}$$

or, in old units:

$$0.2094 \times (760 - 47) = 0.2094 \times 713$$

$$= 149 \text{ mmHg}$$

As a rough approximation, the partial pressure in kPa is close to the percentage concentration at normal barometric pressure. Partial pressure in mmHg may be approximately derived by multiplying the percentage concentration by 7; for example, the Po_2 of air is approximately $21 \times 7 = 147$ mmHg and the tension of 5% carbon dioxide is approximately $5 \times 7 = 35$ mmHg.

In respiratory physiology, gas tensions are almost always considered as being exerted by gas humidified at body temperature. This applies to inspired gas because it cannot participate in gas exchange until after it has been humidified in the upper respiratory tract. Therefore calculations almost always employ the *dry* barometric pressure whether considering inspired, alveolar or expired gas.

Primary factors influencing alveolar oxygen tension

The general equation for the calculation of the alveolar tension of a gas has been stated on pages 110 et seq. In the case of oxygen:

$$\text{alveolar } Po_2 \doteqdot \begin{array}{c}\text{dry} \\ \text{barometric} \\ \text{pressure}\end{array} \left(\begin{array}{c}\text{inspired} \\ \text{oxygen} \\ \text{concentration}\end{array} - \frac{\text{oxygen uptake}}{\text{alveolar ventilation}}\right) \quad \ldots (1)$$

This equation is only approximate and does not include the second order correction factor due to the small difference in volume between the inspired and the expired gas. Normally this factor is small but, during the exchange of a soluble gas such as nitrous oxide, the difference may be quite large.

Various forms of the alveolar air equation may be used to correct for this difference (pages 182 et seq.) . The commonest forms assume that the number of molecules of nitrogen inhaled equals the number exhaled. This, of course, is very seldom true during and after anaesthesia, and in the intensive therapy unit.

Therefore, under these circumstances it is necessary to use a special form of the equation introduced by Filley, MacIntosh and Wright (1954), which makes no assumptions of inert gas equilibrium and is appropriate to most of the varied conditions likely to be encountered in clinical practice:

$$P_{A_{O_2}} = P_{I_{O_2}} - P_{A_{CO_2}} \left(\frac{P_{I_{O_2}} - P\bar{E}_{O_2}}{P\bar{E}_{CO_2}} \right) \qquad \ldots (2)$$

Applications of the equation were discussed by Nunn (1963). A further modification was described by Kelman and Prys-Roberts (1967) which allows for the addition of carbon dioxide to the inspired gas of the patient.

In its more accurate forms (e.g. equation 2), the alveolar air equation is used principally for calculation of the 'ideal' alveolar P_{O_2}, a theoretical entity which was introduced on page 155 and explained in greater detail on pages 182 et seq. 'Ideal' alveolar gas approximates in composition to the mixed gas which is exhaled at the end of expiration from the perfused alveoli. In practice, it is defined as having a P_{CO_2} equal to that of arterial blood and a respiratory exchange ratio equal to that of mixed expired gas. Comparison of 'ideal' alveolar P_{O_2} with arterial P_{O_2} is the standard method of measurement of 'venous admixture' (pages 181 et seq.).

In its simplified form (equation 1), the alveolar air equation is useful for consideration of the important quantitative relationships between barometric pressure, inspired oxygen concentration, oxygen uptake and alveolar ventilation. They are as follows.

Dry barometric pressure. Other factors remaining constant, the alveolar P_{O_2} will be directly proportional to the dry barometric pressure which falls with increasing altitude to become zero at 19 kilometres where the actual barometric pressure equals the saturated vapour pressure of water at body temperature (see *Table 14.1*). The effect of increased pressure is complex (see Chapter 15, page 323). For example, a pressure of 10 atmospheres (absolute) increases the alveolar P_{O_2} by a factor of about 15 if other factors remain constant (see *Table 15.2*).

Inspired oxygen concentration. The alveolar P_{O_2} will be raised or lowered by an amount equal to the change in the inspired gas P_{O_2}, provided that other factors remain constant. Since the concentration of oxygen in the inspired gas should always be under control, it is a most important therapeutic tool which may be used to counteract a number of different factors which may impair oxygenation.

The effect of an increase in the inspired oxygen concentration from 21 to 30 per cent is shown in *Figure 10.6*. For any alveolar ventilation, the improvement of alveolar P_{O_2} will be 8.5 kPa (64 mmHg). This will be of great importance if, for example, hypoventilation while breathing air has reduced the alveolar P_{O_2} to 4 kPa (30 mmHg), a value which is close to the lowest level compatible with life. Oxygen enrichment of inspired gas to 30% will then increase the alveolar P_{O_2} to 12.5 kPa (94 mmHg), which is almost within the normal range. However, at this level of hypoventilation, P_{CO_2} would be about 13 kPa (98 mmHg) and might well have risen further on withdrawal of the hypoxic drive to ventilation. Thus 30% is the maximum concentration of oxygen in the inspired gas which should be required to correct the alveolar P_{O_2} of a patient breathing air, who has become hypoxaemic as a result of hypoventilation. This problem is discussed at some length in Chapter 20 (pages

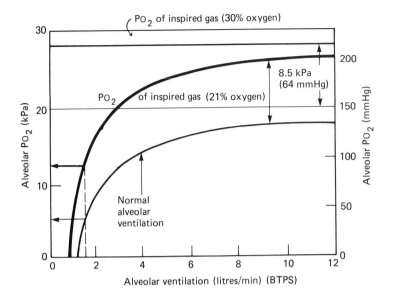

Figure 10.6 The effect on alveolar PO_2 of increasing the inspired oxygen concentration from 21% (thin curve) to 30% (heavy curve). The patient is assumed to have an oxygen consumption of 200 ml/min (STPD). In this example, the alveolar PO_2 is reduced to a dangerously low level when breathing air at an alveolar ventilation of 1.5 l/min. At this point, oxygen enrichment of the inspired gas to 30% is sufficient to raise the alveolar PO_2 almost to within the normal range. All points on the heavy curve are 8.5 kPa (64 mmHg) above the corresponding points on the thin curve at the same ventilation.

388 et seq.). *Figure 5.8* shows ventilation/alveolar PO_2 curves for a wide range of inspired oxygen concentrations, indicating the protection against hypoxaemia (due to hypoventilation) which is afforded by different concentrations of oxygen in the inspired gas.

An entirely different problem is hypoxaemia due to venous admixture. This results in an increased alveolar/arterial PO_2 difference which, within limits, can be offset by increasing the alveolar PO_2. Quantitative aspects are quite different from the problem of hypoventilation and are considered later in this chapter (page 254).

For completeness, it should be mentioned that high concentrations of oxygen may also be used for clearing gas loculi (page 479) and also to provide an increase in the body stores of oxygen (page 271).

Oxygen consumption. The role of oxygen consumption has received insufficient attention and there is an unfortunate tendency to consider that all patients consume 250 ml of oxygen per minute under all circumstances. Oxygen consumption must, of course, be raised by exercise but is often above basal in a patient supposedly 'at rest'. It tends to be just those patients in whom there is a respiratory problem who have oxygen consumptions significantly above basal. A rising oxygen consumption is a factor in the patient who is caught by the pincers of a falling ventilatory capacity and a rising ventilatory requirement (see *Figure 20.5*). Weaning from artificial ventilation may be made unexpectedly difficult by an unsuspected high oxygen consumption. This may be measured directly but is difficult in the circumstances of the intensive therapy unit. Thyrotoxicosis, convulsions and, to a lesser extent, shivering (Bay, Nunn and Prys-Roberts, 1968) cause a very marked rise in oxygen consumption and should, of course, be controlled. The value of measurement of oxygen consumption in the management of tetanus has been stressed by Femi-Pearse et al. (1976).

No less important is the reduction in oxygen consumption which occurs during anaesthesia, hypothermia and myxoedema. Oxygen consumption during anaesthesia tends to be about 15 per cent below basal on the usual standards. This tends to reduce the ventilatory requirement during anaesthesia but the benefit to gaseous homoeostasis is more than offset by other factors (Chapter 19). Hypothermia causes a marked reduction in oxygen consumption with values of about 50 per cent of basal at 31°C. Artificial ventilation of hypothermic patients very commonly results in hypocapnia unless a conscious effort is made to reduce the minute volume or increase the apparatus dead space. *Figure 10.7* shows the effect of different values for oxygen consumption on the relationship between alveolar ventilation and alveolar P_{O_2} for a patient breathing air.

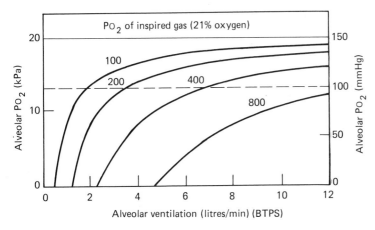

Figure 10.7 The relationship between alveolar ventilation and alveolar P_{O_2} for different values of oxygen consumption for a patient breathing air at normal barometric pressure. The figures on the curves indicate the oxygen consumption in ml/min (STPD). Alveolar ventilation is in l/min (BTPS). A typical value for oxygen consumption by an anaesthetized patient is 200 ml/min; 100 ml/min would be an average figure during hypothermia at 30°C. Higher values may be brought about by restlessness, struggling, pyrexia or shivering. Note that the alveolar ventilation required to maintain any particular alveolar P_{O_2} is directly proportional to the oxygen consumption. (In calculations of this type it is important to make the correction required by the fact that oxygen consumption and alveolar ventilation values are commonly expressed at different temperatures and pressures—see Appendix C.)

Alveolar ventilation. There is a hyperbolic relationship between alveolar P_{O_2} and alveolar ventilation. As ventilation is increased, the alveolar P_{O_2} rises asymptotically towards (but never reaches) the P_{O_2} of the inspired gas (see *Figure 10.6*). It will be seen from the shape of the curves that changes in ventilation *above* normal level have comparatively little effect upon alveolar P_{O_2}. In contrast, changes in ventilation *below* the normal level may have a very marked effect on alveolar P_{O_2}. At very low levels of ventilation, the alveolar ventilation is critical and small changes may precipitate gross hypoxia.

Secondary factors influencing alveolar oxygen tension

Cardiac output. In the short term, cardiac output can influence the alveolar P_{O_2}. For example, if other factors remain constant, a sudden reduction in cardiac output will temporarily increase the alveolar P_{O_2}, since less blood passes through the lungs to remove oxygen from the alveolar gas. However, the reduced cardiac output also causes increased oxygen extraction in the tissues supplied by the systemic circulation, and before long the mixed venous oxygen level is decreased. When that has happened, the removal of oxygen from the alveolar gas returns to its original level as the reduction in blood flow rate is compensated by the greater amount of oxygen which is taken up per unit volume of blood flowing through the lungs. Thus, in the long term, cardiac output does not directly influence the alveolar P_{O_2} and only the oxygen uptake appears in equation (1).

The 'concentration', third gas or Fink effect. The above diagrams and equations have ignored a factor which influences alveolar P_{O_2} during exchanges of large quantities of soluble gases such as nitrous oxide. This effect was mentioned briefly in connection with carbon dioxide on page 224. Its effect on oxygen is probably more important.

During the administration of nitrous oxide, large quantities of the more soluble gas replace smaller quantities of the less soluble nitrogen previously dissolved in body fluids. There is thus a net uptake of 'inert' gas into the body from the alveoli, causing a *temporary* increase in the concentration of both oxygen and carbon dioxide, which will thus *temporarily* exert a higher tension than would otherwise be expected. Conversely, during recovery from nitrous oxide anaesthesia, large quantities of nitrous oxide leave the body to be replaced with smaller quantities of nitrogen. There is thus a net transfer of 'inert' gas from the body into the alveoli causing dilution of oxygen and carbon dioxide, both of which will *temporarily* exert a lower tension than would otherwise be expected.

The alveolar/arterial P_{O_2} difference

The next step in the oxygen cascade is of great clinical relevance. In the healthy young adult breathing air, the alveolar/arterial P_{O_2} difference does not exceed 2 kPa (15 mmHg) but may rise to above 5 kPa (37.5 mmHg) in aged but healthy subjects. These values may be exceeded in any lung disease which causes shunting or mismatching of ventilation and perfusion. Typical examples are pulmonary collapse, consolidation, neoplasm or infection. Extrapulmonary shunting (e.g. Fallot's tetralogy) will also increase the difference. An increased alveolar/arterial P_{O_2} difference is the commonest cause of arterial hypoxaemia in clinical practice and this is a very important step in the oxygen cascade.

Unlike the alveolar P_{O_2}, the alveolar/arterial P_{O_2} difference cannot be predicted from other more easily measured quantities, and there is no simple means of knowing the magnitude of the alveolar/arterial P_{O_2} difference in a particular patient other than by measurement of the arterial blood gas tensions. It is important to understand the factors which influence the difference and the principles of restoration of arterial P_{O_2} by increasing the inspired oxygen concentration.

Factors influencing the magnitude of the alveolar/arterial Po₂ difference

In Chapter 9 it was explained how the alveolar/arterial P_{O_2} difference results from venous admixture (or physiological shunt) which consists of two components: (1) shunted venous blood which mingles with the oxygenated blood leaving the pulmonary capillaries; (2) a component due to scatter of ventilation/perfusion ratios in different parts of the lungs. Any component due to impaired diffusion across the alveolar/capillary membrane is likely to be very small and can probably be ignored (page 195).

Figure 7.10 shows the derivation of the following axiomatic relationship for the first component:

$$\frac{\dot{Q}s}{\dot{Q}t} = \frac{Cc'_{O_2} - Ca_{O_2}}{Cc'_{O_2} - C\bar{v}_{O_2}}$$

Two points should be noted.

1. The equation gives a slightly false impression of precision since it assumes that all the shunted blood is *mixed* venous. This is not the case, thebesian and bronchial venous blood being obvious exceptions.
2. Oxygen content of pulmonary end-capillary blood (Cc'_{O_2}) is, in practice, calculated on the basis of the end-capillary oxygen tension (Pc'_{O_2}) being equal to the 'ideal' alveolar P_{O_2} (see page 182).

The equation may be cleared and solved for the pulmonary end-capillary/arterial oxygen content difference as follows:

$$Cc'_{O_2} - Ca_{O_2} = \frac{\dfrac{\dot{Q}s}{\dot{Q}t}(Ca_{O_2} - C\bar{v}_{O_2})}{\left(1 - \dfrac{\dot{Q}s}{\dot{Q}t}\right)} \qquad \ldots (3)$$

(scaling factors are required to correct for the inconsistency of the units which are customarily used for the quantities in this equation).

$Ca_{O_2} - Cv_{O_2}$ is the arterial/mixed venous oxygen content difference and is a function of the oxygen consumption and the cardiac output thus

$$\dot{Q}t(Ca_{O_2} - C\bar{v}_{O_2}) = \dot{V}_{O_2}\text{(Fick equation)} \qquad \ldots (4)$$

Substituting for ($Ca_{O_2} - C\bar{v}_{O_2}$) in equation (3), we have:

$$Cc'_{O_2} - Ca_{O_2} = \frac{\dot{V}_{O_2}\dfrac{\dot{Q}s}{\dot{Q}t}}{\dot{Q}t\left(1 - \dfrac{\dot{Q}s}{\dot{Q}t}\right)} \qquad \ldots (5)$$

This equation shows the content difference in terms of oxygen consumption ($\dot{V}_{O_2}$), the venous admixture ($\dot{Q}s/\dot{Q}t$) and the cardiac output ($\dot{Q}t$).

The significance of cardiac output has not received due attention until recent years. However, it will be clear that this factor must be of considerable importance, since a reduced cardiac output results in an increased arterial/mixed venous oxygen content difference. This means that the shunted blood will be more desaturated and will therefore cause a greater fall of the arterial oxygen level than would less desaturated blood flowing through a shunt of the same magnitude. This consideration is apart from the fact that an increased cardiac output is usually associated with an increased fraction of the cardiac output flowing through an existing shunt (Cheney and Colley, 1980). This is considered further on page 173.

The final stage in the calculation is to convert the end-capillary/arterial oxygen *content* difference to the *tension* difference. The oxygen content of blood is the sum of the oxygen in physical solution and that which is combined with haemoglobin:

$$\text{oxygen content of blood} = \alpha Po_2 + So_2 \times Hb \times 1.39$$

where: α is the solubility coefficient of oxygen in blood (not plasma); So_2 is the saturation, and varies with Po_2 according to the oxygen dissociation curve, which itself is influenced by temperature, pH and base excess (Bohr effect); Hb is the haemoglobin concentration (g/dl); 1.39 is the volume of oxygen (ml) which can combine with 1 g of haemoglobin. This is the theoretical value based on the molecular weight of haemoglobin, but it is not obtained in practice (see page 260).

Carriage of oxygen in the blood is discussed in detail on pages 258 et seq.

Derivation of the oxygen content from the Po_2 is laborious if due account is taken of pH, base excess, temperature and haemoglobin concentration. Derivation of Po_2 from content is even more laborious, as an iterative approach is required. Tables of tension/content relationships are particularly useful and *Table 10.1* is an extract

Table 10.1 Oxygen content of human blood (ml/100 ml) as a function of Po$_2$ and other variables

	Haemoglobin concentration (g/dl)		
	10	14	18
Po$_2$ at pH 7.4, 37°Ch, base excess zero			
6.7 kPa (50 mmHg)	11.99	16.72	21.45
9.3 kPa (70 mmHg)	13.29	18.53	23.76
13.3 kPa (100 mmHg)	13.85	19.27	24.69
20.0 kPa (150 mmHg)	14.20	19.70	25.20
26.7 kPa (200 mmHg)	14.41	19.94	25.47
Po$_2$ at pH 7.2, 37°C, base excess zero			
6.7 kPa (50 mmHg)	10.45	14.57	18.69
9.3 kPa (70 mmHg)	12.60	17.56	22.52
13.3 kPa (100 mmHg)	13.62	18.94	24.27
20 kPa (150 mmHg)	14.11	19.58	25.04
26.7 kPa (200 mmHg)	14.37	19.87	25.38
Po$_2$ at pH 7.4, 34°C, base excess zero			
6.7 kPa (50 mmHg)	12.81	17.87	22.93
9.3 kPa (70 mmHg)	13.59	18.94	24.30
13.3 kPa (100 mmHg)	13.96	19.43	24.89
20 kPa (150 mmHg)	14.24	19.76	25.28
26.7 kPa (200 mmHg)	14.44	19.98	25.51

The fourth significant figure is not of clinical importance but is useful for interpolation.
(Values from the computer-written tables of Kelman and Nunn, 1968)

from Kelman and Nunn (1968) to show the format and general influence of the several variables.

The principal factors influencing the magnitude of the alveolar/arterial P_{O_2} difference caused by venous admixture may be summarized as follows.

The magnitude of the venous admixture increases the alveolar/arterial P_{O_2} difference with direct proportionality for small shunts, although this is lost with larger shunts (*Figure 10.8*). The resultant effect on arterial P_{O_2} is shown in *Figure 7.11*. Different forms of venous admixture are considered on pages 172 et seq.

$\dot{V}/\dot{Q}$ *scatter.* It was explained in Chapter 7 that scatter in ventilation/perfusion ratios produces an alveolar/arterial P_{O_2} difference for the following reasons.

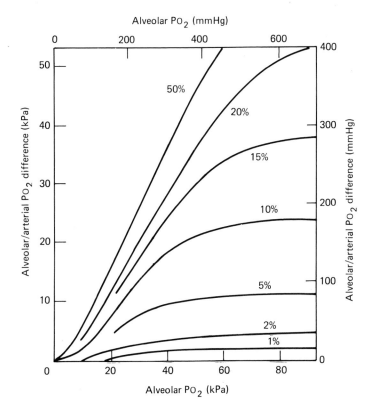

Figure 10.8 Influence of shunt on alveolar/arterial P_{O_2} difference at different levels of alveolar P_{O_2}. For small shunts, the difference (at constant alveolar P_{O_2}) is roughly proportional to the magnitude of the shunt. For a given shunt, the alveolar/arterial P_{O_2} difference increases with alveolar P_{O_2} in non-linear manner governed by the oxygen dissociation curve. At high alveolar P_{O_2}, a plateau of alveolar/arterial P_{O_2} difference is reached but the alveolar P_{O_2} at which the plateau is reached is higher with larger shunts. Note that, with a 50 per cent shunt, an increase in alveolar P_{O_2} produces an almost equal increase in alveolar/arterial P_{O_2} difference. Therefore, the arterial P_{O_2} is virtually independent of changes in alveolar P_{O_2}, if other factors remain constant. Constants incorporated in this diagram: arterial/venous oxygen content difference, 5 ml/100 ml; Hb concentration, 14 g/dl; temperature of blood, 37°C; pH of blood, 7.40; base excess, zero. Figures in the graph indicate shunt as percentage of total pulmonary blood flow.

1. More blood flows through the underventilated overperfused alveoli, and the mixed arterial blood is therefore heavily weighted in the direction of the suboxygenated blood from areas of low $\dot{V}/\dot{Q}$ ratio. The smaller amount of blood flowing through areas of high $\dot{V}/\dot{Q}$ ratio cannot compensate for this (see *Figure 7.12*).
2. Due to the bend in the upper part of the dissociation curve, the fall in saturation in blood from areas of low $\dot{V}/\dot{Q}$ ratio tends to be greater than the rise in saturation in blood from areas of high $\dot{V}/\dot{Q}$ (see *Figure 7.13*). This provides a second reason why blood from alveoli with a high $\dot{V}/\dot{Q}$ ratio cannot compensate for blood from alveoli with a low $\dot{V}/\dot{Q}$ ratio.

The actual alveolar P_{O_2} has a profound but non-linear effect on the alveolar/arterial P_{O_2} gradient (see *Figure 10.8*). The alveolar/arterial oxygen *content* difference for a given shunt is uninfluenced by the alveolar P_{O_2} (equation 5), and the effect on the *tension* difference arises entirely in conversion from *content* to *tension*: it is thus a function of the slope of the dissociation curve at the P_{O_2} of the alveolar gas. For example, a loss of 1 ml/100 ml of oxygen from blood with a P_{O_2} of 93 kPa (700 mmHg) causes a fall of P_{O_2} of about 43 kPa (325 mmHg), most of the oxygen being lost from physical solution. However, if the initial P_{O_2} were 13 kPa (100 mmHg), a loss of 1 ml/100 ml would cause a fall of P_{O_2} of only 4.6 kPa (35 mmHg), most of the oxygen being lost from combination with haemoglobin. Should the initial P_{O_2} be only 6.7 kPa (50 mmHg), a loss of 1 ml/100 ml would cause a very small change in P_{O_2} of the order of 0.7 kPa (5 mmHg), drawn almost entirely from combination with haemoglobin at a point where the dissociation curve is steep. This effect is clearly shown in *Figure 10.8*. The clinical implication is that the alveolar/arterial P_{O_2} difference will be greatest when the alveolar P_{O_2} is highest (other factors being the same). If the alveolar P_{O_2} be reduced (e.g. by underventilation), then the alveolar/arterial P_{O_2} gradient will also be diminished if other factors remain the same. The arterial P_{O_2} thus falls less than the alveolar P_{O_2}. This is fortunate and may be considered as one of the many benefits deriving from the shape of the oxygen dissociation curve. With a 50 per cent venous admixture, the arterial P_{O_2} is almost independent of changes in alveolar P_{O_2} (see *Figure 7.11*).

Cardiac output changes produce inverse changes of the arterial/mixed venous oxygen content difference if the patient's oxygen consumption remains the same (Fick equation: equation 4). Equation (5) shows that there is also an inverse relationship between the cardiac output and the alveolar/arterial oxygen *content* difference if the venous admixture is constant (*Figure 10.9b*). However, when the *content* difference is converted to *tension* difference, the relationship to cardiac output is no longer truly inverse, but assumes a complex non-linear form in consequence of the shape of the oxygen dissociation curve. The relationship between cardiac output and alveolar/arterial P_{O_2} difference shown in *Figure 10.9a* applies only to the conditions specified—particularly the alveolar P_{O_2}, which was assumed to be 24 kPa (180 mmHg) in the preparation of this diagram. In fact, it now appears that a reduction in cardiac output almost always causes a reduction in the shunt fraction. This approximately counteracts the effect of mixed venous desaturation so that arterial P_{O_2} tends to remain much the same (see Chapter 7, page 173). Nevertheless, even if the arterial P_{O_2} is unchanged, the oxygen flux will be reduced in proportion to the change in cardiac output.

The temperature, pH and base excess of the patient's blood influence the dissociation curve (page 263). In addition, temperature affects the solubility coefficient of

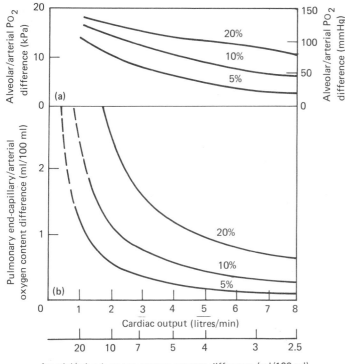

Figure 10.9 Influence of cardiac output on the alveolar/arterial Po₂ difference in the presence of shunts (values indicated for each curve). In this example it is assumed that the patient has an oxygen consumption of 200 ml/min and an alveolar Po₂ of 24 kPa (180 mmHg). Changes in cardiac output produce an inverse change in the pulmonary end-capillary/arterial oxygen content difference (graph b). When converted to tension differences, the inverse relationship is distorted by the effect of the oxygen dissociation curve in a manner which is applicable only to the particular alveolar Po₂ of the patient (graph a). (Alveolar Po₂ is assumed equal to pulmonary end-capillary Po₂.)

oxygen in blood. Thus all three factors influence the relationship between tension and content (see *Table 10.1*), and therefore the effect of venous admixture on the alveolar/arterial Po₂ difference is influenced by these factors although the effect is not usually important except in extreme deviations from normal.

The haemoglobin concentration influences the partition of oxygen between physical solution and chemical combination. While the haemoglobin concentration does not influence the pulmonary end-capillary/arterial oxygen *content* difference (equation 5), it exerts an effect on the *tension* difference. For example, at a cardiac output of 5 l/min and oxygen consumption of 200 ml/min, venous admixture of 20 per cent results in a pulmonary end-capillary/arterial oxygen content difference of 0.5 ml/100 ml. Assuming an alveolar Po₂ of 24 kPa (180 mmHg), the alveolar/arterial Po₂ difference is influenced by haemoglobin concentration as shown in *Table 10.2*. (Different figures would be obtained by selection of a different value for alveolar Po₂.)

Table 10.2 Effect of different haemoglobin concentrations on the arterial P_{O_2} under venous admixture conditions defined in text

Haemoglobin concentration	Alveolar/arterial P_{O_2} difference		Arterial P_{O_2}	
(g/dl)	kPa	mmHg	kPa	mmHg
8	15.0	113	9.0	67
10	14.5	109	9.5	71
12	14.0	105	10.0	75
14	13.5	101	10.5	79
16	13.0	98	11.0	82

Alveolar ventilation. The overall effect of changes in alveolar ventilation on the arterial P_{O_2} presents an interesting problem and serves to illustrate the integration of the separate aspects of the factors discussed above. An increase in the alveolar ventilation may be expected to have the following results.

1. *The alveolar P_{O_2}* must be raised provided the barometric pressure, inspired oxygen concentration and oxygen consumption remain the same (equation 1 and *Figure 10.6*).
2. *The alveolar/arterial P_{O_2} difference* is increased for the following reasons.
   a. The increase in the alveolar P_{O_2} will increase the alveolar/arterial P_{O_2} difference if other factors remain the same (see *Figure 10.8*).
   b. Under many conditions it has been demonstrated that a fall of P_{CO_2} (resulting from an increase in alveolar ventilation) reduces the cardiac output, which will increase the alveolar/arterial P_{O_2} difference if other factors remain the same (equation 5 and *Figure 10.9*).
   c. The change in arterial pH resulting from the reduction in P_{CO_2} causes a small, unimportant increase in alveolar/arterial P_{O_2} difference.

Thus an increase in alveolar ventilation may be expected to raise the alveolar P_{O_2} *and* the alveolar/arterial P_{O_2} difference. The resultant change in arterial P_{O_2} will depend upon the relative magnitude of the two changes. *Figure 10.10* shows the changes in arterial P_{O_2} caused by variations of alveolar ventilation at an inspired oxygen concentration of 30% in the presence of varying degrees of venous admixture, assuming that cardiac output is influenced by P_{CO_2} as described in the legend. Up to an alveolar ventilation of 1.5 l/min, an increase in ventilation will always raise the arterial P_{O_2}. Beyond that, in the example cited, further increases in alveolar ventilation will increase the arterial P_{O_2} only if the venous admixture is less than 3 per cent. For larger values of venous admixture, the increase in the alveolar/arterial P_{O_2} difference exceeds the increase in the alveolar P_{O_2} and the arterial P_{O_2} is thus decreased.

Compensation for increased alveolar/arterial P_{O_2} difference by raising the inspired oxygen concentration

Hypoxaemia is to be expected in patients with most forms of severe respiratory dysfunction. Most patients under treatment in intensive therapy units are

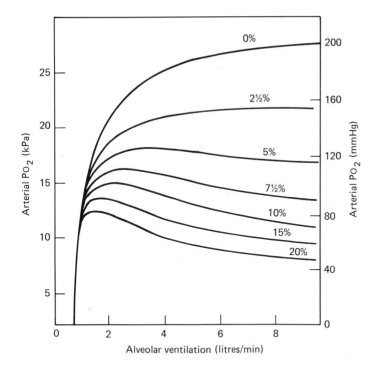

Figure 10.10 The effect of alveolar ventilation on arterial PO_2 is the algebraic sum of the effect upon the alveolar PO_2 (Figure 10.6) and the alveolar/arterial PO_2 difference. When the increase in the latter exceeds the increase in the former, the arterial PO_2 will be diminished. The figures in the diagram indicate the percentage venous admixture. The curve corresponding to zero per cent venous admixture will indicate the alveolar PO_2. Constants incorporated in the design of this figure: inspired O_2 concentration, 30%; O_2 consumption, 200 ml/min; respiratory exchange ratio, 0.8. It has been assumed that the cardiac output is influenced by the PCO_2 according to the equation: $\dot{Q} = 0.039 \times PCO_2$ (mmHg) + 2.23. (Reproduced from Kelman and his colleagues (1967) by permission of the Editor of the British Journal of Anaesthesia)

hypoxaemic while breathing air. The main objective of treatment is clearly to remove the cause of the hypoxaemia but, when this is not immediately possible, it is often possible to relieve the hypoxaemia by increasing the inspired oxygen concentration. The principles for doing so depend upon the cause of the hypoxaemia. As a broad classification, hypoxaemia may be due to hypoventilation or to venous admixture or to a combination of the two. When hypoxaemia is primarily due to hypoventilation and when it is not appropriate or possible to restore the normal ventilation, then the arterial PO_2 may be restored by elevation of the inspired oxygen within the range 21–30% as explained above (page 245 and *Figure 10.6*) and also in Chapter 20 (pages 388 et seq.).

The situation is quantitatively quite different when hypoxaemia is primarily due to venous admixture. It is then only possible to restore the arterial PO_2 by oxygen enrichment of the inspired gas when the venous admixture does not exceed the equivalent of a shunt of 30 per cent of the cardiac output, and this may require up to 100% inspired oxygen (page 171). The quantitative aspects of the relationship are best considered in relation to the iso-shunt diagram (see *Figure 7.11*).

Selection of the optimal arterial P_{O_2} is important to prevent hypoxia on the one hand and pulmonary oxygen toxicity on the other (see Chapter 29). In general, one is reluctant to use concentrations higher than 60–70% for more than a short period. This is sufficient to restore arterial P_{O_2} only when the shunt is less than about 20 per cent, and it is therefore important to ensure that pulmonary function is optimized by careful attention to control of secretions, infection and expansion of areas of collapse. Positive end-expiratory pressure is a particularly valuable method of decreasing the virtual shunt (see page 414).

There is little point in deciding what is the optimal inspired oxygen concentration unless efficient means are available for delivery of the selected oxygen concentration to the patient. This important topic is considered below (page 273).

Transport of oxygen from the lungs to the cell

The most important function of the respiratory and circulatory systems is the supply of oxygen to the cells of the body. The quantity of oxygen transferred in one minute has been termed the 'oxygen flux' (Nunn and Freeman, 1964), and is equal to the following:

$$\text{cardiac output} \times \text{arterial oxygen content}$$

At rest, the numerical values are:

$$5000 \text{ ml/min} \times 20 \text{ ml } O_2/100 \text{ ml blood} = 1000 \text{ ml/min}$$

Of this 1000 ml/min, approximately 250 is utilized by the conscious resting subject. The circulating blood thus loses 25 per cent of its oxygen and the mixed venous blood is approximately 75 per cent saturated. The 75 per cent of unextracted oxygen forms an important reserve which may be drawn upon under the stress of such conditions as exercise, to which additional extraction forms one of the integrated adaptations (see *Figure 12.2*).

The arterial oxygen content consists predominantly of oxygen in combination with haemoglobin and this fraction is given by the following expression:

$$\text{saturation} \times \text{haemoglobin concentration} \times 1.39$$

(1.39 is the theoretical volume of oxygen (ml) which will combine with 1 g of haemoglobin. In practice, this is seldom attained—see below, page 260).

Ignoring the oxygen in physical solution, the expression for the oxygen flux may now be expanded thus:

$$\text{cardiac output} \times \frac{\text{arterial}}{O_2 \text{ saturation}} \times \frac{\text{haemoglobin}}{\text{concentration}} \times 1.39 = \text{oxygen flux}$$

$$5000 \text{ ml/min} \times 95/100 \times 15/100 \text{ g/ml '} \times 1.39 = 1000 \text{ ml/min}$$

Note that three variable factors determine the oxygen flux.

1. *Cardiac output* or, for a particular organ, the regional blood flow. Failure of this factor has been termed 'stagnant anoxia' (Barcroft, 1920).
2. *Arterial oxygen saturation*. Failure of this (for whatever reason) has been termed 'anoxic anoxia'.
3. *Haemoglobin concentration* reduction as a cause of tissue hypoxia, has been termed 'anaemic anoxia'.

The three types of 'anoxia' may be conveniently displayed on a Venn diagram (*Figure 10.11*) which shows the possibility of combinations of any two types of anoxia or all three together. For example, the combination of anaemia and low cardiac output, which occurs in untreated haemorrhage, would be indicated by the

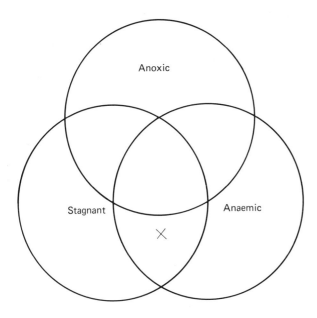

Figure 10.11 *Barcroft's classification of causes of hypoxia displayed on a Venn diagram to illustrate the possibility of combinations of more than one type of hypoxia. The lowest area of overlap, marked with a cross, shows coexistent anaemia and low cardiac output. The central area illustrates a combination of all three types of hypoxia (e.g. a patient with haemorrhage and 'shock lung').*

overlapping area of the stagnant and anaemic circles. If the patient also suffered from 'shock lung', he might then move into the central area, indicating the addition of anoxic anoxia. On a more cheerful note, compensations are more usual. Patients with anaemia normally have a high cardiac output; subjects resident at altitude have polycythaemia, and so on. Such considerations provide a classic example of the importance of viewing a patient as a whole. For example, the question of the lowest permissible haemoglobin concentration for major surgery can be answered only after consideration of the actual and projected cardiac output during surgery, the pulmonary function and so on. No general answer is possible.

It is important to note that the oxygen flux equals the product of three variables and one constant. If one variable is halved, the oxygen flux is halved, but if all three variables are halved, the oxygen flux is reduced to one-eighth of the original value. One-eighth of 1000 is 125 ml/min, and this is a value which, if maintained for any length of time, is incompatible with life, although the reductions of the individual variables are not in themselves lethal. The minimal value of the oxygen flux compatible with survival at rest must vary with circumstances but appears to be of the order of 400 ml/min.

Tissue Po_2. It is often useful to refer to the tissue Po_2 and much of intensive therapy is directed towards increasing tissue Po_2. However, it is almost impossible to quantify tissue Po_2. It is evident that there are differences between different organs, with the tissue Po_2 influenced not only by arterial Po_2 and tissue perfusion but also by oxygen uptake of the organ. However, even greater difficulties arise from the regional variations in tissue Po_2 in different parts of the same organ. They are presumably caused by regional variations in tissue perfusion and oxygen consumption. Nor is this the whole story. An advancing Po_2-sensitive microelectrode detects variations in Po_2 which can be interpreted in relation to the proximity of the electrode to small vessels (see *Figure 8.3*). Very large variations have been demonstratd with exploring electrodes in the brain (Cater et al., 1961). 'Tissue Po_2' is thus an unsatisfactory quantitative index of the state of oxygenation of an organ. Metabolic indicators, such as lactate production, are more useful.

The carriage of oxygen in the blood

Oxygen is carried in the blood in two forms. Much the greater part is in reversible chemical combination with haemoglobin, while a smaller part is in physical solution in plasma and intracellular fluid. The ability to carry large quantities of oxygen in the blood is of great importance to the organism, since without haemoglobin the amount carried would be so small that the cardiac output would need to be increased by a factor of about 20 to give an adequate oxygen flux. This would require a considerable increase in blood volume and, under such handicaps, animals could not have developed to their present extent. The biological significance of the haemoglobin-like compounds is thus immense. It is interesting that the tetrapyrrole ring which contains iron in haemoglobin is also a constituent of chlorophyll which has magnesium in place of iron. The cytochromes also have iron in a tetrapyrrole ring and this structure is thus concerned with production, transport and utilization of oxygen.

Haemoglobin

Haemoglobin was the subject of many years of detailed X-ray crystallographic analysis by the team led by Perutz in Cambridge. Its structure is now well understood and this provides the molecular basis for its remarkable properties (Roughton, 1964; Lehmann and Huntsman, 1966; Perutz, 1969).

The haemoglobin molecule consists of four protein chains, each of which carries a haem group (*Figure 10.12*), the total molecular weight being 64 458.5 (Braunitzer, 1963). The amino acids comprising the chains have been identified and it is known that, in the commonest type of adult human haemoglobin (HbA), there are two types of chain, two of each occurring in each molecule. The two alpha chains each have 141 amino acid residues, with the haem attached to a histidine residue (formula on page 214) occupying position 87. The two beta chains each have 146 amino acid residues, with the haem attached to a histidine residue occupying position 92. *Figure 10.12b* shows details of the point of attachment of the haem in the alpha chain. Similar information for the 'beta' chain is given on page 214.

The four chains of the haemoglobin molecule lie in a ball like a crumpled necklace. However, the form is not random and the actual shape (the quaternary structure) is of critical importance and governs the reaction with oxygen. The shape

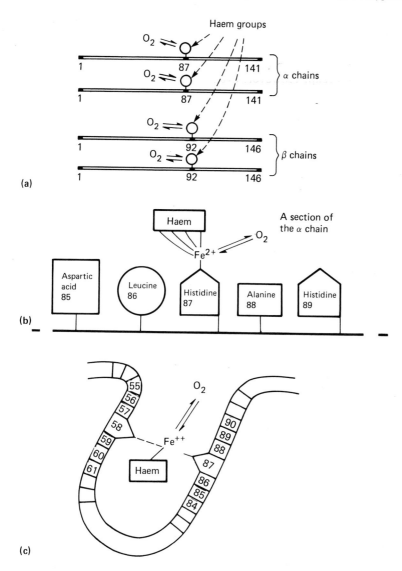

Figure 10.12 The haemoglobin molecule consists of four amino acid chains, each carrying a haem group. (a) Two chains are identical, each with 141 amino acid residues (alpha chains); the other two are also identical and have 146 amino acid residues (beta chains). (b) The attachment of the haem group to the alpha chain. (c) The crevice which contains the haem group.

is maintained by loose bonds between certain amino acids on different chains and also between some amino acids on the same chain. One consequence of these bonds is that the haem groups lie in crevices formed by weak bonds between the haem groups and histidine residues, other than those to which they are attached by normal valency linkages. For example, Figure 10.12c shows a section of an alpha chain with the haem group attached to the iron atom which is bound to the histidine residue in position 87. However, the haem group is also attached by a loose bond to the histidine residue in position 58 and also by non-polar bonds to many other amino acids. This forms a loop and places the haem group in a crevice which limits and controls the ease of access for oxygen molecules.

Bohr Effect? N'est ce pas   (page 263)

Structural basis of the ~~Haldane effect (page 211)~~. The quaternary structure of the is altered by factors which influence the strength of the loose bonds; such factors include temperature, pH, ionic strength and carbon dioxide binding to the N-terminal amino acid residues as carbamate (Kilmartin and Rossi-Bernardi, 1973). This alters the accessibility of the haem groups to oxygen and is believed to be the basis of the mechanism by which the affinity of haemoglobin for oxygen is altered by these factors, an effect which is generally considered in terms of its influence upon the dissociation curve (see *Figure 10.15* below).

Structural basis of the Haldane effect (page 211). The quaternary structure of the haemoglobin molecule is altered by the uptake of oxygen to form oxyhaemoglobin. It is believed that this increases the ionization of certain $-NH_2$ or $=NH$ groups and so reduces their ability to undertake carbamino carriage of carbon dioxide (see *Figure 9.1*).

Oxygen-combining capacity of haemoglobin. There has been some confusion over the oxygen-combining capacity of haemoglobin. Until 1963 the value was taken to be 1.34 ml/g. Following the precise determination of the molecular weight of haemoglobin, the theoretical value of 1.39 ml/g was derived and passed into general use. However, it gradually became clear that this value was not obtained when direct measurements of haemoglobin concentration and oxygen capacity were compared. After an exhaustive study of the subject, Gregory (1974) proposed the values of 1.306 ml/g for human adult blood and 1.312 ml/g for fetal blood. Haemoglobin concentrations are ultimately compared with the International Cyanmethaemoglobin Standard, which is based on iron content and not on oxygen-combining capacity. Since some of the iron is likely to be in the form of haemochromogens, it is not altogether surprising that the observed oxygen-combining capacity is less than the theoretical value of 1.39.

Abnormal forms of haemoglobin

There are a great number of alternative amino acid sequences in the haemoglobin molecule. Most animal species have their own peculiar haemoglobins while, in man, gamma and delta chains occur in addition to the alpha and beta monomers already mentioned. Gamma and delta chains occur normally in combination with alpha chains. The combination of two gamma chains with two alpha chains constitutes fetal haemoglobin (HbF) and the combination of two delta chains for two alpha chains constitutes A_2 haemoglobin (HbA$_2$), which forms 2 per cent of the total haemoglobin in normal adults. Other variations in the amino acid chains can be considered abnormal, and many are associated with disordered oxygen carriage or impaired solubility.

Sickle cell anaemia is caused by the presence of HbS in which valine replaces glutamic acid in position 6 on the two beta chains. This apparently trivial substitution is sufficient to cause critical loss of solubility in the reduced state. It is a hereditary condition and in the homozygous state is a grave abnormality.

Thalassaemia is another hereditary disorder of haemoglobin. It consists of a suppression of formation of HbA with a compensatory production of fetal haemoglobin (HbF) which persists throughout life instead of falling to low levels after birth. The functional disorder thus includes a shift of the dissociation curve to the left (*Figure 10.13*).

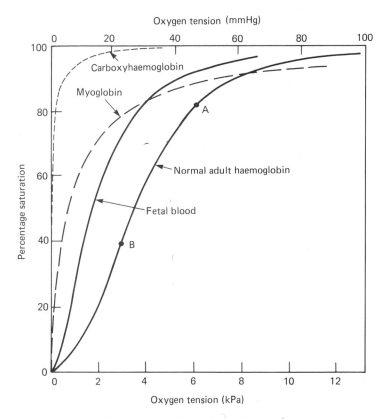

Figure 10.13 Dissociation curves of normal adult haemoglobin compared with fetal blood. Curves for myoglobin and carboxyhaemoglobin are shown for comparison. Note: (1) Fetal blood is adapted to operate at a lower P_{O_2} than adult blood. (2) Myoglobin approaches full saturation of P_{O_2} levels pertaining in voluntary muscle 2–4 kPa (15–30 mmHg); the bulk of its oxygen can be released only at very low oxygen tension. (3) Carboxyhaemoglobin can be dissociated only by the maintenance of very low levels of P_{CO}. After birth, fetal haemoglobin is progressively replaced with adult haemoglobin and the dissociation curve gradually moves across to the position of the adult curve. In a patient with a normal circulation and haemoglobin concentration, point A represents the greatest deterioration of arterial oxygenation which should pass untreated. Arterial blood corresponding to point B is at the threshold of loss of consciousness from hypoxia.

Abnormal ligands. The iron in haemoglobin is able to combine with other inorganic molecules apart from oxygen. The compounds so formed are, in general, more stable than oxyhaemoglobin and therefore block the combination of haemoglobin with oxygen. the most important of these abnormal compounds is carb-oxyhaemoglobin but ligands may also be formed with nitric oxide, cyanide, ammonia and a number of other substances. Apart from the loss of oxygen-carrying power, there is often a shift of the dissociation curve to the left (see below), so that the remaining oxygen is only released at lower tensions of oxygen. This may cause tissue hypoxia when the arterial Po_2 and oxygen content would otherwise appear to be at a safe level.

Methaemoglobin consists of haemoglobin in which the iron has assumed the trivalent ferric form. Methaemoglobin is unable to combine with oxygen but is slowly reconverted to haemoglobin in the normal subject by the action of enzymes which are deficient in familial methaemoglobinaemia (Lehmann and Huntsman, 1966). Alternatively, conversion may be brought about by reducing agents such as ascorbic acid or methylene blue. The nitrite ion is a potent cause of methaemoglobin formation and is a major factor in poisoning by higher oxides of nitrogen (see symposium in May 1967 issue of *British Journal of Anaesthesia*). Methaemoglobin and sulphaemoglobin are a brownish colour and produce a slate-grey colouring of the patient which may be confused with cyanosis.

Kinetics of the reaction of oxygen with haemoglobin

There is now ample experimental proof of Adair's intermediate compound hypothesis (1925) which proposed that the oxidation of haemoglobin proceeds in four separate stages. If the whole haemoglobin molecule, with its four haem groups, is designated as 'Hb$_4$', the reactions may be presented as follows:

$$Hb_4 + O_2 \underset{k_1}{\overset{k_1'}{\rightleftharpoons}} Hb_4O_2 \qquad K_1 = \frac{k_1'}{k_1}$$

$$Hb_4O_2 + O_2 \underset{k_2}{\overset{k_2'}{\rightleftharpoons}} Hb_4O_4 \qquad K_2 = \frac{k_2'}{k_2}$$

$$Hb_4O_4 + O_2 \underset{k_3}{\overset{k_3'}{\rightleftharpoons}} Hb_4O_6 \qquad K_3 = \frac{k_3'}{k_3}$$

$$Hb_4O_6 + O_2 \underset{k_4}{\overset{k_4'}{\rightleftharpoons}} Hb_4O_8 \qquad K_4 = \frac{k_4'}{k_4}$$

the velocity constant of each dissociation is indicated by a small k, while the addition of a prime (′) indicates the velocity constant of the corresponding forward reaction. K'_3 is thus the velocity constant of the reaction of Hb_4O_4 with O_2 to yield Hb_4O_6. The ratio of the forward velocity constant to the reverse velocity constant equals the equilibrium constant of each reaction in the series (represented by capital K).

The separate velocity constants have been measured and it is now known that the last reaction has a forward velocity constant (k'_4) which is much higher than that of the other reactions. During the saturation of the last 75 per cent of reduced haemoglobin, the last reaction will predominate and the high velocity constant counteracts the effect of the ever-diminishing number of oxygen receptors which would otherwise slow the reaction rate by the law of mass action (Staub, Bishop and Forster, 1961). In fact, the reaction proceeds at much the same rate until saturation is completed. The significance of this to oxyen transfer in the lung was presented by Staub (1963a), and its importance in the concept of 'diffusing capacity' is discussed on page 190.

The velocity of the dissociation of oxyhaemoglobin is somewhat slower than its formation. The velocity constant of the combination of carbon monoxide with haemoglobin is of the same order, but the rate of dissociation of carb-oxyhaemoglobin is extremely slow by comparison.

The oxyhaemoglobin dissociation curve

The relationship between Po_2 and percentage saturation of haemoglobin with oxygen is non-linear. It is shown, under standard conditions, in graphical form for adult and fetal haemoglobin and also for myoglobin and carboxyhaemoglobin in *Figure 10.13*. It is displayed as a line chart in *Figure 10.14*.

Displacement of the dissociation curve and the P_{50}. Various factors displace the dissociation curve sideways, and the familiar effect of pH (the Bohr effect) is shown in *Figure 10.15*. Shifts may be defined as the ratio of the Po_2 which produces a particular saturation under standard conditions, to the Po_2 which produces the same saturation with a particular shift of the curve. Standard conditions include pH 7.4, temperature 37°C and zero base excess. In *Figure 10.15*, a saturation of 80% is produced by Po_2 6 kPa (45 mmHg) at pH 7.4 (standard). At pH 7.0 the Po_2 required for 80% saturation is 9.4 kPa (70.5 mmHg). The ratio is 0.64 and this applies to all saturations at pH 7.0. The ratio is indicated on the line chart in *Figure 10.14*, which also shows the ratios (or correction factors) for different values of temperature and base excess.

Since the effects of temperature, pH and base excess are all similar, their influence on the dissociation curve may be considered simultaneously. The usual practice is to derive a factor for the influence of each and then to multiply them together. This combined factor is then multiplied by the observed Po_2 to give the apparent Po_2 which may be entered into the standard dissociation curve to indicate the saturation. The factors may be determined from the line charts in *Figure 10.14*; its use is illustrated by the following example.

	Factor
Blood temperature 33.7°C	1.20
Blood pH 7.08	0.70
Blood base excess −7 mmol/l	1.04
Combined factor = 1.20 × 0.70 × 1.04 =	0.87
Observed Po_2 =	9.3 kPa (70 mmHg)
Apparent Po_2 = observed Po_2 × 0.87 =	8.1 kPa (61 mmHg)
Calculated saturation (from line chart) =	91.3%

This calculation may be expeditiously performed on the slide rule as described by Severinghaus (1966). The factors are also incorporated in the digital computer subroutine described by Kelman (1966) and feature in the tables produced by Kelman and Nunn (1968).

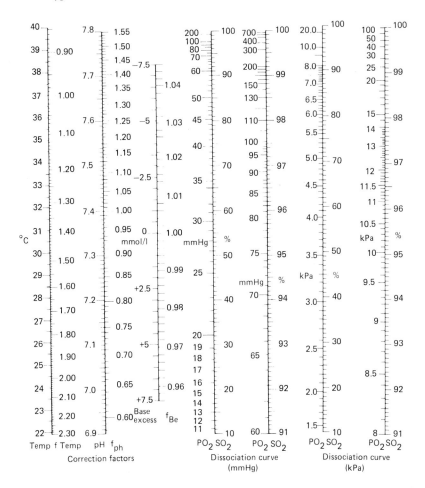

Figure 10.14 The standard oxyhaemoglobin dissociation curve with factors which displace it. The two right-hand line charts give corresponding values of Po_2 and saturation for standard conditions (temperature, 37°C; pH, 7.40; base excess, zero). The remaining lines indicate the factors by which the actual measured Po_2 should be multiplied before entering the standard dissociation curve to determine the saturation. When more than one factor is required, they should be multiplied together as in the example given in the text. (Reproduced from Kelman and Nunn (1966b) by permission of the Editor of the Journal of Applied Physiology, modified in accord with data of Roughton and Severinghaus (1973) and with the addition of kPa scales)

A convenient approach to quantifying a shift of the dissociation curve is to indicate the Po_2 required for 50% saturation. This is known as the P_{50} and, under the standard conditions shown in *Figure 10.14*, is 3.5 kPa (26.3 mmHg). This has become the usual method of reporting shift of the dissociation curve.

Clinical significance of the Bohr effect. There is a good deal of confusion about the clinical significance of the Bohr effect. A shift to the right (caused by low pH) impairs oxygenation in the lungs but aids release of oxygen in the tissue. The overall significance of these two effects in combination is not intuitively obvious. It is

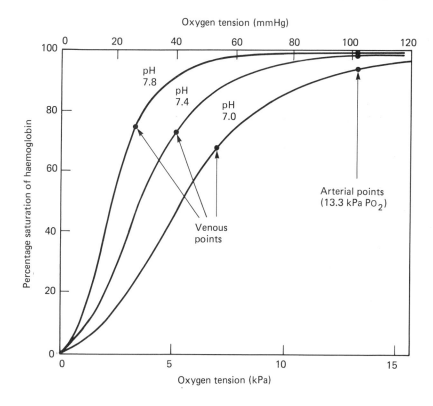

Figure 10.15 The Bohr effect and its effect upon oxygen tension. The centre curve is the normal curve under standard conditions; the other two curves show the displacement caused by the indicated changes in pH, other factors remaining constant. The venous points have been determined on the basis of a fixed arterial/venous oxygen saturation difference of 25% in each case. They are thus 25% saturation less than the corresponding arterial saturation which is equivalent to a Po_2 of 13.3 kPa (100 mmHg) in each case. Under the conditions shown, alkalosis lowers venous Po_2 and acidosis raises venous Po_2. This effect is reversed in severe arterial hypoxaemia. Tissue Po_2 is related to venous Po_2. Temperature, 37°C; base excess, zero.

essential to think in quantitative terms, and an illustrative example is set out in *Figure 10.15*. The arterial Po_2 is assumed to be 13.3 kPa (100 mmHg) and arterial saturation is decreased by a reduction of pH. However, the effect is small except when the arterial Po_2 is very low (less than about 8 kPa or 60 mmHg) or when the pH falls to extremely low values at normal Po_2 (Prys-Roberts, Smith and Nunn, 1967).

At the venous point the position is quite different, and the examples in *Figure 10.15* show the venous oxygen tensions to be very markedly affected. Assuming that the arterial/venous oxygen saturation difference is constant at 25 per cent it will be seen that at low pH the venous Po_2 is raised to 6.9 kPa (52 mmHg), while at high pH the venous Po_2 is reduced to 3.5 kPa (26 mmHg). This is important as the tissue Po_2 is closer to the venous Po_2 than to the arterial Po_2. Over a wide range of conditions it will be found that a shift of the curve to the right will always raise the venous Po_2 provided other factors remain constant. In fact, other factors are unlikely to remain constant, and both cerebral blood flow and cardiac output are likely to be increased by a moderate respiratory acidosis which would further tend to raise the venous and tissue PO_2. Thus, far from being universally harmful as is so often assumed, respiratory acidosis will usually increase the tissue PO_2, particularly in the brain.

Factors which shift the dissociation curve. It is well known that the curve is shifted to the right (P_{50} raised) by an increase of hydrogen ion concentration, PCO_2, temperature, ionic strength or haemoglobin concentration. Certain abnormal haemoglobins (such as San Diego and Chesapeake) have a high P_{50} while others (such as sickle and Kansas) have a low P_{50}.

In 1967 it was found independently by Benesch and Benesch and by Chanutin and Curnish that the presence of certain organic phosphates in the erythrocyte has a pronounced effect on the P_{50}. The most important of these compounds is 2,3-diphosphoglycerate (2,3-DPG), one molecule of which is able to bind preferentially to the beta chains of one tetramer of deoxyhaemoglobin, resulting in a conformational change which reduces oxygen affinity (Arnone, 1972). The percentage occupancy of the 2,3-DPG binding sites governs the overall P_{50} of a blood sample within the range 2–4.5 kPa (15–34 mmHg).

2,3-DPG is formed in the Rapoport–Luebering shunt off the glycolytic pathway (see *Figure 10.3*) and its level is determined by the balance between synthesis and degradation (*Figure 10.16*). Activity of the DPG mutase is enhanced and the DPG phosphatase diminished at high pH, which thus increases the level of 2,3-DPG.

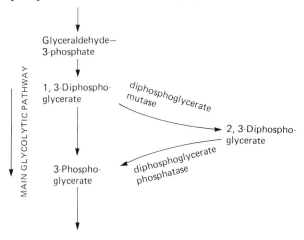

Figure 10.16 Rapoport–Luebering shunt for synthesis of 2,3-diphosphoglycerate.

The relationship between 2,3-DPG levels and P_{50} suggested that 2,3-DPG levels would have a most important bearing on clinical practice and therefore much research effort was devoted to determining those conditions which might result in substantial changes in 2,3-DPG levels.

Storage of bank blood with acid–citrate–dextrose (ACD) preservative results in depletion of all 2,3-DPG within the usual period of 3 weeks' storage, P_{50} being reduced to about 2 kPa (15 mmHg) (McConn and Derrick, 1972). A massive transfusion of old blood shifts the patient's dissociation curve to the left but restoration is usually well advanced within a few hours (see review by Valeri, 1975). Changes in P_{50} of a patient do not usually exceed 0.5 kPa (3.8 mmHg). Storage of blood with citrate–phosphate–dextrose (CPD) substantially reduces the rate of 2,3-DPG depletion (Shafer et al., 1971).

Anaemia results in a raised 2,3-DPG level with P_{50} of the order of 0.5 kPa (3.8 mmHg) higher than control levels (Torrance et al., 1970). This must raise the partial pressure of oxygen delivery to the tissues, and supplements the effect of increased tissue perfusion.

Altitude was reported to cause a 2,3-DPG-mediated shift to the right (Lenfant et al., 1968) with an increase in P_{50} of the order of 0.5 kPa (3.8 mmHg). This has not been confirmed by Weiskopf and Severinghaus (1972) and it should also be noted that, at an altitude of 4000 metres, the arterial Po_2 is of the order of 7 kPa (52.5 mmHg), below which a rightward shift of the dissociation curve is less advantageous since oxygenation in the lung is impaired to a degree which is barely outweighed by improved off-loading in the tissues.

Ventilatory failure does not appear to cause any significant change in either 2,3-DPG levels or the P_{50}. Fairweather, Walker and Flenley (1974) and Flenley et al. (1975) studied a total of 71 patients with arterial Pco_2 ranging from 6.7 to 10.7 kPa (50 to 80 mmHg) and Po_2 4.3–8.7 kPa (32–65 mmHg). P_{50} values (at pH 7.4) ranged from 3 to 4 kPa (22.5–30 mm Hg) and did not appear to differ from the normal value by more than the experimental error of determination. 2,3-DPG levels were widely scattered about the normal value.

Haemorrhagic and endotoxic shock do not appear to be associated with any significant changes of 2,3-DPG or 2,3-DPG-mediated changes in P_{50} (Naylor et al., 1972).

In general it may be said that subsequent research has failed to substantiate the earlier suggestions that 2,3-DPG was of major importance in clinical problems of oxygen delivery. In fact, the likely effects of changes in P_{50} mediated by 2,3-DPG seem to be of marginal significance in comparison with changes in arterial Po_2 and tissue perfusion. Similarly, there has been little application of the suggestions that drug-induced shifts of the dissociation curve would have a major therapeutic role. A valuable review of the subject was presented by Shappell and Lenfant (1972).

Effect of anaesthetics. It has long been known that anaesthetics bind to haemoglobin and this accounts for a substantial part of their carriage in blood (Featherstone et al., 1961). More recently, Barker et al. (1975) have identified specific changes in the nuclear magnetic resonance spectrum for haemoglobin in equilibrium with halothane, methoxyflurane and diethyl ether, suggesting different binding sites for each agent. It is clearly a possibility that hydrophobic binding of anaesthetics to haemoglobin might result in a conformational change which would alter the P_{50}, and certain preliminary reports suggested this possibility. However, a series of carefully controlled studies have established that, even with high concentrations of methoxyflurane, halothane and cyclopropane, there is no measurable change in P_{50} (Cohen and Behar, 1970; Millar, Beard and Hulands, 1971; Weiskopf, Nishimura and Severinghaus, 1971).

Physical solution of oxygen in blood

In addition to combination with haemoglobin, oxygen is carried in physical solution in both erythrocytes and plasma. The total amount carried in normal blood in solution at 37°C is about 0.0225 ml/100 ml per kPa or 0.003/100 ml per mmHg. At normal arterial P_{O_2}, the oxen in physical solution is thus about 0.25 ml/100 ml or rather more than 1 per cent of the total oxygen carried in all forms. However, when breathing 100% oxygen, the level rises to about 2 ml/100 ml. Breathing 100% oxygen at 3 atmospheres pressure absolute (303 kPa), the amount of oxygen in physical solution rises to about 6 ml/100 ml, which is sufficient for the arteriovenous extraction. The amount of oxygen in physical solution rises with decreasing temperature for the same P_{O_2}.

Physical solution in artificial blood substitutes

There are obvious military and civil advantages in the provision of an artificial haemoglobin substitute which would carry oxygen in a synthetic fluid to be used instead of blood. At the present time the best option appears to be large molecular weight fluorocarbons (Faithfull, 1986). Oxygen is highly soluble in these hydrophobic compounds, which are above the critical molecular size to act as anaesthetics.

Being hydrophobic, they are prepared as emulsions and 20% is currently the preferred concentration of fluorocarbon, which will dissolve about 5 ml of oxygen per 100 ml of emulsion on equilibration with 100% oxygen. The use of fluorocarbons thus requires the patient to breathe a very high concentration of oxygen which will just provide sufficient oxygen in physical solution to satisfy the normal mean arteriovenous extraction of 5 ml/100 ml.

Since oxygen is in physical solution in fluorocarbon, its 'dissociation curve' is a straight line, with P_{O_2} directly proportional to the quantity of dissolved oxygen. If, for example, the arterial P_{O_2} is 80 kPa (600 mmHg) and half of the oxygen is extracted in the systemic circulation, the mixed venous P_{O_2} would be 40 kPa (300 mmHg). Even with 90 per cent extraction, mixed venous P_{O_2} would still be well above the normal level. In practice, fluorocarbons would function alongside remaining blood and the relationship between tension and content would depend upon their relative proportions.

Droplet size in the emulsion is of the order of 0.1 μm, compared with the 5 μm diameter of an erythrocyte. The flow resistance is considerably less than that of blood and is virtually unaffected by shear rate so that the rheological properties are particularly favourable at low flow rates. Fluorocarbons may therefore be useful in partial obstruction of the circulation, in myocardial infarction for example.

Carbon monoxide in combination with haemoglobin

Carbon monoxide is well known to displace oxygen from combination with haemoglobin, the affinity being approximately 300 times greater than the affinity for oxygen. The presence of carboxyhaemoglobin also causes a leftward shift of the dissociation curve of the remaining oxyhaemoglobin (Roughton and Darling, 1944), partly mediated by a reduction in 2,3-DPG levels. This is conveniently shown on a plot of oxygen content against P_{O_2} (*Figure 10.17*), the values on the ordinate being the sum of dissolved and combined oxygen. The upper curve is for the normal concentration of haemoglobin without carbon monoxide. The lowest of the three

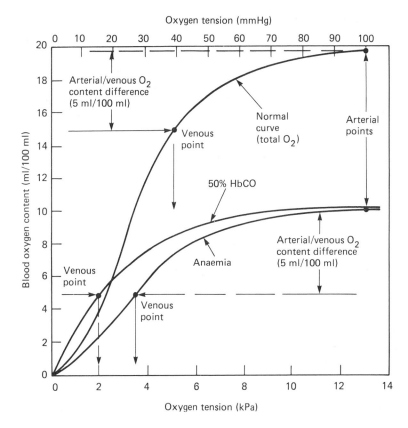

Figure 10.17 Influences of anaemia and carbon monoxide poisoning on the relationship between oxygen tension and content. The normal curve is constructed for a haemoglobin concentration of 14.4 g/dl. Assuming an arterial/venous oxygen content difference of 5 ml/100 ml, the venous P_{O_2} is about 5.3 kPa (40 mmHg). The curve of anaemic blood is constructed for a haemoglobin concentration of 7.2 g/dl. If the arterial/venous oxygen content difference remains unchanged, the venous P_{O_2} will fall to 3.6 kPa (27 mmHg), a level which is low but not dangerously so. The curve of 50% carboxyhaemoglobin is based on a total haemoglobin (incl. carboxyhaemoglobin) of 14.4 g/dl. The curve is interpolated from Roughton (1964). Assuming an arterial/venous oxygen content difference of 5 ml/100 ml, the venous P_{O_2} is only 1.9 kPa (14 mmHg), a level which is dangerously low as it must be associated with a greatly reduced tissue P_{O_2}. Arterial P_{O_2} is assumed to be 13.3 kPa (100 mmHg) in all cases.

curves applies to a patient with haemoglobin at half the normal concentration. At each P_{O_2}, the oxygen concentration is approximately half that of the patient with a normal concentration of haemoglobin. The intermediate curve applies to blood with normal haemoglobin concentration but with half of the haemoglobin bound to carbon monoxide, resulting in a displacement of the dissociation curve of the remaining haemoglobin. It will be seen that, in comparison with the anaemic blood, this displacement has little effect on the oxygen content of the arterial blood provided that it is in excess of about 8 kPa (60 mmHg). However, the effect on the venous P_{O_2}, after unloading of oxygen in the tissues, is very great. Assuming an arterial P_{O_2} of 13.3 kPa (100 mmHg) and an arterial venous oxygen content difference of 5 ml/100 ml, the venous points are as follows:

Normal haemoglobin concentration	5.3 kPa (40 mmHg)
Half normal haemoglobin concentration	3.6 kPa (27 mmHg)
50 per cent carboxyhaemoglobin	1.9 kPa (14 mmHg)

The disappearance of coal gas from domestic use in many countries has decreased the popularity of carbon monoxide for attempted suicide. However, carbon monoxide is still to be found in the blood of patients, in trace concentrations as a result of its production in the body but mainly as a result of the internal combustion engine and smoking. Jones, Commins and Cernik (1972) reported levels of 0.4–9.7 per cent in London taxi drivers but the highest level in a non-smoking driver was 3.0 per cent. Levels up to 10 per cent of carboxyhaemoglobin were also found in smokers by Castleden and Cole (1974). Maternal smoking results in appreciable levels of carboxyhaemoglobin in fetal blood (Longo, 1970), and smoking prior to blood donation may result in levels of carboxyhaemoglobin up to 10 per cent in the blood. This level appears to persist throughout the usual 3 weeks of storage (Millar and Gregory, 1972). Smoking is considered in Chapter 17.

The 'normal' arterial oxygen tension

In contrast to the arterial P_{CO_2}, the arterial P_{O_2} shows a progressive decrease with age. Marshall and Whyche (1972) analysed 12 studies of healthy subjects and from the pooled results suggested the following relationship in subjects breathing air:

$$\text{mean arterial } P_{O_2} = 13.6 - 0.044 \text{ (age in years) kPa}$$

$$\text{or } 102 - 0.33 \text{ (age in years) mmHg}$$

About this regression line there are 95 per cent confidence limits (2 s.d.) of ± 1.33 kPa (10 mmHg) (*Table 10.3*). Five per cent of normal patients will lie outside these limits and it is therefore preferable to refer to this as the reference range rather than the normal range.

It seems likely that some of the scatter of values for P_{O_2} is due to transient changes in ventilation, perhaps associated with arterial puncture. Because of the meagre body oxygen stores, such changes have a greater effect on P_{O_2} than on P_{CO_2}.

When breathing oxygen the most important factor causing scatter of values for arterial P_{O_2} is failure to exclude air from the breathing system. Provided that great care is taken to prevent dilution with air, very high values of arterial P_{O_2} may be obtained in the healthy subject. A number of studies of normal conscious subjects were reviewed by Raine and Bishop (1963) and by Laver and Seifen (1965). Mean values for arterial P_{O_2} in these studies range from 80 to 86.7 kPa (600 to 650 mmHg), but individual values range from 73.3 kPa (550 mmHg) to values which are (no doubt erroneously) in excess of the alveolar P_{O_2}.

Reports of 'abnormalities' of oxygenation must be interpreted against the high degree of scatter in normal subjects under normal conditions.

Table 10.3 Normal values for arterial P_{O_2}

	Mean and range	
Age (years)	kPa	mmHg
20–29	12.5 (11.2–13.9)	94 (84–104)
30–39	12.1 (10.8–13.5)	91 (81–101)
40–49	11.7 (10.4–13.1)	88 (78–98)
50–59	11.2 (9.9–12.5)	84 (74–94)
60–69	10.8 (9.5–12.1)	81 (71–91)

Oxygen stores and the steady state

It is a fact of great clinical importance that the body oxygen stores are small and, if replenishment ceases, are normally insufficient to sustain life for more than a few minutes. The principal stores are shown in *Table 10.4.*

Table 10.4 Principal stores of body oxygen

	While breathing air	While breathing 100% oxygen	
In the lungs (FRC)	450 ml		3 000 ml
In the blood	850 ml		950 ml
Dissolved in tissue fluids	50 ml	?	100 ml
In combination with myoglobin	? 200 ml	?	200 ml
Total	1 550 ml		4 250 ml

While breathing air, not only are the total oxygen stores very small but also, to make matters worse, only part of the stores can be released without an unacceptable reduction in P_{O_2}. Reference to the dissociation curves in *Figure 10.13* shows that blood will not release substantial quantities of oxygen until the P_{O_2} falls below 5.3 kPa (40 mmHg). Myoglobin is even more reluctant to part with its oxygen and very little can be released above a P_{O_2} of 2.7 kPa (20 mmHg).

Breathing oxygen causes a substantial increase in total oxygen stores. Most of the additional oxygen is accommodated in the alveolar gas where 80 per cent of it may be withdrawn without causing the P_{O_2} to fall below the normal value. With 2400 ml of easily available oxygen after breathing oxygen, there is no difficulty in breath holding for as long as 8 minutes without becoming hypoxic.

The small size of the oxygen stores means that changes in factors affecting the alveolar or arterial P_{O_2} will produce their full effects very quickly after the change. This is in contrast to carbon dioxide where the size of the stores buffers the body against rapid changes. *Figure 10.18* compares the time course of changes in P_{O_2} and P_{CO_2} produced by the same changes in ventilation. *Figure 9.11* showed how the time course of changes of P_{CO_2} is different for falling and rising P_{CO_2}.

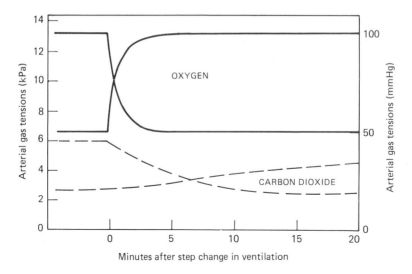

Figure 10.18 The upper pair of curves indicates the rate of change of arterial P_{O_2} following step changes in ventilation. Half of the total change occurs in about 30 seconds. The rising curve could be produced by an increase of alveolar ventilation from 2 to 4 l/min while breathing air (see Figure 10.6). The falling curve could result from the corresponding reduction of alveolar ventilation from 4 to 2 l/min. The lower pair of curves indicates the time course of changes in P_{CO_2} which are very much slower than for oxygen. These changes are shown in greater detail in Figure 9.11.

Factors which reduce the P_{O_2} always act rapidly, but the following is the order of rapidity of changes which produce anoxia.

1. *Circulatory arrest.* When the circulation is arrested, hypoxia supervenes as soon as the oxygen in the tissues and stagnant capillaries has been exhausted. In the case of the brain, with its high rate of oxygen consumption, there is only about 10 seconds before consciousness is lost. If the eyeball is gently compressed with a finger to occlude its vessels, vision commences to be lost at the periphery within about 6 seconds (a convincing experiment suggested by Rahn, 1964). Circulatory arrest also differs from other forms of hypoxia in the failure of clearance of products of anaerobic metabolism (e.g. lactic acid) which, with the exception of the brain, should not occur in arterial hypoxaemia.

2. *Exposure to a barometric pressure of less than 6.3 kPa (47 mmHg).* At a pressure of less than 6.3 kPa (47 mmHg), body fluids boil and alveolar gas is replacd with 100% water vapour (page 310). the P_{O_2} rapidly falls to zero and consciousness is lost within one circulation time, which is of the order of 15 seconds (Ernsting and McHardy, 1960).

3. *Inhalation of nitrogen.* Washing out the alveolar oxygen by hyperventilation with nitrogen results in a very rapid fall of arterial P_{O_2}, which reached 4 kPa (30 mmHg) in 30 seconds in a series of dogs (Cater et al., 1963). Even more rapid changes were obtained in human volunteers by Ernsting (1963).

4. *Inhalation of nitrous oxide.* Alveolar wash-out with a soluble gas such as nitrous oxide causes a slower fall of P_{O_2} because of the loss of the flushing gas into the tissues. This delays the decrease in alveolar P_{O_2} (page 248).

5. *Apnoea.* The rate of onset of anoxia is dependent upon the initial alveolar P_{O_2}, the lung volume and the rate of oxygen consumption. It is, for example, more

rapid while swimming underwater than while breath holding in the laboratory. Generally speaking, after breathing air, 90 seconds of apnoea results in a substantial fall of Po_2 to a level which threatens the subject with loss of consciousness. If a patient has previously inhaled a few breaths of oxygen, the arterial Po_2 should remain above 13.3 kPa (100 mmHg) for at least 3 minutes of apnoea (Heller and Watson, 1961), and this is the basis of the usual method of protection against hypoxia during any deliberate interference with ventilation, as for example during tracheal intubation. If the patient is preoxygenated and then connected to a supply of oxygen while apnoeic, the arterial Po_2 is well maintained for a long time by the process of 'apnoeic mass-movement oxygenation' (see pages 228 et seq.)

Since a steady state for oxygen is very rapidly attained, it follows that oxygen uptake is seldom appreciably different from oxygen consumption. Therefore, measurement of oxygen uptake usually gives a satisfactory estimate of the oxygen consumption. In contrast, measured values of carbon dioxide output may be very different from the simultaneous level of carbon dioxide production if the ventilation is unsteady. During the irregular and depressed breathing of anaesthesia with spontaneous respiration, values for carbon dioxide output may range widely, while values for oxygen consumption are reasonably steady (Nunn and Matthews, 1959; Nunn, 1964).

Control of the inspired oxygen concentration

Much of this chapter has been devoted to the problem of selection of the optimal inspired oxygen concentration for a particular pathophysiological state. It now remains to be considered how this should be put into effect.

Interface with the patient's airway

A crucial factor in oxygen therapy is the nature of the seal between the patient's airway and the external breathing apparatus. Airtight seals may be obtained with cuffed endotracheal or tracheostomy tubes, and these should give complete control over the composition of the inspired gas. An anaesthetic facemask will usually provide an airtight seal with the face, but it must be held by a trained person and is at best a temporary measure. Physiological mouthpieces with a noseclip are satisfactory for short-term use with co-operative subjects but cannot be tolerated for long periods. Lightweight masks can be glued to the face but there is no mask generally available for clinical use which can be guaranteed to provide an airtight fit to a patient's face unless it is actually held onto the face by trained staff. Most disposable oxygen masks do not attempt to provide an airtight fit. An alternative solution to the problem of the airtight seal is to provide a high flow of gas which can vent to atmosphere between the mask and the face (see below).

Gas mixing

The most satisfactory technique for delivery of a designated inspired oxygen concentration is to mix the required proportions of air and oxygen. Gas mixtures are conveniently obtained from air and oxygen pipeline installations with appropriate humidification. A pair of rotameters may be used, and *Figure E.7* in Appendix E shows a wall chart to facilitate the calculation of flow rates. A simpler arrangement is to employ a mixing device with separate controls for total flow rate and oxygen concentration. It is important that such devices have a visible indication of oxygen flow (Richardson, Chinn and Nunn, 1976).

Air/oxygen mixtures can be delivered to ventilators, passed over a T-piece for patients breathing spontaneously with a cuffed endotracheal tube or passed to the patient by means of a non-rebreathing system. They can also be passed to loose-fitting disposable masks but, under these circumstances, high flow rates are required, preferably in excess of the peak inspiratory flow rate (page 67).

Use of venturi devices

Oxygen may be passed through the jet of a venturi to entrain air. This is a convenient and highly economical method of preparing oxygen mixtures in the range 25–40% concentration. For example, 1 l/min of oxygen passed through the jet of a venturi with an entrainment ratio of 8:1 will deliver 9 l/min of 30% oxygen. Higher oxygen concentrations require a lower entrainment ratio and therefore a higher oxygen flow in order to maintain an adequate total delivered flow rate. The familiar venturi mask was introduced by Campbell (1960b) on the suggestion of the author who had used a venturi to provide the oxygen-enriched carrier gas for an anaesthetic apparatus designed for use in the Antarctic (Nunn, 1961b).

With the availability of an ample flow rate of the air/oxygen mixture, the venturi mask need not fit the face with an airtight junction. The high flow rate escapes round the cheeks and room air is effectively excluded. Numerous studies have indicated that the venturi mask gives excellent control over the inspired oxygen concentration with an accuracy of $\pm 1\%$ unaffected by variations in the ventilation of the patient (Leigh, 1973). There is no doubt that this is the most satisfactory method of controlling the inspired oxygen concentration of a patient who is breathing spontaneously without tracheal intubation.

Control of the patient's gaseous environment

Oxygen tents have been in use for many years but suffer from the disadvantages of the large volume and high rate of leakage which make it difficult to attain and maintain a high oxygen concentration, unless the volume is reduced and a high gas flow rate is used (Wayne and Chamney, 1969). In addition, the fire hazard cannot be ignored. These problems are minimized when the patient is an infant, and oxygen control within an incubator is a satisfactory method of administering a precise oxygen concentration. Largely because of the danger of retrolental fibroplasia (page 494), it is mandatory to monitor the oxygen concentration in the incubator.

Spectacles, nasal catheters, simple disposable oxygen masks, etc.

A wide range of simple devices aim to blow oxygen at or into the air passages. This oxygen is mixed with inspired air to give an inspired oxygen concentration which is a complex function of the geometry of the device, the oxygen flow rate, the patient's ventilation and whether the patient is breathing through his mouth or nose. The effective inspired oxygen concentration is impossible to predict and may vary within very wide limits (Leigh, 1973). These devices cannot be used for oxygen therapy when the exact inspired oxygen concentration is critical (e.g. ventilatory failure), but may be useful in less critical situations such as recovery from routine anaesthesia. Nasal prongs are the preferred method for delivering 'sleeping oxygen' (Flenley, 1985). Fairly high oxygen concentrations may be obtained with a combination of two techiques such as nasal catheters used under a simple mask, an arrangement with which Down and Castleden (1975) obtained an arterial Po_2 of 51.7 kPa (388 mmHg). Administration by transtracheal catheter appears to be effective at about half the flow rate required for nasal catheters (Banner and Govan, 1986).

With a device such as a nasal catheter or prongs, the lower the ventilation, the greater will be the fractional contribution of the fixed flow of oxygen to the inspired gas mixture. There is thus an approximate compensation for hypoventilation, with greater oxygen concentrations being delivered at lower levels of ventilation. However, this may result in ventilatory depression with progressive hypercapnia but no hypoxia, a potentially dangerous situation.

Hyperbaric oxygenation

Two systems are in use. One-man chambers are filled with 100% oxygen and the patient is entirely exposed to 100% oxygen at high pressure: no mask is required. Larger chambers are pressurized with air which is breathed by staff; 100% oxygen is made available to the patient by means of a well fitting facemask. The quality of the airtight fit is obviously crucial and has caused considerable difficulties in the past.

Monitoring oxygen concentrations

When the inspired gas has a fixed composition (e.g. in oxygen tents and with venturi masks), there is no problem in sampling inspired gas and measuring the oxygen concentration with devices such as paramagnetic analysers (see below). With variable performance devices (e.g. oxygen spectacles, nasal catheters, simple masks, etc.), it is extremely difficult to determine the inspired oxygen, which may not be constant throughout the duration of inspiration. Furthermore, the measured oxygen concentration may be highly dependent on the point from which the sample was taken and whether the patient is breathing through his nose or his mouth. In the face of these difficulties it may be preferable to measure the end-expiratory oxygen concentration or even the arterial blood Po_2. However, if such measures are necessary it would be wiser to use a device with a fixed performance.

Supply of oxygen

Choice of the best method for supplying oxygen depends on consumption and convenience. For a large hospital, the most economical provision of oxygen is by bulk deliveries of liquid oxygen with the evaporated oxygen distributed by a pipeline, usually at 4 atmospheres pressure. For a smaller hospital it may be more economical to use a bank of cylinders of oxygen, also distributed by pipeline. With only occasional and small scale use of oxygen, it may be cheaper to use cylinders at the point of consumption. This avoids the cost of installing a pipeline but the logistic costs are considerable and there is always the fear of a cylinder running empty unnoticed. Domestic pipelines can be installed for provision of oxygen in the home. The patient then plugs into various strategically located outlets as required. Small cylinders are available which are suitable for 'walking oxygen'. Miniature liquid oxygen dispensers are used in military aircraft.

An entirely different approach is the oxygen concentrator which removes most of the nitrogen from air, providing an oxygen concentration in the range 90–95%, the remainder being a mixture of argon and residual nitrogen. Nitrogen is removed at high pressure by Zeolite acting as a molecular sieve with pore size of 0.5 nm (5 Å). Its activity is regenerated by exposure to vacuum or by purging with air at atmospheric pressure. Thus a pair of sieves can be used alternately to provide a continuous supply. It is difficult to imagine any clinical condition which requires administration of 100% oxygen rather than the 90–95% oxygen provided by an oxygen concentrator and the contaminating argon is harmless.

It appears that oxygen concentrators can compete economically with traditional methods of oxygen supply for both large and small levels of consumption. However, the method would seem to have outstanding advantages in remote locations (Ezi-Ashi, Papworth and Nunn, 1983) and small units are now extensively used for domestic oxygen.

Cyanosis

The commonest method of detection of hypoxia is by the appearance of cyanosis, and the change in colour of haemoglobin on desaturation affords the patient a safeguard of immense value. Indeed, it is interesting to speculate on the additional hazards to life if gross hypoxia could occur without overt changes in the colour of the blood. There must have been countless occasions in which the appearance of cyanosis has given warning of hypoventilation, pulmonary shunting, stagnant circulation or decreased oxygen concentration of inspired gas.

Central and peripheral cyanosis

If shed arterial blood is seen to be purple, this is a reliable indication of arterial desaturation. However, when skin or mucous membrane is inspected, most of the blood which colours the tissue is lying in veins (i.e. subpapillary venous plexuses) and its oxygen content is related to the arterial oxygen content as follows:

$$\begin{matrix} \text{venous oxygen} \\ \text{content} \end{matrix} = \begin{matrix} \text{arterial oxygen} \\ \text{content} \end{matrix} - \begin{matrix} \text{arterial/venous oxygen} \\ \text{content difference} \end{matrix}$$

The last term may be expanded in terms of the tissue metabolism and perfusion:

$$\begin{matrix} \text{venous oxygen} \\ \text{content} \end{matrix} = \begin{matrix} \text{arterial oxygen} \\ \text{content} \end{matrix} - \frac{\text{tissue oxygen consumption}}{\text{tissue blood flow}}$$

The oxygen consumption by the skin is usually low in relation to its circulation, so the quantity in parentheses is generally small. Therefore the cutaneous venous oxygen content is close to that of the arterial blood and inspection of the skin gives a reasonable indication of arterial oxygen content. However, when circulation is reduced in relation to skin oxygen consumption, cyanosis may occur in the presence of normal arterial oxygen levels. This occurs typically in patients with low cardiac output, in cold weather and in the face of a patient in the Trendelenburg position.

The influence of anaemia

Lundsgaard and Van Slyke (1923) stressed the importance of anaemia in appearance of cyanosis. Much credence is attached to their statement that cyanosis is apparent when there are 5 g of reduced haemoglobin per dl of capillary blood. They defined capillary blood as having a reduced haemoglobin concentration which was the mean of the levels in arterial and venous blood. If, for example, the arterial blood contained 3 g/dl of reduced haemoglobin (80% saturation at normal haemoglobin concentration) and the arterial/venous difference for the skin were 4 ml/100 ml of oxygen (corresponding to the reduction of a further 3 g/dl of haemoglobin), the 'capillary' blood would contain 4.5 g/dl of reduced haemoglobin and the degree of hypoxaemia would be just below the threshold at which cyanosis should be evident. In cases of severe anaemia, it might be impossible for the reduced haemoglobin concentration of the capillary blood to attain the level of 5 g/dl, which is said to be required for the appearance of cyanosis and, clearly, cyanosis could never occur if the haemoglobin concentration were only 5 g/dl.

There seems little doubt that qualitatively the views of Lundsgaard and Van Slyke are sound. There has been little quantitative confirmation of their theory but it is generally found that cyanosis can be detected at an arterial oxygen saturation of about 85% although there is much variation (Comroe and Botelho, 1947). Such a level would probably correspond to a 'capillary' saturation of more than 80% and a reduced haemoglobin of about 3 g/dl.

Sites for detection of cyanosis

Kelman and Nunn (1966a) carried out a comparison of the appearance of cyanosis in different sites with various biochemical indices of hypoxaemia of arterial blood. Best correlations were obtained with cyanosis observed in the buccal mucosa and lips, but there was no significant correlation between the oxygenation of the arterial blood and the appearance of cyanosis in the ear lobes, nail bed or conjunctivae.

The importance of colour-rendering properties of source of illumination

Kelman and Nunn also compared the use of five types of fluorescent lighting in use in hospitals. There was no significant difference in the correlation between hypoxaemia and cyanosis for the different lights. None was therefore more *reliable* than the others for the detection of hypoxaemia. However, there was a striking difference in the *degree* of cyanosis with the different lights, some tending to make the patient pinker and others imparting a bluer tinge to the patients. The former gave false negatives (no cyanosis in the presence of hypoxaemia), while the latter gave false positives (cyanosis in the absence of hypoxaemia). However, the total number of false results was approximately the same with all tubes.

It is potentially dangerous for patients to be inspected under lamps of different colour-rendering properties, particularly if the medical and nursing staff do not know the characteristics of each type of lamp. It would be too much to suggest that the staff should calibrate their impressions of cyanosis for a particular lamp by relation to arterial oxygen levels, but it is not too much to expect that hospitals will standardize their lighting and acquaint staff with the colour-rendering properties of the type which is finally chosen.

Sensitivity of cyanosis as an indication of hypoxaemia

It has been stressed above that the appearance of cyanosis is considerably influenced by the circulation, haemoglobin concentration and lighting conditions. Even when all these are optimal, cyanosis is by no means a precise indication of the arterial oxygen level and it should be regarded as a warning sign rather than a measurement. Kelman and Nunn (1966a) detected cyanosis in about 50 per cent of patients who had a saturation of 93%. Cyanosis was detected in about 95 per cent of patients who had a saturation of 89%. It should be remembered that 89% saturation corresponds to about 7.7 kPa (58 mmHg) Po_2, a level which many would consider unacceptable. Absence of cyanosis does not necessarily mean normal arterial oxygen levels.

Principles of measurement of oxygen levels

Oxygen concentration in gas samples

For many years the use of the Haldane apparatus, or its modification by Lloyd (Cormack, 1972), has been the standard method of measurement of oxygen concentrations in physiological gas samples. However, analysers working on the paramagnetic properties of oxygen (Pauling, Wood and Sturdivant, 1946) many years ago attained a degree of accuracy and reliability which has enabled them to supplant the older chemical methods of analysis (Nunn et al., 1964; Ellis and Nunn, 1968). A particularly attractive feature of the method is that interference by other gases likely to be present does not cause major inaccuracies and, if particularly high accuracy is required, correction factors may be employed. Fuel cells and polarographs may also be used and are particularly suitable as monitors.

Measurement of breath-to-breath changes in oxygen concentrations of respired gases requires an instrument with a response time of less than about 300 ms. Formerly the only suitable technique for oxygen measurement was the mass spectrometer (Fowler and Hugh-Jones, 1957). However, a number of alternative methods have been described although their use has remained limited. The first of these was a modification of the polarograph (Severinghaus, 1963), followed by a fast-response version of the Servomex DCL 83 paramagnetic oxygen analyser (Cunningham, Kay and Young, 1965). A hitherto unapplied principle was employed in the oxygen-sensitive solid electrochemical cell described by Elliot, Segger and Osborn (1966). Only the mass spectrometer is capable of following the full range of respiratory frequencies likely to be encountered in clinical practice.

Oxygen content of blood samples

The older chemical methods are those of Van Slyke and Neill (1924) and Haldane (1920). Gregory (1973) described a technique for assessment of the accuracy of the Van Slyke apparatus against hydrogen peroxide. There was no significant systematic error, but random error was in the range of ± 0.3 ml/100 ml. The Natelson apparatus (1951) appears to be a simpler alternative to the Van Slyke manometric apparatus but many have found it unexpectedly difficult to obtain reliable results for oxygen content.

Still more recently, the polarographic method of measurement of Po_2 (see below) has been utilized to measure oxygen content. Chemically combined oxygen is liberated from blood by saponin-ferricyanide solution and the P_{O_2} of the resultant solution is proportional to the oxygen content of the blood sample (Linden, Ledsome and Norman, 1965). This method is uninfluenced by the presence of inhalational anaesthetic agents, and has proved to be simple, accurate and reliable.

An alternative technique for determination of content uses a fuel cell for measurement of evolved oxygen. Satisfactory results were reported by Kusumi, Butts and Ruff (1973), but Selman, White and Tait (1975) obtained 95 per cent confidence limits of ± 2 ml/100 ml in comparison with the Van Slyke.

Blood oxygen saturation

The classic method of measurement of saturation is in the form of the ratio of content to capacity (with dissolved oxygen subtracted from each):

$$\text{saturation} = HbO_2/(Hb + HbO_2)$$
$$= \frac{\text{oxygen content} - \text{dissolved oxygen}}{\text{oxygen capacity} - \text{dissolved oxygen}}$$

Oxygen capacity is determined as the content after saturation of the blood by exposure to oxygen.

Nowadays, it is more usual to measure saturation photoelectrically. Methods are based on the fact that the absorption of monochromatic light of wavelength 805 nm is the same for reduced and oxygenated haemoglobin. At other wavelengths (particularly 650 nm) there is a marked difference between the absorption of transmitted or reflected light by the two forms of haemoglobin (Zijlstra, 1958). Various devices are marketed which depend upon the simultaneous absorption of light at these two wavelengths and so indicate the saturation directly. These instruments tend to be used uncritically and their calibration is seldom checked for the simple reason that such a check is a difficult and time-consuming operation.

Saturation may be derived from P_{O_2}. This is reasonably accurate above a P_{O_2} of about 7.3 kPa (55 mmHg) where the dissociation curve is flat. However, it is inaccurate at lower tensions since, on the steep part of the curve, the saturation changes by 3% for a tension change of only 0.13 kPa (1 mmHg).

At a superficial glance the concept of saturation appears simple enough. However, on further consideration there are seen to be difficulties which cannot easily be overcome. They arise chiefly from the presence of abnormal forms and compounds of haemoglobin. Methaemoglobin is usually present as about 5 per cent of total haemoglobin, and carboxyhaemoglobin may be as high as 10 per cent of total haemoglobin in smokers. Optical methods do not then necessarily give the same value as for the equation above.

Blood P_{O_2}

Four methods of measurement are·available.

1. A tiny bubble of gas may be equilibrated with blood at the patient's body temperature and then analysed quantitatively for oxygen (Riley, Campbell and Shepard, 1957). P_{O_2} is derived from the oxygen concentration of the bubble. The technique is difficult and inaccurate when the P_{O_2} is more than 12.7 kPa (95 mmHg). It cannot be used in the presence of anaesthetic gases.

2. If the dissociation curve is known, the P_{O_2} may be derived from the saturation (see above). This method is quite accurate on the steep part of the dissociation curve, but is of limited value when the P_{O_2} is greater than about 11.3 kPa (85 mmHg).

3. P_{O_2} of blood is directly proportional to the oxygen content of the plasma. This relationship may be used for deriving P_{O_2} from content, provided that blood can be separated anaerobically without change in the distribution of oxygen between plasma and erythrocytes. The solubility of oxygen in the patient's plasma must be accurately known. The method is difficult because of the small quantities of oxygen dissolved in plasma. However, Stark and Smith (1960) successfully used the method of Smith and Pask (1959) for measuring plasma oxygen content and derived values for blood P_{O_2} in a pioneer study.

4. Since 1960, polarography has virtually displaced all other methods of measurement of blood P_{O_2}. This technique is now widely used both for research and for the management of patients who present problems of oxygenation. It has been of immense value in anaesthesia since it is uninfluenced by the presence of anaesthetic agents. The apparatus consists essentially of a cell formed by a silver anode and a platinum cathode, both in contact with an electrolyte in dilute solution. If a potential difference of about 700 mV is applied to the cell, a current is passed which is directly proportional to the P_{O_2} of the electrolyte in the region of the cathode. In use, the electrolyte is separated from the sample by a thin membrane which is permeable to oxygen. The electrolyte thus attains the same P_{O_2} as the sample and the current passed by the cell is proportional to the P_{O_2} of the sample, which may be gas, blood or other liquids.

A important source of error in the polarographic measurement of blood P_{O_2} is the difference in reading between blood and gas of the same P_{O_2}. Estimates of the ratio very between 1.0 and 1.17 but it may change unexpectedly due to changes in the position of the membrane. This error may be avoided by calibration with tonometer-equilibrated blood, but some workers prefer to calibrate on gas and then use a correction factor. A third approach is to calibrate with a solution of 30% glycerol in water. This solution gives the same reading as blood of the same P_{O_2}. Additional errors arise from a current due to the polarographic reduction of anaesthetic gases at the cathode. This may be minimized by selection of the appropriate polarizing voltage. Automated blood gas analysers are used extensively and can give satisfactory results even when used by untrained staff (Minty and Barrett, 1978).

The major errors in the measurement of blood oxygen levels usually arise from faulty sampling and handling of the sample (Nunn, 1962b) and from failure to correct for differences in temperature between the patient and the measurement system. The following points require attention:

1. The blood sample must be collected without exposure to air.
2. Oxygen is consumed by blood (Greenbaum et al., 1967b), and avoidance of error due to the consequent fall in P_{O_2} after sampling requires one of the following actions:
   a. immediate analysis after sampling;
   b. storage of sampled blood at 0°C;
   c. application of a correction factor for oxygen consumed during the interval between sampling and analysis (see Appendix E, *Figure E.1*).
   (The first is the most satisfactory method.)

3. If blood P_{O_2} is measured at a lower temperature than the patient, the measured P_{O_2} will be less than the P_{O_2} of the blood while it was in the patient. It is not usual to maintain the measuring apparatus at the patient's body temperature, and significant error results from a temperature difference of more than about 1°C. Correction is possible but the factor is variable depending upon the saturation (Nunn et al., 1965a). A convenient nomogram was described by Kelman and Nunn (1966b) and is included in Appendix E as *Figure E.2*.

Cutaneous oximetry

Saturation may be measured photometrically *in vivo* as well as *in vitro* as described above for blood. Light at the appropriate wavelengths is either transmitted through a finger or an ear lobe or else is reflected from the skin, usually on the forehead. The blood which is visualized is venous or capillary rather than arterial and the method therefore depends on there being a brisk cutaneous blood flow to minimize the arterial/venous oxygen difference (see above in relation to cyanosis). New equipment using pulsed light beams gives excellent results and, after many decades of development, oximetry now seems to have reached a level at which it can become a practical clinical monitor. As with blood oximetry, calibration presents a problem. Optical filters are used for routine calibration but a fundamental check of accuracy against arterial blood P_{O_2} or saturation is seldom undertaken. An indirect method of calibration suggested by Campbell (unpublished) was described by Nunn et al. (1965b). It involves rebreathing air and relating the decreasing alveolar P_{O_2} to the saturation simultaneously displayed. When oxygenation is critical, there is no substitute for direct measurement of arterial P_{O_2}.

Measurement of mixed venous P_{O_2}

The usual method of measurement of mixed venous P_{O_2} (or oxygen content) is to sample blood from the right ventricle or pulmonary artery and analyse it according to the methods described above. It has, however, been suggested that a rebreathing technique might be used to derive mixed venous P_{O_2} indirectly, along the same lines as the Campbell and Howell technique for measurement of mixed venous P_{CO_2} (page 233). The technique for oxygen was described by Cerretelli et al. (1966) and requires the rebreathing of a mixture of carbon dioxide in nitrogen. This procedure causes a reduction of the arterial P_{O_2} which, although of short duration, may be unacceptable for some patients. There is, however, a more serious objection to the method. Calculations show that the cardiac output in most patients will not be sufficiently high for the alveolar P_{O_2} to be brought into equilibrium with the mixed venous P_{O_2} in one circulation time (Spence and Ellis, 1971). Furthermore, the change in alveolar P_{O_2} is likely to be so slow that there may be a false impression that equilibrium has been attained.

Indirect methods of measurement of arterial P_{O_2}

Unfortunately, indirect methods of measurement of arterial P_{O_2} are of limited value. The arterial/venous P_{O_2} difference is so large that the rebreathing method of measurement of mixed venous P_{O_2} (see above) is valueless for indirect assessment of the arterial P_{O_2}. The end-expiratory P_{O_2} differs from the ideal alveolar P_{O_2} in patients with increased alveolar dead space, for reasons identical to those producing a difference in the P_{CO_2} (page 158). End-expiratory P_{O_2} is not, therefore, a reliable indicator of arterial P_{O_2}, particularly in the presence of respiratory disease, although it may give some indication of changes.

Cutaneous venous or capillary blood P_{O_2} may, under ideal conditions, be close to the arterial P_{O_2}, but a modest reduction in skin perfusion will cause a substantial fall in P_{O_2} since the oxygen is consumed at a point on the dissociation curve where small changes in content correspond to large changes in tension. Unsatisfactory correlation between arterial and 'arterialized' venous P_{O_2} was reported by Forster et al. (1972).

Tissue P_{O_2}

Clearly the tissue P_{O_2} is of greater significance than the P_{O_2} at various intermediate stages higher in the oxygen cascade. It would therefore appear to be logical to attempt the measurement of P_{O_2} in the tissues, but this has proved difficult both in technique and in interpretation. Difficulties of measurement arise from the extremely small size of the polarographic electrode which is needed to avoid excessive damage to the tissues. Difficulties of interpretation arise from the fact that P_{O_2} varies from one cell to another and from one part of a cell to another, the most important factor being the relation of the elecrode to the capillaries (*Figure 8.3*). Thus the significance of measurements of tissue P_{O_2} depends upon the precise location of the electrode and the degree of damage caused by its insertion: this requires meticulous attention to detail. Cater et al. (1961) inserted electrodes by a stereotaxic technique, fixed the tissues before removal and then examined serial sections cut along the track of the electrode to determine its position in relation to blood vessels and to exclude the possibility of a haematoma around the tip of the electrode.

Such are the difficulties of measurement of tissue P_{O_2} that it may be preferable to measure the venous P_{O_2} of blood draining a particular tissue. Even the significance of this measurement is not entirely clear, but the venous P_{O_2} is roughly related to the mean pressure head of oxygen for diffusion into the cells of the area drained by the blood.

Transcutaneous P_{O_2}

Polarographic estimation of P_{O_2} of skin has been advocated as a non-invasive method of determination of P_{O_2}. A polarographic electrode is applied to the skin which must be heated to at least 44°C to maximize cutaneous blood flow (Severinghaus, 1981). The resultant P_{O_2} does not equal arterial P_{O_2} in all circumstances but is nevertheless one of the most useful indirect determinations of the adequacy of the overall oxygenation of a patient, particularly infants. It has the added advantage of providing a continuous record. Transcutaneous P_{O_2} is probably best considered as a measurement in its own right and not as a substitute for arterial P_{O_2}.

Oxygen consumption

Oxygen consumption may be measured either as the loss of oxygen from a closed rebreathing system or, more accurately, by the subtraction of the quantity of oxygen exhaled from the quantity inhaled. Measurement of the minute volume and the concentration of oxygen in the inspired and expired gas presents no great difficulty and the main problem centres on the measurement of the difference between the inspired and expired minute volumes. This is easy enough when a patient is in equilibrium with the nitrogen in ambient air but, when he is breathing an artificial gas mixture, the difficulties increase (Nunn and Pouliot, 1962).

Chapter 11

Non-respiratory functions of the lung

The lungs are not concerned solely with gas exchange but have other very important functions. Their significance largely derives from the fact that the lungs are so placed in the circulatory system that the entire blood volume passes through it within a single circulation time. The location of the lungs, which is optimal for gas exchange, is also no less suitable for its function as a filter as well as for a large number of metabolic functions.

These non-respiratory functions have been extensively reviewed in volume 4 of *Lung Biology in Health and Disease*, edited by Bakhle and Vane (1977), the Ciba Foundation Symposium on *Metabolic Activities of the Lung* (1980) and in the *Handbook of Physiology* of the American Physiological Society, section 3, volume I edited by Fishman (1985).

The relationship of pulmonary ultrastructure to non-respiratory function has been reviewed by Ryan and Ryan (1977), Simionescu (1980), Ryan (1982) and Weibel (1985).

Filtration

Sitting astride the whole output of the right ventricle, the lung is ideally situated to filter out particulate matter from the venous return. Without such a filter, there would be a constant risk of particulate matter entering the arterial system where the coronary and cerebral circulations are particularly vulnerable. Its position and function are closely analogous to the oil filter of the internal combustion engine. Desirable though this function appears at first sight, it cannot be regarded as essential to life since it is bypassed in patients with a right-to-left intracardiac shunt.

Pulmonary capillaries have a diameter of about 7 μm but this cannot be regarded as the effective pore size of the pulmonary circulation considered as a filter. There is no clear agreement on the maximal diameter of particles which can traverse the pulmonary circulation. Tobin and Zariquiey (1950) demonstrated the passage through perfused animal lungs of glass beads up to 500 μm. Niden and Aviado (1956) observed the passage of glass beads up to 420 μm following embolization of dog's lungs. It is well known that gas and fat emboli may gain access to the systemic circulation in patients without intracardiac shunting. The pathway for the passage of emboli into the systemic circulation has not been identified but may result from the opening of 'sperr' arteries (page 119). The geometry of the pulmonary microcirculation is particularly well adapted to maintaining perfusion in the face of microembolization (page 20). Embolization blocks the circulation to parts of the lungs and it is not surprising that the alveolar component of the physiological dead space is increased.

Thrombi are cleared more rapidly from the lungs than from other organs. The lung possesses well developed proteolytic systems not confined to the removal of fibrin. Pulmonary endothelium is known to be rich in plasmin activator (Warren, 1963). This converts plasminogen into plasmin which itself converts fibrin into fibrin degradation products. However, the lung is also rich in thromboplastin which converts prothrombin to thrombin. To complicate the position further, the lung is a particularly rich source of heparin and bovine lung is used in its commercial preparation. The lung can thus produce high concentrations of substances necessary to promote or delay blood clotting and also for fibrinolysis. The interplay of these activities is not fully understood. Apart from the lung's ability to clear itself of thromboemboli, it may play a role in controlling the overall coagulability of the blood.

Oxidative metabolism of the lung

It is not easy to measure the oxygen consumption of the lung but it has its own oxygen consumption for which estimates range from 3 to 15 ml/min. In relation to its weight of metabolically active tissue, the lung ranks below kidney, brain, heart and liver but above the average for the body as a whole (Fisher and Forman, 1985). The oxygen consumption of the lung constitutes a systematic error in the measurement of cardiac output by the direct Fick method (page 135).

Oxidative phosphorylation. The major part of the oxygen consumption of the lung is in the mitochondria for the production of high energy phosphate compounds by the process of oxidative phosphorylation (page 236). There seems no reason to believe that this is essentially different from the process in other tissues except that the tissue P_{O_2} must be higher in the lungs. However, when ventilation of part of the lung fails (e.g. in consolidation or collapse), the P_{O_2} of the lung tissue must depend on the P_{O_2} of the mixed venous blood. Substrates consumed by the lungs include glucose, lactate, pyruvate and amino acids (Datta, Stubbs and Alberti, 1980; Tierney and Young, 1985)

Cytochrome P-450 systems. The lung is one of the major extrahepatic sites of mixed function oxidation by the cytochrome P-450 systems (page 241). However, gram-for-gram the lung is considerably less active than the liver and its weight of metabolically active tissue is much less than that of the liver. Therefore the total contribution of the lung is quite small in relation to the liver. Furthermore, the lung has only limited capacity for induction of the cytochrome P-450 enzymes.

The role of the cytochrome P-450 system in the lung is not immediately obvious. Biotransformation of drugs has been demonstrated but the total contribution to the body cannot be large. Fisher and Forman (1985) do not think it likely to provide a mechanism for the active transport of oxygen (Gurtner and Burns, 1975), which was considered at some length in the previous edition of this book. It has, however, been considered more recently as a possible mechanism in hypoxic pulmonary vasoconstriction (page 127). There may be a role in the metabolism of steroids or fatty acids, and pulmonary cytochrome P-450 systems may be important in the detoxification of inhaled substances.

Formation of oxygen-derived free radicals. Neutrophils, macrophages and certain other cells of the lung are active in the formation of oxygen-derived free radicals for bacterial killing. Substantial quantities of oxygen may be consumed and the mechanism is described elsewhere (page 487) in relation to oxygen toxicity.

Miscellaneous forms of oxygen consumption include inactivation of vasoactive amines and synthesis of eicosanoids (see below).

Protease transport system

The activity of neutrophils and other phagocytes in the lungs leads to the release of dangerous proteases, particularly elastase and trypsin. These enzymes may destroy the alveolar septa and there are at least two mechnisms to protect against this eventuality. Firstly, the proteases are swept towards the larynx by the flow of mucus. Secondly, they are conjugated by α_1-antitrypsin, present in plasma. Conjugated proteases are then removed in the pulmonary circulation and lymph and transferred to conjugation with α_2-macroglobulin, which is then destroyed in the liver.

In 1963 Laurell and Eriksson described patients whose plasma proteins were deficient in α_1-antitrypsin and who had developed emphysema. The enzyme deficiency is inherited as an autosomal recessive gene and the incidence of homozygous patients is about 1:3000 of the population, with perhaps a higher incidence in Scandinavia. Homozygotes form a higher proportion of patients with emphysema and estimates range from 3 to 26 per cent. These patients tend to have basal emphysema, onset at a younger age and a severe form of the disease (Hutchison et al., 1971). It thus appears that α_1-antitrypsin deficiency is an aetiological factor in a small proportion of patients with emphysema. There may be a family history and heterozygotes may have a slightly increased incidence of the disease.

Synthesis of surfactant

The role of surfactant in the control of alveolar surface tension was considered in Chapter 2 (page 26). This subject has recently been reviewed by King and Clements (1985). The most important constituents are phospholipids of the general structure shown in *Figure 11.1*. The fatty acids are hydrophobic while the other end of the molecule is hydrophilic, the whole thus comprising a detergent. It is believed that the surfactant is concentrated on the surface of the alveolar lining fluid, with the fatty acid chains projecting into the alveolar gas, perpendicular to the interface, with the rest of the molecule in solution.

Lecithins are a series of phospholipids in which the nitrogenous base is choline. Dipalmitoyl lecithin is the most important constituent of the pulmonary surfactant. Palmitic acid is saturated and the fatty acid chains are therefore straight. Harlan and Said (1969) advanced the attractive theory that lipids with straight chain fatty acids will pack together more closely during lung deflation than would be the case with lipids with unsaturated fatty acids (e.g. oleic acid) which are bent at the double bond.

It seems likely that surfactant is both formed in and liberated from the alveolar epithelial type II cell (page 18). Pulmonary surfactant is formed relatively late

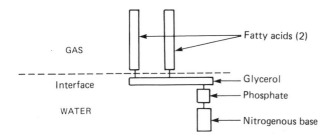

Figure 11.1 General structure of phospholipids.

in the process of maturation of the fetus. The concentration of lecithin in the amniotic fluid reflects the quantity in the alveoli and it increases sharply late in gestation. In contrast, the quantity of sphingomyelin remains fairly constant, and the lecithin/sphingomyelin (L/S) ratio in the amniotic fluid has been used as an indication of pulmonary maturity.

Processing of hormones and other vasoactive compounds

As long ago as 1925, Starling and Verney observed that passage of blood through the lungs was essential for maintenance of adequate circulation through an isolated perfused kidney. It was later found that the 'detoxification of a serum vasoconstrictor substance' in the blood was due to removal of 5-hydroxytryptamine (serotonin) in the pulmonary circulation. Much recent research has now shown that certain hormones pass through the lung unchanged while others may be almost entirely removed from the blood during a single pass: some may be secreted in the lung while others are chemically changed during transit (*Table 11.1*). Vane (1969) suggested that substances with local vasomotor effects (e.g. noradrenaline, bradykinin and 5-hydroxytryptamine) are removed in the pulmonary circulation so that their effects are not broadcast by recirculation. In contrast, generally active circulating hormones, such as adrenaline, pass unchanged through the pulmonary circulation. Somewhat similar arguments have been adduced in relation to the highly selective removal of eicosanoids by the pulmonary circulation (Said, 1982). Teleological though this argument may be, it focuses the mind and the theme has been developed in many reviews.

Endogenous vasoactive amines
(see reviews by Gillis and Pitt, 1982; and Junod, 1985)

Noradrenaline (norepinephrine). There is a striking difference in the handling of noradrenaline and adrenaline. Although each catecholamine has a half-life of about

Table 11.1 Summary of metabolic changes in the lungs

Substances largely removed from the circulation
Noradrenaline
5-Hydroxytryptamine
Bradykinin
ATP, ADP, AMP
PGE_2, PGE_1, $PGF_{2\alpha}$
Leukotrienes

Substances largely unaffected by passage through the lung
Adrenaline
Angiotensin II
Vasopressin
Isoprenaline
Dopamine
Histamine
PGI_2, PGA_2

Substances biotransformed by the lung
Angiotensin I (into angiotensin II)

---

20 seconds in blood, some 30 per cent of noradrenaline is removed in a single pass through the lungs in animals (Ginn and Vane, 1968) and also in man (Sole et al., 1979), while adrenaline (and isoprenaline and dopamine) are unaffected. Noradrenaline is taken up by the endothelium, mainly in the microcirculation, including arterioles and venules.

In contrast to neuronal uptake, noradrenaline is rapidly metabolized after uptake in the lung. Uptake is not inhibited by monoamine oxidase or catechol-*o*-methyl transferase inhibitors but has been reported to be inhibited by inhalational anaesthetics in laboratory animals (Naito and Gillis, 1973; Bakhle and Block, 1976). Extraneuronal uptake of noradrenaline is not confined to the endothelium of the lungs, but uptake by the pulmonary circulation differs in some respects from extraneuronal uptake (uptake 2) in other tissues (Junod, 1985).

5-Hydroxytryptamine (5-HT, serotonin) is very effectively removed by the lungs, up to 98 per cent being removed in a single pass (Thomas and Vane, 1967). There are considerable similarities to the processing of noradrenaline. Uptake is in the endothelium, mainly in the capillaries (see Junod, 1985). Following uptake, 5-HT is rapidly metabolized by monoamine oxidase. Uptake is not blocked by monoamine oxidase inhibitors but unchanged 5-HT then accumulates in the lung (Alabaster, 1980). The half-life of 5-HT in blood is about 1–2 minutes and pulmonary clearance plays the major role in the prevention of its recirculation. If the uptake of 5-HT is inhibited (e.g. by cocaine or tricyclic antidepressant drugs), its pulmonary clearance is greatly reduced (Said, 1982).

Histamine is not removed from the pulmonary circulation although histamine is inactivated by chopped lung. It thus appears that removal of histamine from the circulation is limited by its transport mechanism across the blood/endothelium barrier. The lung is a major site of synthesis of histamine, and mechanisms for its release from mast cells are considered elsewhere (page 56).

Acetylcholine is rapidly hydrolysed in blood where it has a half-life of less than 2 seconds. This tends to overshadow any changes attributable to the lung, which nevertheless does contain acetylcholinesterases and pseudocholinesterases.

Angiotensin, bradykinin and other peptides. It has long been known that angiotensin I (a decapeptide formed by the action of renin on a plasma α_2-globulin) was converted into the vasoactive octapeptide angiotensin II by incubation with plasma (*Figure 11.2*). In 1967, Ng and Vane found greatly increased conversion in the pulmonary circulation, some 80 per cent being converted in a single pass. Enhanced conversion of angiotensin is not peculiar to the pulmonary circulation but the lung is certainly a major site for angiotensin conversion.

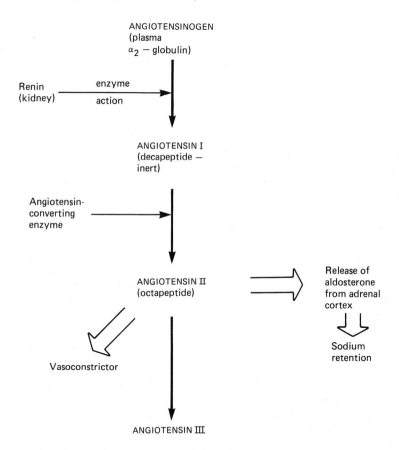

Figure 11.2 Renin–angiotensin–aldosterone axis. Angiotensin-converting enzyme is present on the vascular surface of the pulmonary endothelium.

Angiotensin-converting enzyme (ACE) is free in the plasma but is also bound to the surface of endothelium. This appears to be a general property of endothelium but ACE is present in abundance on the vascular surface of pulmonary endothelial cells, also lining the inside of the caveolae and extending onto the projections into the lumen (Ryan, 1982).

Bradykinin, a vasoactive nonapeptide, is also very effectively removed during passage through the lung and other vascular beds. The half-life in blood is about 17 seconds but less than 4 seconds in various vascular beds (Ryan, 1985). Bakhle (1968) reported that bradykinin and angiotensin I were both cleaved by the same fraction of lung homogenate, and it transpired that ACE was the enzyme responsible in both cases. Thus angiotensin I may act as a competitive inhibitor of the bradykininase activity. There is evidence that other enzymes are capable of metabolizing both angiotensin I and bradykinin but they have not yet been characterized. It is likely that these other enzymes are also located on the endothelial surface.

ACE is inhibited by many substances, some of which (e.g. captopril and enlapril) have a clinical role in the treatment of hypertension. However, this also decreases the degradation of bradykinin by ACE, although other enzymes are capable of handling bradykinin. Even with total inhibition of ACE there is thought to be an adequate reserve for bradykinin metabolism (Bakhle, 1980). Angiotensin II itself passes through the lung unchanged, as do vasopressin and oxytocin.

Prostaglandins and thromboxanes. The lung is a major site of synthesis, metabolism, uptake and release of arachidonic acid metabolites (see Bakhle and Ferreira, 1985). The group as a whole are 20-carbon carboxylic acids, generically known as eicosanoids. The initial stages of metabolism of arachidonic acid are oxygenations with two main pathways for which the enzymes are respectively cyclo-oxygenase and lipoxygenase. The cyclo-oxygenase pathway (*Figure 11.3*) commences with oxygenation and cyclization to form the prostaglandin PGG_2, the enzyme being microsomal and found in most cells. (The subscript $_2$ indicates two double bonds in the carbon chain.) A non-specific peroxidase then converts PGG_2 to PGH_2, which is the parent compound for synthesis of many important derivatives shown in *Figure 11.3*.

$PGF_{2\alpha}$, PGD_2, PGG_2, PGH_2 and thromboxane TXA_2 are bronchial and tracheal constrictors, $PGF_{2\alpha}$ and PGD_2 being much more potent in asthmatics than in normal subjects. PGE_1 and PGE_2 are bronchodilators, particularly when administered by aerosol. Prostacyclin (PGI_2) has different effects in different species. In man, it has no effect on airway calibre in doses which have profound cardiovascular effects (Hardy et al., 1985). PGI_2 and PGE_1 are pulmonary vasodilators. PGH_2 and $PGF_{2\alpha}$ are pulmonary vasoconstrictors.

Eicosanoids are not stored preformed but are synthesized as required by many cell types in the lung, including endothelium, airway smooth muscle, mast cells, epithelial cells and vascular muscle. Activation of the complement system is a potent stimulus to the metabolism of arachidonic acid. Synthesis from endogenous arachidonic acid in the lung appears to be limited by the rate of formation of arachidonic acid from parent lipids. Steroids decrease the availability of endogenous arachidonic acid. Infusion of exogenous arachidonic acid bypasses this stage and results in both bronchoconstriction and vasoconstriction, mediated by its metabolites and depending on the dose. This effect can be blocked by high dose aspirin and some other non-steroidal anti-inflammatory drugs which inhibit cyclo-oxygenase. Release of eicosanoids, particularly TXA_2, occurs in anaphylactic reactions in response to complement activation. However, release of cyclo-oxygenase products does not seem to be a major factor in allergic asthma, which is not significantly relieved by inhibition of cyclo-oxygenase. This may well be explained by increased availability of arachidonic acid for the lipoxygenase pathway (see below). PGI_2 appears to be continuously released from the lungs of certain anaesthetized labora-

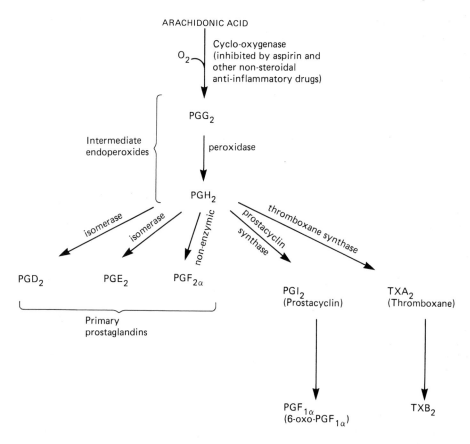

Figure 11.3 The cyclo-oxygenase pathway of metabolism of arachidonic acid to form the prostaglandins and thromboxane. See text for metabolism taking place in the lungs.

tory animals. In anaesthetized man, blood levels of PGI_2 are subthreshold, but artificial ventilation or extracorporeal circulation causes a tenfold increase (Edlund et al., 1981).

Various specific enzymes in the lung are responsible for extensive metabolism of PGE_2, PGE_1 and $PGF_{2\alpha}$. However, PGA_2 and PGI_2 pass through the lung unchanged, but are metabolized on passing through the portal circulation (see review by Bakhle and Ferreira, 1985).

Leukotrienes are also eicosanoids derived from arachidonic acid but by the lipoxygenase pathway (*Figure 11.4*). The leukotrienes LTC_4 and LTD_4 are mainly responsible for the bronchoconstrictor effects of what was formerly known as slow-reacting substance A or SRS-A (Morris et al., 1980; Piper et al, 1981). SRS-A also contains LTB_4, which is a less powerful bronchoconstrictor but increases vascular permeability. These compounds, which are synthesized by the mast cell, could have an important role in asthma, and the mechanism of their release is discussed in Chapter 3 (page 57).

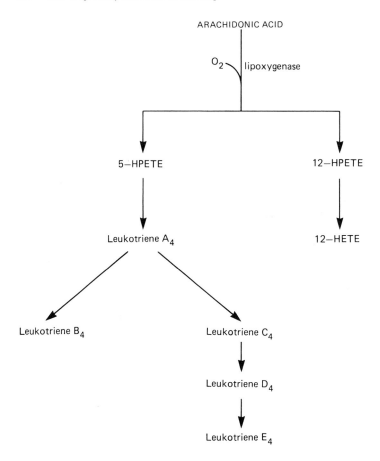

Figure 11.4 The lipoxygenase pathway of metabolism of arachidonic acid to form the leukotrienes. See text for metabolism taking place in the lungs.

Handling of foreign substances by the lungs

The lungs have considerable ability to take up, store or detoxify foreign substances (Bend, Serabjit-Singh and Philpot, 1985). This includes a wide range of drugs which bind reversibly although most of them are not metabolized. Drugs which are taken up in the pulmonary circulation include propranolol (Geddes et al., 1979), lignocaine (Jorfeldt et al., 1979), chlorpromazine, imipramine and nortriptyline (Gillis, 1973). Basic drugs tend to be taken up in the pulmonary circulation while acidic drugs preferentially bind to plasma proteins (Bakhle, 1986, personal communication).

Accumulation of toxic substances in the lung may cause dangerous local toxicity, and paraquat is an outstanding example (page 488). Chronic exposure to a number of amphiphilic drugs may induce phospholipidosis (Philpot, Anderson and Eling, 1977).

The cytochrome P-450 system is active in the lung (see above) and Philpot, Anderson and Eling (1977) list an impressive number of compounds which are detoxified in this manner. It is also known that certain anaesthetics undergo biotransformation (Blitt et al., 1979). Mixed function oxidase systems have been identified in the microsomes of alveolar macrophages and bronchial epithelium. As outlined at the beginning of this chapter, the microsomal systems of the lung cannot be induced as effectively as in the liver. It will be of special interest to know how well the lung can detoxify inhaled substances. Unfortunately, there is little information on this subject at present.

Conclusion

Processing of substances in the lungs has many important implications. Firstly, there will be a substantial difference between arterial and venous plasma concentrations of various substances. Therefore analyses are meaningful only if the appropriate sampling site is used and specified. Secondly, the route of administration and the dosage of relevant drugs must be influenced. Thirdly, bypassing the pulmonary circulation must have substantial effects on the levels of many substances liberated into the systemic circulation. It always seems to the author remarkable how well this is tolerated.

The last word should perhaps be by John Vane (1969): 'It is intriguing to think that venous blood may be full of noxious, as yet unidentified, chemicals released from the peripheral vascular beds, but removed by the lungs before they can cause effects in the arterial circulation'.

Part II

The Applications

Chapter 12

Respiratory aspects of exercise

Levels of exercise

The respiratory response to exercise depends on the level of exercise, which can be conveniently divided into three grades (Whipp, 1981):

1. *Moderate exercise* is below the subject's anaerobic threshold and the arterial blood lactate is not raised. He is able to transport all the oxygen required and is in a steady state. This would correspond to work levels up to about 100 watts (600 kg m min^{-1}).
2. *Heavy exercise* is above the anaerobic threshold but the arterial blood lactate elevation remains constant. This too may be regarded as a steady state.
3. *Severe exercise* is well above the anaerobic threshold and the arterial blood lactate continues to rise. This is an unsteady state and the level of work cannot long be continued.

Oxygen consumption

There is a close relationship between the external power which is produced and the oxygen consumption of the subject (*Figure 12.1*). The oxygen consumption at rest (the basal metabolic rate) is of the order of 200–250 ml/min. As work is done, the oxygen consumption increases by about 12 ml/min per watt (2 ml/min per kg m min^{-1}). A consumption of about 1 l/min is required for walking briskly on the level. About 3 l/min is needed to run at 12 km/hour (7.5 miles/hour). A fit and healthy young adult of 70 kg should be able to maintain a maximal oxygen consumption of about 3 l/min, but this decreases with age to about 2 l/min at the age of 70. A sedentary existence without exercise can reduce maximal oxygen consumption to 50 per cent of the expected value. Conversely, it can be increased by regular exercise, and athletes commonly achieve consumptions of 5 l/min. The highest levels (over 6 l/min) are attained in rowers who utilize a greater muscles mass than other athletes. Clark, Hagerman and Gelfand (1983) have reported an elite group of oarsmen who, for a brief period, attained a mean oxygen consumption of 6.6 l/min on the treadmill. This required a minute volume of 200 l/min (tidal volume 3.29 litres at a frequency of 62 b.p.m.).

Oxygen consumption rises rapidly to a steady level at the onset of a period of continuous light or moderate exercise. If the level of exercise exceeds 60 per cent of the maximal oxygen consumption, there is usually a secondary slow increase in oxygen consumption which has been observed between the 5th and 20th minutes

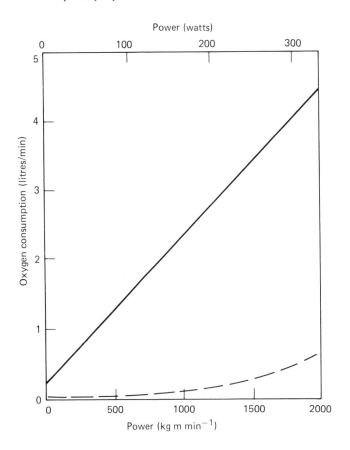

Figure 12.1 The upper curve denotes whole-body oxygen consumption as a function of the level of power developed. The lower curve indicates a typical estimate of the oxygen cost of breathing, but widely different values have been reported by various laboratories (Otis, 1964).

of exercise. This has been attributed to lactacidosis but Hagberg, Mullin and Nagle (1978) adduced evidence to suggest that it could be explained by increased temperature and the oxygen cost of breathing which is disproportionately high as minute volume increases (*Figure 12.1*).

At the end of moderate exercise below the anaerobic threshold, the oxygen consumption rapidly returns within a few minutes to the resting level. However, after heavy exercise there is a delay in the return of oxygen consumption to basal levels as the oxygen debt is discharged (see below).

Anaerobic metabolism

During heavy work, the total work exceeds the capacity for aerobic work which is limited by oxygen transport (see below). The difference is made up by anaerobic metabolism, of which the principal product is lactic acid (see *Figure 10.3*) which is almost entirely ionized to lactate and hydrogen ions. An increase in blood lactate level is therefore taken as the indication that there is a significant anaerobic contribution to metabolism. This defines the anaerobic threshold, which depends not only on the power produced but also on many other factors including altitude, environmental temperature and the fitness of the subject. An additional factor is the muscle groups which are used to accomplish the work. Thus it was found that lactate began to rise when oxygen consumption exceeded about 2 l/min during leg exercise but at less than 1 l/min during arm exercise (Asmussen and Neilsen, 1946). 1946).

During steady state heavy anaerobic exercise, the lactate level reaches a plateau within the first 5–10 minutes. The level is influenced by the factors described above in relation to the anaerobic threshold but is of the order of 100 mg/dl at 200 watts (1200 kg m min^{-1}).

During severe exercise the lactate level continues to rise and begins to cause distress at levels above about 100 mg/dl, a tenfold increase above the resting level. Trained athletes can tolerate levels of 200 mg/dl. Lactate accumulation appears to be the limiting factor for sustained heavy work, and the progressive increase in blood lactate results in the level of work being inversely related to the time for which it can be maintained. Thus there is a reciprocal relationship between the record time for various distances and the speed at which they are run (Asmussen, 1965).

Oxygen debt

The difference between the total work and the aerobic work is achieved by anaerobic metabolism of carbohydrates to lactate which is ultimately converted to citrate, enters the citric acid cycle and is then fully oxidized. Like glucose, lactate has a respiratory quotient of 1.0. Although this process continues during heavy exercise, lactate accumulates and the excess is oxidized in the early stages of recovery. Oxygen consumption remains above the resting level during recovery, the excess above the resting level being used for this purpose. This constitutes the 'repayment of the oxygen debt' and is related to the lactate level attained by the end of exercise.

Repayment of the oxygen debt is especially well developed in the diving mammals such as seals and whales. During a dive, their circulation is largely diverted to heart and brain and the metabolism of the skeletal muscles is almost entirely anaerobic (page 329). On regaining the surface, very large quantities of lactate are suddenly released into the circulation and are rapidly metabolized while the animal is on the surface between dives.

There is considerable evidence that some of the early part of the repayment of the oxygen debt is not only concerned with clearing lactate. Apart from oxidation of other products of anaerobic metabolism, there is the restoration of both oxygen stores and levels of high energy phosphate compounds to their normal resting levels (Asmussen, 1965).

Response of the oxygen delivery system

A ten- or twentyfold increase in oxygen consumption requires a complex adaptation of both circulatory and respiratory systems. Oxygen flux (page 256) is the product of cardiac output and arterial oxygen content, which is the total delivery of oxygen to the body. The arterial oxygen content cannot be significantly increased and

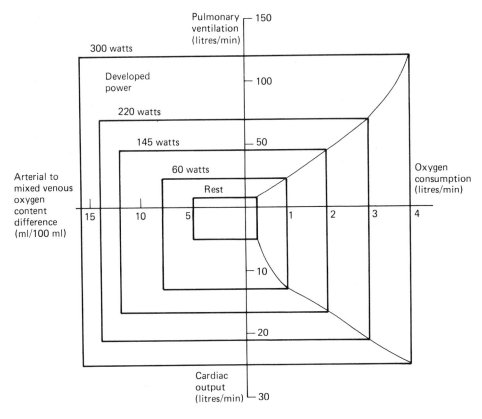

Figure 12.2 Changes in ventilation, oxygen consumption, cardiac output and oxygen extraction at different levels of power developed.

therefore an increase in cardiac output is essential. However, the cardiac output does not increase in proportion to the oxygen consumption. For example, an oxygen consumption of 4 l/min is a 16-fold increase compared with the resting state. A typical cardiac output at this level of exercise would be only 25 l/min (*Figure 12.2*), which is only a fivefold increase above the resting value. Therefore, there must also be increased extraction of oxygen from the blood.

In the resting state, blood returns to the right heart with haemoglobin 70% saturated. This provides a substantial reserve of oxygen and the arterial to mixed venous oxygen content difference is markedly increased in heavy exercise (*Figure 12.2*). Since the resting mixed venous point is at the top of the steep part of the dissociation curve, a considerable amount of additional oxygen can be extracted without resulting in an undue fall in tissue P_{O_2}. However, the additionally desaturated blood returning to the lungs and the greater volume of blood require that the respiratory system transport a larger quantity of oxygen to the alveoli. If there were no increased oxygen transport to the alveoli, then the reserve oxygen in the mixed venous blood could be exhausted in a single circulation time. In fact, the respiratory system adapts with great rapidity to increase the oxygen consumption at the beginning of exercise (see below).

The essential adaptation of the respiratory system is an increase in the respiratory minute volume, and this is normally very well matched to the increased oxygen consumption (*Figure 12.2*). The relationship between minute volume and oxygen consumption is approximately linear up to an oxygen consumption of about 3 l/min. At higher levels of oxygen consumption the minute volume is proportionately higher.

There is an immediate increase in ventilation at the start or even before exercise commences (phase I). During moderate exercise, there is then a further increase (phase II) to reach an equilibrium level of ventilation (phase III) within about 3 minutes (Wasserman, 1978). With heavy exercise there is a secondary increase in ventilation which may reach a plateau, but ventilation continues to rise in severe work.

Minute volumes as great as 200 l/min have been recorded during exercise although the normal subject cannot maintain a minute volume approaching his maximal breathing capacity (MBC) for more than a very short period. It has been variously estimated that 50 per cent of the MBC can be voluntarily maintained for 15 minutes, or 70–80 per cent for 15 minutes during maximal work (Shepard, 1967). Wasserman (1978) observed that ventilation approximates to 60 per cent of MBC at maximal oxygen consumption. The usable fraction of the maximal breathing capacity can be increased by training.

Diffusion across the membrane does not limit the increased oxygen consumption at sea level but this is a limiting factor at altitude (see Chapters 8 and 14).

Control of ventilation
(see reviews by Asmussen, 1965; Wasserman, 1978; Whipp, 1981)

Arterial blood gas tensions

There is a large body of evidence that, during exercise at sea level with oxygen consumption up to about 3 l/min, there is no significant change in either Pco_2 or Po_2 of arterial blood. Asmussen and Neilsen (1960) found that even at the point of exhaustion for their subjects (oxygen consumption 3.5 l/min), the arterial Po_2 was the same as the resting value and Pco_2 was actually reduced. Blood gas tensions are clearly not a limiting factor during exercise at sea level although they are critically important at great altitude (see Chapter 14). These crucial observations indicate that arterial blood gas tensions, which are the main factors in the control of resting ventilation, cannot explain the increase of ventilation during exercise. Other factors are clearly operative and their elucidation has presented physiologists with a continuing challenge for many years.

Neural factors

It has long been evident that neural factors play an important role, particularly since ventilation normally increases *before* the start of exercise when no other physiological variable has changed except cardiac output. Kao (1963) and his colleagues showed that virtually all of the hyperventilation of exercise can be explained by afferents arising from the exercising muscles of anaesthetized dogs. This was convincingly shown in crossed-circulation studies. The essential observation was that an anaesthetized dog in neurological continuity with electrically stimulated limb muscles hyperventilated, while another dog receiving the venous drainage from the exercising muscles did not. It was established that afferent traffic from the stimulating electrode was not the explanation (Tibes, 1977).

Humoral mechanisms

Humoral factors play a comparatively minor role in moderate exercise but are more important in heavy and severe exercise when lactacidosis is an important factor. Exercise at high altitude ls a special case when oxygen transport becomes a limiting factor (see Chapter 14).

Metabolic acidosis drives ventilation during heavy and severe exercise and there is usually a slight reduction in arterial Pco_2. However, study of arterial pH may be misleading since the very short transit time from lungs to carotid body during exercise (of the order of 4–6 seconds) is insufficient for the change in Pco_2 in the lungs to result in an equilibrium change in plasma pH by the time the blood reaches the chemoreceptors. The limiting step is the dehydration of carbonic acid (equation 2 in Chapter 9), which takes an appreciable time even in the presence of carbonic anhydrase. However, there is ample time for equilibration to occur in arterial blood sampled for analysis. Therefore the peripheral chemoreceptors see a different pH from that indicated by the pH meter, and blood perfusing the carotid bodies may be 0.02–0.03 pH units more acid, and the Pco_2 slightly higher than indicated by analysis of an arterial blood sample by conventional methods (Crandall, Bidani and Forster, 1977).

Another humoral factor is the oscillation of arterial pH and Pco_2 (page 83). This is detectable at rest but becomes very much more prominent during exercise, due to the greater desaturation and acidaemia of the mixed venous blood. Oscillating discharge in the sinus nerve is believed to increase the gain of the central chemoreceptors (see *Figure 4.4*). In spite of the apparent absence of a direct role for arterial hypoxia in regulating the ventilation during exercise, studies of asthmatic patients after carotid body resection have shown a slowing of the rate of increase of ventilation during exercise (Wasserman, 1978). Less surprising is the absence of response to lactacidosis in these patients.

It has been observed many times that the hyperventilation of exercise accords with the blood gas changes of the mixed venous blood. However, there is no evidence of any chemoreceptor in the great veins, the right heart or the input side of the lungs. There is some evidence that there may be metabolic chemoreceptors in the muscles (see review by Whipp, 1981). There is, however, no general agreement on the importance of this factor (Dejours, 1964).

Humoral factors are likely to be relatively more important for exercise in hypoxaemic patients. Inhalation of 30% oxygen has pronounced beneficial effects on exercise in patients with chronic respiratory failure (King et al., 1977).

Chapter 13

Respiratory aspects of sleep

This book contains numerous references to the effects of sleep on various aspects of respiration. The purpose of this chapter is to gather the information in one place and provide a general review of the effects of sleep on respiration. Normal sleep in healthy subjects is accompanied by only minor changes in respiratory function. The muscles of respiration, including those concerned with the patency of the upper airway, continue their rhythmic discharge during normal sleep but there are special circumstances in which their function is deranged. First, however, it is useful to consider normal sleep.

Normal sleep

Sleep is classified on the basis of the electroencephalogram (EEG) and electro-oculogram (EOG) into non-REM (stages 1–4) and REM (rapid eye movement) sleep.

Stage 1 is dozing from which arousal easily takes place. The EEG is low voltage and the frequency is mixed but predominantly fast. This progresses to stage 2 in which the background EEG is similar to stage 1 but with episodic sleep spindles (frequency 12–14 Hz) and K complexes (large biphasic waves of characteristic appearance). Slow, large amplitude (delta) waves start to appear in stage 2 but become more dominant in stage 3 in which spindles are less conspicuous and K complexes become difficult to distinguish. In stage 4, which is often referred to as deep sleep, the EEG is mainly high voltage (more than 75 µV and more than 50 per cent slow (delta) frequency.

REM sleep has quite different characteristics. The EEG pattern is the same as in stage 1 but the EOG shows frequent rapid eye movements which are easily distinguished from the rolling eye movements of non-REM sleep. Other forms of activity are manifest in REM sleep and dreaming occurs.

The stage of sleep changes frequently during the night, and the pattern varies between different individuals and on different nights for the same individual (*Figure 13.1*). Sleep is entered in stage 1 and usually progresses through 2 to 3 and sometimes into 4. Episodes of REM sleep then alternate with non-REM sleep throughout the night. On average there are four or five episodes of REM sleep per night, with a tendency for the duration of the episodes to increase towards morning. Conversely, stages 3 and 4 predominate in the early part of the night. The sleeper can pass from

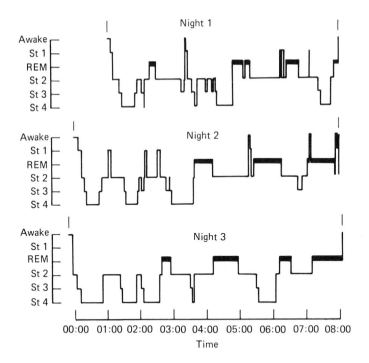

Figure 13.1 Patterns of sleep on three consecutive nights in a young fit man aged 20. The thick horizontal bars indicate rapid eye movement (REM) sleep. (Record kindly supplied by Miss Christine Thornton)

any stage to any other stage but it is unusual for him to pass from stage 1 or REM into either 3 or 4 or from stage 3 or 4 into REM. However, it is not uncommon for the sleeper to pass from any stage into stage 1 or full consciousness.

Respiratory changes

The metabolic rate decreases during sleep to about 10 per cent below the conventional basal level. This corresponds to the basal level as defined by Robertson and Reid (1952) and is similar to levels encountered during anaesthesia (page 366). The oxygen consumption tends to be highest in REM sleep and lowest in stages 3 and 4.

In sleep stages 3 and 4, the slope of the P_{CO_2}/ventilation response curve is little different from the conscious state. However, it is markedly depressed in REM sleep in the dog (Phillipson, 1977). The P_{O_2}/ventilation response curve is unaffected in all levels of sleep, in marked contrast to what happens during anaesthesia (page 353). Tidal volume decreases with deepening levels of non-REM sleep and is minimal in REM sleep when it is about 25 per cent less than in the awake state (Douglas et al., 1982). Respiratory frequency increases slightly in all stages of sleep but the minute volume is progressively reduced in parallel with the tidal volume. Arterial P_{CO_2} is usually slightly elevated by about 0.4 kPa (3 mmHg).

In the young healthy adult, arterial P_{O_2} decreases by about the same amount as the P_{CO_2} is increased, and therefore the oxygen saturation remains reasonably steady, usually within the range 95–98%. However, as age advances, episodes of transient hypoxaemia occur in subjects who are otherwise healthy. Saturation may fall to 75%, usually in association with hypoventilation and irregular breathing in REM sleep (Flenley, 1985b). Such changes must be regarded as a normal part of the ageing process.

Snoring

Snoring may occur at any age, but the incidence is bimodal, peaking in the first, fifth and sixth decades of life. It is commoner in males than females, and obesity is an additional factor. It may occur in any stage of sleep, becoming more pronounced as non-REM sleep deepens, though usually attenuated in REM sleep (Lugaresi et al, 1984). It has been suggested that about 25 per cent of the population are habitual snorers.

Snoring originates in the oropharynx and in its mildest form is due to vibration of the soft palate and posterior pillars of the fauces. However, in its more severe forms, the walls of the oropharynx collapse as a result of the subatmospheric pressure generated during inspiration against more upstream airway obstruction (Jennett, 1984). This may be at the level of the palate as described above or may be the result of nasal polyps, nasal infection or adenoids which are the commonest cause of snoring in children. The tongue may be drawn back during inspiration until it obstructs against the posterior pharyngeal wall although, in contrast to anaesthesia, the tone of the genioglossus is not normally lost during sleep (page 4). As obstruction develops, the inspiratory muscles greatly augment their action and intrathoracic pressure may fall as low as 7 kPa (70 cmH$_2$O). Posture is not a major factor in the production of snoring (Sullivan, Berton-Jones and Issa, 1983).

Apart from the annoyance to conjugal partners and others, there are strong associations between snoring and a wide range of pathological conditions, including hypertension, heart and chest disease, rheumatism, diabetes and depression (Norton and Dunn, 1985). In addition, these authors confirmed the association with obesity, smoking and alcoholism. However, perhaps the most serious aspect of snoring is that it may be a precursor of the sleep apnoea syndrome, which is considered below.

The sleep apnoea syndrome

This syndrome is characterized by periods of apnoea lasting more than 10 seconds and recurring at least 11 times per hour during sleep (Guilleminault, van der Hoed and Mitler, 1978). In fact, durations of apnoea may be as long as 90 seconds and the frequency of the episodes as high as 160 hour. Typically, 50 per cent of sleep time may be spent without tidal exchange. Apnoea may be central (absence of all respiratory movements—*Figure 13.2a*) or obstructive. Both types may occur in the same patient. Differentiation between central and obstructive apnoea is conveniently made by continuous recording of rib cage and abdominal movements. Inductance plethysmography permits calculation of the tidal volume attributable to each component and, if these are equal but opposite in phase, there is total obstructive apnoea (*Figure 13.2b*). Obstructive apnoea may occur in REM or non-REM sleep but the longest periods of apnoea tend to occur in REM sleep. The syndrome can occur at any age but is commonest in obese male snorers.

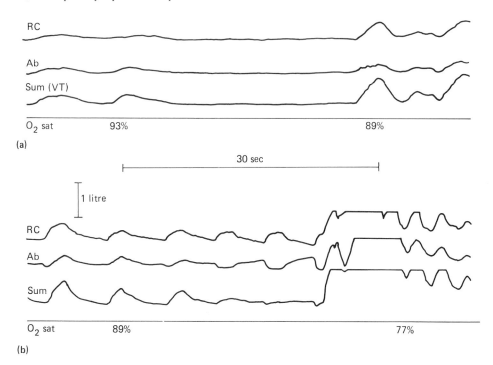

Figure 13.2 Continuous records of breathing showing a central (a) and an obstructive (b) apnoea in a patient sleeping after surgery. 'RC' indicates the cross-sectional area of rib cage and 'Ab' that of the abdomen. 'Sum' indicates the arithmetic sum of RC and Ab. Note the absence of all movements in (a) and out-of-phase movements in (b), indicating obstruction. Note that the desaturation is much greater in the obstructive apnoea. (Record kindly supplied by C. Jordan)

Obstructive apnoea is commoner than central apnoea and now appears to account for many cases of the primary hypoventilation syndrome. It is usually associated with much more severe arterial hypoxaemia than is central apnoea. A typical pattern of recurrent hypoxaemia in the obstructive type of sleep apnoea is shown in *Figure 13.3*. In many patients the changes are not trivial and the recurrent hypoxaemia is considered to be responsible for both intellectual deterioration and pulmonary hypertension.

There is no sharp dividing line between snoring and nocturnal obstructive apnoea. The one may lead into the other and many of the risk factors are similar for both conditions. There are many possible causes of obstruction but perhaps the most important is temporary loss of tone in the genioglossus muscles, causing the tongue to fall back against the posterior pharyngeal wall (Remmers et al., 1978; Harper and Sauerland, 1978). Whatever the primary cause of obstruction, attempted inspiration against obstruction causes collapse of the pharynx, which tends to make the obstruction complete. Computerized tomography has shown pharyngeal narrowing in patients with obstructive sleep apnoea, even while awake (Haponik et al., 1983).

Episodes of irregular breathing with hypoventilation that do not amount to true apnoea are very common in otherwise healthy subjects over the age of 55. These episodes, which often result in temporary hypoxaemia, occur most frequently during REM sleep in patients with chronic bronchitis.

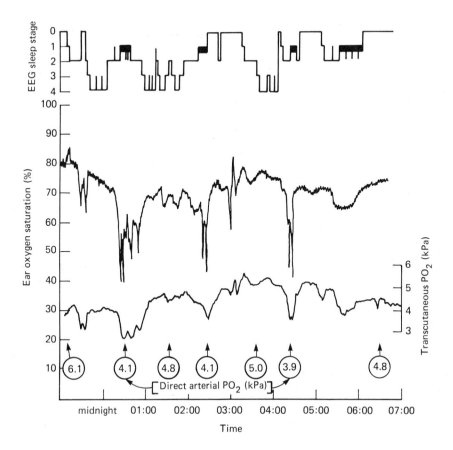

Figure 13.3 EEG sleep stage, ear oximetry and transcutaneous P_{O_2} and arterial P_{O_2} in a 'blue bloater' throughout a night while breathing air. Note that the worst episodes of desaturation occur during REM sleep (indicated by closed bars in the EEG record). (Reproduced from Flenley (1985c) by permission of the author and the publishers)

Arousal

Obstruction normally results in arousal, and this is clearly important for survival. Hypoxia is a major factor in arousal, and studies in dogs have demonstrated a normal threshold for arousal at about 85% saturation in non-REM sleep and 70% in REM sleep (Bowes and Phillipson, 1984). This mechanism appears to be dependent on the peripheral chemoreceptors and the arousal thresholds are significantly reduced by carotid body denervation. It is not entirely clear whether mechanical obstruction can result in arousal other than as a result of hypoxaemia. In the postoperative period arousal was observed following obstruction when hypoxaemia had been prevented by administration of oxygen (Catley et al., 1985).

Chronic bronchitis

Transient nocturnal hypoxaemia is particularly dangerous in patients with chronic bronchitis who have lost much of their hypoxic drive to respiration. These patients ('blue bloaters') fare very much worse than 'pink puffers' and tend to have more frequent and more severe episodes of desaturation, particularly during REM sleep (Wynne, 1984). Although the prognosis is grave in such patients, the condition can be ameliorated by the administration of sleeping oxygen. The new French respiratory stimulant almitrine has also been found effective in preventing transient hypoxaemia in these patients (Connaughton et al., 1985). Combination of chronic bronchitis and true obstructive sleep apnoea syndrome in the same patient has been termed the 'overlap' syndrome (see Flenley, 1985b, c).

Oxygen

Oxygen can easily be provided during sleep by techniques such as nasal catheters or prongs. These methods have the advantage of increasing the inspired oxygen concentration as minute volume decreases. In fact, oxygen does not decrease the incidence of sleep apnoea but it does reduce the desaturation which results. It does not appear to delay arousal from obstruction and neither does it result in hypercapnia. Provision of sleeping oxygen is important for preventing the sequelae of the recurrent bouts of hypoxaemia—in particular, pulmonary hypertension and intellectual deterioration.

Treatment of obstruction

The first approach is the removal of any pathological obstruction such as nasal polyps which cause the development of subatmospheric pressure in the pharynx during inspiration. If this is not feasible, it is possible to prevent collapse of the pharyngeal airway by the application of constant positive airway pressure (Sullivan, Berton-Jones and Issa, 1983). This is conveniently achieved with soft plastic tubes which fit inside the external nares and do not interfere unduly with sleep. However, there are logistic hurdles in providing the requisite gas flow and humidification in the home.

A more radical approach is uvulo-palato-pharyngoplasty (Fujita et al., 1980), which corrects anatomical abnormalities in the oropharynx. Finally, tracheostomy (opened only at night) has been used in some cases as a last resort.

The postoperative period

Continuous monitoring has shown that transient apnoeas occur very frequently during sleep in the postoperative period (Catley et al., 1985). Both central and obstructive apnoeas occur but hypoxaemia is more pronounced in the obstructive type (see *Figure 13.2*). Stage 3 and 4 and REM sleep were not observed in the first 24 hours after operation and apnoeas were therefore restricted to stages 1 and 2. Avoidance of opiates greatly reduced the incidence of episodes of hypoxia, which were seldom seen in patients whose postoperative pain was controlled only with regional analgesia.

Relationship to sudden infant death syndrome (SIDS)

Healthy infants do not have apnoeic episodes exceeding 15 seconds during sleep. However, severe attacks of hypoxaemia (Po_2 2–4 kPa, 15–30 mmHg) have been described by Southall et al. (1985), predominantly during sleeping and feeding in infants under 2 months old. The hypoxaemia developed very rapidly, usually within about 20 seconds of the start of apnoea. The attacks were characterized by expiratory muscle activity and reduced lung volume. Although there appeared to be glottic closure, episodes continued after tracheostomy in two children. Apnoea terminated spontaneously even when administration of oxygen prevented hypoxaemia.

Apnoeic episodes have also been observed in infants with relatively mild illnesses such as upper respiratory tract infections, stridor, metabolic alkalosis and also in infants who have had a 'near miss' from SIDS (Abreu e Silva et al., 1985). It seems very likely that something resembling the adult apnoea sydrome may account for some cases of SIDS but it is unlikely to be the sole cause. It will be extremely difficult to determine in what proportion of deaths ascribed to SIDS apnoea has in fact played a role.

Chapter 14

Respiratory aspects of high altitude

This chapter is concerned with the respiratory effects of high altitude as it affects the aviator and the mountaineer. With increasing altitude, the barometric pressure falls but the fractional concentration of oxygen in the air and the saturated vapour pressure of water at body temperature remain constant (6.3 kPa or 47 mmHg). The P_{O_2} of the inspired air falls with the barometric pressure according to the usual relationship:

Inspired gas P_{O_2} = 0.21 (Barometric pressure − 6.3)   kPa
Inspired gas P_{O_2} = 0.21 (Barometric pressure − 47)   mmHg

The influence of the saturated vapour pressure of water becomes relatively more important until, at an altitude of approximately 19 000 metres or 63 000 feet, the barometric pressure equals the water vapour pressure, the body fluids boil and the alveolar P_{O_2} and P_{CO_2} rapidly fall to zero.

For the purpose of standardization of altitude in aviation there is a standard table relating altitude and barometric pressure (*Table 14.1*). However, there are important deviations from the predicted barometric pressure under certain circumstances, particularly at low latitudes. For example, on the summit of Everest, the difference between predicted and actual barometric pressure is crucial to reaching the summit without oxygen. In *Figure 14.1*, expected P_{O_2} of air is shown as a function of altitude by the uppermost curve. Crosses indicate observed values which have always been higher than expected in the Himalayas.

Equivalent oxygen concentration

The acute effect of altitude on inspired P_{O_2} may be simulated by reduction of the oxygen concentration of gas inspired at sea level (*Table 14.1*). This provides the basis for much experimental work. Conversely, up to certain limits of altitude, it is possible to restore the inspired P_{O_2} to the sea level value by increasing the oxygen concentration of the inspired gas (also shown in *Table 14.1*). The first limitation occurs at 10 000 metres (33 000 ft), above which it is no longer possible to maintain the sea level value even if the subject breathes 100% oxygen. The second limitation occurs at 19 000 metres (63 000 ft) when body fluids boil and it is impossible to raise the alveolar P_{O_2} above zero.

Table 14.1 Barometric pressure relative to altitude

Altitude		Barometric pressure		Inspired gas P_{O_2}		Equivalent oxygen % at sea level	Percentage oxygen required to give sea level value of inspired gas P_{O_2}
feet	metres	kPa	mm Hg	kPa	mm Hg		
0	0	101	760	19.9	149	20.9	20.9
2 000	610	94.3	707	18.4	138	19.4	22.6
4 000	1 220	87.8	659	16.9	127	17.8	24.5
6 000	1 830	81.2	609	15.7	118	16.6	26.5
8 000	2 440	75.2	564	14.4	108	15.1	28.8
10 000	3 050	69.7	523	13.3	100	14.0	31.3
12 000	3 660	64.4	483	12.1	91	12.8	34.2
14 000	4 270	59.5	446	11.1	83	11.6	37.3
16 000	4 880	54.9	412	10.1	76	10.7	40.8
18 000	5 490	50.5	379	9.2	69	9.7	44.8
20 000	6 100	46.5	349	8.4	63	8.8	49.3
22 000	6 710	42.8	321	7.6	57	8.0	54.3
24 000	7 320	39.2	294	6.9	52	7.3	60.3
26 000	7 930	36.0	270	6.3	47	6.6	66.8
28 000	8 540	32.9	247	5.6	42	5.9	74.5
30 000	9 150	30.1	226	4.9	37	5.2	83.2
35 000	10 700	23.7	178	3.7	27	3.8	—
40 000	12 200	18.8	141	2.7	20	2.8	—
45 000	13 700	14.8	111	1.8	13	1.9	—
50 000	15 300	11.6	87	1.1	8	1.1	—
63 000	19 200	6.3	47	0	0	0	—

100% oxygen restores sea level inspired P_{O_2} at 10 000 metres (33 000 ft)

Acute exposure to altitude

Acute exposure to potentially dangerous altitudes will seldom occur when the climber relies upon his own exertions to gain altitude. Some degree of acclimatization will usually take place during the early part of the ascent, which would seldom exceed 2000 metres (6500 ft) per day from sea level, decreasing to only 300 metres (1000 ft) per day at very high altitudes. However, rail, cable car or motor transport may take the passenger within a few hours from near sea level to as high as 4000 metres (13100 ft) or even 5000 metres (16400) ft) in certain exceptional locations. Aircraft, helicopters and balloons can take the traveller very much higher but, for commercial operations, passengers in unpressurized aircraft are not normally exposed to an altitude of more than 3700 metres (12 000 ft). Pressurized aircraft normally maintain the cabin pressure equivalent to about 2000–2500 metres (6500–8200 ft) but only 1500 metres (5000 ft) in Concorde. The most acute exposure to altitude occurs after rupture of the pressurized hull of an aircraft. Subsonic jet airliners have an operational ceiling of 13000 metres (43000 ft) but Concorde operates up to 18300 metres (60000 ft). Military aircraft can fly very much higher with an external pressure well below that at which body fluids boil.

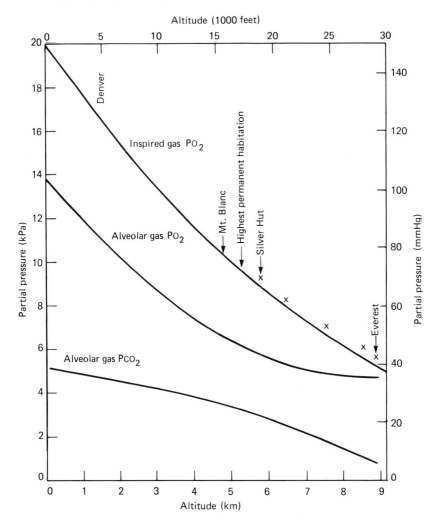

Figure 14.1 Inspired and alveolar gas tensions as a function of altitude. The continuous curve for inspired
P_{O_2} *is taken from the data in* Table 14.1 *but the crosses show measured values for* P_{O_2}.

At high altitude the decrease in inspired gas P_{O_2} causes an inevitable decrease in alveolar and therefore arterial P_{O_2}. The actual decrease in alveolar P_{O_2} is mitigated by hyperventilation caused by the hypoxic drive to ventilation (page 81). However, the hyperventilation results in a reduction of arterial P_{CO_2} which, in the acute situation, substantially reduces the full ventilatory response to hypoxia which would otherwise occur if P_{CO_2} remained constant. *Figure 14.1* compares the alveolar gas tensions measured on acute exposure and after acclimatization at various altitudes. The negative feedback from hypocapnia on the ventilatory response to hypoxia is clearly disadvantageous and is a major factor in acute exposure to altitude. We shall see below that offsetting the respiratory depressant effect of hypocapnia by buffering of the cerebrospinal fluid (CSF) pH is a most important acclimatization to altitude, taking place within the first two or three days at altitude. It is essential to survival at extreme altitudes.

   Impairment of night vision is the earliest sign of hypoxia and this may be detected as low as 1200 metres (4000 ft). Although this is important for pilots, the most serious aspect of acute exposure to altitude is impairment of mental performance culminating in loss of consciousness, which usually occurs on acute exposure to altitudes in excess of 6000 metres (about 20000 ft). The time to loss of consciousness varies with altitude and is of great practical importance to pilots of aircraft in the event of loss of pressurization (*Figure 14.2*). The limiting minimal time of about 15 seconds is governed by lung-to-brain circulation time and the capacity of high energy phosphate stores in the brain (page 471). This applies above about 16000 metres (52000 ft).

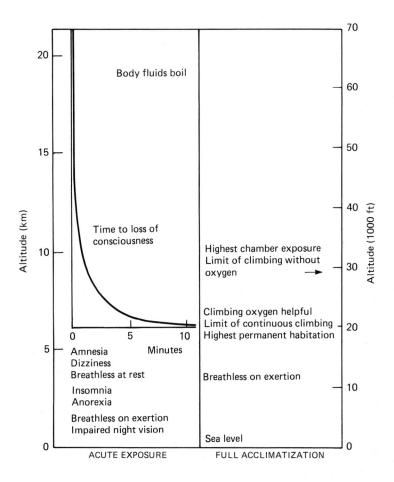

Figure 14.2 Symptomatology of acute and chronic exposure to altitude.

The use of oxygen

Oxygen must be provided for passengers if unpressurized aircraft operate above 3700 metres (12000 ft), while the pilots are required to use oxygen above 3000 metres (10000 ft) to ensure proper handling of the aircraft. Oxygen provides adequate protection from loss of consciousness up to an altitude of about 12000 metres (40000 ft) where the atmospheric pressure is about equal to the sea level atmospheric Po_2. This covers the maximal cruising altitude of subsonic transports. Concorde, however, operates above the altitude at which oxygen would be effective and has therefore been designed to minimize the rate at which accidental depressurization would be likely to occur in the event of, for example, breakage of a window (Mills and Harding, 1983a). Precautions include the small size of the windows, reserve capacity for pressurization, and pressure breathing equipment for the flight crew. This equipment supplies oxygen at 4 kPa (40 cmH$_2$O) and is essential equipment for all pilots flying above 12200 metres (40000 ft) (*Medical Aspects of Supersonic Flight*, published by British Airways Medical Services).

Manned spacecraft rely on a sealed closed circuit environment. The American Gemini and Mercury projects used 100% oxygen at a total pressure of 34.5 kPa (259 mmHg). Because of the tragic fire in 1967, the composition was changed to 64% oxygen/36% nitrogen at the same pressure, which still gives an inspired Po_2 in excess of the normal sea level value. The Russian approach has been more conservative and they have employed a cabin atmosphere of the same pressure and composition as sea level air (Mills and Harding, 1983b).

Acute mountain sickness

The mountaineer is affected by altitude in a manner which differs from that of the aviator because his physical exertion is much greater and the time course of exposure is different. Acute mountain sickness has been categorized into benign and malignant forms (Dickinson, 1985), but the relationship between the two forms is not clear. Benign manifestations may progress to the malignant forms, pulmonary, cerebral and mixed.

The unacclimatized mountaineer usually first becomes aware of increased breathlessness on exertion at about 2000 metres (6600 ft) and above that level, new arrivals at altitude often have headache, nausea, anorexia, difficulty in sleeping and their climbing performance may be impaired (*Figure 14.2*). At about 5000 metres (or approximately 16000 ft), there are feelings of unreality (often enhanced by the environment!), amnesia and dizziness. The unacclimatized person has extreme dyspnoea on exertion at this level and usually has dyspnoea at rest.

Sleep apnoea is common above about 4000 metres (13000 ft) and may take many forms. The commonest is classic Cheyne–Stokes breathing with periodic apnoeas and a cycle time of about 20 seconds. Apnoeas may result in considerable additional hypoxaemia at high altitude, saturation changing by a mean value of 10% at 6300 metres (21000 ft) (West et al., 1986). The incidence of Cheyne–Stokes breathing was found by Lahiri (1984) to be related to the strength of the subject's hypoxic ventilatory drive, and it is seldom seen in high altitude residents who have a much attenuated hypoxic drive.

Pulmonary oedema may occur during acute exposure to altitudes in excess of about 3000 metres (10 000 ft). It is most commonly seen in the unacclimatized but overambitious climber. However, it is difficult to predict who will be affected and it may occur in subjects who have previously attained higher altitudes without mishap. Several fatalities have been recorded, the first being on Mont Blanc in 1891.

The aetiology of high altitude pulmonary oedema is far from clear. Various theories have been advanced and the condition may well be multifactorial. Fluid retention probably occurs in susceptible subjects when exercise is taken at altitude (Milledge, 1985) but this is unlikely to be the only cause. Many different theories are discussed by Hultgren (1978) but the most credible are based on pulmonary hypertension caused by hypoxic pulmonary vasoconstriction. Firstly, it has been suggested that this may cause an opening of the tight endothelial junctions in the pulmonary arterial tree allowing transudation to occur. Secondly, Hultgren has suggested that regional failure of vasoconstriction in some parts of the lung may lead to a localized hyperdynamic circulation with high intravascular pressure resulting in localized transudation. Dickinson et al. (1983) have stressed that in some cases oedema has been found to be associated with bronchopneumonia, pulmonary thrombosis and infarction.

Cerebral oedema is also potentially lethal and is manifest in the early stages by ataxia, irritability and irrational behaviour. It may progress to hallucinations, drowsiness and coma; papilloedema has been observed. Postmortem studies have shown that cerebral oedema may be accompanied by intracranial thrombosis and haemorrhage (Dickinson et al., 1983). Pulmonary and cerebral forms of malignant acute mountain sickness may both be present in the same patient.

Treatment of the malignant forms of mountain sickness includes relief of hypoxaemia and dehydration. Administration of oxygen and descent to a lower altitude are the first essentials. Diuretics may be used, and acetazolamide may improve the arterial P_{O_2} (see below).

Adaptation to altitude

It has long been known that the human body is capable of a remarkable degree of adaptation to altitude. Thus Everest has been climbed without oxygen (as predicted in the previous edition of this book) at a pressure which results in loss of consciousness in the untrained subject within less than 2 minutes (*Figure 14.2*).

Changes in alveolar gas tensions with altitude are shown for acclimatized mountaineers at rest in *Figure 14.1*. Alveolar P_{O_2} was unexpectedly well preserved at extreme altitude (West et al., 1983b) and above 8000 metres (26 000 ft) tended to remain at about 4.8 kPa (36 mmHg). This was slightly higher than the values observed just below this altitude by Pugh et al. (1964). In part this was due to the fact that the barometric pressure on the summit of Everest was higher than the predicted value: the P_{O_2} of the inspired gas was 5.7 kPa (43 mmHg), shown by a cross in *Figure 14.1*, instead of the expected 5.2 kPa (39 mmHg). Secondly, extreme hyperventilation reduced the alveolar P_{CO_2} to about 1 kPa (7.5 mmHg). (The apparent discrepancy in the values is explained by the high respiratory quotient (1.49) in the gas sample collected on the summit, which cannot be satisfactorily explained.) A brisk hypoxic ventilatory response is an essential attribute for the high altitude climber.

Limits of adaptation

Temporary residence by lowlanders at very high altitudes results in a characteristic pattern of deterioration to which anorexia, sleeping difficulties and polycythaemia all contribute. The Himalayan Scientific and Mountaineering Expedition of 1960/61 (Pugh et al., 1964) set up temporary residence in the 'Silver Hut' at 5800 metres (19 000 ft), the same altitude as the highest Andean mine. Several members of the expedition completed 3 months' residence. During forays to higher altitudes there were two cases of pneumonia, one probable mild cerebral thrombosis and a pulmonary thrombosis with infarction (Pugh, 1962). Climbing to very high altitudes requires a careful balance between acclimatization and deterioration. The ascent of Everest without oxygen appears to be close to the limit of human achievement.

For those who live permanently at great altitude, the upper limit for sustained work seems to be about 5800 metres (19000 ft) in a silver mine in the Andes. The upper limit for elective permanent habitation is lower and the Andean miners declined to live in accommodation built for them near the silver mine, preferring to live at 5330 metres (17500 ft) and climb every day to their work. Those who live at very high altitude acquire a markedly attenuated ventilatory response to hypoxia. Nevertheless, their capacity for work is usually superior to that of acclimatized lowlanders.

A small minority of those who dwell permanently at very high altitude in certain locations develop a characteristic condition known as Monge's syndrome or chronic mountain sickness. The condition is well recognized in miners living above 4000 metres in the Andes. It is characterized by an exceptionally poor ventilatory response to hypoxia resulting in low arterial Po_2 and high Pco_2. There is cyanosis, high haematocrit, finger clubbing, pulmonary hypertension, dyspnoea and lethargy.

Mechanisms of adaptation

Ventilatory control. It has been explained above that the hypoxic drive to ventilation on acute exposure to altitude is to a large extent offset by the resultant respiratory alkalosis. In the course of 2 or 3 days' residence at altitude, ventilation increases as a result of increased drive from the central chemoreceptors. This is caused by a restoration of CSF pH towards its normal value of 7.32, and the resultant favourable change in alveolar Po_2 is shown in *Figure 14.3*.

Michel and Milledge (1963) suggested that the restoration of CSF pH, by means of bicarbonate transport, might explain the acclimatization of ventilation to altitude, a hypothesis which they based on observations of Merwarth and Sieker (1961). Later in 1963, Severinghaus and his colleagues measured their own CSF pH during acclimatization to altitude and showed that this was indeed the case. The improvement in Po_2 is substantial (*Figures 14.2* and *14.3*) and a similar effect may be achieved by the administration of acetazolamide during acute exposure to altitude. This is a carbonic anhydrase inhibitor and interferes with the transport of carbon dioxide out of cells. It therefore causes an intracellular acidosis which includes the cells of the medullary chemoreceptors and so drives respiration (Cotev,

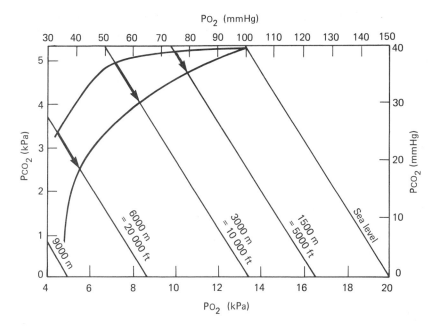

*Figure 14.3 Alveolar gas tension changes during early acclimatization to altitude. Straight lines represent-
ing the respiratory exchange ratio (R) have been drawn for various altitudes through the inspired gas point
at the bottom of the graph. At equilibrium, alveolar Po_2 and Pco_2 values must lie on the corresponding R
line. (Data from Rahn and Otis, 1949, and West et al., 1983b)*

Lee and Severinghaus, 1968; Milledge, 1985a). The mechanism of the shift in CSF
bicarbonate is considered on page 87.

The initial ventilatory response to hypoxia is also opposed by the resultant
alkalaemia of the arterial blood. This is counteracted over the course of a few days
by renal excretion of bicarbonate, resulting in a metabolic acidosis which increases
respiratory drive (see *Figure 4.8*). This was formerly thought to be the main factor
in the ventilatory adaptation to altitude but it now appears to be of secondary
importance to the change in CSF pH.

Polycythaemia. It has long been known that chronic residence at altitude increased
the haemoglobin concentration of the blood. During residence in the Silver Hut at
5800 metres (19000 ft), alveolar Po_2 stabilized at about 6 kPa (45 mmHg) corresponding to about 80% saturation of haemoglobin (Pugh, 1962). Haemoglobin
concentration increased from a mean sea level value of 14.1 to 19.6 g/dl after 4
weeks. Thus the oxygen content of the arterial blood would actually have increased
by about 15 per cent. Haematocrit values reached 55.8% (sea level controls were
43.2%) and blood viscosity would inevitably have been increased. Andean miners
living at 5300 metres (17500 ft) have even higher haemoglobin concentrations (22.9
g/dl).

The renin–angiotensin–aldosterone system. Frayser et al. (1975) observed that the
greatly enhanced plasma renin activity seen at altitude is not accompanied by a
corresponding increase in plasma aldosterone concentration (see *Figure 11.2*).

Milledge (see review—1984) found that at altitude the aldosterone response to an exercise-induced rise in renin activity was also blunted in comparison with the response at sea level. This has been confirmed by Shigeoka, Colice and Ramirez (1985). It was originally thought that this might be due to a reduction in the activity of angiotensin-converting enzyme brought about by hypoxia. However, it has now become clear that hypoxia has no effect on this enzyme and the mechanism for the reduced aldosterone response and the low resting levels found at altitude is not clear.

The major mechanisms of acclimatization have their maximal effect within 6 weeks.

Exercise at high altitude

The summit of Everest was attained without the use of oxygen in 1978 by Messner and Habeler, and by many other climbers since that date. Detailed physiological observations have been made at various altitudes up to and including the summit (West et al., 1983a, b). These complement the extensive observations made between 4650 and 7440 metres (15 300 and 24 400 ft) by Pugh et al. (1964). Of necessity these observations are largely confined to very fit and acclimatized mountaineers and Sherpas. The difficulties of making the observations increased with altitude, and the range and number of the measurements decreases sharply above 7500 metres (24 600 ft). West et al. (1983a) simulated very high altitudes by reduction of inspired oxygen concentration at an altitude of 6300 metres (20 700 ft), using acclimatized subjects.

Apart from the beauty of the surroundings, there appears to be only one factor which assists in the performance of work at high altitude. The density of air is reduced in proportion to the barometric pressure at altitude and therefore the work of breathing at a particular minute volume of respiration is decreased. Maximum breathing capacity is increased by about 40 per cent at an altitude of 8200 metres (27 000 ft) (Miles, 1957) and minute volumes (measured at body temperature and pressure, saturated) during maximal exercise at 4650–6400 metres (15 300–21 000 ft) were well above those at sea level (Pugh et al., 1964; West et al., 1983a).

During exercise at altitude, alveolar P_{CO_2} falls and P_{O_2} rises (*Figure 14.4*). However, oxygenation of the pulmonary end-capillary blood is diffusion-limited during exercise at high altitude (West et al., 1962) and the alveolar/arterial P_{O_2} difference increases more than the alveolar P_{O_2} rises (Pugh et al., 1964). There is a resultant decrease in arterial P_{O_2}, the lowest measured value being 2.7 kPa (20 mmHg) in the case of John West himself (*Figure 14.4*). Similar degrees of hypoxaemia occur at higher altitudes where the maximal work output is lower (West et al., 1983a). Arterial haemoglobin saturation values in the range 50–60% were observed during maximal exercise at simulated altitudes above 6300 metres (20 700 ft). This more than offset the rise of haemoglobin concentration, which was about 20 g/dl. However, the limiting factor would appear not to be the arterial oxygen content but the tension at which it was delivered and the respiratory minute volume that was required.

The oxygen cost of different work rates appears to be the same at altitude as at sea level (Pugh et al., 1964; West et al., 1983). Similarly, cardiac output bears the

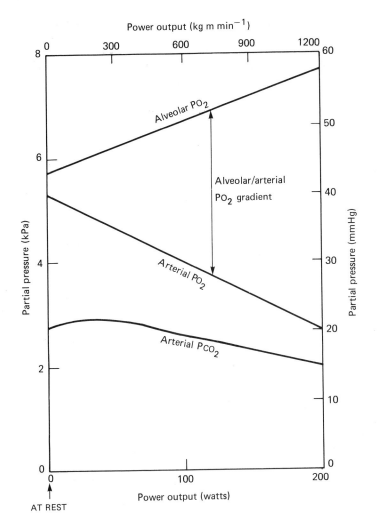

Figure 14.4 *PO₂ and PCO₂ changes during exercise in a single subject (John West) at 5800 metres (19 000 feet). (Data from Pugh et al. (1964).*

same relationship to work rate and oxygen uptake at altitude as at sea level (Pugh, 1964). Capacity for work is progressively reduced with increasing altitude (*Figure 14.5*). Although ergometry studies have not been carried out on the summit of Everest, it is likely that the maximal oxygen uptake for an acclimatized and exceptionally fit mountaineer at that altitude would be about 1 l/min corresponding

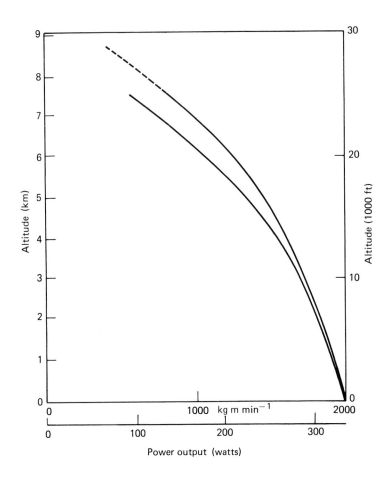

Figure 14.5 Maximal power output by acclimatized mountaineers at different altitudes.

to a work rate of the order of about 400 kg m min^{-1}, although this could be maintained for only about 3 minutes. This level of power (about 65 watts) corresponds approximately to walking on the level at a normal pace but, at that altitude, it required a minute volume in excess of 150 l/min. This clearly explains the immense achievement of climbing to the summit of Everest without oxygen.

Chapter 15

Respiratory aspects of high pressure and diving

Man has sojourned temporarily in high pressure environments since the introduction of the diving bell. The origin of this development is lost in antiquity but Alexander the Great was said to have been lowered to the sea bed in a diving bell in 320 BC.

The environment of the diver is often, but not invariably, aqueous. Saturation divers spend most of their time in a gaseous environment in chambers which are held at a pressure close to that of the depth of water at which they will be working. Tunnel and caisson workers may also be at high pressure in a gaseous environment. Workers in both environments share the physiological problems associated with increased pressures and partial pressures of respired gases. However, those in an aqueous environment also have the additional effect of different gravitational forces applied to their trunks, which influence the mechanics of breathing and other systems of the body. Further problems arise as a result of any change in the composition of the inspired gas, which is standard practice at pressures of more than about 6 atmospheres.

The aim of this chapter is to review the salient features of those aspects of high pressure which concern the respiratory system, together with an outline of the effects of inhalation of the various inspired gas mixtures which are used at high pressure. In this field, as in others, we cannot escape from the multiplicity of units, and some of these are set out in *Table 15.1*. Note particularly that 'atmosphere gauge' is relative to ambient pressure. Thus 2 atmospheres absolute (ATA) equals 1 atmosphere gauge relative to sea level. Throughout this chapter atmospheres of pressure mean absolute and not gauge.

Exchange of oxygen and carbon dioxide

Oxygen consumption

The relationship between power output and oxygen consumption at high pressure is not significantly different from the relationship for comparable work at normal pressure: neither does immersion appear to have any effect (Lundgren, 1984). The relationship between power output and oxygen consumption shown in *Figure 12.1* applies equally well to work at pressures up to at least 66 ATA (Salzano et al., 1984). Oxygen consumption is expressed under standard conditions of temperature and pressure, dry (STPD—see page 497) and therefore represents an absolute quantity of oxygen. However, this volume, when expressed at the diver's environ-

Table 15.1 Pressures and Po$_2$ values at various depths of sea water

Depth of sea water		Pressure (absolute)		Po$_2$ (breathing air)				Percentage oxygen to give sea level inspired Po$_2$
				inspired		alveolar		
metres	feet	atm.	kPa	kPa	mmHg	kPa	mmHg	
0	0	1	101	19.9	149	13.9	104	20.9
10	32.8	2	203	41.2	309	35.2	264	10.1
20	65.6	3	304	62.3	467	56.3	422	6.69
50	164	6	608	126	945	120	900	3.31
		Usual limit for breathing air						
100	328	11	1 110					1.80
200	656	21	2 130					0.94
		Usual limit for saturation dives						
		Threshold for high pressure nervous syndrome						
500	1 640	51	5 170					0.39
1000	3 280	101	10 200					0.20
		Depth reached by sperm whale						
2000	6 560	201	20 400					0.098
2500	8 200	251	25 400					0.078
		Pressure reached by non-aquatic mammals with pharmacological amelioration of the high pressure nervous syndrome						

Notes
1 metre = 3.28 feet; 10 metres sea water = 1 atmosphere (gauge); 1 atmosphere = 101.3 kPa = 760 mmHg; air is 20.94% oxygen.
Alveolar Po$_2$ is assumed 6 kPa (45 mmHg) less than inspired Po$_2$.
Saturated water vapour pressure at body temperature assumed to be 6.3 kPa (47 mmHg).
All values are rounded to three significant figures.

mental pressure, is inversely related to the pressure. Thus, an oxygen consumption of 1 l/min (STPD) at a pressure of 10 atmospheres would be only 100 ml/min when expressed at the pressure to which the diver was exposed.

Oxygen consumption may reach very high values during free swimming and are of the order of 2–3 l/min (STPD) for a swimming speed of only 2 km/h (Lanphier and Camporesi, 1982). Maximal oxygen consumptions in the range 2.4–3.3 l/min have been attained at pressures of 66 atmospheres (Salzano et al. 1984).

Ventilatory requirement

The ventilatory requirement for a given oxygen consumption is also not greatly different at increased pressure provided that the oxygen consumption is expressed at STPD and minute volume is expressed at body temperature, saturated with water vapour, and at the pressure to which the diver is exposed. It is, in fact, usual to express pulmonary ventilation at body temperature and pressure saturated with water vapour (BTPS—see page 497). Considerable confusion is possible as a result of the different methods of expressing gas volumes. The difference is trivial at sea level but becomes very important at high pressures. As an example, specimen calculations are set out in *Table 15.2* comparing certain respiratory volumes and gas tensions at sea level and at 10 atmospheres. Oxygen consumptions, minute volume and dead space/tidal volume ratios are taken from the data of Salzano et al. (1984). Conversions of gas volumes for different pressures are described in Appendix B. It will be seen that volumes at STPD are the same at both pressures while volumes at BTPS are greatly different. Although it clarifies the problem to consider conditions at 10 atmospheres, air would not nowadays be considered an appropriate inspired gas at this pressure, for reasons which are discussed below.

Table 15.2 Respiratory variables at sea level and pressure

		Sea level		10 ATA	
		Rest	Exercise 220 watts	Rest	Exercise 220 watts
Oxygen consumption (ml/min)	STPD	250	3000	250	3000
	BTPS	303	3630	28.5	342
Minute volume (l/min)	BTPS	7	70	7	70
Inspired oxygen concentration (%)		20.9	20.9	20.9	20.9
Inspired P_{O_2}	kPa	19.9	19.9	210	210
	mmHg	149	149	1575	1575
Alveolar oxygen concentration (%)		14.3	14.4	20.2	20.1
Alveolar P_{O_2}	kPa	13.6	13.7	203	202
	mmHg	102	103	1523	1515
Carbon dioxide output (ml/min)	STPD	200	2400	200	2400
	BTPS	242	2904	22.8	274
Alveolar ventilation (l/min)	BTPS	4.55	56.0	4.06	42.0
Alveolar carbon dioxide concentration (%)		5.3	5.2	0.56	0.65
Alveolar P_{CO_2}	kPa	5.1	4.9	5.6	6.5
	mmHg	38	37	42	49

Assumptions are listed in the text.
This Table is for illustrative purposes only and is not a recommendation to expose divers to 10 atmospheres pressure of air.

Effect of pressure on alveolar P_{CO_2} and P_{O_2}

Pressure has quite complicated effects on P_{CO_2} and P_{O_2}. The carbon dioxide output for a given level of work at 10 atmospheres is similar to the value at sea level when expressed as STPD but is only a little more than one-tenth of this value when expressed at BTPS. However, the pulmonary ventilation is virtually the same at both pressures when correctly expressed at BTPS. Therefore it follows that the fractional concentration of carbon dioxide in the expired (and alveolar) air at 10 atmospheres, derived from the equation on page 221 will be only about one-tenth of the sea level value. The example in *Table 15.2* shows an alveolar fractional concentration of CO_2, at rest, of 5.3% at sea level and 0.56% at 10 atmospheres. However, when these values are converted to partial pressures, the P_{CO_2} at 10 atmospheres is within the normal sea level range (5.6 kPa or 42.3 mmHg). Thus, as a rough approximation, F_{CO_2} decreases inversely to the environmental pressure, but the P_{CO_2} remains at its sea level value.

Effects on the Po_2 are slightly more complicated. The difference between the inspired and alveolar oxygen *concentration* equals the ratio of oxygen uptake to alveolar ventilation (see the universal alveolar air equation, page 110). This fraction behaves like the alveolar concentration of carbon dioxide and decreases inversely with the environmental pressure. However, the difference between the inspired and alveolar oxygen *tension* will remain close to the sea level value, again as does the alveolar Pco_2 (*Figure 15.1*). In the example shown in *Table 15.2*, at rest, the difference between inspired and alveolar oxygen concentration is 6.6% at sea level but only 0.7% at 10 atmospheres. However, the tension differences are similar at both pressures.

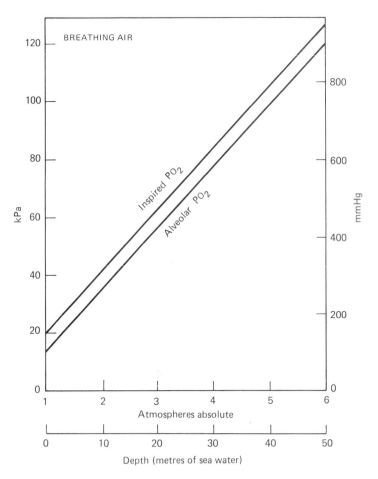

Figure 15.1 Inspired and alveolar Po_2 values as a function of increasing pressure, while breathing air at rest.

As pressure increases, so the inspired Po_2 increases, the proportional change being slightly greater than that of the total pressure, because the saturated vapour pressure of water is unchanged (see *Table 15.1*). If the inspired/alveolar tension difference is unchanged (as explained above), then the alveolar Po_2 will increase by the same absolute amount as the inspired P_{O_2}, and not in proportion to the change in total pressure (*Figure 15.1*). In the example in *Table 15.2*, at 10 atmospheres pressures while breathing air, the inspired P_{O_2} at rest is increased from a sea level value of 19.9 kPa (149 mmHg) to 210 kPa (1579 mmHg), which is slightly more than a tenfold increase. Meanwhile the corresponding change in the alveolar P_{O_2} is from 13.6 kPa (102 mmHg) to 203 kPa (1523 mmHg), which is an increase by a factor of almost 15. This may not be intuitively obvious.

The above considerations only take into account the direct effect of pressure on gas tensions. There are other and more subtle effects on respiratory mechanics and gas exchange which must now be considered.

Effect on mechanics of breathing

Two main factors must be considered. Firstly, there is the increased density of gases at pressure. This, of course, may be affected by changing the composition of the inspired gas. Helium, which is used at depths greater than 50 metres, has only one-seventh of the density of air and so is easier to breathe. The second factor is the pressure of water on the body, which alters the gravitational effects to which the respiratory system is normally exposed.

Gas density is increased in direct proportion to pressure. Thus air at 10 atmospheres has ten times the density of air at sea level. It is very well established that maximal breathing capacity (MBC) is decreased as pressure is increased. For example, breathing air, a subject with an MBC of 200 l/min at sea level can attain only about 100 l/min at 5 atmospheres and 50 l/min at 15 atmospheres (Lanphier and Camporesi, 1982). In fact, it is usual to breathe a helium/oxygen mixture at pressures in excess of about 6 atmospheres because of nitrogen narcosis (see below). Furthermore, lower inspired oxygen concentrations are both permissible and indeed desirable as the pressure increases (see *Table 15.1*). Therefore, at 15 atmospheres it would be reasonable to breathe a mixture of 98% helium and 2% oxygen. This would more than double the MBC which the diver could attain while breathing air at that pressure (Lanphier and Camporesi, 1982).

The effect of immersion is additional to any change in the density of the respired gases. In open-tube snorkel breathing, the alveolar gas is close to normal atmospheric pressure but the trunk is exposed to a pressure depending on the depth of the subject which is limited by the length of the snorkel tube. This is equivalent to a standing subatmospheric pressure applied to the mouth and it is difficult to inhale against a 'negative' pressure loading of more than about 5 kPa (50 cmH$_2$O). This corresponds to a mean depth of immersion of only 50 cm. It is virtually impossible to use a snorkel tube at a depth of 1 metre. The normal length of a snorkel tube assures that the swimmer is barely more than awash and so the problem does not normally arise.

'Negative' pressure loading is avoided by supplying gas at a pressure which is close to the hydrostatic pressure surrounding the diver. This is achieved by providing an excess flow of gas with a pressure relief valve controlled by the surrounding water pressure. Such an arrangement was used for the traditional helmeted diver supplied by an air pump on the surface. Free-swimming divers carrying their own compressed gas supply rely on inspiratory demand valves which are also balanced by the surrounding water pressure.

These arrangements supply gas which is close to the hydrostatic pressure surrounding the trunk. However, minor differences result from the various postures which the diver may assume. Thus, if he is 'head-up', the pressure surrounding the trunk is higher than the airway pressure by a mean value of about 3 kPa (30 cmH$_2$O). If he is 'head-down', airway pressure is greater than the pressure to which the trunk is exposed. The 'head-up' position thus corresponds to 'negative pressure' breathing and the 'head-down' position to positive pressure breathing (Lundgren, 1984).

Negative pressure breathing causes a reduction of functional residual capacity (FRC) of about 20–30 per cent in the head-up diver. Effects of a decrease in FRC are considered elsewhere (page 360) but include increased airway resistance, reduced compliance and an increased alveolar/arterial PO_2 difference. In general, breathing is easier head-up than head-down and this would accord with the changes in FRC (Lanphier and Camporesi, 1982).

Apart from these considerations, immersion has relatively little effect on respiratory function and the additional work of moving extracorporeal water does not add appreciably to the work of breathing. Other effects of immersion include a relative increase in central blood volume, a tendency to gastric/oesophageal regurgitation and diuresis.

Effect on efficiency of gas exchange

The efficiency of gas exchange can be assessed only by measurement of arterial blood gas tensions and there are formidable technical difficulties at high pressures. However, Salzano and his colleagues (1984) have obtained measurements of the physiological dead space at pressures of 47 and 66 atmospheres. The dead space/tidal volume (VD/VT) ratio at rest averaged 42 per cent compared with 35 per cent at sea level. However, the decrease observed with exercise at sea level was much less marked at depth, values remaining close to 40 per cent, compared with 20 per cent at sea level. Therefore, for the same minute volume, alveolar ventilation would be less at depth in comparison with sea level. This factor has been taken into account in the preparation of *Table 15.2*, although data at 10 atmospheres are not currently available.

The best measure of the efficiency of oxygenation of the arterial blood is the alveolar/arterial PO_2 gradient, and this has not been rigorously quantified at high pressures. Nevertheless, arterial PO_2 values reported by Salzano et al. (1984) are not greatly different at 1, 47 and 66 atmospheres with similar inspired oxygen tensions.

Arterial blood gas tensions

Since it is customary to supply deep divers with an inspired oxygen tension of at least 0.5 atmosphere, arterial hypoxaemia is unlikely to occur either from hypoventilation or from maldistribution of pulmonary ventilation and perfusion. In the study of Salzano and his colleagues (1984), when inspired oxygen tensions were in the range 47–50 kPa (353–375 mmHg) arterial PO_2 values were in the range 33–41 kPa (248–308 mmHg) at pressures of 47 and 66 atmospheres, both at rest and at work.

The position as regards arterial PCO_2 is less satisfactory. Salzano et al. (1984) found values within the normal range at pressures of 47 and 66 atmospheres when the subjects were at rest and performing exercise up to about 200 watts in one of his subjects. However, the remaining four subjects, although normocapnic at rest, became hypercapnic at exercise levels ranging from 100 to 200 watts. Maximal values of arterial P_{CO_2} at exercise and pressure were in the range 6.2–8.3 kPa (46.7–62.2 mmHg). This cannot be regarded as satisfactory since 9 kPa is approaching the level at which there may be some clouding of consciousness, and that is potentially dangerous at depth. It seems likely that the increased dead space during exercise at pressure compared with the value at sea level plays a significant role in causing hypercapnia by reducing the alveolar ventilation.

In addition to hypercapnia, some of Salzano's subjects showed a metabolic acidosis in association with an increased arterial lactate concentration. Lactate levels were consistently higher at pressure than at sea level, not only at all rates of exercise but also at rest.

Effects attributable to the composition of the inspired gas

Air

Up to about 50 years ago, helmeted divers worked up to pressures of about 10 atmospheres breathing air. Nowadays with the increased use of helium, it is unusual to breathe air at pressures of more than 6 atmospheres (depths of 50 metres of sea water). The effects of increased partial pressures of oxygen and nitrogen will be considered separately.

Oxygen. When breathing air at a pressure of 6 atmospheres, the inspired P_{O_2} will be about 126 kPa (945 mmHg) and the alveolar P_{O_2} about 120 kPa (900 mmHg). This is below the threshold for oxygen convulsions (see below), but probably above the threshold for pulmonary oxygen toxicity if exposure is continued for more than a few hours (see Chapter 29).

Nitrogen. It is actually nitrogen which limits the depth at which air can be breathed. There are three separate effects to be considered.

Nitrogen is an anaesthetic and, in accord with its lipid solubility, can cause full surgical anaesthesia at a partial pressure of about 30 atmospheres. The narcotic effect of nitrogen is first detectable when breathing air at about 4 ATA and there is usually serious impairment of performance at 10 atmospheres (Bennett, 1982a). This effect is known as nitrogen narcosis or 'the rapture of the deep'. It is believed that there is some cross-tolerance with alcohol and it has been suggested that divers accustomed to regular alcohol intake are capable of better performance under these conditions. It is a general rule that nitrogen narcosis precludes the use of air at depths greater than 100 metres of sea water (11 ATA pressure) and, in fact, air is not used today at pressures greater than 6 atmospheres. Helium is the preferred substitute at higher pressures and has no detectable narcotic properties up to at least 100 atmospheres.

The second problem attributable to nitrogen is increased solution of the gas in body tissues at high pressures. This creates no problem during compression but, if decompression is too rapid, gas bubbles may be evolved causing a range of disabilities variously known as 'bends', 'chokes' or caisson disease (Vann, 1982). Detailed and elaborate tables have been prepared to indicate the safe rate of decompression depending on the pressure and time of exposure. Other inert gases, particularly helium, are less soluble in body tissues and this is the second reason for the use of helium at high pressures.

The third problem with nitrogen at high pressures is its density, which causes greatly increased hindrance to breathing at high pressure (see above). Helium has only one-seventh of the density of nitrogen and this is the third reason for its choice.

Helium/oxygen mixtures (Heliox)

For the three reasons outlined in the previous section, helium is the preferred diluent inert gas at pressures above about 6 atmospheres. The concentration of oxygen required to give the same inspired gas P_{O_2} as at sea level is shown in *Table 15.1*. In fact, it is usual practice to provide an inspired P_{O_2} of about 0.5 atmosphere (50 kPa or 375 mmHg) to give a safety margin in the event of error in gas mixing and to provide protection against hypoventilation or defective gas exchange. It seems likely that this level of P_{O_2} is below the threshold for pulmonary oxygen toxicity, even during prolonged saturation dives.

Even with an inspired P_{O_2} of 0.5 atmosphere, the concentration of oxygen in the gas mixture is very low at high pressures (e.g. 2.5% oxygen at 20 atmospheres pressure). Clearly such a mixture would be lethal if breathed at a total pressure of 1 atmosphere. Therefore the inspired oxygen concentration must be very carefully monitored as it is changed during compression and decompression.

A special problem of helium is its very high thermal conductivity, which tends to cause hypothermia unless the diver's environment is heated. It is usual for chambers to be maintained at temperatures as high as 30–32°C during saturation dives on helium/oxygen mixtures. An additional problem arises from its low density, which causes a considerable increase in the pitch of the voice, sometimes resulting in difficulty in communication.

Helium/oxygen/nitrogen mixtures (Trimix)

The pressure which can be attained while breathing helium/oxygen mixtures is currently limited by the high pressure nervous syndrome (Halsey, 1982). This is a hyperexcitable state of the central nervous system which appears to be due to hydrostatic pressure *per se* and not to any changes in gas tensions. It becomes a serious problem for divers at pressures in excess of about 50 atmospheres, but is first apparent at about 20 atmospheres.

Various treatments can mitigate this effect and so increase the depth at which a diver can safely operate. At the time of writing, the most practicable is the use of partial nitrogen narcosis. Not only does the nitrogen mitigate the high pressure nervous syndrome but also the high pressure reverses the narcosis which would be caused by the nitrogen (Halsey, Wardley-Smith and Green, 1978). Various concentrations of nitrogen have been used in the range 4–10% (Bennett, 1982b).

Oxygen

The use of oxygen as inspired gas permits the use of closed circuit apparatus, which does not leave a trail of bubbles to reveal the presence of a clandestine diver. While this requirement may be of overwhelming importance in warfare, sabotage and espionage, it carries the grave hazard of oxygen convulsions (page 491). The lowest threshold for convulsions in man is a P_{O_2} of 2 ATA and this limits diving on oxygen to a depth of 10 metres (Donald, 1947).

Special circumstances of exposure to pressure

Breath holding dives

The earliest method of diving is by breath holding and this is still used for pearl and sponge diving. After breathing air, breath holding time is normally limited to 60–75 seconds, and the changes in alveolar gas tensions are shown in *Figure 4.9*. Astonishingly, the depth record is 102 metres (Bachrach, 1982). Duration of breath hold can be increased by previous hyperventilation but this carries the danger of syncope from hypoxia before the breaking point is reached. Duration can be more safely increased by preliminary oxygen breathing, and a time of 14 minutes has been attained (page 97).

During a breath hold dive, the lung volume is decreased as the pressure rises, according to Boyle's law. Thus, starting with a maximal inspiration and a total lung capacity of 6 litres, the lung volume would be reduced to 1 litre at a total pressure of 6 ATA (50 metres of sea water). This would result in loss of buoyancy of about 5 kg. The lung volume would re-expand on ascent and the buoyancy would be regained. Reduction of lung volume below residual volume is unpleasant and interferes with oxygenation of the arterial blood.

The diving mammals rely on breath holding for dives and have adaptations which permit remarkably long times under water and the attainment of great depths. Sperm whales, for example, can attain depths of 1000 metres (Halsey, 1982). For shallower dives they are able to remain underwater for as long as an hour. Such feats depend on a variety of biochemical and physiological adaptations discussed by Hempleman and Lockwood (1982). During a dive the circulation is directed almost exclusively through heart and brain, which rely on the meagre oxygen stores in the lungs and the blood (see *Table 10.4*). Intense vasoconstriction severely limits flow through other organs and the voluntary muscles. Muscle contraction is based on anaerobic metabolism and there is extreme lactacidosis which is confined to the muscle beds and so is not sensed by the peripheral chemoreceptors. After surfacing, the vasoconstriction is relaxed and there is generalized acidaemia. While on the surface, the excess lactate is metabolized and the arterial $P\text{CO}_2$ returns to normal. This process takes only a few minutes and the animal is then ready for another dive.

The diving reflex in man. The diving reflex is less well developed in man than in the diving mammals but it may nevertheless be detected. The primary stimulus is immersion of the face in water, the most effective temperature being 10–20°C (Gooden, 1982). However, in addition, breath holding seems to be an essential adjunct. It is possible to demonstrate vasoconstriction in skin, muscle, kidney and intestines but the main effect in man is bradycardia. The latter effect has been proposed for treatment of paroxysmal tachycardia.

Limited duration dives

Most dives are of relatively brief duration and involve a rapid descent to operating depth, a period spent at depth, followed by an ascent, the rate of which is governed by the requirement to avoid release of inert gas dissolved in the tissues. The profile and the duration of the ascent are governed by the depth attained, the time spent at depth and the nature of the diluent inert gas.

The diving bell. The simplest and oldest technique was the diving bell. Air was trapped on the surface but the internal water level rose as the air was compressed at depth. Useful time at depth was generally no more than 20–30 minutes. Crude though this technology appears, it was used to recover most of the guns from the Wasa in Stockholm harbour in 1663 and 1664 from a depth of 34 metres. It seems unlikely that the salvage operators left the bell. At a later date, additional air was introduced into the bell under pressure from the surface and divers could leave the bell.

The helmeted diver. From about 1820 until recent times, the standard method of diving down to 100 metres has been by a helmeted diver supplied with air pumped from the surface into the helmet and escaping from a relief valve controlled by the water pressure. This gave much greater mobility than the old diving bell and permitted the execution of complex tasks. The system was used with helium/oxygen mixtures in 1939 for the salvage of the USS *Squalus* from a depth of 74 metres.

SCUBA diving. Since about 1930 there has been a progressive move towards free-swimming divers carrying their own gas supply (SCUBA—self-contained under-water breathing apparatus). The system is based on a demand valve which is controlled by both the ambient pressure and the inspiration of the diver. Air-breathing SCUBA dives are usually restricted to depths of 30 metres. Greater depths are possible but special precautions must then be taken to avoid 'bends'. SCUBA divers are far more mobile than helmeted divers and can also work in any body position. They also avoid the hazard of suit inflation, which was caused by a helmeted diver lowering his head below the rest of his body. This resulted in a rapid ascent to the surface and the danger of 'bends'.

Caisson and tunnel working

Since 1839, tunnel and bridge foundations have been constructed by pressurizing the work environment to exclude water. This does not normally require a pressure greater than 4 ATA and air is usually breathed. The work environment is maintained at pressure with staff entering and leaving by air locks. Shifts normally last 8 hours. Entry is rapid but exit requires adherence to the appropriate decompression schedule if the working pressure is in excess of 2 ATA. Workers can be rapidly transferred from the working pressure to atmosphere and then, within 5 minutes, transferred to a separate chamber where they are rapidly recompressed to the working pressure and then follow the decompression schedule (Walder, 1982). This process, known as decanting, has obvious logistic advantages. Apart from the danger of 'bends', working in compressed air carries the additional hazard of bone necrosis for which the aetiological factors are not yet clearly established (Walder, 1982).

Saturation dives

When prolonged and repeated work is required at great depths, it is more convenient to hold the divers in a dry chamber, kept on board a ship or oil rig, and held at a pressure close to the pressure of their intended working depth. Divers then transfer to a smaller chamber at the same pressure which is lowered to depth as and when required. The divers then leave the chamber for work without any major change in pressure. They then return to the chamber which can be raised to the surface where they wait, still at pressure, until they are next required. A normal tour of duty is about 3 weeks, the whole of which is spent at operating pressure, currently up to about 20 atmospheres breathing helium/oxygen mixtures.

During the long period at pressure, tissues are fully saturated with inert gas at the chamber pressure and prolonged decompression is then required which may last for several days.

Free submarine escape

It is possible to escape from a submarine by free ascent from depths down to about 100 metres. The submariner first enters an escape chamber which is then pressurized to equal the external water pressure. He then opens a hatch communicating with the exterior and leaves the chamber. His natural buoyancy is sufficient to take him to the surface but he may be helped with additional buoyancy or an apron which traps gas leaving the escape chamber. During the ascent, the gas in his lungs expands according to Boyle's law. It is therefore imperative that he keeps his glottis and mouth open, allowing gas to escape in a continuous stream. If gas is not allowed to escape, lung rupture is almost certain to occur. Buoyancy is not changed by the loss of gas during ascent. In an uneventful escape, the time spent at pressure is too short for there to be any danger of 'bends'. Thorough training is necessary and all submariners are trained in a vertical tank of 100 feet depth.

Avoidance of exposure of man to pressure

The maintenance of a diver at great depths is both very expensive and dangerous although his economic importance is great. The future may well lie either with remotely controlled non-manned devices, such as were used for the discovery of the *Titanic*, or with solutions which maintain man underwater at a pressure of 1 atmosphere, under so-called 'shirt sleeve conditions'. There are three possibilities for exploiting the last option. Firstly, there are armoured diving suits (manufactured under the names JIM or WASP) with an internal pressure of 1 atmosphere and capable of operating down to 700 metres of sea water. It is possible for a diver in a JIM to walk short distances and carry out very simple manipulations by means of pincers mounted on the arms. Secondly, there is the minisubmarine, capable of free movement but severely limited in the manipulations which can be carried out by the crew. Thirdly, a habitat can be constructed at the base of an oil rig which encompasses the working area and is maintained at 1 atmosphere and can be entered as the work schedule requires.

All of these solutions have their limitations. Divers in a JIM or WASP and minisubmariners can do little more than make an inspection or carry out the simplest tasks. The major limiting factor is the difficulty in providing torque as for fastening a nut. While the habitat is an attractive option for pipeline tie-ins and work on the well head, it is clearly useless for structural work on underwater parts of the rig itself or for attention to a pipeline at some distance from the rig. The future position is by no means clear at the time of writing and it is likely that, in the foreseeable future, different options will be employed for particular tasks.

Chapter 16

Drowning

The incidence of drowning differs greatly between different countries and is related to aquatic sports and particularly swimming pools in the home. At least in the USA, it has become a major cause of accidental death. It is particularly disturbing that most of the victims are below 20 years, many being unable to swim. Alcohol is a major aetiological factor, particularly in older victims (Mackie, 1979). In addition to death by drowning, there are substantial numbers who are resuscitated and others who recover spontaneously. 'Near-drowning' is defined as survival for 24 hours but death may occur a considerable time after the accident from pulmonary complications (secondary drowning). There may be residual brain damage but this is happily rare (Modell, Graves and Ketover, 1976).

The essential feature of drowning is asphyxia but the physiological responses depend on whether aspiration of water occurs and upon the substances which are dissolved or suspended in the water. The temperature of the water is crucially important and hypothermia following drowning in very cold water is a major factor influencing survival. In addition, much depends on the state of the victim at the time of the accident. Important factors include his state of health, his gastric contents, blood alcohol, exhaustion and lung volume at the time of immersion. Furthermore, drowning may be murder, accident or suicide, which may have an important bearing on the outcome.

Drowning without aspiration

The larynx is firmly closed during submersion and some victims will lose consciousness before water is aspirated. Modell (1984) cites the evidence for believing that this applies in approximately 10 per cent of cases. It is particularly likely to occur if there has been previous hyperventilation (Craig, 1961). The breaking point then occurs at lower values of both P_{O_2} and P_{CO_2} (see *Figure 4.9*). Because the alveolar/mixed venous gas tension gradient is much greater for oxygen than for carbon dioxide, arterial P_{O_2} falls initially at almost ten times the rate of rise of arterial P_{CO_2}. The subsequent rate of decrease is mainly dependent on the lung volume and the oxygen consumption. Oxygen stored in the alveolar gas after a maximal inspiration is unlikely to exceed 1 litre and an oxygen consumption of 2 l/min would not be unusual in a subject either swimming (page 322) or struggling. The 'diving reflex' is probably not a major factor in human drowning and is considered on page 329.

Loss of consciousness from decreased alveolar Po_2 usually occurs very suddenly and without warning. The critical level is probably in the range 4–6 kPa (30–45 mmHg).

If a swimmer who has lost consciousness from hypoxia can be removed from the water before aspiration occurs, the situation is no different from other forms of simple asphyxia and restoration of pulmonary ventilation (spontaneous or artificial) should result in a near-normal arterial Po_2. The outcome will then depend upon the intensity and duration of hypoxia. Apart from the extremes of full recovery and death, there may be any degree of residual cerebral damage, and details of assessment are described by Conn and Barker (1984).

Although comparatively little water is directly inhaled by human victims, a great deal is swallowed. Vomiting occurs in over 50 per cent of resuscitation procedures (Harries, 1981) and inhalation may occur as a result.

Aspiration of fresh water

Two-thirds of all fatal immersion incidents in the USA, Britain, Australia, Canada and New Zealand occur on inland waters (Harries, 1981). This is the basis for the belief that fresh water is inherently more dangerous. However, it seems likely that a major factor is the relative lack of rescue services in inland locations. This contrasts with the very high success rate of the rescue services on beaches used for surfing (Simcock, 1986).

Most victims will eventually aspirate water either before or after the loss of consciousness, although, relatively, the quantity of water is usually much less than in experimental studies of anaesthetized laboratory animals. Aspiration of fresh water results in a temporary reflex bronchospasm although this is not the most important pulmonary factor. There is, in addition, a loss of compliance due to effects on the pulmonary surfactant (Giammona and Modell, 1967).

In fresh water drowning, almost none of the water which enters the lungs can be aspirated because it rapidly enters the circulation (Modell and Moya, 1966). Nevertheless, there is always a significant shunt which responds favourably to positive end-expiratory pressure (PEEP) or continuous positive airway pressure (CPAP). This may be compared with the effect of these measures in pulmonary oedema. Modell (1984) draws attention to the possibility that neurogenic pulmonary oedema due to cerebral hypoxia may coexist with alveolar flooding due to aspirated water. The distinction would clearly be difficult. The pulmonary changes appear to be reversible, with good prospects of return to normal pulmonary function in those who survive near-drowning (Butt et al., 1970).

Absorption of fresh water from the lungs results in haemodilution. This becomes significant when the aspirated water approaches 800 ml for a 70 kg man (Modell and Moya, 1966). However, redistribution rapidly corrects the blood volume and there may even be hypovolaemia if pulmonary oedema supervenes. Haemodilution can theoretically result in haemolysis but Modell (1984) gives the opinion from his extensive experience that dangerous changes in plasma electrolytes and free haemoglobin are very unusual and he suggests that the importance of these changes has been overrated. Nevertheless, profound hyponatraemia (less than 100 mmol/l) may occur in infants drowned in fresh water.

Sea water drowning

Sea water, like fresh water, causes reflex bronchospasm after aspiration. However, there are major differences on other aspects of lung function which are attributable to the tonicity of the water which enters the lungs. Sea water is hypertonic, having more than three times the osmolarity of blood. Consequently, sea water in the lungs is not initially absorbed and, on the contrary, draws fluid from the circulation into the alveoli. Thus, in laboratory animals that have aspirated sea water, it is possible to recover from the lungs 50 per cent more than the original volume which was aspirated (Modell et al., 1974). This clearly maintains the proportion of flooded alveoli and results in a persistent shunt and reduction in arterial P_{O_2}. However, surprisingly, sea water has less effect than fresh water on the surfactant which remains (Giammona and Modell, 1967). Haemoconcentration and hypernatraemia seldom occur to any significant extent in human victims.

Other material contaminating the lungs

It is not unusual for drowning persons to swallow large quantities of water and then to regurgitate or vomit. Material aspirated into the lungs may then be contaminated with gastric contents and the drowning syndrome complicated with features of the acid-aspiration sydrome.

Aspiration of solid foreign bodies is a frequent complication of near-drowning in shallow rivers and lakes.

Tests of drowning

There appears to be no conclusive test for aspiration of either fresh or sea water. Modell (1984) reviews and dismisses the use of tests based on differences in specific gravity and chloride content of plasma from the right and left chambers of the heart. He is also unimpressed by the value of demonstration of diatoms in the tissues and concludes that there is still no definitive test. He cites a remarkable case of a patient with severe pulmonary oedema who was thought to be a near-drowned victim but who, on careful enquiry, was found to have fractured his skull in a misjudged dive without having actually entered the water.

The role of hypothermia

Some degree of hypothermia is usual in near-drowned victims and body temperature is usually in the range 33–36°C (Pearn, 1985). In cold water, temperature may fall very rapidly under drowning conditions and rates of 1°C/min have been reported (Conn and Barker, 1984). There have been reports of survival of near-drowned children trapped for periods as long as 40 minutes beneath ice. It is clear that reduction in cerebral metabolism is protective (Conn, Edmonds and Barker, 1978) but, on the other hand, consciousness is lost at about 32°C and ventricular fibrillation may occur at temperatures below 28°C. Current practice is to rewarm the patient over a few hours and then to maintain normal temperature, except when hypothermia is indicated for treatment of brain damage.

Principles of treatment of near-drowning

There is a high measure of agreement on general principles in three recent reviews (Conn and Barker, 1984; Modell, 1984; Pearn, 1985).

Immediate treatment

At the scene of the drowning, it can be very difficult to determine whether there has been cardiac or even respiratory arrest. However, there are many records of apparently dead victims who have recovered without evidence of brain damage after long periods of total immersion. It is therefore essential that cardiopulmonary resuscitation be undertaken in all victims until fully assessed in hospital, no matter how hopeless the outlook may appear.

Early treatment of near-drowning is crucial and this requires efficient instruction in resuscitation for those who may be available in locations where drowning is likely to occur. The normal priorities of airway clearance, artificial ventilation and chest compression (cardiac massage) should be observed. Mouth-to-mouth ventilation is the method of choice but high inflation pressures are usually required when there has been flooding of the lungs. In sea water drowning it may be possible to drain water from the lungs by gravity but this is less important than the prompt institution of ventilation (Modell, 1984). Many authorities do not believe that it is practicable to drain water from the lungs. Care should be taken to avoid squeezing swallowed water out of the stomach, since this may be inhaled. Oxygen is clearly valuable if available and should be continued until hospital is reached. Most survivors will breathe spontaneously within 1–5 minutes after removal from the water. The decision to discontinue resuscitation should not be taken until assessment in hospital, particularly if the state of consciousness is confused by hypothermia.

Circulatory failure and loss of consciousness may occur when a patient is lifted from the water in a vertical position, as for example by a helicopter winch. This is probably due to the loss of water pressure resulting in relative redistribution of blood volume into the legs.

Hospital treatment

On arrival at the accident and emergency department of a hospital, patients should be triaged into the following categories:

1. Awake.
2. Blunted (but conscious).
3. Comatose.

There should be better than 90 per cent survival in the first two categories but they should be admitted for observation and followed up after discharge. Patients who are comatose will require admission to intensive care. Treatment follows the general principles for hypoxic cerebral damage and aspiration lung injury. Pulmonary shunting may be as high as 70 per cent of pulmonary blood flow and this may only slowly resolve. Late deterioration of pulmonary function may occur and is known as 'secondary drowning', which is a form of the adult respiratory distress syndrome (see Chapter 26). If spontaneous breathing does not result in satisfactory levels of arterial Po_2 and Pco_2, continuous positive airway pressure (CPAP) may be tried, but it is now more usual to institute artificial ventilation with or without positive end-expiratory pressure (PEEP) (Simcock, 1986). If severe, metabolic acidosis should be corrected, as should abnormal electrolyte levels. Steroids have been used in high dosage but there is no clear evidence for their efficacy (Modell, Graves and Ketover, 1976; Simcock, 1986).

Chapter 17

Smoking

Smoking and lung function

Smoking was introduced from the New World into Europe in the sixteenth century. Although first used for supposedly medicinal purposes, Sir Walter Raleigh made it an essential fashionable activity of every gentleman. Thereafter the practice steadily increased in popularity until the explosive growth of the habit following the First World War (1914–1918). Particularly in the Second World War (1939–1945), large numbers of women adopted the habit and, more recently, there seems to have been a relative increase in young smokers.

There have always been those opposed to smoking and King James I (1603–1625) described it as 'a custom loathsome to the eye, hateful to the nose, harmful to the brain and dangerous to the lungs'. However, firm evidence to support his last conclusion was delayed by some 350 years. Only relatively recently did it become clear that smokers had a higher mortality (Doll and Peto, 1976) and that the causes of the excess mortality included lung cancer (Doll and Hill, 1950), chronic bronchitis, emphysema and cor pulmonale (Anderson and Ferris, 1962).

Constituents of tobacco smoke

More than 2000 potentially noxious constituents have been identified in tobacco smoke, some in the gaseous phase and others in the particulate phase. The particulate phase is defined as the fraction eliminated by passing smoke through a Cambridge filter of pore size 0.1 μm. This is not to be confused with the 'filter tip' which allows passage of considerable quantities of particulate matter.

The quantities of the various compounds yielded by a burning cigarette are determined by the use of a smoking machine. This simulates a typical human smoking pattern and normally draws air through the cigarette in a series of 'puffs' of 35 ml, each lasting 2 seconds and repeated every minute until the cigarette is reduced to a length of 2 cm from the butt. Constituents are then expressed in units of milligrams per cigarette. Values so obtained exclude components of 'sidestream smoke' which escape from the smouldering cigarette between puffs. This is somewhat in excess of half of the total products of the burning cigarette.

There is great variation in the yields of the various constituents between different brands and different types of cigarettes. This is achieved by using leaves of different species of plants, varying the conditions of curing and cultivation and by the use of filter tips. Ventilated filters have a ring of small holes in the paper between the filter tip and the tobacco. These holes admit air during a puff and dilute all constituents of the smoke. By these various means, it is possible to have wide variations in the different constituents of smoke, which do not bear a fixed relationship to one another. Quantities of constituents retained by the smoker are influenced by the pattern of smoking (see below).

The gaseous phase

Yields of carbon monoxide generally vary from 15 to 25 mg (12–20 ml) (Borland et al., 1983) but levels as low as 1.8 mg have been achieved. The concentration issuing from the butt of the cigarette during a puff is in the range 1–5%, which is far into the toxic range. A better indication of the extent of carbon monoxide exposure is the percentage of carboxyhaemoglobin in blood. For non-smokers, the value is normally less than 1.5% but is influenced by exposure to traffic because automobile exhaust contains carbon monoxide. Typical values for smokers range from 2 to 12%. The value is influenced by the number of cigarettes smoked, the type of cigarette and the pattern of inhalation of smoke. Nevertheless, it remains the most reliable objective indication of smoke exposure and correlates well with most of the harmful effects of smoking (see below).

Tobacco smoke also contains a mixture of nitric oxide and trace concentrations of nitrogen dioxide, the former being slowly oxidized to the latter in the presence of oxygen. The toxicity of these compounds is well known. Nitrogen dioxide hydrates in alveolar lining fluid to form an equimolecular mixture of nitrous and nitric acid. Both ionize, liberating hydrogen ions. In addition, the nitrite ion converts haemoglobin to methaemoglobin. It is not clear whether these factors are harmful in the concentrations inhaled in tobacco smoking, but higher oxides of nitrogen may be lethal in concentrations in excess of 1000 p.p.m. (Greenbaum et al., 1967a). Industrial environmental contamination is limited in the UK to 25 p.p.m. of nitric oxide and 3 p.p.m. of nitrogen dioxide for long-term exposure.

Other constituents of the gaseous phase include hydrocyanic acid, cyanogen, aldehydes, ketones and volatile polycyclic aromatic hydrocarbons and nitrosamines which have been shown to be carcinogenic and mutagenic in animals.

The particulate phase

The material removed by a Cambridge filter is known as the 'total particulate matter', with aerosol particle size in the range 0.2–1 μm. The particulate phase comprises water, nicotine and 'tar'. Nicotine ranges from 0.05 to 2.5 mg per cigarette and 'tar' from 0.5 to 35 mg per cigarette. The means of both levels have declined progressively by about 50 per cent between 1954 and 1980 (Report of the US Surgeon General, 1981). Yields of the main constituents of cigarette smoke are currently classified in the UK as set out in *Table 17.1*.

Individual smoke exposure

Individual smoke exposure is a complex function of the quantity of cigarettes which are smoked and the pattern of inhalation.

Table 17.1 Classification of tar content of British cigarettes (Department of Health and Social Security, 1982) (yields in mg per cigarette)

	Tar	Nicotine	Carbon monoxide
Low tar	<4–10	<0.3–1	<3–14
Low to medium tar	11–16	0.6–1.6	10–19
Medium tar	17–22	1.1–1.9	10–19
Medium to high tar	24–26	1.3–2.6	14–19

The quantity of cigarettes smoked

Exposure is usually quantified in 'pack years'. This equals the product of the number of packs (20 cigarettes) smoked per day, multiplied by the number of years that that pattern was maintained. The totals for each period are then summated for the lifetime of the subject.

There is good evidence that the habituated smoker adjusts his smoking pattern to maintain a particular blood level of nicotine (Russell et al., 1975; Ashton, Stepney and Thompson, 1979). For example, after changing to a brand with a lower nicotine yield, it is common practice to modify the pattern of inhalation to maximize nicotine absorption.

The pattern of inhalation

There are very wide variations in patterns of smoking. Air is normally drawn through the cigarette in a series of 'puffs' with a volume of about 25–50 ml per puff. The puff may be simply drawn into the mouth and rapidly expelled without appreciable inhalation. However, the habituated smoker will either inhale the puff directly into the lungs or, more commonly, pass the puff from the mouth to the lungs by inhaling air either through the mouth or else through the nose while passing the smoke from the mouth into the pharynx by apposing the tongue against the palate and so obliterating the gas space in the mouth (see *Figure 1.1b*). The inspiration is often especially deep, to flush into the lung any smoke remaining in the dead space.

It will be clear that the quantity of nicotine, 'tar' and carbon monoxide obtainable from a single cigarette is highly variable and the number and type of cigarettes smoked are not the sole determinants of effective exposure. Furthermore, retention is different for different constituents, being about 60 per cent for carbon monoxide but as much as 90 per cent for nicotine.

Passive smoking

The non-smoker is exposed to all constituents of smoke when he is indoors in the presence of smokers (Report of the US Surgeon General, 1984). Exposure varies with many factors, including size and ventilation of the room, number of people smoking and absorption of smoke constituents on soft furnishings and clothing. Carbon monoxide concentrations of 20 p.p.m. have been reported, which is above the recommended environmental concentration (9 p.p.m. in the USA). It has been estimated that non-smokers are exposed to quantities of 'tar' ranging from zero to

14 mg/day (Rapace and Lowrey, 1982). 'Side-stream smoke' from a smouldering cigarette stub produces greater quantities of potentially noxious substances than 'main-stream smoke' produced when a cigarette burns in a stream of air drawn through it during a puff. On average, 'side-stream smoke' is generated during 58 seconds in each minute and this is not included in the measured yield of a cigarette. There is conflicting evidence as to whether passive smoking increases the incidence of smoking-related diseases.

Respiratory effects of smoking

Cigarette smoking has most extensive effects on respiratory function and is clearly implicated in the aetiology of a number of respiratory diseases, particularly emphysema, chronic bronchitis and bronchial carcinoma. The progress of emphysema is usually accelerated in smokers, who also have an increased susceptibility to respiratory infection.

Ventilatory capacity

The Report of the US Surgeon General (1984) reviews a large number of publications indicating that there is a greater decline in indices of ventilatory capacity with increasing age in smokers, compared with non-smokers. For example, FEV_1 reached a mean value of 2.22 litres in American male smokers at the age of 65–74, compared with 2.86 in a comparable group of non-smokers. Somewhat larger differences were found for the mean expiratory flow rate at 25 per cent of a forced vital capacity. The Report of the US Surgeon General (1984) concludes that cigarette smoking is the major cause of morbidity in chronic obstructive lung disease in the USA and that 80–90 per cent of cases are attributable to cigarette smoking.

Alveolar/capillary barrier function

The most sensitive indication of impaired respiratory function in smokers is the clearance of ^{99m}Tc DTPA from the alveoli into the blood (Jones et al., 1980). The mean half-time of clearance was 59 minutes in non-smokers but only 20 minutes in smokers, with almost total separation of the two groups. This change occurs in all smokers, including young and asymptomatic smokers in whom all other pulmonary function tests are normal. Clearance is increased within days of starting smoking and returns to a plateau value about 70 per cent of normal within a week of cessation of smoking (Minty, Jordan and Jones, 1981). This contrasts with changes of other pulmonary function tests which tend to be irreversible. It was already known that horseradish peroxidase (molecular weight 40000 daltons) penetrates the alveolar epithelium in guinea-pigs exposed to cigarette smoke (Simani, Inoue and Hogg, 1974).

Clearance of DTPA is closely related to carboxyhaemoglobin levels in the blood (Jones et al., 1983) but this appears to be an indication of smoke exposure rather than the cause, since filtration of the particulate matter prevented the change in rats, despite the development of very high levels of carboxyhaemoglobin (Minty and Royston, 1985).

Bronchoalveolar lavage in man has shown that smokers have larger numbers of macrophages and also significant numbers of neutrophils which are not normally present in non-smokers (Hunninghake and Crystal, 1983). These authors have also demonstrated that it is the particulate component of smoke which is responsible for the recruitment and activation of the neutrophils in the alveoli. This suggests that the interaction of particulate matter and alveolar macrophages releases a neutrophil chemattractant and that subsequently neutrophils are activated to release either proteases or oxygen-derived free radicals (page 488). Any of these could impair the integrity of the alveolar/epithelial barrier.

Other effects on respiratory function

Distribution of inspired gas as indicated by the single breath nitrogen test (page 149) is often abnormal in asymptomatic smokers but there is no good evidence that this is predictive of the development of chronic obstructive airway disease. There is usually increased production of mucus in smokers, and there is also impairment of the normal mechanisms of mucus clearance, such as ciliary activity (Dalhamn and Rylander, 1965). There is almost always increased coughing which is often productive.

Reference has been made above to the accelerated decline in indices of ventilatory capacity with age in smokers. This change is attributable to narrowing of small airways and there is usually increased reactivity of the airways. The concentration of inhaled histamine required to reduce specific airway conductance by 35 per cent in smokers is less than 40 per cent of that required in non-smokers (Gerrard et al., 1980). Carbon monoxide diffusing capacity is slightly reduced in heavy smokers (Tockman et al., 1976).

Postoperative respiratory complications

There is ample evidence that smokers have an increased incidence of postoperative respiratory complications (see review by Pearce and Jones, 1984). This is attributable both to increased secretion of mucus and impaired clearance and to small airway narrowing. Apart from changes in respiratory function considered above, there is an impairment of many aspects of the response to infection in smokers, and this may contribute further to postoperative morbidity.

Chapter 18

Respiration in neonates and children

The lungs before birth

Embryologically, the lungs develop as an outgrowth from the foregut and first appear about the 24th day of gestation. The lungs begin to contain surfactant and are first capable of function by approximately 24–26 weeks, this being a major factor in the viability of premature infants. At full term all major elements of the lungs are fully formed but the respiratory tract is filled with some 40 ml of fluid approximating to a transudate of plasma. Its volume corresponds approximately with the functional residual capacity (FRC) after breathing is established (Strang, 1965). The fluid is continuously formed in the lungs and passes upwards to be swallowed or discharged into the amniotic fluid.

There is excellent evidence that respiratory movements are present *in utero* for about 40 per cent of the time in the last third of gestation in the lamb (Dawes et al., 1972). These movements occur predominantly during rapid eye movement (REM) sleep (see Chapter 13). Chernick (1981) has reviewed the evidence supporting similar respiratory activity in the human fetus.

The fetal circulation

The fetal circulation differs radically from the postnatal circulation (*Figure 18.1*). Blood from the right heart is deflected away from the lungs, partly through the foramen ovale and partly through the ductus arteriosus. Less than 10 per cent of the output of the right ventricle reaches the lungs, the remainder passing to the systemic circulation and the placenta. Right atrial pressure exceeds left atrial pressure and this maintains the patency of the foramen ovale. Furthermore, since the vascular resistance of the pulmonary circulation exceeds that of the systemic circulation before birth, pressure in the right ventricle exceeds that in the left ventricle and these factors control the direction of flow through the ductus arteriosus. The direction may be reversed in abnormal circumstances if the pressure gradient between the ventricles is reversed.

The umbilical veins drain via the ductus venosus into the inferior vena cava which therefore contains better oxygenated blood than the superior vena cava. The anatomy of the atria and the foramen ovale is such that the better oxygenated blood from the inferior vena cava passes preferentially into the left atrium and thence to the left ventricle and so to the brain. (This is not shown in *Figure 18.1*.) Overall

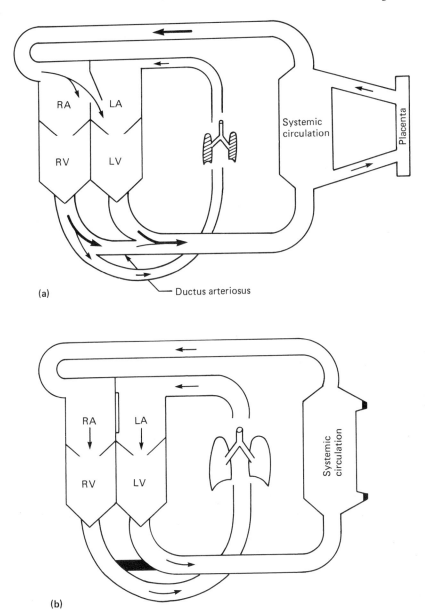

Figure 18.1 Fetal circulation (a) compared with adult circulation (b). The foramen ovale is between right atrium (RA) and left atrium (LA). RV and LV, right and left ventricles.

gas tensions in the fetus are of the order of 6.4 kPa (48 mmHg) for P_{CO_2} and 2.9 kPa (22 mmHg) for P_{O_2} (Chernick, 1981). It is surprising that the fetus remains apnoeic for most of the time *in utero* with these levels.

Events at birth

Changes in the circulation

The geometry of the circulation changes radically and quickly at birth. These changes are initiated by three events. Firstly, passage through the pelvis normally expels much of the fluid from the lungs, although this does not occur at caesarean section. Secondly, the child takes its first breath. Thirdly, the placental circulation ceases.

The establishment of spontaneous breathing causes a decrease in the vascular resistance of the pulmonary circulation, due partly to mechanical factors and partly to reduction of hypoxic pulmonary vasoconstriction following the first breath. Simultaneously there is an increase in the resistance of the systemic circulation, due partly to vasoconstriction and partly to cessation of the placental circulation. As a result, the right atrial pressure falls below the left atrial pressure, to give the relationship which is then maintained throughout life. This normally results in closure of the foramen ovale (*Figure 18.1*) which is followed by closure of the ductus arteriosus as a result of active vasoconstriction of its smooth muscle layer. The circulation is thus converted from the fetal mode in which the lungs and the systemic circulation are essentially in parallel to the adult mode in which they are in series (*Figure 18.1*).

Factors in the initiation of breathing

Most normal infants take their first breath within the first 20 seconds after delivery and rhythmic respiration is usually established within 90 seconds. Many factors combine in the stimulation to breathing. Following thoracic compression during delivery, the recoil of the rib cage tends to cause air to be drawn passively into the lungs (Rees, 1980). However, the major stimuli to breathing are probably the cooling of the skin and mechanical stimulation. Hypoxaemia, resulting from apnoea or clamping of the cord, is unlikely to be a reliable respiratory stimulus at this time. Ceruti (1966) studied the effect of hypoxia in normal infants during the first 3 days of life. Inhalation of 12% oxygen in a warm environment induced only transient hyperventilation lasting barely a minute and this was followed by respiratory depression. A lowered environmental temperature resulted in ventilation being increased by about 30 per cent. Hypoxia in this cool environment caused only depression of breathing. A ventilatory response to 3% CO_2 of about 15 per cent was observed which was not related to temperature. There was limited evidence to suggest that the hypoxic drive to ventilation became more sustained by the seventh day of life.

The Apgar score

The scoring system devised many years ago by Virginia Apgar is still widely accepted as an assessment of the overall condition of the neonate. This is based on scoring of a scale of 0–2 for five attributes, two of which are related to respiration (*Table 18.1*). The total score is the sum of each of the five constituent scores and is best undertaken 1 and 5 minutes after delivery. Scores of 8–10 are regarded as normal.

Table 18.1 The Apgar scoring system

Score	0	1	2
Heart rate	Absent	Less than 100/min	More than 100/min
Respiratory effort	Absent	Slow, irregular	Good, crying
Colour	Blue, pale	Body pink, extremities blue	Completely pink
Reflex irritability	Absent	Grimace	Cough, sneeze
Muscle tone	Limp	Some flexion of extremities	Active motion

Add together scores for each section (maximum possible 10).
Score at 1 and 5 minutes after delivery.
(After Gregory, 1981)

Neonatal asphyxia

Asphyxia may occur *in utero* from partial detachment of the placenta, maternal hypoxia or any reduction in uterine perfusion. After delivery, it has been reported in various studies that 13 per cent of infants were still apnoeic 2 minutes after birth and 4.7 per cent after 3 minutes (Davenport and Valman, 1980). This constitutes primary apnoea and, if prolonged for 5–10 minutes, characteristically leads to a gasp which is then followed by secondary or terminal apnoea (Dawes, 1968). Brain damage commences after about 10 minutes of apnoea. Various stimuli may initiate breathing and usually do so during primary apnoea. However, in secondary apnoea, only artificial ventilation is effective. There are many causes of fetal asphyxia and these include the administration of respiratory depressant drugs to the mother before delivery (Davenport and Valman, 1980).

In view of the short time scale of events, active measures should be instituted if breathing has not commenced by 30 seconds after delivery, and intermittent positive pressure ventilation (IPPV) may be started with oxygen using a well-fitting facemask. If there is no response after 1 minute, the trachea should be intubated, since this permits more effective suction to remove mucus and also more effective IPPV.

Neonatal lung function

A good deal is known about lung function immediately after birth (Nelson, 1966; Cotes, 1975).

Mechanics of breathing

Functional residual capacity is about 30 ml/kg and total respiratory compliance 50 ml/kPa (5ml/cmH$_2$O). Most of the impedance to expansion is due to the lung and depends primarily on the presence of surfactant in the alveoli. The chest wall of the neonate is highly compliant. This contrasts with the adult where compliance of lung and chest wall are approximately equal (see *Figure 2.7*). Total respiratory resistance is of the order of 7 kPa l^{-1} s (70 cmH$_2$O l^{-1} s), most of which is in the bronchial tree. Thus compliance is about one-twentieth that of an adult and resistance about 15 times greater. The time constant (product of compliance and resistance—see page 398) is thus rather less than in the adult and is about 0.3 second. At the first breath the infant is capable of generating a subatmospheric pressure of the order of 7 kPa (70 cmH$_2$O).

Ventilation and gas exchange

The minute volume is about 0.5 litre, depending on weight, and this is achieved with a high respiratory frequency (25–40 b.p.m.) and a tidal volume ranging from 14 ml at 2 kg to 20 ml at 4 kg. Dead space is variously reported as between a third and a half of tidal volume, giving a mean alveolar ventilation of about 250–335 ml for a neonate of average size. There is a shunt of about 10 per cent immediately after birth. However, distribution of gas is better than in the adult and there is, of course, a negligible hydrostatic pressure gradient in the vertical axis of the tiny lungs of an infant (compare with *Figure 6.4*). Diffusing capacity for carbon monoxide per square metre of body area is about half the corresponding value in the adult (Nelson, 1966).

Oxygen consumption is of the order of 20–30 ml/min depending on weight in the range 2–4 kg. Arterial P$_{CO_2}$ is close to 4.5 kPa (34 mmHg) and P$_{O_2}$ 9 kPa (68 mmHg). Due to the shunt of 10 per cent, there is an alveolar/arterial P$_{O_2}$ gradient of about 3.3 kPa (25 mmHg) compared with less than half of this in a young adult. Arterial pH is within the normal adult range.

Control of breathing (see reviews by Chernick, 1981; Fleming and Ponte, 1983). In contrast to the poorly developed ventilatory response to hypoxia, outlined above, ventilation is immediately depressed by the inhalation of 100% oxygen (Brady, Cotton and Tooley, 1964), indicating a tonic drive from the peripheral chemo-receptors. Chemoreceptor drive is probably the mechanism of the periodic breathing which is often seen in infants. Ventilatory response to carbon dioxide appears to be similar to that in the adult if allowance is made for body size.

Haemoglobin

Children are normally born polycythaemic with a mean haemoglobin of about 18 g/dl and a haematocrit of 53% (Delivoria-Papadopoulos, Roncevic and Oski, 1971). Seventy per cent of the haemoglobin is HbF and the resultant P$_{50}$ is well below the normal adult value (see *Figure 10.13*). The haemoglobin concentration decreases rapidly to become less than the normal adult value by 3 weeks of life. HbF gradually disappears from the circulation to reach negligible values by 6 months, by which time the P$_{50}$ has already attained the normal adult value.

Development of lung function during childhood

The lungs continue to develop during childhood. Between birth and adult life there is an approximately tenfold increase in the number of airways. Cotes (1975) has provided tables and graphs showing the gradual assumption of adult values of lung volumes and various indices of ventilatory capacity in relation to the height of the subject. Ventilatory capacity at the age of 7–8 was studied by Strang (1959), and

Figure 18.2 summarizes some of his results. It is not practicable to determine ventilatory capacity in very young children.

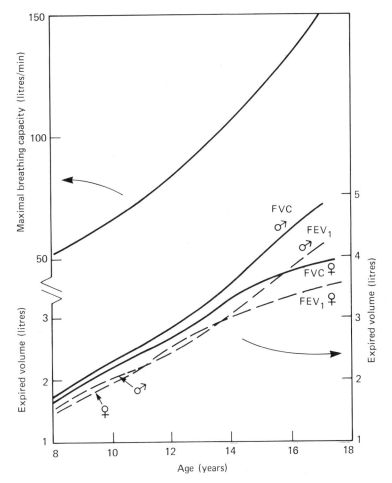

Figure 18.2 Indices of ventilatory capacity as a function of age. FVC, forced vital capacity; FEV₁, forced expiratory volume (1 second). (Drawn from data of Strang (1959))

Various indices of respiratory function are independent of age and body size so that adult values can be used. These include forced expiratory volume (1 second) as a fraction of vital capacity, FRC and peak expiratory flow rate as a fraction of total lung capacity, specific airway conductance and compliance divided by FRC and probably dead space/tidal volume ratio (Cotes, 1975).

Arterial P_{CO_2} and alveolar P_{O_2} do not change appreciably during childhood but arterial P_{O_2} increases from the neonatal value to reach a maximum of about 13 kPa (98 mmHg) at young adulthood. Much of this increase occurs during the first year of life (Mansell, Bryan and Levison, 1972). There are obvious difficulties in determining the normal arterial P_{O_2} in children.

Respiratory distress syndrome

(see review by Swyer, 1975)

The essential lesion is a deficiency of surfactant and it occurs in 1 per cent of all live births but with a greatly increased incidence in premature infants. Surfactant is first detectable in the fetal lung at 20–24 weeks of gestation but the concentration increases rapidly after the 30th week. Not only does the total concentration change but also there is a shift from sphingomyelin (S) to lecithin (L) which can be detected as a change in the L/S ratio in the amniotic fluid. In view of these changes late in pregnancy, it is not surprising that prematurity is a major factor in the aetiology of respiratory distress syndrome (RDS).

The disease presents with difficulty in inspiration against the decreased compliance due to the high surface tension of the alveolar lining fluid deficient in surfactant. This progresses to ventilatory failure, alveolar collapse, hyaline membrane deposit and severe interference with gas exchange with severe hypoxaemia. Increased pulmonary vascular resistance may raise right atrial pressure and reopen the foramen ovale, so increasing the shunt.

The essential features of treatment are artificial ventilation and very careful titration of inspired oxygen concentration to avoid hypoxaemia on the one hand and the danger of pulmonary oxygen toxicity on the other. This condition is best treated in a special neonatal intensive care unit, where the mortality may be brought below 20 per cent in comparison with 60 per cent without effective treatment.

Artificial ventilation of the neonate and young child

Artificial ventilation is most commonly required for the neonate with RDS. The usual choice is for time-cycled square-wave pressure generators (page 396), but operating at much higher respiratory frequencies than in the adult. Inspiratory and expiratory durations may be as little as 0.3 second, but inflation pressures are of the same order as those used in adults and do not usually exceed 3 kPa (30 cmH$_2$O). Positive end-expiratory pressure (PEEP) is widely used and spontaneous respiration is often undertaken with continuous positive airway pressure (CPAP). Bronchopulmonary dysplasia appears to be a form of barotrauma in the ventilated infant and is considered on page 416. Normal humidification and monitoring of airway pressure are important. Many ventilators are available but the choice of ventilator is probably less important than the skill and experience of its operator.

Both the compressible volume of the ventilator circuit and the apparatus dead space tend to be large in relation to the size of very small children. It is for this reason that pressure generators are preferable to volume generators. Furthermore, there is considerable practical difficulty in measuring the very small imposed tidal volumes or minute volumes. For this reason, close monitoring of PO_2 and PCO_2 is essential and transcutaneous PCO_2 will probably prove to be satisfactory for the latter. High frequency ventilation (page 406) may well have a place here but has not yet been fully evaluated. Detailed management of ventilation of neonates has been described by Llewellyn and Swyer (1975).

Treatment by CPAP with preservation of spontaneous respiration was described by Gregory et al. (1971). Much thought has been given to the possibility of raising airway pressure without the necessity of tracheal intubation. Gastight facemasks are described by Llewellyn and Swyer and it is also possible to obtain a seal around the head. However, these techniques are not generally used as a first line of treatment, although they may have some role in weaning from artificial ventilation.

Chapter 19

Respiratory aspects of anaesthesia

It has long been recognized that anaesthesia has profound effects upon the respiratory system. It is now clear that the effects are diverse and highly specific, some aspects of respiratory function being profoundly modified while others are scarcely affected at all.

Much of this chapter is concerned with anaesthesia without paralysis and with spontaneous breathing preserved. However, it will also describe the effects of the combination of anaesthesia, paralysis and artificial ventilation.

Control of breathing
(see reviews by Hornbein, 1985; Pavlin and Hornbein, 1986)

Effect on P_{CO_2}/ventilation response curve

It has long been known that anaesthesia may diminish pulmonary ventilation. The first aspect of the problem to be elucidated was the effect of anaesthetics on the P_{CO_2}/ventilation response curve. This has been discussed on pages 89 et seq. as the most informative way of describing the interaction of P_{CO_2}, ventilation and a wide range of stimulant and depressant drugs.

In *Figure 19.1*, the flat curve rising to the left represents the starting points for various P_{CO_2}/ventilation response curves. Without added carbon dioxide in the inspired gas, deepening anaesthesia is associated with a decreasing ventilation and a rising P_{CO_2}, starting points moving progressively down and to the right along the flat curve. At intervals along this curve are shown P_{CO_2}/ventilation response curves resulting from adding carbon dioxide to the inspired gas. Progressive increases in the alveolar concentration of all inhalational anaesthetic agents decrease the slope of the P_{CO_2}/ventilation response curve and, at deep levels of anaesthesia, there may be no response at all to P_{CO_2}. Deepening anaesthesia also increases the intercept on the P_{CO_2} axis. Furthermore, the anaesthetized patient, as opposed to the awake subject, always becomes apnoeic if the P_{CO_2} is reduced below this intercept which is known as the apnoeic threshold P_{CO_2} (see Chapter 4, page 90). These changes appear to be attributable in part to the effect of anaesthetics on the pattern of contraction of the inspiratory muscles (see below).

Anaesthetics differ quantitatively in their capacity to depress the response of ventilation to P_{CO_2}. This is conventionally shown by plotting the slope of the P_{CO_2}/ventilation response curve against equi-anaesthetic concentrations of different

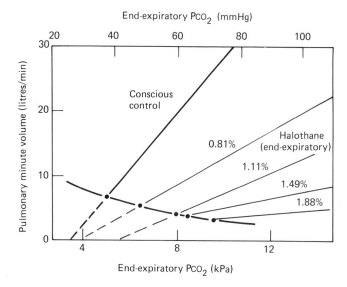

Figure 19.1 Displacement of P_{CO_2}/ventilation response curve with different end-expiratory concentrations of halothane. The curve sloping down to the right indicates the pathway of P_{CO_2} and ventilation change resulting from depression without the challenge of exogenous carbon dioxide. The dotted lines indicate extrapolation of apnoeic threshold P_{CO_2}. The curves have been constructed from the data of Munson et al. (1966). A rather similar set of curves was obtained for methoxyflurane by Dunbar, Ovassapian and Smith (1967) except that these workers did not observe the same degree of displacement to the right of the initial P_{CO_2} at different depths of anaesthesia before the carbon dioxide challenge. Roughly similar changes in slope were reported for equipotent concentrations of the two agents.

anaesthetics. This may be conveniently expressed as multiples of the minimal alveolar concentration (MAC) required for anaesthesia (*Figure 19.2*) although there is considerable doubt as to the validity of using MAC values in this way. The halogenated agents do not differ greatly from one another but diethyl ether is exceptional in having little effect up to 1.0 MAC. Thereafter the effect increases markedly with increasing concentrations until, at 2.5 MAC, the extrapolated value appears to be comparable to the halogenated agents. Anaesthesia with diethyl ether causes an increase in the level of circulating catecholamines and it is thought that this may counteract the depressant effect of the anaesthetic. Noradrenaline is known to increase the slope of the P_{CO_2}/ventilation response curve (Cunningham et al., 1963). Ether, furthermore, blocks neuromuscular transmission in high dosage and its irritant vapour may have a stimulant effect on ventilation.

Surgical stimulation antagonizes the effect of anaesthesia on the P_{CO_2}/ventilation response curve (*Figure 19.3*). It may easily be observed that a surgical incision increases the ventilation whatever the depth of anaesthesia, provided that spontaneous breathing is still present. During prolonged anaesthesia without surgical stimulation, there is no progressive change in the response curve up to 3 hours, but some return towards the preanaesthetic position has been reported after 6 hours (Fourcade et al., 1972). Depression of ventilation by anaesthesia is relatively greater in patients with chronic obstructive airway disease (Pietak et al., 1975).

Barbiturates have little effect on ventilation in sedative or light sleep dosage. However, anaesthetic doses have similar effects to the inhalational anaesthetics

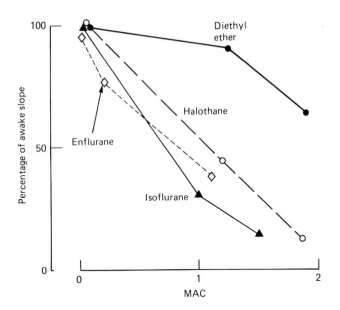

Figure 19.2 Relative respiratory depression of different anaesthetics as a function of multiples of minimal alveolar concentration (MAC) required for anaesthesia. (Based on a review by Eger (1981))

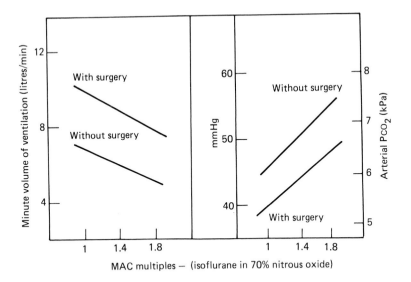

Figure 19.3 Respiratory depression of isoflurane with and without surgery at different multiples of minimal alveolar concentration (MAC) required for anaesthesia. (Drawn from data of Eger et al. (1972))

(Bellville and Seed, 1960). Ketamine has little effect. Opiates are well known to depress ventilation, and a reduction in respiratory frequency is often observed. Small doses have been reported to increase the intercept of the P_{CO_2}/ventilation response curve on the P_{CO_2} axis without changing the slope (Loeschcke et al., 1953) but there is certainly a marked change in slope at higher dosage. With very large doses (of the order of 2 mg/kg) there is a plateau of effect on slope, with a reduction to about 20 per cent of the value in the conscious state. Apnoea does not normally occur when doses of this order are given to the conscious subject.

Effect on P_{O_2}/ventilation response curve

The normal relationship between P_{O_2} and ventilation has been described on pages 81 et seq. It was long believed that this reflex was the *ultima moriens* and, unlike the P_{CO_2}/ventilation response curve, unaffected by anaesthesia. This doctrine was a source of comfort to many generations of anaesthetists in the past. No one seemed to notice the observation of Gordh in 1945 that ether anaesthesia nearly abolished the ventilatory response to hypoxaemia while the response to carbon dioxide was still present.

Nearly 30 years later Weiskopf, Raymond and Severinghaus (1974) showed depression of the P_{O_2}/ventilation response curve in anaesthetized dogs. Then Duffin, Triscott and Whitwam (1976) showed that halothane anaesthesia reduced the ventilatory response to oxygen in man. Shortly afterwards, Knill and Gelb (1978) showed that not only was the hypoxic response affected by inhalational anaesthetics but it was also, in fact, exquisitely sensitive (*Figure 19.4*). Hypoxic drive was markedly attenuated at 0.1 MAC, a level of anaesthesia which would continue for

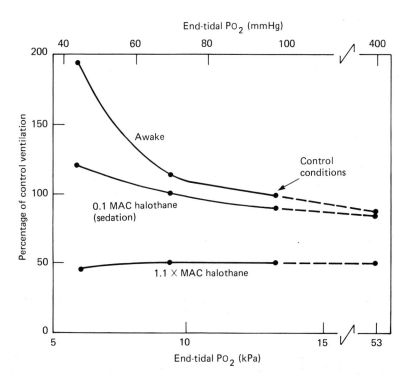

Figure 19.4 Effect of halothane anaesthesia on ventilatory response to hypoxia. MAC is the minimal alveolar concentration required for anaesthesia. (Redrawn from data of Knill and Gelb (1978))

a considerable time during recovery from anaesthesia. This effect has now been amply confirmed and shown to occur with at least six inhalational anaesthetics including even nitrous oxide (Knill and Clement, 1982). The responses to halothane and isoflurane are very similar. It seems likely that the effect is on the carotid body chemoreceptor itself (Davies, Edwards and Lahiri, 1982; Knill and Clement, 1984) and there is evidence that the effect can be reversed with almitrine (Clergue et al., 1984). Anaesthesia also impairs the ventilatory response to doxapram, which acts on the peripheral chemoreceptors (Knill and Gelb, 1978).

There are four important practical implications of the loss of the hypoxic ventilatory response in anaesthesia. Firstly, the patient cannot act as his own hypoxia alarm by responding with hyperventilation. Secondly, the patient who has already lost his sensitivity to PcO$_2$ (e.g. 'the blue bloater' category of patient with chronic bronchitis) may stop breathing after induction of anaesthesia has abolished his hypoxic drive. This effect was, in fact, well known in the past but the significance was not realized at the time. Thirdly, anaesthesia may be dangerous at very high altitude or in other situations where survival depends on hyperventilation in response to hypoxia. In contrast to anaesthesia, sleep has no effect on the hypoxic drive and this is important for survival of high-altitude mountaineers. Finally, since the hypoxic drive is obtunded at subanaesthetic concentrations, this effect will persist into the early postoperative period after the patient has regained consciousness and is apparently able to fend for himself.

Response to metabolic acidaemia

The ventilatory response to non-respiratory changes in arterial PcO$_2$ has been described on page 91. This response is also obtunded by anaesthesia and even by subanaesthetic concentrations of anaesthetics (Knill and Clement, 1985). The sensitivity of this response to anaesthesia is no less than that of the hypoxia response (*Figure 19.5*).

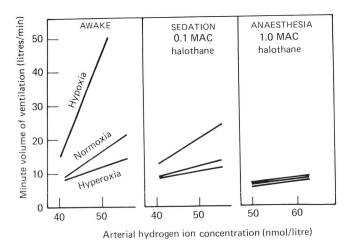

Figure 19.5 Effect of halothane anaesthesia on the ventilatory response to acidaemia. MAC is the minimal alveolar concentration required for anaesthesia. (Redrawn, with permission, from data of Knill and Clement (1985))

Response to added resistance

The paragraphs above would lead one to expect that anaesthesia would cause grave impairment of the ability of a patient to increase his work of breathing in the face of added resistance. Surprisingly, this is not the case and anaesthetized patients preserve a remarkable ability to overcome added resistance (Nunn and Ezi-Ashi, 1961). The anaesthetized patient responds to inspiratory loading in two phases. Firstly, there is an instant augmentation of the force of contraction of the inspiratory muscles, mainly the diaphragm, during the first loaded breath (Muller et al., 1979). This has the appearance of a typical spindle reflex, and the same authors have reported the existence of spindles in the human diaphragm. The second response is much slower and overshoots when the loading is removed (Nunn and Ezi-Ashi, 1961). The time course suggests that this is mediated by an increase in P_{CO_2}. In combination, these two mechanisms enable the anaesthetized patient to achieve good compensation with inspiratory loading up to about 0.8 kPa (8 cmH$_2$O). Moote, Knill and Clement (1986) have confirmed the ability of the anaesthetized patient to compensate for respiratory loading. Even more remarkable is the preservation of the elaborate response to expiratory resistance (see *Figure 3.14*) which is described on page 67.

Anaesthetics and pulmonary stretch receptors

It has been shown in cats that the common inhalational anaesthetics, particularly trichloroethylene, sensitize the pulmonary stretch receptors and so would be expected to cause an enhancement of the inflation reflex (Whitteridge and Bulbring, 1944). This is in contrast to Head's conclusion (1889) that ether and chloroform paralysed vagal endings. Whitteridge and Bulbring concluded that the sensitization of the stretch receptor was largely responsible for the shallow breathing seen in trichloroethylene anaesthesia, but observed that trichloroethylene and cyclopropane could have opposite effects on respiratory rate while both agents were causing sensitization of stretch receptors. They further stated that these agents 'must exert another action on a second set of pulmonary endings, or on the respiratory centre, or on extrapulmonary endings'. Ngai, Katz and Farhi (1965) showed that, in midcollicular decerebrate cats, the marked tachypnoea produced by trichloroethylene was not prevented by bilateral vagotomy and carotid denervation. It would therefore seem that there is no solid foundation for the oft repeated view that trichloroethylene causes tachypnoea as a result of sensitization of the pulmonary stretch receptors.

Pattern of contraction of respiratory muscles

One of the most remarkable examples of the specificity of anaesthetic action is their action on the muscles associated with respiration. There appears to be no logic in the pattern of change which has been elucidated.

The inspiratory muscles

In the very early days of anaesthesia John Snow (1858) observed that deepening anaesthesia was associated with a decrease in thoracic respiratory excursion. This change has always been used as an indication of deepening surgical anaesthesia.

The effect was quantified by Miller (1925) and more precisely related to depth of anaesthesia by Jones and his colleagues (1979). Abdominal respiratory excursion is well preserved. This is normally interpreted as progressive failure of the intercostal muscles with preservation of the action of the diaphragm although there is no obvious reason why there should be this differential response of the inspiratory muscles. In contrast, there is an increased thoracic component of ventilation during IPPV of the anaesthetized paralysed patient (Vellody et al., 1978).

These changes appear to play a major part in the effect of anaesthesia on the ventilatory response to P_{CO_2}. Tusiewicz, Bryan and Froese (1977) showed that the major part of the ventilatory response to P_{CO_2} was in the rib cage rather than in the abdominal component of the total respiratory excursion. Since the former was largely obliterated during anaesthesia, it was not surprising that it was unable to respond to a carbon dioxide challenge. The abdominal excursion still responded but was feeble as in the awake state. The implication of this study is that much of the reduced ventilatory response to P_{CO_2} observed during anaesthesia is due to inactivation of intercostal muscle activity. Thus a major part of the effect of anaesthesia on the P_{CO_2}/ventilation response curve is mediated peripherally rather than centrally as had hitherto been assumed. Relative loss of the rib cage component of breathing may present a hazard during anaesthesia in a patient with an impediment to abdominal breathing such as abdominal distension. It is also potentially dangerous in a patient with hyperinflated lungs and a flattened diaphragm.

The second major change in the pattern of contraction of the inspiratory muscles during anaesthesia is in the diaphragm itself. During normal breathing by the conscious subject in the supine position, the diaphragm retains considerable tone at the end of expiration. This holds the lung volume above that which it would attain if determined solely by the equilibration of elastic forces. This may well be a special mechanism to prevent the weight of the viscera pushing the diaphragm too far into the chest in the supine position. Muller and his colleagues (1979) have used diaphragmatic electromyography to demonstrate that this residual end-expiratory tone is lost during anaesthesia with halothane. Under these circumstances, the end-expiratory position of the diaphragm is the same as in the paralysed patient. The altered end-expiratory position of the diaphragm confirmed what had long been suspected from the change in functional residual capacity during anaesthesia (see below).

The expiratory muscles

Freund, Roos and Dodd (1964) first demonstrated that general anaesthesia caused phasic activity of the expiratory abdominal muscles which are normally silent in the conscious supine subject. This would probably have come as no surprise to the generation of abdominal surgeons who worked in the days before the introduction of neuromuscular blocking drugs. The observations were extended by Kaul, Heath and Nunn (1973) who found that in some patients it was very difficult to abolish this activity as long as spontaneous breathing persisted. This activation of expiratory muscles seems to serve no useful purpose and it does not appear to have any significant effect on the change in functional residual capacity (Hewlett et al., 1974b). It is, however, undoubtedly a nuisance for the abdominal surgeon operating on an anaesthetized patient without paralysis.

Other muscles

The genioglossus muscle contracts rhythmically in phase with breathing (Remmers et al., 1978). At least in the cat, there is interference with its activity during anaesthesia (Nishino et al., 1984). Extrapolating this observation to man, it is reasonable to believe that anaesthesia may interfere with activity of the genioglossus (as in the intercostal muscles) and this causes the tongue to fall back against the posterior pharyngeal wall. This results in airway obstruction which almost always occurs when anaesthesia is induced. The anatomy of this effect and the usual methods of overcoming it are shown in *Figure 1.2*. It has recently been suggested by Boidin (1985) that the epiglottis may be involved in obstruction at this site during anaesthesia.

Changes in lung and trunk volumes
(see reviews by Rehder, 1985; Froese, 1985)

Change in functional residual capacity

Bergman (1963) was the first to report a decrease of functional residual capacity (FRC) during anaesthesia. This was followed by many studies which have established the following characteristics of the change.

1. FRC is reduced during anaesthesia with all anaesthetic drugs which have been investigated, by a mean value of about 16–20 per cent of the FRC (in the supine position). However, there is considerable individual variation and changes range from about +19 per cent to −50 per cent.
2. FRC does not seem to fall progressively during anaesthesia and appears to reach its final value within the first few minutes of anaesthesia. It does not return to normal until some hours after the end of anaesthesia.
3. Inhalation of high concentrations of oxygen does not appear to be a factor in the change and does not usually result in progressive changes.
4. FRC is reduced to the same extent during anaesthesia whether the patient is paralysed or not (*Table 19.1*).
5. Expiratory muscle activity has no significant effect on the change in FRC.
6. The reduction in FRC has a weak but significant correlation with the age of the patient.
7. Artificial ventilation of the conscious subject causes only a small reduction in FRC.
8. Anaesthesia does not change FRC in the sitting position.
(References: Don et al., 1970; Rehder et al., 1971; Don, Wahba and Craig, 1972; Hewlett et al., 1974b, c; Rehder and Marsh 1986.)

The cause of the reduction in FRC remained a mystery for many years. Froese and Bryan (1974) in a classic study of lateral chest radiographs during anaesthesia clearly showed that the diaphragm ascended into the chest by about 2 cm during anaesthesia with or without paralysis and this change accorded roughly with the decrease in FRC (*Figure 19.6*). The loss of end-expiratory diaphragmatic tone was then demonstrated by Muller and his colleagues (1979). However, Jones and his colleagues (1979) found no decrease in abdominal volume to correspond with the ascent of the diaphragm, suggesting that the changes might be complicated by a

Table 19.1 Values for functional residual capacity

Conscious subjects

Seated	3.0 litres	(normalized for body height of 170 cm; mean of normal values from Cotes, 1975, and Bates, Macklem and Christie, (1971)
Supine mean	2.2 litres	(mean of 125 values in volunteers and patients prior to surgery, reported in studies cited in this chapter)
SD	0.64 litre	

Anaesthetized patients (supine) mean percentage reductions in FRC following induction of anesthesia

Spontaneous breathing	31.4%	(Don et al., 1970)
	19.0%	(Don, Wahba and Craig, 1972)
	23.3%*	(Westbrook et al., 1973)
	12.6%	(Hickey et al., 1973)
	16.1%	(Hewlett et al., 1974b)
Mean	20.5%	
Artificial ventilation	9.0%	(Laws, 1968)
	14.0%*	(Rehder et al., 1971)
	25.0%*	(Westbrook et al., 1973)
	15.4%	(Hewlett et al., 1974c)
Mean	15.9%	

*These studies were of healthy volunteers and not patients.

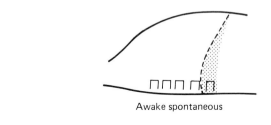

Awake spontaneous

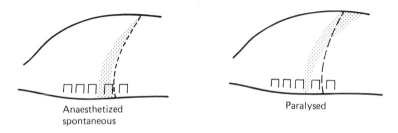

Anaesthetized spontaneous

Paralysed

Figure 19.6 Position of the diaphragm in the awake and anaesthetized states. The broken line is the end-expiratory position in the awake state (supine position) and is reproduced for comparison in all three figures. The shaded area indicates the respiratory excursion of the diaphragm. (Reproduced from Froese and Bryan (1974) by permission of the authors and the Editors of Anesthesiology)

change in the distribution of blood volume. Following induction of anaesthesia and paralysis in the supine position, there is a small decrease in the anteroposterior and a small increase in the lateral diameter of the chest wall (Vellody et al., 1978). Reduction in lung compliance (see below), probably secondary to reduction in FRC, may play a role in maintaining the reduction in FRC.

Changes in thoracic and abdominal volumes

The next generation of studies used new imaging techniques to make more precise measurements of geometric changes and to relate these to observed changes in FRC and central blood volume. Hedenstierna and his colleagues (1985) used computerized tomography to indicate the changes following anaesthesia and paralysis which are summarized in *Figure 19.7*. The ascent of the diaphragm was found to correspond to slightly more than the observed decrease in FRC (450 ml).

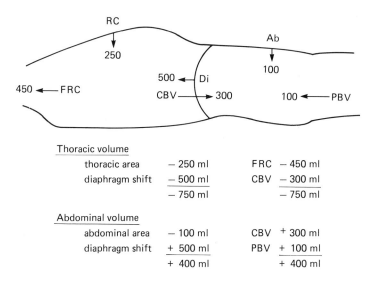

Thoracic volume				
thoracic area	− 250 ml		FRC	− 450 ml
diaphragm shift	− 500 ml		CBV	− 300 ml
	− 750 ml			− 750 ml

Abdominal volume				
abdominal area	− 100 ml		CBV	+ 300 ml
diaphragm shift	+ 500 ml		PBV	+ 100 ml
	+ 400 ml			+ 400 ml

Figure 19.7 Mean changes in volume (ml) of rib cage (RC) and abdomen (Ab) and movement of central blood volume (CBV) and peripheral blood volume (PBV). 'FRC' indicates the change in functional residual capacity. 'Di' indicates the volume change resulting from the ascent of the diaphragm. (Reproduced from Hedenstierna et al. (1985) by permission of the authors and the Editors of Anesthesiology)

However, there was also a decrease in the volume of the rib cage of 250 ml which was more than offset by a shift of blood volume from thorax to abdomen. The decrease in diameter of the rib cage corresponding to a volume change of 250 ml would be only about 2 mm and it is not surprising that this had been missed by earlier investigators. Abdominal blood volume increased by a total of 400 ml which almost entirely offset the ascent of the diaphragm. The resultant decrease in abdominal volume was only 100 ml which would be very difficult to measure by conventional methods.

Consequences of the change in FRC

In the supine position, the expiratory reserve has a mean value of only 1 litre in males and 600 ml in females (Whitfield, Waterhouse and Arnott, 1950). Therefore, the reduction in FRC following the induction of anaesthesia will bring the lung volume close to residual volume. This has major effects on lung function, particularly in respect to airway closure, airway calibre, compliance and gas exchange.

Airway closure

A reduction of FRC, such as follows the induction of anaesthesia, might be expected to reduce the end-expiratory lung volume below the closing capacity (CC), at least in older patients (see *Figure 2.12*), and so result in airway closure, absorption collapse of lung and shunting. Pulmonary collapse can easily be demonstrated in conscious subjects who voluntarily breathe oxygen close to residual volume (Nunn et al., 1965b; Nunn et al., 1978). *Figure 19.8* shows the effect on arterial P_{O_2} of

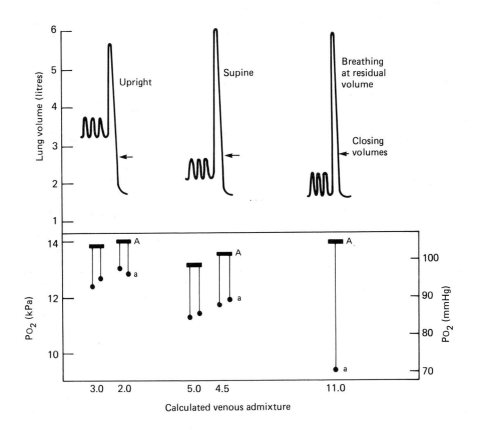

Figure 19.8 Changes in tidal excursion relative to vital capacity in the author when aged 45: arrows indicate the closing volume. Ideal alveolar (A) P_{O_2} is shown by the horizontal bar and arterial (a) P_{O_2} by the black circles. Venous admixture was calculated on the assumption of an arterial/mixed venous oxygen content difference of 5 ml/100 ml. (Reproduced from Nunn (1978) by permission of the Editors of Acta Anaesthesiologica Scandinavica)

breathing air at different lung volumes in the author at the age of 45. 'Miliary atelectasis' was put forward by Bendixen, Hedley-Whyte and Laver (1963) as an explanation of the increased alveolar/arterial Po_2 difference during anaesthesia. This view is reinforced by the recent demonstration, using computerized tomography, of what appears to be absorption collapse in dependent zones of the lung following the induction of anaesthesia (Brismar et al., 1985). For technical reasons, it would be extremely difficult to define these areas with conventional radiography. Observed changes in distribution of ventilation/perfusion ratios also support the view that airway closure is a major factor during anaesthesia in older patients (see below).

However, there is also evidence against the theory that atelectasis occurs to any significant effect during anaesthesia. The pulmonary shunt during anaesthesia seems to be much the same whether the patient breathes oxgyen, nitrous oxide/oxygen mixtures, or nitrogen/oxygen mixtures, although these different gas mixtures might be expected to have different effects on the development of pulmonary collapse (see below). Furthermore, many workers have been unable to show that the Po_2 gradient can be reduced by hyperinflation of the lung (Panday and Nunn, 1968). Restoration of FRC, either by PEEP (Bindslev et al., 1981) or by change of posture (Heneghan, Bergman and Jones, 1984) does not entirely restore the pulmonary shunt to the value before anaesthesia. It seems likely that the residual defect in gas exchange may be attributable to the effect of anaesthetics on hypoxic pulmonary vasoconstriction.

An important aspect of the problem is whether CC remains constant during anaesthesia or whether it changes with FRC. Earlier studies suggested that CC remained constant (Hedenstierna, McCarthy and Bergstrom, 1976), but more recently Juno et al. (1978) have provided convincing evidence that both FRC and CC are reduced during anaesthesia. (CC − FRC) showed a positive correlation with age, the relationship being similar while anaesthetized and paralysed to the control values in the conscious patient. In both conditions the mean value of (CC − FRC) was zero at about the age of 45. Bergman and Tien (1983) obtained very similar values for (CC − FRC) as a function of age during anaesthesia. Since the relationship was the same as in the conscious subject (see *Figure 2.12*), Bergman and Tien concluded that CC had decreased in parallel with FRC following the induction of anaesthesia. There is thus rather convincing evidence that the reduction in FRC during anaesthesia does not alter the relationship between FRC and CC. It is likely that bronchodilatation caused by the anaesthetic counteracts the reduction in airway calibre which would be expected to result from the reduction in FRC (see below). As a result, it would appear that the tendency to airway closure is not increased during anaesthesia, and this point is considered further below in relation to airway resistance.

Airway calibre

Figure 19.9 shows the hyperbolic relationship between lung volume and airway resistance. This is due to the fact that the airways participate in the overall change in lung volume and, other things being equal, as the lung volume decreases, the airway calibre is reduced and the airway resistance increased. *Figure 19.9* clearly shows that the curve is steep in the region of FRC in the supine position and therefore the reduction in FRC which occurs during anaesthesia should result in a marked increase in airway resistance.

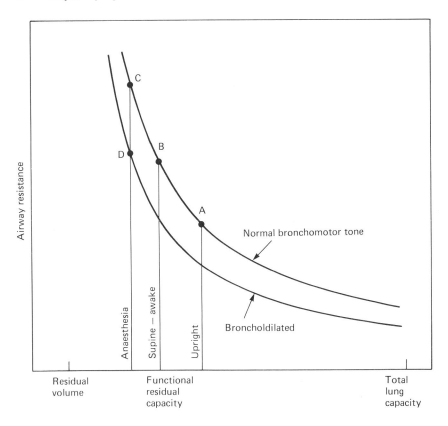

Figure 19.9 Airway resistance as a function of lung volume with normal bronchomotor tone and when bronchodilated. A = upright and awake; B = supine and awake; C = supine and anaesthetized without bronchodilatation; D = supine, anaesthetized and with the degree of bronchodilatation which normally occurs during anaesthesia. Note that the airway resistance is similar at B and D with bronchodilatation approximately compensating for the decrease in FRC.

The effect of decreased lung volume is to a large extent offset by the bronchodilator effect which seems to be shared by most of the inhalational anaesthetics: this causes an increase in specific airway conductance (Lehane, Jordan and Jones,1980; Heneghan et al., 1986). Typical changes are summarized in *Figure 19.9*. In the past there have been a great number of studies of the effect of anaesthesia on airway resistance in which the effect on lung volume was not recorded (*Table 19.2*). In general these have shown little change or a moderate increase in airway resistance although the individual variation is very large.

Other causes of increased airway resistance. Changes resulting from reduced lung volume and bronchodilatation may be regarded as normal consequences of any anaesthetic. However, there are in addition many other possible causes of increased airway resistance. These may be serious and threaten life. Excessive resistance or obstruction may arise in apparatus such as breathing circuits, valves, connectors and tracheal tubes. The tubes may be kinked, the lumen may be blocked or the cuff may herniate and obstruct the lower end, which may also abut against the

Table 19.2 Pulmonary resistance studies in healthy anaesthetized patients

	$kPa\ l^{-1}\ s$	$cmH_2O/l/sec$
Newman, Campbell and Dinnick (1959)	0.05–0.3	0.5–3.0
Bodman (1963)*	0.12–0.32	1.2–3.2
Bergman (1966)	0.55–0.60	5.5–6.0
Bergman (1969)* at 1.5 l/s	0.50–0.57	5.0–5.7
at 1.0 l/s	0.44–0.49	4.4–4.9
at 0.5 l/s	0.36–0.39	3.6–3.9
Hedenstierna and McCarthy (1975)	0.4–0.6	4.0–6.0
Bergman and Waltemath (1974)	0.4–0.6	4.0–6.0

Values exclude apparatus resistance.
*These series also report patients with physical and radiographic evidence of pulmonary disease, who showed much greater levels of resistance.

carina or the side wall of the trachea. A reduction in diameter of a tracheal tube increases the resistance inversely to the fourth or fifth power of the radius of the tube (*Figure 19.10*).

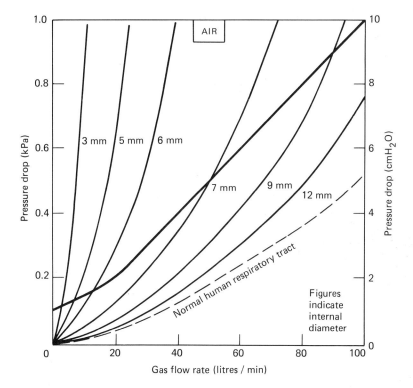

Figure 19.10 Flow rate/pressure drop plots of a range of endotracheal tubes, with their connectors and catheter mounts. The heavy line is the author's suggested upper limit of acceptable resistance for an adult. Pressure drop does not quite increase according to the fourth power of the diameter (inverse) because the catheter mount offered the same resistance throughout the range of tubes. With 70% N_2O/30% O_2, the pressure drop is about 40 per cent greater for the same gas flow rate when flow is turbulent, but little different when the flow is chiefly laminar.

The pharynx is commonly obstructed by the tongue as a result of relaxation of the genioglossus muscles, as described earlier in this chapter and on page 4. The large airways may be blocked with foreign material such as blood, tumour, pus or inhaled gastric contents. Bronchospasm may result from the causes outlined on pages 54 et seq.

Compliance

Figure 19.11, based on the work of Westbrook et al. (1973) and Butler and Smith (1957), summarizes the effect of anaesthesia on the pressure/volume relationships of the lung and chest wall. The diagram shows the major differences between the conscious state and anaesthesia. There are, however, only minor differences between anaesthesia with and without paralysis.

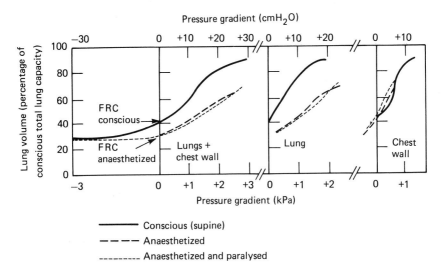

Figure 19.11 Pressure/volume relationships in supine volunteers before and after the induction of anaesthesia and paralysis. The first section shows the relationship for lungs plus chest wall where the relevant pressure gradient is alveolar minus ambient. The second section represents lungs alone where the pressure gradient is alveolar minus intrathoracic (transmural). The third section relates to chest wall alone for which the pressure gradient is intrathoracic minus ambient. There are only insignificant differences between observations during anaesthesia with and without paralysis. There are, however, major differences in pressure/volume relationships of the lung and whole system following the induction of anaesthesia. Arrows indicate the FRC while conscious and during anaesthesia. The curves meet at a lung volume close to the residual volume. (Redrawn from the data of Westbrook et al. (1973), except that the subatmospheric extensions of the curves for the lungs plus chest wall have been derived from other sources)

The left-hand section shows the relationship for the whole respiratory system comprising lungs plus chest wall. The curves obtained during anaesthesia clearly show the reduction in FRC (lung volume with zero pressure gradient from alveoli to ambient). The subatmospheric section of the curve also shows the very small volume change which can be achieved by application of a subatmospheric pressure to the airway of an anaesthetized patient. This implies a very low expiratory reserve volume. Application of a positive pressure as high as 3 kPa (30 cmH$_2$O) to the airways expands the lungs to barely 70 per cent of the preoperative total lung capacity, which implies a reduced overall compliance. The two sections of *Figure 19.11* on the right show that the major changes are in the lung rather than the chest wall.

The reduction in total respiratory compliance during anaesthesia has been known for many years and *Table 19.3* lists consensus values based on the review of Rehder, Sessler and Marsh (1975). Compliance appears to be reduced very early in anaesthesia and the change is not progressive. The change appears to be due to a reduction in pulmonary compliance, the cause of which has been difficult to explain.

Table 19.3 Values for compliance in anaesthetized and paralysed subjects

		l/kPa	*ml/cmH$_2$O*
Lungs	static	1.5	150
	dynamic	1.0	100
Chest wall		2.0	200
Total compliance	static	0.85	85
	dynamic	0.6	60

These values represent a reasonable mean from a large number of studies in anaesthetized patients reviewed by Rehder, Sessler and Marsh (1975).

There is no general agreement on a direct effect of anaesthetics on the pulmonary surfactant. The study of Pattle, Schock and Battensby (1972) suggested that anaesthesia does not alter pulmonary compliance although Forrest (1972) demonstrated decreased surfactant activity in the lung of the hyperventilated guinea-pig. Woo, Berlin and Hedley-Whyte (1969) showed that ventilation of excised dogs' lungs with air containing 1.2% halothane produced small but significant decreases of compliance. They showed that no such changes occurred when the lungs were filled with liquid, and concluded that the anaesthetic might have altered surfactant function. Stanley, Zikria and Sullivan (1972) found that halothane and cyclopropane increased the minimal surface tension of tracheobronchial aspirations from a series of patients. None of this evidence is entirely convincing.

An alternative explanation is that the reduced lung compliance is the consequence of breathing at reduced lung volume (Schmidt and Rehder, 1981). Caro, Butler and DuBois (1960) and also Scheidt, Hyatt and Rehder (1981) strapped the chest of volunteers, thereby decreasing their lung volume, and found that this resulted in a decrease in pulmonary compliance which could be restored to normal by taking a maximal inspiration. The latter observation raised the question that pulmonary collapse may have played a part in their experiment. The conflicting evidence for the existence of pulmonary collapse during anaesthesia is reviewed above under the heading of airway closure.

A third view is that the reduction in pulmonary compliance is the primary cause and not the effect of the reduction in FRC. The change in the end-expiratory electrical activity of the diaphragm (see above) would seem to refute this hypothesis.

Metabolic rate

During anaesthesia, the metabolic rate is reduced about 15 per cent below basal according to the conventional standards of Aub and DuBois (1917) and Boothby and Sandiford (1924). However, these standards do not stipulate sedation or any period of rest. Robertson and Reid proposed new standards for metabolic rate in 1952, based on three hours' rest, with or without sedation. Their values are about 15 per cent below the conventional standards and so correspond fairly closely to those of the anaesthetized patient (Nunn and Matthews, 1959). *Table 19.4* lists expected values for oxygen consumption and carbon dioxide output during uncomplicated anaesthesia at normal body temperature (mean 36.5°C). In comparison with the conscious subject there are major reductions in cerebral and cardiac oxygen consumptions during anaesthesia.

Table 19.4 Predicted values for oxygen consumption and carbon dioxide output during uncomplicated anaesthesia (ml/min) (STPD)

Age	Oxygen consumption			Carbon dioxide		
	Small patient	*Average patient*	*Large patient*	*Small patient*	*Average patient*	*Large patient*
Male						
14–15		190			152	
16–17		200			160	
18–19	168	210	252	134	168	202
20–29	162	203	243	130	162	194
30–39	162	203	243	130	162	194
40–49	158	198	237	126	158	190
50–59	155	194	233	124	155	186
60–69	150	187	224	120	159	179
Female						
14–15		174			139	
16–17		188			150	
18–19	156	194	233	125	155	186
20–29	152	190	228	122	152	182
30–39	150	187	224	120	150	179
40–49	148	184	221	118	147	177
50–59	144	180	216	115	144	173
60–69	140	175	210	112	140	168

Values for CO_2 output will apply only in a steady respiratory state.
Values are probably about 6 per cent lower during artificial ventilation.
Figures are based on 85 per cent of basal according to data of Aub and Dubois (1917) and Boothby and Sandiford (1924).

Gas exchange

There can be no doubt that, in all except very young patients, uncomplicated anaesthesia produces abnormalities of gas exchange. Under normal circumstances these changes pose no threat to the patient since their effects can easily be overcome by such simple means as increasing the concentration of oxygen in the inspired gas. These normal changes may be contrasted with a range of pathological alterations in gas exchange which may arise during anaesthesia from such circumstances as bronchial intubation, tension pneumothorax, gross hypotension and apnoea. These may be life threatening and require urgent action for their correction.

The major changes which adversely affect gas exchange during anaesthesia are:

1. Reduced minute volume of ventilation.
2. Increased dead space.
3. Increased shunt.

The first will be considered separately while the last two will be considered in relation to the three-compartment model of gas exchange.

Minute volume of ventilation

During anaesthesia with spontaneous breathing, the minute volume may remain normal but it is usually decreased. This is due partly to the reduction in oxygen consumption but mainly to the interference with chemical control of breathing as described above in this chapter. In an uncomplicated anaesthetic, there should not be sufficient resistance to breathing to affect the minute volume. However, the minute volume may be much decreased if there is overt respiratory obstruction. Causes of respiratory obstruction are outlined in Chapter 3 and will not be considered further here.

If the patient is permitted to breathe spontaneously during anaesthesia, the minute volume may decrease to very low levels, particularly in the absence of surgical stimulation. Thus, for example, Nunn (1964) reported 3 patients out of 27 with a minute volume of less than 3 l/min. This will inevitably result in hypercapnia which, in the various studies of the author, has ranged up to almost 10 kPa (75 mmHg). Clearly there is no limit to the rise which may occur if the anaesthetist is prepared to tolerate gross hypoventilation, and Birt and Cole (1965) reported arterial P_{CO_2} values up to 20 kPa (150 mmHg) during closed circuit halothane anaesthesia (not administered by the authors!).

There are anaesthetists in many parts of the world, including the UK, who do not believe that temporary hypercapnia during anaesthesia is harmful to a healthy patient. Under normal circumstances, arterial P_{CO_2} rapidly returns to normal in the postoperative period (Nunn and Payne, 1962). Vast numbers of patients have been subjected to this transient physiological insult since 1846 and there seems to be no convincing evidence of harm resulting from it, except perhaps increased bleeding from the incision. In other parts of the world, particularly the USA, the departure from physiological normality is regarded with concern and it is usual to assist spontaneous respiration by manual compression of the reservoir bag.

Quite different conditions apply during anaesthesia with artificial ventilation. The minute volume can then be set at any level which seems appropriate to the anaesthetist. Values up to 17.5 l/min were recorded during routine anaesthesia with manual ventilation (Nunn, 1958a). Hypocapnia almost invariably results from hyperventilation during anaesthesia. Observed values extend from the normal range down to about 2.4 kPa (18 mmHg) in the course of routine anaesthesia. Without measurement of P_{CO_2}, there is a natural tendency to hyperventilate the patient. Again it has proved difficult to demonstrate that hypocapnia does any significant harm during anaesthesia but most anaesthetists tend to avoid extreme hypocapnia because of its effects on cerebral blood flow (page 462). There is some consensus that one should aim for an arterial Pco_2 of about 4.5 kPa (34 mmHg). Hypothermia, either intentional or accidental, may result in severe hypocapnia unless the minute volume is reduced in accord with the reduced metabolic rate.

The three-compartment model of gas exchange

This model has been described on pages 154 et seq. It is a favourite of the author, not because he is under any illusions that it is a correct representation of affairs, but because it is capable of precise definition and it is of direct relevance to therapy.

In essence this model (see *Figure 7.7*) presents the lung as though it comprised three compartments—ideally perfused and ventilated alveoli, alveolar dead space and shunt. Physiological dead space is quantified by the Bohr equation (page 163) and shunt by the shunt equation (page 168), with or without direct measurement of the mixed venous oxygen content.

Physiological dead space

The increase in physiological dead space during anaesthesia was first observed by Campbell, Nunn and Peckett in 1958 and subsequently confirmed in many studies. With allowance for the apparatus dead space of the tracheal tube and its connections, the dead space/tidal volume ratio from carina downwards averages 32 per cent during anaesthesia with either spontaneous or artificial ventilation (Nunn and Hill, 1960). This corresponds closely to the ratio for the normal conscious subject *including* trachea, pharynx and mouth (approximately 70 ml) (Nunn, Campbell and Peckett, 1959). Therefore, it follows that the subcarinal dead space must increase by about 70 ml during anaesthesia. It was then shown that this was in the physiological, but not the anatomical, dead space and must therefore be in the alveolar component (Nunn and Hill, 1960). There is no measurable difference between physiological and anatomical dead space in the normal conscious subject.

Figure 19.12 shows the physiological dead space approximating to a third of tidal volume over a wide range of tidal volumes. Anatomical dead space was always significantly less than physiological, reaching a maximum of about 70 ml at a tidal volume above 350 ml. This roughly accords with the expected geometric dimensions of the lower respiratory tract. At smaller tidal volumes, the anatomical dead space was less than the expected geometric volume. Values of less than 30 ml were recorded in some patients with a tidal volume less than 250 ml. This is attributed to axial streaming and the mixing effect of the heart beat (page 161), and is clearly an important and beneficial factor in patients with depressed breathing.

For practical purposes the apparatus dead space of the tracheal tube and its connections must be added for the purpose of calculating alveolar ventilation during anaesthesia. The total dead space then increases to a mean of 50 per cent of tidal volume (*Figure 19.13*). If the trachea is not intubated, it is necessary to add the volume of the facemask and its connections to the physiological dead space, which now includes trachea, pharynx and mouth. The total dead space then amounts to about two-thirds of the tidal volume (Kain, Panday and Nunn, 1969). Thus, a seemingly adequate minute volume of 6 l/min may be expected to result in an

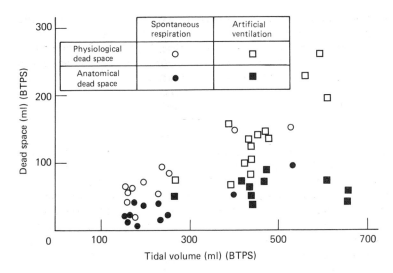

Figure 19.12 Anatomical and physiological dead space as a function of tidal volume in anaesthetized patients with tracheal intubation. (Reproduced from Nunn and Hill (1960) by permission of the Editors of the Journal of Applied Physiology)

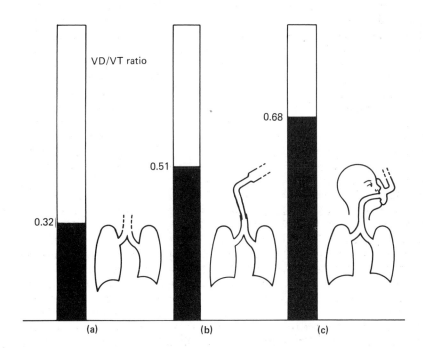

Figure 19.13 Physiological plus apparatus dead space (where applicable) as a fraction of tidal volume in anaesthetized patients: (a) from carina downards; (b) including tracheal tube and connector; and (c) including upper airway, facemask and connector.

alveolar ventilation of only 2 l/min, which would almost inevitably result in hypercapnia.

The cause of the increase in alveolar dead space during anaesthesia is not immediately obvious. There is no evidence that it is due to pulmonary hypotension causing development of a zone 1 (page 131) and the supine position would militate against this. The alternative explanation is relative maldistribution with overventilation of underperfused alveoli. Studies of ventilation/perfusion relationships (see below) lend support to this view but the evidence is not wholly convincing.

Compensation for increased dead space may be made by increasing the minute volume to maintain the alveolar ventilation. In practice, the problem hardly exists. The artificially ventilated anaesthetized patient may have a large dead space but the high minute volume usually provides more than adequate compensation, so that the alveolar ventilation is commonly greater than necessary for carbon dioxide homoeostasis. In the case of the hypoventilating patient who is allowed to breathe spontaneously during anaesthesia, the reduction in dead space (see *Figure 19.12*) prevents some of the expected reduction in alveolar ventilation. This, together with the reduced metabolic rate, results in the hypercapnia being very much less than the figures for minute volume might lead one to expect. No doubt, over the years, many patients have owed their lives to these factors.

Shunt

In the conscious healthy subject, the shunt or venous admixture amounts to only 1–2 per cent of cardiac output and this results in an alveolar/arterial P_{O_2} gradient of less than 1 kPa (7.5 mmHg) in the young healthy subject breathing air but the gradient increases with age. During anaesthesia, the alveolar/arterial P_{O_2} difference is usually increased to a value which corresponds to a shunt of about 10 per cent. *Figure 19.14* shows the mean values of a large number of different studies plotted on the iso-shunt diagram which is explained in detail on page 170. In fact, formal measurements of pulmonary venous admixture have been made (*Table 19.5*) and these show that the shunts really are of the order of 10 per cent. This provides an acceptable basis for predicting arterial P_{O_2} during an uncomplicated anaesthetic and also to calculate the concentration of oxygen in the inspired gas which will provide an acceptable arterial P_{O_2}. Some 30–40% inspired oxygen is usually adequate in an uncomplicated anaesthetic.

The cause of the venous admixture has long been debated and is still not definite. The likelihood of pulmonary collapse occurring during anaesthesia was discussed earlier in this chapter and, in the section on ventilation/perfusion relationships, it will be seen that there is evidence for the development of areas of relative as well as absolute underventilation during anaesthesia. Another factor is interference with the pulmonary hypoxic vasoconstrictor reflex which would impair the matching of perfusion to ventilation. It is quite likely that all of these mechanisms play a part to a varying extent in different patients.

Effect of age. There is minimal change of shunt or alveolar/arterial P_{O_2} gradient following induction of anaesthesia in young adults (Taylor, Scott and Donald, 1964). Progressively larger changes occur as age increases (Nunn, Bergman and Coleman, 1965; Hewlett et al., 1974c). It is tempting to believe that this is related to the increased closing capacity in older patients.

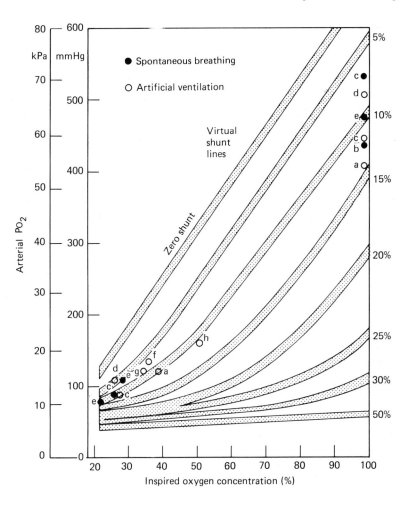

Figure 19.14 Mean values for arterial PO$_2$ are plotted against inspired oxygen concentrations for 15 published studies of anaesthetized patients, using the same co-ordinates as in Figure *7.11. (a) Michenfelder, Fowler and Theye, 1966; (b) Marshall et al., 1969; (c) Price et al., 1969; (d) Nunn, Bergman and Coleman, 1965; (e) Nunn, 1964; (f) Hewlett et al., 1974c; (g) Theye and Tuohy, 1964a; (h) Gold and Helrich, 1967.*

Effect of positive end-expiratory pressure (PEEP). It has long been known that, in contrast to the situation in intensive care, PEEP does little to improve the arterial PO$_2$ during anaesthesia (Nunn, Bergman and Coleman, 1965). The work of Colgan, Barrow and Fanning (1971) in dogs suggested that, although the shunt might be reduced, the associated decrease in the cardiac output reduced the saturation of the blood traversing the remaining shunt and so the arterial PO$_2$ was unaltered. This was in fact demonstrated in anaesthetized man by Bindslev and his colleagues (1981)—see below. The essential difference from the patient undergoing intensive care is probably the lack of protection from intrathoracic pressure changes which are afforded by stiff lungs in most patients undergoing therapy in intensive care.

Table 19.5 Values for pulmonary venous admixture measured during anaesthesia in man

Reference	Circumstances	F_{IO_2} (%)	$\dot{Q}s/\dot{Q}t$ (%)
Michenfelder, Fowler and Theye (1966)	Artificial ventilation	40*	10.2
	Inhalational anaesthesia	100*	13.7
Price et al. (1969)	Conscious controls	25	5.9
	before anesthesia	100	3.1
	Halothane anaesthesia	25	18.9
	spontaneous respiration	98.5	6.1
	Halothane anaesthesia	25	15.1
	artificial ventilation	98.5	11.1
	Conscious controls	25	2.5
	before anesthesia	80	2.0
	Cyclopropane anesthesia	25	11.3
	(spont. and artif. vent.)	80	7.9
	Halothane + N_2O anaesth.	28	10.0
	(spont. and artif. vent.)		
Marshall et al. (1969)	Conscious controls	100	4.4
	before anesthesia		
	Halothane anesthesia:		
	30 minutes after induction	100*	12.1
	3 1/2 hours after induction	100*	14.8
	30 minutes after anaesthesia	100	6.5
	3 hours after anaesthesia	100	5.2

*These values were slightly reduced by the addition of unspecified concentrations of halothane or other inhalational anaesthetics.

Ventilation/perfusion relationships

The three-compartment model of the lung provides a definition of lung function in terms of dead space and shunt, parameters which are reproducible and provide a basis for corrective therapy. Nevertheless, it does not pretend to provide a true picture of what is going on in the lung. It simply presents gas and blood gas data in terms of the dead space and shunt which would be required to yield the same results.

A far more sophisticated approach is provided by the analysis of the distribution of pulmonary ventilation and perfusion in terms of ventilation/perfusion ratios. This complex and challenging technique is outlined on pages 181 et seq., and the present section describes the changes which have been reported during anaesthesia. At the time of writing, there have been three studies, conducted respectively in young fit subjects (Rehder et al., 1979), typical surgical patients (Bindslev et al., 1981) and elderly patients with respiratory pathology (Dueck et al., 1980). In addition, Prutow et al. (1982) have presented a study of young surgical patients in abstract.

Rehder's group studied young healthy volunteers and both ventilation and perfusion were found to be distributed to a wider range of ventilation/perfusion ratios after induction of anaesthesia and paralysis (*Figure 19.15*). The true intrapulmonary shunt had a mean value of less than 1 per cent during anaesthesia but the alveolar/arterial P_{O_2} gradient was slightly increased and this was attributed to the increased spread of the distribution of perfusion to areas of poorer ventilation (lower

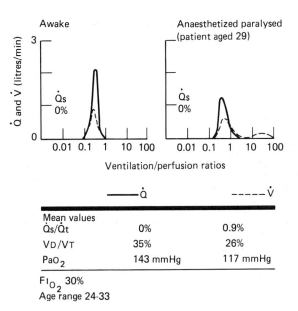

Mean values	$\dot{Q}$	$\dot{V}$
$\dot{Q}s/\dot{Q}t$	0%	0.9%
V_D/V_T	35%	26%
PaO_2	143 mmHg	117 mmHg

FI_{O_2} 30%
Age range 24-33

Figure 19.15 Distribution of ventilation and perfusion as a function of ventilation/perfusion ratios in the awake and anaesthetized paralysed subject. (Adapted from Rehder et al. (1979) and reproduced from Nunn (1985a) by permission of the publishers)

ventilation/perfusion ratio). Anatomical dead space was reduced, largely because of tracheal intubation, but alveolar dead space was increased, partly due to increased spread of distribution of ventilation to areas of poorer perfusion (higher ventilation/perfusion ratio). In a group of surgical patients of similar age range to Rehder's volunteers, Prutow et al. (1982) found an average increase in shunt of 8 per cent during anaesthesia. Pulmonary blood flow to areas of zero and low $\dot{V}/\dot{Q}$ correlated with the reduction in FRC.

Bindslev's group studied typical surgical patients with ages ranging from 37 to 64. They were studied awake, anaesthetized and breathing spontaneously, anaesthetized paralysed and ventilated artificially and finally with PEEP (*Figure 19.16* and *Table 19.6*). In this group of older patients, they found that the true intrapulmonary shunt was increased during anaesthesia. However, the shunt calculated from the alveolar/arterial PO_2 gradient according to the three-compartment lung model would be larger still and the difference would be due to perfusion of areas of low ventilation/perfusion ratio. The dead space/tidal volume ratio was increased during anaesthesia in spite of the tracheal tube bypassing the upper airway. PEEP reduced the shunt but also reduced the cardiac output and therefore the mixed venous oxygen content. The decreased admixture of more desaturated blood resulted in virtually no change in arterial PO_2.

Dueck's group studied elderly patients (mean age 60) who all had some deterioration in pulmonary function. His results can most easily be appreciated by considering the patients in three groups (*Figure 19.17*). In the first, there was only a small increase in the true shunt following the induction of anaesthesia but there appeared a 'shelf' of perfusion of regions of very low ventilation/perfusion ratios in the range 0.01–0.1. In the second group, this 'shelf' was less prominent but there

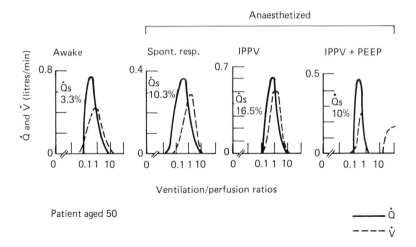

Figure 19.16 Typical changes in distribution of ventilation and perfusion as a function of ventilation/ perfusion ratios during anaesthesia in a middle-aged patient. IPPV, intermittent positive pressure ventilation; PEEP, positive end-expiratory pressure: Q̇, perfusion; V̇, ventilation; Q̇s, shunt. (Adapted from Bindslev et al. (1981) and reproduced from Nunn (1985a) by permission of the publishers)

TAble 19.6 Changes in factors influencing gas exchange after induction of anaesthesia

	Awake	Anaesthesia		
		Spont. vent.	IPPV	IPPV + PEEP
F_{IO_2}	0.21	0.4	0.4	0.4
$\dot{Q}s/\dot{Q}t$ (%)	1.6	6.2	8.6	4.1
V_D/V_T (%)	30	35	38	44
Cardiac output (l/min)	6.1	5.0	4.5	3.7
Pa_{O_2} (kPa)	10.5	17.6	18.8	20.5
V − mean $\dot{V}/\dot{Q}$	0.81	1.30	2.20	3.03
Q − mean $\dot{V}/\dot{Q}$	0.47	0.51	0.83	0.55

(Adapted from Bindslev et al. (1981) and reproduced from Nunn (1985a) by permission of the publishers)

was a substantial increase in true shunt. Finally, in the third group, there was both a 'shelf' and an increase in true shunt. All of these changes are compatible with a decrease in FRC below closing capacity.

These three studies of ventilation/perfusion relationships during anaesthesia complement one another and give us greatly increased insight into the effect of anaesthesia on gas exchange. We are now in a position to summarize the effect of anaesthesia on gas exchange as follows:

1. Changes in alveolar/arterial P_{O_2} gradient are markedly affected by age, being minimal in the young.

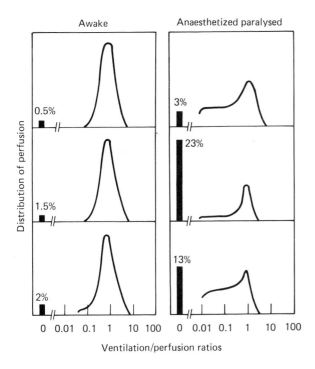

Figure 19.17 Changes in pulmonary perfusion as a function of ventilation/perfusion ratios following induction of anaesthesia in elderly patients. Numbers to the left of each block indicate the shunt. (Adapted from Dueck et al. (1980) and reproduced from Nunn (1985a) by permission of the publishers

2. The increase in alveolar/arterial P_{O_2} gradient is due partly to an increase in true intrapulmonary shunt and partly to increased distribution of perfusion to areas of low (but not zero) ventilation/perfusion ratios.
3. The increase in alveolar dead space appears to be due to increased distribution of ventilation to areas of high (but not usually infinite) ventilation/perfusion ratios.
4. The major differences are between the awake and the anaesthetized states. Paralysis and artificial ventilation do not greatly alter the parameters of gas exchange in spite of the quite different spatial distribution of ventilation.
5. PEEP reduces the shunt but the beneficial effect on arterial P_{O_2} is offset by the decrease in cardiac output which reduces the mixed venous oxygen content.

All of these main conclusions had been tentatively drawn from studies of the effect of anaesthesia on the parameters of the three-compartment lung model. However, these direct studies of ventilation/perfusion relationships have permitted inference to be replaced by direct observation and we can now speak with a level of certainty which was not previously possible.

Effect of hypoxic pulmonary vasoconstriction

Hypoxia causes an increase in pulmonary vascular resistance (see Chapter 6, pages 127 et seq.). When confined to a single lung or localized areas of lung, hypoxic pulmonary vasoconstriction (HPV) appears to be an important mechanism for reducing the perfusion of inadequately ventilated lung and so, within limits, optimizes the relative distribution of ventilation and perfusion. When HPV is abolished by vasodilators, shunting and arterial P_{O_2} are worsened (Marshall and Marshall, 1985).

Thilenius (1966), working with dogs, suggested that anaesthetics might interfere with HPV. Several inhalational anaesthetics were then found to inhibit HPV in the isolated lungs of both dog and cat (Sykes et al., 1972). These observations were amply confirmed in many laboratories throughout the world, but no such effect was found with intravenous anaesthetics (Bjertnaes, 1977).

Further studies in the intact animal followed and are reviewed by Sykes (1986). Intravenous anaesthetic agents were again found to be without effect but studies with inhalational anaesthetics gave results which were apparently conflicting. Some studies showed that inhalational anaesthetics increased the pulmonary blood flow through hypoxic areas of lung (i.e. blocking of HPV), while others showed no change. Some even showed a decrease in flow through hypoxic lung, suggesting that the anaesthetics had actually augmented HPV. The confusion appears to be due to the concomitant effect of anaesthetics on cardiac output. In Chapter 6 (pages 127 et seq.) it was explained how pulmonary vascular resistance is governed not only by the alveolar P_{O_2} but also, in part, by the mixed venous P_{O_2}. A reduction in cardiac output must decrease the mixed venous P_{O_2} if oxygen consumption remains unchanged, and this would intensify pulmonary vasoconstriction. Thus an inhalational anaesthetic will inhibit HPV by direct action on the one hand while, on the other hand, it may intensify HPV by reducing mixed venous P_{O_2} as a result of decreasing cardiac output. Marshall and Marshall (1985) have analysed the results of studies by many different authors and shown that their results are consistent with the view that inhalational anaesthetics depress HPV provided that allowance is made for the effect of concomitant changes of cardiac output.

Special conditions arising during anaesthesia

Lateral position

In Chapter 7 it was explained that, in the lateral position, there is preferential distribution of inspired gas to the lower lung (see *Table 7.1*) and this accords approximately with the distribution of pulmonary blood flow. This favourable distribution of inspired gas is disturbed by anaesthesia whether respiration is spontaneous or artificial in the paralysed patient (Rehder et al., 1972; Rehder and Sessler, 1973). The dependent lung volume is much reduced (see *Figure 5.2*) and is often below its closing capacity. It is therefore liable to absorption collapse (Potgieter, 1959).

Thoracotomy
(see review by Gothard and Branthwaite, 1984)

In the early days of thoracic surgery it was commonplace to maintain spontaneous respiration. This resulted in pendulum breathing between the two lungs and routine arterial P_{CO_2} values were recorded in excess of 30 kPa (225 mmHg) apparently without evidence of overt harm to the patients (Ellison, Ellison and Hamilton, 1955). Spontaneous breathing with an open chest but without pendulum breathing can be achieved by collapse of the exposed lung, but at the cost of severe shunting.

It took many years to realize that the solution to the open chest was IPPV. However, when one side of the chest is opened, the exposed lung may receive a very large proportion of the total ventilation during IPPV (Nunn, 1961a). Since the patient is commonly in the lateral position, there will then be a gross mismatch between the overventilated upper and exposed lung and the overperfused lower lung. However, surgical intervention will commonly restrict the ventilation of the upper exposed lung, either by retraction of the lung or by obstruction of the bronchi.

One-lung anaesthesia. The surgeon may find his task is simplified by total collapse of the upper (exposed) lung. This is usually achieved by the use of a double-lumen tracheal tube, with the lumen connecting to the exposed lung left open to atmosphere. Although pulmonary blood flow through the collapsed lung is reduced, it is not zero (page 130) and there is inevitably a substantial shunt (Khanam and Branthwaite, 1973; Kerr et al., 1974; Katz et al., 1982). There is seldom difficulty in maintaining a satisfactory P_{CO_2} but oxygenation is usually compromised. Hypoxia may be minimized by restricting the duration of one-lung anaesthesia and by increasing the inspired oxygen concentration. However, the use of even 99% oxygen does not always guarantee a normal arterial P_{O_2}, and PEEP applied to the ventilated lung usually reduces the arterial P_{O_2} further (Katz et al., 1982). A better solution seems to be the application of oxygen at continuous positive pressure to the non-ventilated lung (Benumof, 1982).

Haemorrhagic hypotension

Physiological dead space is increased in haemorrhagic hypotension (Gerst, Rattenborg and Holaday, 1959; Freeman and Nunn, 1963) and also when hypotension is induced by ganglion blockade (Eckenhoff et al., 1963). The obvious explanation is pulmonary hypotension causing failure of perfusion of the uppermost parts of the lung fields. However, this has not yet been convincingly demonstrated. Both Gerst and colleagues and Freeman and Nunn found no evidence of increased shunting during haemorrhagic hypotension. This is one of the examples of pulmonary shunting being in direct proportion to cardiac output (page 173).

The postoperative period

The increased alveolar/arterial P_{O_2} gradient observed during anaesthesia usually returns to normal during the first few hours after minor operations (Nunn and Payne, 1962). In the first few minutes of recovery, alveolar P_{O_2} may be reduced by elimination of nitrous oxide which dilutes alveolar oxygen and carbon dioxide (page 224). Shivering in the early postoperative period causes a large increase in oxygen consumption, which requires a corresponding increase in minute volume (Bay, Nunn and Prys-Roberts, 1968).

Following major surgery, the restoration of a normal alveolar/arterial P_{O_2} gradient may take a few days and this is associated with a continued reduction in FRC (Alexander et al., 1973).

Note added in proof

An important paper by Tokics and his colleagues (*Anesthesiology*, 1987, **66**, 157) related lung opacities, visualized by computerized tomography, to the distribution of ventilation/perfusion ratios measured by the multiple inert gas wash-out technique. Following induction of anaesthesia, paralysis and artificial ventilation, mean shunt increased from 1.2 per cent to 6.5 per cent. The magnitude of the shunt correlated significantly with the size of opacities in the dependent parts of the lung field ($r = 0.84$). It was concluded that the development of collapse in dependent lung regions was a major cause of gas exchange impairment during halothane anaesthesia, with both spontaneous breathing and mechanical ventilation. PEEP decreased the areas of collapse but not necessarily the shunt, and did not improve arterial P_{O_2}. Lung collapse was present but less marked during anaesthesia with spontaneous breathing. Under these conditions there was substantial distribution of ventilation to areas of high ventilation/perfusion ratios (>10), and dead space (including apparatus) was 71.6 per cent of tidal volume before tracheal intubation.

Chapter 20

Ventilatory failure

Ventilatory failure is defined as a pathological reduction of the alveolar ventilation below the level required for the maintenance of normal arterial blood gas tensions. Mean of the normal arterial P_{CO_2} is 5.1 kPa (38.3 mmHg) with 95 per cent limits (2 s.d.) of $\pm$ 1.0 kPa (7.5 mmHg)(page 225). The normal arterial P_{O_2} is more difficult to define since it decreases with age (page 270). Furthermore, the arterial P_{O_2} is strongly influenced by the concentration of oxygen in the inspired gas and therefore cannot be interpreted unless the inspired oxygen concentration is known. Arterial P_{O_2} is also strongly influenced by shunting (page 172) and the adequacy of ventilation is therefore best defined by the arterial P_{CO_2}.

Pattern of changes in arterial blood gas tensions

Figure 20.1 shows, on a P_{O_2}/P_{CO_2} diagram, the typical pattern of deterioration of arterial blood gas tensions in ventilatory failure. The shaded area indicates the normal range of tensions with increasing age corresponding to a leftward shift. Pure ventilatory failure in a young person with otherwise normal lungs would result in changes along the broken line. However, chronic obstructive airway disease, the commonest cause of ventilatory failure, has been observed to result in blood gas changes within the upper arrow in *Figure 20.1* (Refsum, 1963; McNicol and Campbell, 1965). The limit of survival, while breathing air, is reached at a P_{O_2} of about 2.7 kPa (20 mmHg) and P_{CO_2} 11 kPa (83 mmHg). The limiting factor is not P_{CO_2} but P_{O_2}. This prevents the rise of P_{CO_2} to higher levels except when the patient's inspired oxygen concentration is increased. It may also be raised above 11 kPa by the inhalation of carbon dioxide. In either event, a P_{CO_2} in excess of 11 kPa may be considered an iatrogenic disorder. *Figure 20.1* also shows the pattern of blood gas changes in the case of shunting or pulmonary venous admixture. This is explained and discussed in detail on pages 249 et seq.

In general the arterial P_{O_2} indicates the severity of respiratory failure (assuming that the patient is breathing air), while the P_{CO_2} indicates the differential diagnosis between ventilatory failure and shunting as shown in *Figure 20.1*. It is, of course, possible to have coexistence of ventilatory failure and shunting in the same patient.

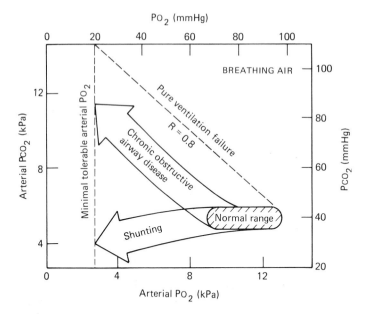

Figure 20.1 Pattern of deterioration of arterial blood gases in chronic obstructive airway disease and pulmonary shunting. The shaded area indicates the normal range of arterial blood gas tensions in which Po_2 *decreases with age. The oblique broken line shows the theoretical changes in alveolar* Po_2 *and* Pco_2 *resulting from pure ventilatory failure. In chronic obstructive airway disease, the arterial* Po_2 *is always less than the value which would be expected in pure ventilatory failure at the same* Pco_2 *value. Discussion of shunting is to be found in Chapter 7.*

Time course of changes in blood gas tensions in acute ventilatory failure

Although the upper arrow in *Figure 20.1* shows the effect of chronic ventilatory failure on arterial blood gas tensions, short-term deviations from this pattern occur in acute ventilatory failure. This is because the time courses of changes of Po_2 and Pco_2 in response to acute changes in ventilation are entirely different.

Body stores of oxygen are small amounting to about 1550 ml, while breathing air, which corresponds to only 6 minutes' consumption at basal metabolic rate. Therefore, following a step change in the level of alveolar ventilation, the arterial Po_2 rapidly assumes its new value (as shown in *Figure 5.8*) and the half-time for the change is only 30 seconds (see page 271 and *Figure 10.18*). In contrast, the body stores of carbon dioxide are very large and of the order of 120 litres or about 600 minutes of the basal output. Therefore, following a step change in the level of alveolar ventilation, the arterial Pco_2 only slowly assumes the new value indicated in *Figure 5.8*. The time course is slower following a reduction of ventilation than an increase (see page 226 and *Figure 9.11*) and the half-time of rise of Pco_2 following a step reduction of ventilation is of the order of 16 minutes.

The practical point is that, during this transient phase of acute hypoventilation, there may be a low Po_2 while the Pco_2 is still within the normal range. This breaks the rule that the Pco_2 is the essential index of alveolar ventilation and it may be erroneously believed that the diagnosis is shunting rather than hypoventilation. Note that, during the acute phase of hypoventilation, the respiratory exchange ratio may fall far below its metabolic level as the carbon dioxide production is partly diverted into the body carbon dioxide stores and so does not appear in the expired air.

Acid–base changes

An acute increase in arterial P_{CO_2} results in respiratory acidosis with the relationship between P_{CO_2} and pH defined by the whole-body CO_2 equilibration curve which approximates to that of blood with a haemoglobin concentration of 10 g/dl (see page 216 and *Figure 9.5*). Chronic respiratory acidosis results in partial compensation of blood pH by increase in the plasma bicarbonate level which is best quantified as the base excess.

Causes of failure of ventilation

Most of the causes of failure of ventilation have been mentioned in the first part of this book. This section reviews and classifies the causes of failure. They may be conveniently considered under the headings of the anatomical sites where they arise.These sites are indicated in *Figure 20.2*. Lesions or malfunctions at sites A to E result in a reduction of input to the respiratory muscles. Dyspnoea may not be apparent and the diagnosis of ventilatory failure may be overlooked on clinical inspection of the patient. Lesions or malfunctions at sites G to I result in evident dyspnoea and no one is likely to miss the diagnosis of hypoventilation. The various sites will now be considered individually.

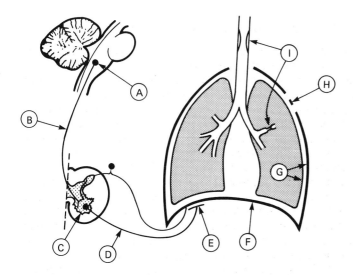

Figure 20.2 Summary of sites at which lesions, drug action or malfunction may result in ventilatory failure. (A) The 'respiratory centre'. (B) Upper motoneurone. (C) Anterior horn cell. (D) Lower motoneurone. (E) The neuromuscular junction. (F) The respiratory muscles. (G) Altered elasticity of lungs or chest wall. (H) Loss of structural integrity of chest wall and pleural cavity. (I) Increased airway resistance.

A: The respiratory neurones of the medulla are depressed by hypoxia and also by very high levels of P_{CO_2}, probably of the order of 40 kPa (300 mmHg) in the healthy unanaesthetized subject but at a lower P_{CO_2} in the presence of anaesthetics or narcotic drugs. Reduction of P_{CO_2} below the apnoeic threshold results in apnoea in the unconscious subject but usually not in the conscious subject (page 75). Loss of respiratory sensitivity to carbon dioxide occurs in various types of chronic ventilatory failure, particularly chronic bronchitis (the 'blue bloater'). Such patients tend to rely on their hypoxic drive to maintain ventilation. If this is abolished, as, for example, by the administration of 100% oxygen or anaesthesia, gross hypoventilation or apnoea may result (*Figure 20.3*).

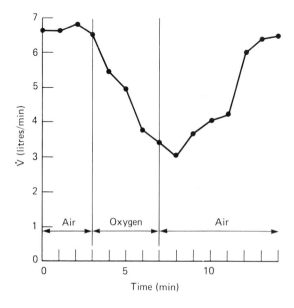

Figure 20.3 Rapid onset of hypoventilation when a patient with chronic hypercapnia and loss of chemoreceptor sensitivity to carbon dioxide breathed 100% oxygen. (Nunn, unpublished data)

A wide variety of drugs may cause central apnoea or respiratory depression and these include opiates, barbiturates and all anaesthetic agents. Reflex apnoea may follow noxious stimuli but the Hering–Breuer inflation reflex is weak in man and lung inflation does not normally cause apnoea (Widdicombe, 1961).

Finally, it should be noted that the respiratory neurones may be affected by anything which affects their blood supply, including pressure, trauma, neoplasm or vascular catastrophe.

B: The upper motoneurones serving the respiratory muscles are most likely to be interrupted by trauma. Only lesions above cervical 3–4 will affect the phrenic nerve and result in total apnoea. However, fracture dislocations of the lower cervical vertebrae are relatively common and result in loss of action of the intercostal and expiratory muscles while sparing the diaphragm. Upper motoneurones may be involved in various disease processes, including tumours, demyelination and, occasionally, in syringomyelia.

C: The anterior horn cell may be affected by various disease processes, of which the most important is poliomyelitis. Happily this condition is now rare in the developed world but it can produce any degree of respiratory involvement up to total paralysis of all respiratory muscles. Anterior horn cells are reversibly depressed by the drug mephenesin (Myanesin) which was formerly used to obtain relaxation in anaesthesia.

D: Lower motoneurones supplying the respiratory muscles are prone to normal traumatic risks and, in former times, the phrenic nerves were surgically interrupted for the treatment of pulmonary tuberculosis. Polyneuritis (e.g. Guillain–Barré syndrome) and motoneurone disease are the main conditions which may cause ventilatory failure at this level.

E: The neuromuscular junction is affected by myasthenia gravis and botulism. Drugs acting at this site include all the neuromuscular blocking agents used in anaesthesia and certain organophosphorus compounds and nerve gases. Procaine acts by preventing the synthesis of acetylcholine.

F: The respiratory muscles themselves are unlikely to be involved in any disease process which results in ventilatory failure. However, the efficiency of contraction of the diaphragm may be severely affected by 'splinting' due to abdominal distension or by flattening of the domes due, for example, to tension pneumothorax. The respiratory muscles may also become fatigued as a result of working against excessive impedance (Roussos and Macklem, 1983; Moxham, 1984). In dogs it has been shown that the administration of *Escherichia coli* endotoxin causes ventilatory failure in the presence of increased electrical activity in the respiratory muscles and unaltered respiratory impedance (Hussain, Simkus and Roussos, 1985). These authors concluded that ventilatory failure in endotoxic shock is due to enhanced fatigue in the respiratory muscles.

G: Loss of elasticity of the lungs or chest wall is a potent cause of ventilatory failure. It may arise within the lungs (e.g. pulmonary fibrosis, Hamman–Rich syndrome and respiratory distress syndrome), in the pleura (e.g. chronic empyema with fibrinous covering of the pleura), in the chest wall (e.g. kyphoscoliosis) or in the skin (e.g. contracted burn scars in children). However, it is frequently forgotten that seemingly mild pressures applied to the outside of the chest may seriously embarrass the breathing and even result in total apnoea. A sustained pressure of only 6 kPa (45 mmHg or a depth of 2 feet of water) is sufficient to prevent breathing. This is prone to occur when crowds get out of control on a staircase and people fall on top of one another. It may also occur when workers on a building site become buried under a load of sand or rubble.

H: Loss of structural integrity of the chest wall may result in ventilatory failure in the case of open pneumothorax where the reduction in overall minute volume is further complicated by pendulum breathing between the two lungs. Even if the parietal pleura is intact, ventilatory failure may result from multiple fractured ribs, a condition known as flail chest. This condition, resulting from impact on the steering wheel, was commonplace in the UK before the use of seat belts became compulsory. The condition was particularly amenable to treatment by artificial ventilation with intermittent positive pressure although some centres preferred conservative treatment with rib fixation.

Closed pneumothorax causes interference with ventilation in proportion to the quantity of air in the chest. Tension pneumothorax is a condition in which the pressure rises above atmospheric, collapsing the ipsilateral lung, displacing the mediastinum and partially collapsing the contralateral lung. Convexity of the diaphragm is lost and ventilation may be critically impaired. The diagnosis and correction of the condition is a matter of great urgency. Gross dyspnoea with deviation of trachea and displacement of the apex beat should always alert staff to the possibility of this condition.

I: Airway resistance remains the commonest and most important cause of ventilatory failure. The causes of increased airway resistance have been described in Chapter 3 (pages 54 et seq.) and will not be discussed any further here. However, the relationship between airway resistance and ventilatory failure is a complex subject which is considered further below. In the clinical field, airway resistance is seldom measured but is most often inferred from measurement of ventilatory capacity.

Increased dead space

Very rarely, a large increase in the respiratory dead space may be the cause of ventilatory failure. Minute volume will be increased but the alveolar ventilation is reduced and the patient presents with a high Pco_2 accompanied by a high minute volume. This may be distinguished from a hypermetabolic state either by measurement of carbon dioxide output or by measurement of the dead space (page 177). The dead space/tidal volume ratio should be above 65 per cent in this condition. An increase in the arterial/end-expiratory Pco_2 gradient (more than 2 kPa or 15 mmHg) indicates an increase in the alveolar dead space. This condition is caused by ventilation of large unperfused areas of the lungs, such as may be caused by air cysts communicating with the bronchus, pulmonary emboli or pulmonary hypotension. External or apparatus dead space also tends to reduce alveolar ventilation and may be added either intentionally or accidentally.

Relationship between ventilatory capacity and ventilatory failure

Appropriate tests for the measurement of ventilatory capacity are described on pages 115 et seq. A reduction in ventilatory capacity does not necessarily mean that a patient will be in ventilatory failure, and *Figure 20.4* drawn from data obtained by the author shows the lack of correlation between $FEV_{1.0}$ and Pco_2 in the range of $FEV_{1.0}$ 0.3–1.0 litre, a range which is grossly abnormal. Most of the patients represented in *Figure 20.4* have chronic obstructive airway disease and they may be very conveniently classified into 'pink puffers' and 'blue bloaters'. Those in the former category, predominantly with emphysema, maintain a considerable degree of respiratory sensitivity to carbon dioxide and struggle to keep a normal arterial Pco_2 for as long as possible. They are in evident dyspnoea and no one is likely to overlook the fact that they have a respiratory problem. Nevertheless, in spite of the distressing appearance of their respiratory exertions, their general condition is far more favourable than that of blue bloaters. Most of these patients suffer from chronic bronchitis but the author has seen at least one in whom the condition was related to poliomyelitis 20 years previously. The essential feature of the blue bloater is that he has lost his ventilatory sensitivity to carbon dioxide and

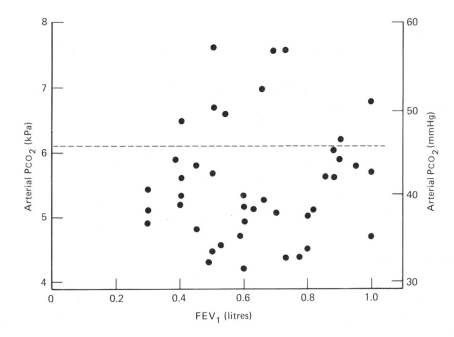

Figure 20.4 Lack of correlation between arterial P_{CO_2} and forced expiratory volume (1 second) in 44 patients with chronic obstructive airway disease. The broken line indicates the upper limit of normal for P_{CO_2}. (Nunn, unpublished data)

has allowed his P_{CO_2} to drift upwards. These patients rely on hypoxic drive for the maintenance of ventilation and are in a precarious state. Nevertheless, in the absence of dyspnoea, their appearance is deceptively tranquil and it is not immediately obvious that they are in ventilatory failure, yet their condition is more serious than that of the pink puffer.

Asthmatic patients tend to behave like pink puffers and, even in quite severe attacks of bronchospasm, maintain a normal or subnormal arterial P_{CO_2}. In an asthmatic, ventilatory failure, indicated by a rising P_{CO_2}, is a grave sign, indicating that he is no longer able to overcome the added airway resistance by increased work of breathing.

It should perhaps be stressed that the usual tests of ventilatory capacity depend on the expiratory muscles while the work of breathing is normally achieved by the inspiratory muscles. However, expiratory resistance is usually more important than inspiratory resistance because of the factors illustrated in *Figure 3.7*.

The relationship between metabolic demand and ventilatory failure

In renal failure, protein intake is a major factor in the onset of uraemia. Similarly, in ventilatory failure, the onset of hypoxia and hypercapnia is directly related to the metabolic demand. Just as a patient with renal failure may benefit from a low protein diet, so a patient with a severe reduction of ventilatory capacity protects himself by limiting the exercise which he takes.

As chronic obstructive airway progresses, the ventilatory capacity decreases and the minute volume of breathing for a particular level of activity increases. The latter change is because both the dead space and the oxygen cost of breathing increase. The patient is thus trapped in a pincer movement of decreasing ventilatory capacity and increasing ventilatory requirement. As the jaws of the pincer close, there is first a limitation on heavy exercise, then on moderate exercise and so on until the patient is dyspnoeic at rest. At any time his metabolic capacity is limited by the ratio of his ventilatory capacity to the minute volume which he must maintain for a given level of oxygen uptake.

The complex interaction between these factors is shown in *Figure 20.5*, where the upper part shows the normal state. Assuming that an untrained subject can sustain a minute volume equal to about 30 per cent of his maximal breathing capacity (MBC) without dyspnoea, he has a reserve of ventilatory capacity which is adequate for rest and a power output of 100 watts. However, a power output of 200 watts requires a ventilation which exceeds a third of his MBC and he becomes aware of his breathing at this level of exercise.

The middle section of the Figure shows moderately severe obstructive airway disease with the following changes:

1. MBC reduced to 60 l/min.
2. Dead space/tidal volume ratio increased from 30 per cent to 40 per cent.
3. Oxygen cost of breathing increased by 10 per cent for each level of activity.
4. Factors 2 and 3 together result in an increased minute volume for each level of activity.

Again, on the assumption that dyspnoea will not be apparent until the minute volume is 30 per cent of MBC, the reserve of ventilation is now sufficient for rest, but 100 watts of power output will result in dyspnoea.

Finally, in *Figure 20.5c*, the changes have progressed to the point where resting minute volume exceeds 30 per cent of MBC and the patient is dyspnoeic at rest.

Breathlessness

Breathlessness or dyspnoea has been defined by Campbell and Guz (1981) as 'undue awareness of breathing or awareness of difficulty in breathing'. This definition would apply to both the awareness of breathing during severe exercise in the healthy subject and the dyspnoea of the patient with respiratory failure or heart failure. In the first case the sensation is normal and to be expected. However, in the latter, it is pathological and should be considered as a symptom.

The origin of the sensation

Hypoxia and hypercapnia may force the patient to breathe more deeply but they are not *per se* responsible for the sensation of dyspnoea which arises from the ventilatory response rather than the stimulus itself. Dyspnoea is usually more prominent in the 'pink puffer' who keeps his blood gases relatively normal than in the 'blue bloater' who is both hypoxic and hypercapnic. Patients with respiratory paralysis caused by poliomyelitis are not usually dyspnoeic in spite of abnormal blood gas tensions.

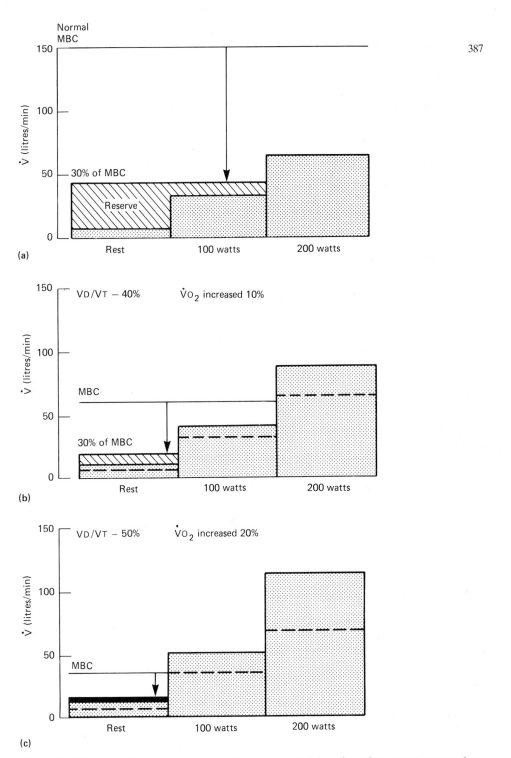

Figure 20.5 Relationship between maximal breathing capacity (MBC) and ventilatory requirements of rest and work at 100 and 200 watts. The tips of the arrows indicate 30 per cent of MBC which can usually be maintained without dyspnoea. Ventilatory reserve is between this level and the various ventilatory requirements. (a) Normal. (b) Moderate loss of ventilatory capacity with some increase in oxygen cost of breathing. (c) Severe loss of ventilatory capacity with considerable increase in the oxygen cost of breathing.

Campbell and Guz (1981) advanced their reasons for believing that dyspnoea is not akin to pain and neither is it strictly related to the work of breathing. In different patients there may be dyspnoea at relatively low levels of work of breathing or, conversely, no dyspnoea at high levels of work. Fatigue of the respiratory muscles (page 383) may be a factor in some cases but is clearly not the only cause of dyspnoea.

Campbell and Howell (1963) suggested that a major factor in the origin of dyspnoea was an 'inappropriateness' between the tension generated in the respiratory muscles and the resultant shortening of the muscle fibres. This might arise in obstructed breathing and would tend to increase with hyperventilation when the efficiency of breathing is less.

Breath holding

Breath holding (reviewed on pages 95 et seq.) provides many clues to the origin of the sensation of breathlessness. It has been shown that blood gas tensions are by no means the only factor limiting breathing holding time although Po_2 is more important than Pco_2. The sensation which terminates breath holding can be relieved by ventilation without change of blood gas tensions, by bilateral vagal block and by curarization. Diaphragmatic afferents appear to be more important than those from the intercostals.

It cannot be said that the problem of breathlessness is completely understood at the present time. It is, however, clear that there is no single and simple mechanism comparable to the sensations of touch, pain or temperature. The origin may well be multifactorial and the mechanisms of its generation are clearly complex.

Treatment of ventilatory failure

Many patients go about their business with arterial Pco_2 levels as high as 8 kPa (60 mmHg). Higher levels are associated with increasing disability, largely due to the accompanying hypoxaemia when the patient is breathing air (see *Figure 20.1*). Treatment may be divided into symptomatic relief of hypoxaemia and attempts to improve the alveolar ventilation.

Treatment of hypoxaemia due to hypoventilation by administration of oxygen

Oxygen usually does nothing to improve the ventilation or reduce the arterial Pco_2 which may, in fact, rise further. Thus it is important to be certain that relief of hypoxaemia, important though it may be, does not result in hypercapnia.

The relationship between alveolar Po_2, alveolar ventilation and inspired oxygen concentration is explained on pages 110 et seq. and illustrated in *Figure 5.8*. If other factors remain constant, an increase in inspired gas Po_2 will result in an equal increase in alveolar gas Po_2. Therefore only small increases in inspired oxygen concentration are required for the relief of hypoxia due to underventilation. *Figure 20.6* shows the rectangular hyperbola relating Pco_2 and alveolar ventilation (as in *Figure 5.8*) but superimposed are the concentrations of inspired oxygen required to restore a normal alveolar Po_2 for different degrees of ventilatory failure. It will be seen that 30% is sufficient for the degree of alveolar hypoventilation which will result in an alveolar Pco_2 of 13 kPa (almost 100 mmHg). Clearly this is a level

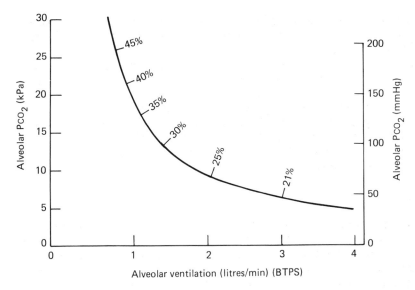

Figure 20.6 The curve indicates the alveolar PO₂ as a function of alveolar ventilation at rest. The percentages indicate the inspired oxygen concentration which is then required to restore normal alveolar PO₂.

of ventilatory failure which requires active intervention to increase the alveolar ventilation and thus 30% can be regarded as the upper limit of inspired oxygen concentration to be used in the palliative relief of hypoxia due to ventilatory failure. This limit is, in fact, recognized by the range of venturi masks which is available. It is also the level attainable with 'walking' oxygen equipment and domiciliary oxygen.

The use of very high concentrations of inspired oxygen will prevent hypoxia even in gross alveolar hypoventilation which carries the risk of dangerous hypercapnia. Although this is itself a strong contraindication to the use of high concentrations of oxygen under these circumstances, an even graver risk exists in patients who have lost their ventilatory sensitivity to carbon dioxide and rely upon their hypoxic drive to maintain ventilation. High concentrations of oxygen will abolish the hypoxic drive and may precipitate acute-on-chronic ventilatory failure. This is particularly liable to occur with blue bloaters (see above) but *Figure 20.3* shows an alarming example of the effect of administration of 100% oxygen to a patient with chronic ventilatory failure due to old poliomyelitis.

The rule is that hypoxia must be treated first, because hypoxia kills quickly while hypercapnia kills slowly. However, it must be remembered that administration of oxygen to a patient with ventilatory failure will do nothing to improve the PCO_2 and may make it worse. It is therefore essential to ensure that palliative relief of hypoxia does not result in hypercapnia and arterial PCO_2 should be checked if there is any doubt.

Improvement of alveolar ventilation

The only way to reduce the arterial PCO_2 is to improve the alveolar ventilation and this is the first consideration. In many cases of ventilatory failure, particularly the outpatient with chronic obstructive airway disease, there is very little that can be done, although in other situations there is a wide range of therapeutic possibilities.

The first line of therapy is to improve ventilatory capacity by such measures as bronchodilators, control of infections and secretions, stabilization of the chest wall, closure of an open pneumothorax, relief of pain, careful control of oxygen therapy and avoidance of drugs which depress breathing. The second line is chemical stimulation of breathing. This was never very satisfactory when nikethamide was the best drug available but the position has been radically altered by the introduction of doxapram which is capable of prolonged stimulation of breathing with little tachyphylaxis. This drug stimulates breathing via the peripheral chemoreceptors (Mitchell and Herbert, 1975) and is further discussed on page 84. It may be conveniently administered by a continuous intravenous infusion at a dose of 2–8 mg/min. The third line of treatment is by tracheal intubation or tracheostomy which may improve alveolar ventilation by reducing dead space and facilitating the control of secretions.

The fourth line of therapy is the institution of artificial ventilation considered in detail in Chapter 21. It is difficult to give firm guidelines for the institution of artificial ventilation and the arterial P_{CO_2} should not be considered in isolation. However, a P_{CO_2} in excess of 10 kPa (75 mmHg) which cannot be reduced by other means in a patient who is deemed recoverable is generally considered as a firm indication. However, artificial ventilation may be required at much lower levels of P_{CO_2} if there is actual or impending respiratory fatigue as a result of increased work of breathing. This may be difficult to diagnose or predict. Neverthless, it is now recognized that intense activity by the respiratory muscles results in low frequency fatigue, as in the case of other skeletal muscles under similar conditions (Moxham, 1984). Response to high frequency stimulation is unaltered but the central nervous system is unable to maintain high frequency output for long periods of time. Dyscoordinated breathing with thoracic and abdominal movements out of phase is a valuable indication of fatigue. It has been mentioned above that the P_{CO_2} rises late in asthma, and artificial ventilation may be required before the arterial P_{CO_2} has risen much above the normal range.

Artificial ventilation may also be useful for treatment of hypoxaemia, even if the P_{CO_2} is normal. The benefit is probably related to the increased tidal volume opening up closed airways and alveoli. This effect can be augmented by the use of positive end-expiratory pressure (page 414).

It may be useful to ventilate a patient with chronic obstructive airway disease to tide him over a period of infection which has resulted in acute-on-chronic ventilatory failure. However, in the absence of a transient factor of this nature, it is unlikely that a period of artificial ventilation can influence the long-term progress of the disease (Nunn, Milledge and Sigaraya, 1979; Petheram and Branthwaite, 1980). Similar considerations apply to pulmonary fibrosis (Hamman–Rich syndrome). A difficult decision may be required whether to ventilate patients with untreatable progressive ventilatory failure. Great difficulties and much distress may arise from instituting artificial ventilation from which it proves impossible to wean the patient.

For many years it has been accepted that artificial ventilation is the treatment of choice in severe crushed chest injury. However, there remains a school of thought which favours conservative management (Trinkle et al., 1975). Opinions differ on the management of acute epiglottitis in children. One school favours expectant treatment with antibiotics, steroids, sedation and high humidity of the inspired gas, while the other favours prophylactic intubation when the diagnosis is confirmed by lateral radiography of the larynx.

In an emergency it is frequently necessary to institute artificial ventilation to save life without consideration of the long-term aspects of the case. Under such circumstances, it may be very difficult to distinguish between acute, chronic and acute-on-chronic ventilatory failure. Resuscitation may well commit the intensive care unit to artificial ventilation of a patient who is not recoverable. It is virtually impossible to devise a system which will avoid this situation.

Chapter 21

Artificial ventilation

Artificial ventilation is defined as the provision of the minute volume of respiration by external forces when there is impaired action of the patient's respiratory muscles. It is used in four main situations:

1. Resuscitation following acute apnoea.
2. Anaesthesia with paralysis.
3. Intensive care with failure of one or more vital functions.
4. Prolonged treatment of chronic ventilatory failure.

Extracorporeal gas exchange cannot really be considered as artificial ventilation and is presented separately in Chapter 22.

Artificial ventilation of the apnoeic patient during resuscitation was formerly carried out by application of direct force to the chest in an attempt to produce either inhalation or exhalation, or both. These methods have been shown to be largely ineffective and are therefore considered only briefly below. It is now universally agreed that the best method of artificial ventilation during resuscitation is inflation of the lungs with the expired air of the rescuer and the physiology of this technique is considered in some detail below.

Much the commonest application of artificial ventilation is during anaesthesia with paralysis. It would normally be applied to some 2–5 per cent of the population of a developed country each year. Almost without exception it is achieved by the application of intermittent positive pressure to the airway of the patient, either manually or by means of one of a large range of mechanical devices, which can be of a comparatively simple design.

Artificial ventilation during intensive therapy is also undertaken almost exclusively by intermittent positive pressure ventilation (IPPV). However, in this environment, a proportion of patients present problems in ventilation and there is a requirement for more sophisticated ventilators with increased control of the manner and pattern of ventilation. In this field there is sometimes recourse to positive end-expiratory pressure (PEEP) and it is now usual for ventilators to permit the patient to breathe spontaneously in between artificial breaths, a technique which permits intermittent mandatory ventilation (IMV). Finally there is a new generation of ventilators which have the capacity to interact with any spontaneous breathing of the patient. These include devices to synchronize artificial with spontaneous breaths (a development of the old triggered ventilators) and apparatus which adjusts the minute volume of artificial ventilation in accord with the spontaneous ventilation which the patient is able to achieve. The latter permits maintenance of a constant minimal minute volume and has been termed mandatory minute volume (MMV).

Treatment of chronic ventilatory failure has been achieved by phrenic nerve stimulation although the technique is not commonly used. The commonest methods are by the intermittent development of a positive pressure gradient between airways and the air surrounding the trunk. At the present time this is most commonly achieved by IPPV as in anaesthesia or intensive care. However, this requires tracheostomy to ensure the necessary airtight fit to the airways without the possibility of inflation of the stomach. This difficulty can be avoided by generating the intermittent pressure differential by phasic reduction of pressure in the air around the trunk, and this may be achieved by means of a tank or cuirass ventilator.

Methods used for resuscitation

Artificial ventilation by application of mechanical forces directly to the trunk

Until about 1960, the usual methods were based on the rescuer manipulating the trunk and arms of the victim. These methods, which undoubtedly saved many lives in the past, are now largely obsolete. They can be classified into those with an active expiratory phase, those with an active inspiratory phase and those with both (push–pull).

Active expiratory phase. It would appear intuitively obvious that exerting pressure on the chest wall or the abdomen would result in a passive exhalation. This would be followed by inspiration as elastic forces restored the lung volume to functional residual capacity (FRC) when the distorting force was removed. This was the basis of the back pressure method (Schafer, 1904) and the Paul–Bragg Pneumobelt. However, neither method can be relied upon to guarantee an adequate tidal volume even if the airway is unobstructed. This is mainly because tidal exchange must take place within the expiratory reserve volume which is much reduced in the supine position (page 40). Lower limits of normal expiratory reserve volume in the supine position reported by Whitfield, Waterhouse and Arnott (1950) are of the order of 200 ml and clearly there is no possibility of obtaining a satisfactory tidal volume by this method in such a patient.

Active inspiratory phase. In an attempt to achieve tidal exchange within the inspiratory capacity, techniques have been developed which seek to expand the chest by traction on the arms or lifting of the hips. Somewhat similar is the cuirass respirator which applies an intermittent subatmospheric pressure to the epigastrium. Although these methods have the advantage of operating above FRC as in normal breathing, they cannot be relied upon to produce an adequate tidal volume in all patients.

Both active inspiratory and expiratory phases (push–pull). Of all the manual methods, these are the most efficient. The imposed tidal volume is partly above and partly below FRC. The rocking stretcher (Eve, 1932) relies on the fact that lung volume is markedly affected by posture (page 40) and phasic tilting 40 degrees on either side of horizontal can achieve a satisfactory tidal volume (Comroe and Dripps, 1946). The other push–pull methods include the arm lift, back pressure method applied to the prone victim (Holger Nielsen, 1932) and the arm lift, chest pressure method applied to the supine victim (Silvester, 1857). Safar (1959) obtained mean tidal volumes of 619 and 503 ml respectively in studies of these two methods in curarized subjects with tracheal tubes in place.

The significance of airway obstruction. Studies in curarized subjects with tracheal tubes in place do not reflect the usual circumstances of resuscitation. Virtually all unconscious patients will have some degree of airway obstruction which will be severe in many cases (page 4). Performance of the techniques described above requires the use of both hands, making it very difficult for the rescuer to protect the patency of the airway by the methods described on page 5. Recognition of the critical role of airway obstruction led to a major investigation of this factor by Safar (1959). His results (*Table 21.1*) clearly demonstrate that effective artificial ventilation by the manual methods can be guaranteed only if the trachea is intubated.

Table 21.1 Curarized anaesthetized patients—artificial ventilation by back pressure, arm lift method (Holger Nielsen method, 1932)

Airway	Mean tidal volume (ml)	Percentage of patients with tidal volume less than dead space
Natural (head in flexion)	126	75
Oropharyngeal airway (head in flexion)	178	71
Natural (head in extension)	328	31
Oropharyngeal airway (head in extension)	351	20
Endotracheal tube	619	0

Even if a normal tidal volume is obtained, it does not guarantee that arterial P_{O_2} will be satisfactory. Considerable arterial desaturation has been found during artificial respiration using Schafer's method, which could not be entirely explained by hypoventilation. It is likely that reduction of lung volume below FRC resulted in sufficient airway closure to cause appreciable shunting.

Expired air resuscitation

Recognition of the inadequacy of the manual methods of artificial ventilation led directly to a radical new approach to artificial ventilation in the emergency situation. Around 1960 there was vigorous re-examination of the concept of the rescuer's expired air being used for inflation of the victim's lung. Elisha has been credited with use of this technique on the son of the Shunammite woman (2 Kings 4:32) but the first clear and unequivocal account of the method was by Herholdt and Rafn in 1796.

At first sight, it might appear that expired air, being 'vitiated', would not be a suitable inspired air for the victim. However, if the rescuer doubles his ventilation he is able to breathe for two. If neither party had any respiratory dead space, the simple relationship shown in *Table 21.2* would apply. In fact, the rescuer's dead space improves the situation. At the start of inflation, the rescuer's dead space is filled with fresh air and this is the first gas to enter the victim's lungs. If the rescuer's dead space is artificially increased by apparatus dead space, this will improve the freshness of the air which the victim receives and it will also prevent hypocapnia in

Table 21.2 Alveolar gas concentrations during expired air resuscitation

	Normal spontaneous respiration	*Expired air resuscitation with doubled ventilation*	
		Donor	*Recipient*
Alveolar CO_2	6%	3%	6%
Alveolar O_2	15%	18%	15%

(Doubling the donor's ventilation increases his alveolar O_2 concentration to a value midway between the normal alveolar oxygen concentration and that of room air.)

the rescuer. This concept has been exploited in certain instrumental aids (Elam, 1962).

Expired air resuscitation has now displaced the manual methods in all except the most unusual circumstances and its success depends on the following factors:

1. It is normally possible to achieve adequate ventilation for long periods of time without fatigue (Greene et al., 1957; Cox, Woolmer and Thomas, 1960).
2. The hands of the rescuer are free to control the patency of the victim's airway.
3. The rescuer can monitor the victim's chest expansion visually and he can also hear any airway obstruction and sense the tidal exchange from the proprioceptive receptors in his own chest wall.
4. The method is extremely adaptable and has been used, for example, before drowning victims have been removed from the water, and by linesmen electrocuted while working on pylons. No manual method would have any hope of success in such situations.
5. The method seems to come naturally, and many rescuers have achieved success with the minimum of instruction.

Expired air resuscitation was extensively reviewed by Elam and Greene (1962) and Elam (1962). There have been few new developments in recent years. Essential features of the technique are as follows:

1. The airway must be cleared, firstly by removal of any foreign matter and secondly by opening the pharynx either by extension of the head or by protrusion of the mandible (page 5).
2. The rescuer should employ a tidal volume about double normal and most people do this intuitively.
3. The first few breaths should be delivered as fast as possible; thereafter a normal respiratory rate should be employed.
4. Alternative variants of the technique should be taught as no one method is applicable to all circumstances. For example, mouth-to-nose may be preferable to mouth-to-mouth with trismus or injuries to the mouth.
5. No potential rescuer should be led to believe that success depends on the use of ancillary apparatus such as the Brooke airway. A rescue is such a rare event in the lives of all except those with professional involvement, that there is little chance of having apparatus to hand.

Intermittent positive pressure ventilation (IPPV)

Phases of the respiratory cycle

Inspiration. During IPPV, the mouth (or airway) pressure is intermittently raised above ambient pressure. The inspired gas then flows into the respiratory system in accord with the resistance and compliance of the respiratory system, which are discussed in detail in Chapters 2 and 3. If inspiration is slow, the distribution is governed solely by regional compliance. If inspiration is fast, the regional time constants of the system become the major factor. Different temporal patterns of pressure may be applied and are discussed below. The anatomical pattern of distribution of inspired gas is different from that of spontaneous breathing, there being a relatively greater expansion of the rib cage (Vellody et al., 1978).

Expiration. During IPPV, expiration results from allowing mouth pressure to fall to ambient. Expiration is then passive and differs from expiration during spontaneous breathing only in the absence of residual diaphragmatic tone (page 356). Expiration may be retarded by the application of positive end-expiratory pressure (PEEP) or by the addition of external resistance to gas flow (an expiratory retard). Alternatively, expiration can be accelerated by the application of a subatmospheric pressure. This may be termed negative end-expiratory pressure (NEEP). Expiration to ambient pressure is also termed zero end-expiratory pressure (ZEEP).

If the inflating pressure is maintained for several seconds, the resulting tidal volume will be indicated by the following relationship:

tidal volume = sustained inflation pressure × total compliance

Thus, for example, a sustained inflation pressure of 1 kPa (10 cmH$_2$O) with a compliance of 0.5 l/kPa (0.05 l/cmH$_2$O) would result in a lung volume 500 ml above functional residual capacity (FRC).

Time course of inflation and deflation

Equilibration according to the above equation usually takes several seconds. When the airway pressure is raised during inspiration, it is opposed by the two forms of impedance which have already been considered, the elastic resistance of lungs and chest wall (Chapter 2) and resistance to air flow (Chapter 3). At any instant, the inflation pressure equals the sum of the pressures required to overcome these two forms of impedance. The pressure required to overcome elastic resistance equals the lung volume above FRC divided by the total compliance, while the pressure required to overcome air flow resistance equals the air flow resistance multiplied by the instantaneous flow rate (assuming for the moment that air flow is entirely laminar).

The effect of applying a constant pressure (or square wave inflation) is shown in *Figure 21.1*. The two components of the inflation pressure vary during the course of inspiration while their sum remains constant. The component overcoming air flow resistance is maximal at first and declines exponentially with air flow as inflation proceeds. The component overcoming elastic resistance increases with the lung volume. With normal respiratory mechanics in the unconscious patient, the change in lung volume should be 95 per cent complete in about 1.5 seconds, as in *Figure 21.1*.

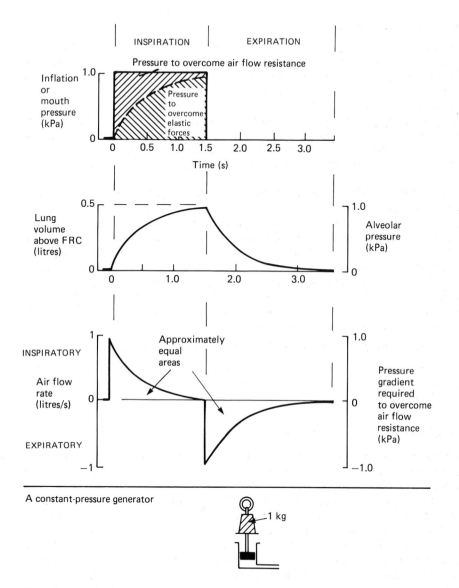

Figure 21.1 Artificial ventilation by intermittent application of a constant pressure (square wave). Passive expiration. Inspiratory and expiratory flow rates are both exponential. Assuming that air flow resistance is constant, it follows that flow rate and pressure gradient required to overcome resistance may be shown on the same graph. Lung volume and alveolar pressure may be shown on the same graph if compliance is constant. Values are typical for an anaesthetized supine paralysed patient: total dynamic compliance, 0.5 l/kPa (50 ml/cmH$_2$O); pulmonary resistance, 0.3 kPa l^{-1} s) (3 cmH$_2$O/l/sec); apparatus resistance, 0.7 kPa l^{-1} s (7 cmH$_2$O/l/sec); total resistance, 1 kPa l^{-1} s (10 cmH$_2$O/l/sec); time constant, 0.5 s.

The approach of the lung volume to its equilibrium value is according to an exponential function of the wash-in type (see Appendix F). The time constant, which is the time required for inflation to 63 per cent of the equilibrium value, equals the product of resistance and compliance. Normal values for an unconscious patient are as follows:

$$\text{time constant} = \text{resistance} \times \text{compliance}$$

$$0.5 \text{ second} = 1 \text{ kPa l}^{-1} \text{ s} \times 0.5 \text{ l kPa}^{-1}$$

(or, in non–SI units, $10 \text{ cmH}_2\text{O/l/s} \times 0.05 \text{ l/cmH}_2\text{O}$, which also equals 0.5 second)

The time constant is the time which would be required to reach equilibrium if the initial inspiratory flow rate were maintained. It is sometimes more convenient to use the half-time, which is 0.69 times the time constant. The inflation curve is shown in full with further mathematical detail in Appendix F.

It is clearly not usual for equilibrium of lung volume to occur during IPPV, and it is normal practice for the inspiratory phase to be terminated after 1 or 2 seconds at which time the lung volume will still be increasing. Inflation pressure is not then the sole arbiter of tidal volume but must be considered in relation to the duration of the inspiratory phase.

If expiration is passive and mouth pressure remains at ambient, the driving force is the elevation of alveolar pressure above ambient, caused by elastic recoil of lungs and chest wall. This pressure is dissipated in overcoming air flow resistance during expiration. In *Figure 21.1*, during expiration the alveolar pressure (proportional to the lung volume above FRC) is directly proportional to expiratory flow rate, and all three quantities change according to a wash-out exponential function with a time constant which is again equal to the product of compliance and resistance.

The effect of changes in inflation pressure, resistance and compliance

This is best considered during the application of constant, or 'square wave', positive airway pressure during the inspiratory phase. Many ventilators operate on this principle. The heavy line in *Figure 21.2* shows the inflation curve for the normal parameters of an unconscious paralysed patient as listed in *Table 21.3*. These are

Table 21.3

	Basic curve	Pulmonary resistance doubled	Inflation pressure doubled	Compliance doubled	Compliance halved
Inflation pressure					
(kPa)	1	1	2	1	1
(cmH$_2$O)	10	10	20	10	10
Compliance					
(l/kPa)	0.5	0.5	0.5	1	0.25
(ml/cmH$_2$O)	50	50	50	100	25
Ultimate tidal volume (l)	0.5	0.5	1	1	0.25
Pulmonary resistance					
(kPa l^{-1} s)	1	2	1	1	1
(cmH$_2$O/l/sec)	10	20	10	10	10
Time constant					
(s or sec)	0.5	1	0.5	1	0.25

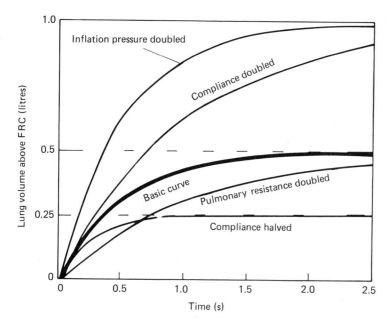

Figure 21.2 Effect of changes in various factors on inflation of the lungs. Fixed relationships: ultimate tidal volume = inflation pressure × compliance; time constant = compliance × resistance. (See also Table 21.3)

63% of inflation completed in 1 time constant
86.5% of inflation completed in 2 time constants
95% of inflation completed in 3 time constants
98% of inflation completed in 4 time constants
99% of inflation completed in 5 time constants

the same values which were considered above. The basic curve is a single exponential approaching a lung volume 0.5 litre above FRC with a time constant of 0.5 second.

Changes in inflation pressure do not alter the time constant of inflation, but directly influence the amount of air introduced into the lungs in a given number of time constants. In *Figure 21.2*, each point on the curve labelled 'inflation pressure doubled' is twice the height of the corresponding point on the basic curve for the same time.

If the compliance is doubled, the equilibrium tidal volume is also doubled. However, the time constant (product of compliance and resistance) is also doubled and therefore the equilibrium volume is approached more slowly (*Figure 21.2*). Conversely, if the compliance is halved, the equilibrium tidal volume is also halved and so is the time constant.

Changes in resistance have a direct effect on the time constant of inflation but do not affect the equilibrium tidal volume. Thus the effect of an increased resistance on tidal volume is through the reduction in inspiratory flow rate. Within limits, this can be counteracted by prolonging inspiration or by increasing the inflation pressure and the degree of overpressure. These effects, shown in *Figure 21.2*, apply not only to the whole lung but also to regions which may have different compliances, resistances and time constants (page 144).

Increasing the inflation pressure has a major effect on the time required to achieve a particular lung volume above FRC. In *Figure 21.3*, the lung characteristics are the same as for the basic curve in *Figure 21.2*. If the required tidal volume is 475 ml, this is achieved in 1.5 seconds with an inflation pressure of 1 kPa (10 cmH₂O). However, the same lung volume is achieved in only 0.3 second by doubling the inflation pressure. The application of a pressure which, if sustained, would give a tidal volume higher than that which is intended, is known as overpressure and is

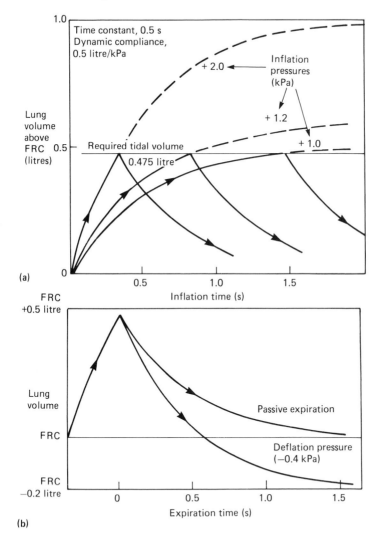

Figure 21.3 (a) How the duration of inflation may be shortened by the use of overpressure. Inflation curves are shown for +2 kPa (+20 cmH₂O) (equilibrium 1 litre), +1.2 kPa (+12 cmH₂O) (equilibrum 0.6 litre and +1 kPa (+10 cmH₂O) (equilibrium 0.5 1 litre). With a required tidal volume of 0.475 litre note the big reduction in duration of inflation needed when the inflation pressure is increased from 1 to 2 kPa (10 to 20 cmH₂O). (b) How expiration is influenced by the use of a subatmospheric pressure or 'negative phase'. Expiration may be terminated at the FRC after 0.6 s, or may be prolonged, in which case the lung volume will fall to 0.2 litre below the FRC.

extensively used to increase the inspiratory flow rate and so to permit a shorter duration of the inspiratory phase. The use of a subatmospheric pressure to increase the rate of passive expiration is similar but may be complicated by airway trapping (*Figure 21.3*).

Deviations from true exponential character of expiration

It is helpful to assume that the patterns of air flow described above are exponential in character since this greatly assists our understanding of the situation. However, there are many reasons why air flow should not be strictly exponential in character. Air flow is normally partly turbulent (see Chapter 3) and therefore resistance cannot be considered as a constant. Furthermore, as expiration proceeds, the calibre of the air passages decreases and there is also a transition to more laminar flow as the instantaneous flow rate decreases. Approximation to a single exponential function is nevertheless good enough for many practical purposes.

Alternative patterns of application of inflation pressure

Constant pressure or square wave inflation has been considered above because it is the easiest for mathematical analysis. There are, however, an almost infinite number of pressure profiles which may be applied for IPPV. There is no very convincing evidence of the superiority of one over the other except that distribution of inspired gas is improved if there is a prolongation of the period during which the applied pressure is maximal. This permits better ventilation of the 'slow' alveoli (page 32) and is not very important in patients with relatively healthy lungs. It is probably best achieved by an inspiratory pause.

Constant flow rate ventilators are extensively used, and *Figure 21.4* shows pressure, volume and flow changes in a manner analogous to *Figure 21.2*. This pattern of air flow is conveniently achieved with electronically controlled ventilators such as the CPU-1 (Nunn and Lyle, 1986).

Sine wave generators were popular in the days of mechanical (as opposed to electronic) ventilators, and the pattern of inspiratory flow rate was a direct consequence of the mechanical linkage in ventilators such as the original Engstrom or the Smith-Clark. *Figure 21.5* shows the pattern of pressure, volume and flow rate changes with a sine wave generator.

Control of duration of inspiration

Three methods are in general use.

Time cycling terminates inspiration after a preset time. With mechanical ventilators delivering a sine pressure wave, the inspiratory time usually derives directly from the pressure generator itself. However, with constant pressure generators and constant flow generators, a separate and variable timing device is incorporated. With constant flow generators, inspiratory time has a direct effect on the tidal volume. With constant pressure generators the relationship is more complex, as described above (see *Figure 21.3*).

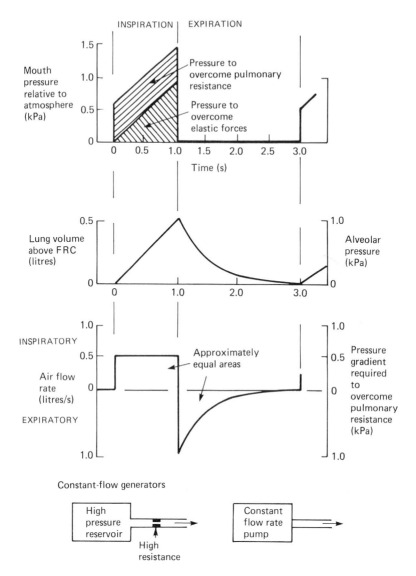

Figure 21.4 Artificial ventilation by intermittent application of a constant-flow generator with passive expiration. Note that inspiratory flow rate is constant. Assuming that pulmonary resistance is constant, it follows that a constant amount of the inflation pressure is required to overcome flow resistance. Lung volume and alveolar pressure may be shown on the same graph if compliance is constant. Values are typical of an anaesthetized supine paralysed patient: total dynamic compliance, 0.5 l/kPa (50 ml/cmH$_2$O); pulmonary resistance, 0.3 kPa l^{-1} s (3 cmH$_2$O/l/sec); apparatus resistance, 0.7 kPa l^{-1} s (7 cmH$_2$O/l/sec); total resistance, 1 kPa l^{-1} s (10 cmH$_2$O/l/sec); time constant, 0.5 s.

Volume cycling terminates inspiration when a preset volume has been delivered. In the absence of a leak this should guarantee the tidal volume even if the compliance or resistance of the patient changes within limits. Formerly, volume-cycled ventilators were usually based on a reciprocating pump of preset tidal volume. Now-

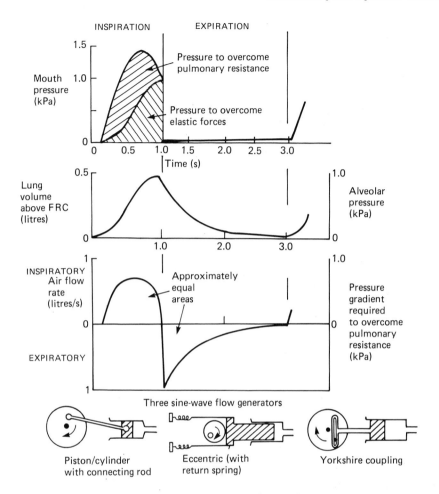

Figure 21.5 Artificial ventilation with inspiratory gas flow conforming to a sine wave. Passive expiration. Note that inspiratory gas flow rate is out of phase with the change in lung volume. (The latter conforms to a sine wave and the former to the differential of the sine which is the cosine.) Assuming that air flow resistance is constant, it follows that flow rate and pressure gradient required to overcome resistance may be shown on the same graph. Lung volume and alveolar pressure may be shown on the same graph if compliance is constant. Peak inspiratory flow rate $=\pi \times$ the minute volume $\times 1.5$. (The factor 1.5 is inserted because in this example inspiration does not last half the respiratory cycle.) Values are typical of an anaesthetized supine paralysed patient: total dynamic compliance, 0.5 l/kPa (50 ml/cmH$_2$O); pulmonary resistance, 0.3 kPa l^{-1} s (3 cmH$_2$O/l/sec); apparatus resistance, 0.7 kPa l^{-1} s (7 cmH$_2$O/l/sec); total resistance, 1 kPa^{-1} s (10 cmH$_2$O/l/sec)/ time constant, 0.5 s.

adays they are more likely to be flow generators with an inspiratory flow sensor which terminates inspiration when the required volume has entered the lungs.

Pressure cycling terminates inspiration when a particular mouth pressure is achieved. This in no way guarantees the tidal volume. Increased airway resistance, for example, would limit inspiratory flow rate and cause a more rapid increase in mouth pressure, thus terminating the inspiratory phase. Pressure-cycled ventilators are almost invariably flow generators.

Limitations on inspiratory duration. Whatever the means of cycling, it is possible to add a limitation on inspiratory duration, usually as a safety precaution. For example, a pressure limitation can be added to a time cycled or a volume cycled ventilator. This can either function as a pressure relief valve or it can terminate the inspiratory phase.

The inspiratory/expiratory ratio

For a given minute volume of ventilation, it is possible to vary within wide limits the duration of inspiration and expiration and the ratio between the two. The commonest pattern is about 1 second for inspiration, followed by 2–4 seconds for expiration, giving respiratory frequencies in the range 12–20 breaths per minute. The problem is whether changes from this pattern confer any appreciable benefit in terms of gas exchanges. There is no guarantee that studies in animals or healthy anaesthetized patients are relevant to patients with pulmonary dysfunction in whom some benefit might be expected to accrue. Watson (1962b) demonstrated a substantial increase in dead space in patients in an intensive therapy unit when the duration of inspiration was reduced below one second. A similar but less marked change was found in anaesthetized patients with healthy lungs by Bergman (1967) and Fairley and Blenkarn (1966). Sykes and Lumley (1969) reported the same effect during cardiac surgery. However, the changes have mostly been too small to be of much clinical significance except in the study of Watson. The consensus view seems to be that 1 second is a reasonable minimal time for inspiration.

There seems to be no convincing evidence in any of the studies cited above that the duration of inspiration (in the range 0.5–3 seconds) has any appreciable effect on the alveolar/arterial P_{O_2} gradient.

Inverse inspiratory/expiratory ratio ventilation has the effect of increasing the mean lung volume and so may be expected to achieve some of the advantages of positive end-expiratory pressure (PEEP) as considered below. It may be achieved either by slowing the inspiratory flow rate (shallow ramp) or by holding the lung volume at the end of inspiration (top hat), the latter appearing to be more logical. Inspiratory/ expiratory ratios as high as 4:1 have been used but 2:1 is generally preferable. A limiting factor is the time available for expiration. If this is unduly curtailed, FRC will be increased as with the use of PEEP.

Gas redistribution during an inspiratory hold reduces the dead space (page 161) and so results in a lower P_{CO_2} for the same minute volume (Fuleihan, Wilson and Pontoppidan, 1976). This permits the use of a lower peak inflation pressure. Shunting is also reduced (Perez-Chada et al., 1983), presumably because of the increased fraction of the respiratory cycle during which airways tend to be patent. Clinical applications have been described by Cole, Weller and Sykes (1984).

Interaction of ventilator controls

The commonest controls which are provided on an artificial ventilator are drawn from the following list:

tidal volume
inspiratory flow rate
duration of inspiration
duration of expiration

inspiratory/expiratory ratio
respiratory frequency
minute volume

It will be found that the maximum possible number of independent controls is three. A setting of any three on this list will determine the values for all the remaining variables. Opinion is divided on which of these controls the clinician likes to operate directly. However, an excellent compromise is to display computed values corresponding to the variables which are not available as controls. For example, the CPU-1 ventilator, in the volume cycled IPPV mode, provides controls for duration of inspiration, duration of expiration and inspiratory flow rate (it is a constant flow rate ventilator). Although other controls on the list are not available, there is a display of the imposed inspiratory/expiratory ratio, tidal volume, respiratory frequency and minute volume, which are computed from the setting of the three controls (Nunn and Lyle, 1986).

Special techniques for IPPV

Non-mechanical methods

Expired air resuscitation has been considered above under emergency methods of resuscitation.

Glossopharyngeal respiration (frog breathing) is a technique which may be helpful for short periods in patients with paresis of the respiratory muscle who retain the use of the muscles used in swallowing. Gulps of air are taken into the mouth and passed into the lungs which are thus inflated stepwise. After a number of swallows, a passive expiration takes place (Dail, Affeldt and Collier, 1955).

Venturis and jets

Venturis and jets can be used to generate a positive pressure which can be applied intermittently during bronchoscopy to maintain ventilation without any mechanical barrier to obstruct the line of vision. If oxygen is used as the driving gas, air is entrained to provide an inspired gas mixture of appropriate oxygen concentration (Sanders, 1967).

The same principle has been used in a simple, convenient and highly controllable artificial ventilator which can also provide positive pressure during expiration (Whitwam et al., 1983). Jet ventilators are essentially T-piece circuits. Fresh gas is supplied by the afferent limb while the efferent limb contains four jets. The three facing the patient can provide any required pressure during inspiration or expiration while the fourth, facing away from the patient, can provide subatmospheric pressure if required during expiration. By setting the timing and the profile of the flow rates through the various jets it is possible to provide total control of the airway pressures throughout the respiratory cycle. The system operates as a time-phased pressure generator but one which is particularly easy to control and is particularly suitable for feedback control and servo operation. An important feature is that jet ventilators can operate at very high frequencies.

High frequency ventilation

Öberg and Sjöstrand (1967, unpublished) made the surprising observation that effective respiration could be maintained in dogs during artificial ventilation at a respiratory frequency of 80 b.p.m. with a tidal volume which did not appear to be sufficient to wash out the dead space (Sjöstrand, 1980). It was soon found that similar techniques could be applied to patients (Heijman et al., 1972).

High frequency ventilation may be classified into the following.

High frequency positive pressure ventilation (HFPPV) is applied in the frequency range 1–2 Hz (60–120 b.p.m.) and can be considered as an extension of conventional IPPV techniques.

High frequency jet ventilation (HFJV) covers the frequency range 1–5 Hz. The essential difference from HFPPV is that the use of jets permits a higher operating frequency.

High frequency oscillation (HFO) covers the frequency range 3–50 Hz and the flows are usually generated by an oscillating pump or diaphragm making a fourth connection to a T-piece with a low pass filter on the open limb (*Figure 21.6*).

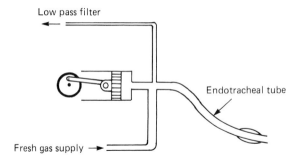

Figure 21.6 Circuit for provision of high frequency oscillation.

The waveform is usually sinusoidal. Tidal volumes are inevitably small at these frequencies but are exceedingly difficult to measure. Studies in dogs have shown that satisfactory gas exchange may be maintained by this technique, for periods up to at least 36 hours, with oscillator frequencies in the range 13–28 Hz. Small pleural effusions were found in dogs ventilated at high frequency but otherwise there were no important differences in respiratory or cardiovascular function when high frequency was compared with conventional artificial ventilation (Rehder, Schmidt and Knopp, 1983). However, in another study by the same group it was shown that oxygenation and the uniformity of distribution of ventilation and perfusion were somewhat better at 5.8 Hz than at 15 or 29.8 Hz or with conventional artificial ventilation (Brusasco et al., 1984).

Satisfactory results have been obtained in anaesthetized man (Crawford and Rehder, 1985). Butler et al. (1980), using oscillator frequencies of 15 Hz (900 b.p.m.) with volume settings in the range 50–150 ml, have obtained satisfactory levels of P_{CO_2} and P_{O_2} in 12 patients requiring artificial ventilation for respiratory failure. Cardiac output was much the same for both IPPV and HFO. Mean shunt was decreased with HFO in all 8 patients in whom the measurement was made, the benefit being greatest in those patients thought to have an extensive mismatch of ventilation and perfusion.

The relationship between tidal volume and dead space during high frequency ventilation is crucial to an understanding of the technique. It is useless to infer values for tidal volume and dead space from measurements made under other circumstances and yet it is very difficult to make direct measurements of these variables under the actual conditions of high frequency ventilation, especially in man. Chakrabarti, Gordon and Whitwam (1986) studied anaesthetized man during HFPPV up to frequencies of 2 Hz, holding arterial P_{CO_2} approximately constant at about 5 kPa (37.5 mmHg). As frequency increased from conventional ventilation at 15 b.p.m. to HFPPV at 2 Hz it was necessary to double the minute volume (*Table 21.4*). The actual volume of the physiological dead space decreased with decreasing tidal volume to reach a minimal value of about 90 ml at about 1 Hz.

Table 21.4 Gas exchange during high frequency ventilation

		Respiratory frequency		
		15 b.p.m. *0.25 Hz*	*60 b.p.m.* *1 Hz*	*120 b.p.m.* *2 Hz*
Arterial P_{CO_2}	kPa	4.8	4.8	4.9
	mmHg	36	36	37
$\dot{V}$	l/min	6.8	10.2	14
V_T	ml	454	170	117
V_D (physiol.)	ml	165	96	88
V_D/V_T ratio	%	36	56	75

(Data from Chakrabarti, Gordon and Whitwam, 1986)

However, the normal proportionality between dead space and tidal volume (page 164) was not maintained. Dead space/tidal volume ratio increased from 37 per cent at 15 b.p.m. to 75 per cent at 2 Hz, which explains the requirement for the increased minute volume. The situation is more complex at higher frequencies. However, the study of Butler et al. (1980) suggests that tidal volumes of at least 100 ml are still required at frequencies of 15 Hz, corresponding to an *applied* minute volume of 90 l/min which would indicate a dead space/tidal volume ratio of over 90 per cent. There are severe technical difficulties in the measurement of the actual delivered tidal volumes which, though undoubtedly less than the pump settings, are probably much larger than the external movements of the thorax would suggest.

End-expiratory pressure is inevitably raised at high frequencies because the duration of expiration will be inadequate for passive exhalation to FRC, since the time constant of the normal respiratory system is about 0.5 second (see above). Therefore, the use of respiratory frequencies above about 2 Hz will usually be associated with PEEP and an increased end-expiratory lung volume. This effect has been called 'auto-PEEP' (Beamer et al., 1984) and is likely to be a major factor promoting favourable gas exchange (see page 414).

Gas mixing and streaming is likely to be modified at high frequencies. The sudden reversals of flow direction are likely to set up eddies which blur the boundary between dead space and alveolar gas, thus improving the efficiency of ventilation. It has been suggested that such 'enhanced diffusion' or 'augmented dispersion' plays a major role in gas exchange during HFO (Butler et al., 1980; Rossing et al., 1981). Air passages dilated by PEEP may contribute to this effect. Furthermore, cardiac mixing of gases becomes relatively more important at small tidal volumes (Nunn and Hill, 1960).

The clinical indications for high frequency ventilation are still not clear at the time of writing. There is no doubt that effective gas exchange is possible with high frequency ventilation but the advantages over conventional artificial ventilation are not fully clarified. Although there are enthusiasts, others believe that it is merely a technique in search of an application. There is agreement on its special role for patients with bronchopleural fistula and the technique is particularly convenient when there is no airtight junction between ventilator and the tracheobronchial tree at laryngoscopy, for example. However, there is little agreement on its benefits in relation to conventional ventilation in other situations. The most attractive feature is the avoidance of high *peak* inspiratory pressures. However, *mean* airway pressure may still be high if exhalation is impeded, as it must be at very high frequencies. Whether high frequency ventilation is less likely to produce pulmonary barotrauma than conventional techniques of ventilation will be difficult to determine in man but animal experiments suggest this may be so (Kolton et al., 1982). It may prove valuable to combine high frequency ventilation with conventional artificial ventilation.

Perhaps the major difficulty lies in the prediction of efficiency of gas exchange in a particular patient. Tidal volume cannot easily be measured and reliance must be placed on arterial blood gas tensions. Recent reviews include those of Kolton (1984), McEvoy (1985) and Smith and Hanning (1986).

Differential lung ventilation

There are many circumstances, such as posture, surgery and disease, which require a different ventilatory pattern for the two lungs (Nunn, 1961a; Hedenstierna, 1985). Techniques are now available for use of selective tidal volumes and selective PEEP for the two lungs. Such techniques are complex and require double-lumen tracheal intubation. Neverthless, there is no question that they can optimize gas exchange (Hedenstierna et al., 1984). A similar problem is considered in relation to 'one-lung anaesthesia' (page 377).

Application of subatmospheric pressure to the trunk

Cabinet ventilators differ from conventional IPPV in reducing the pressure surrounding the trunk rather than raising the airway pressure. However, in terms of the airway-to-ambient pressure gradient they are identical in principle (*Figure 21.7*). The special attraction of the technique is that it can be used for patients without tracheostomies or tracheal tubes. However, vomiting or regurgitation of gastric contents exposes the patient to the danger of aspiration during the inspiratory phase, and fatalities have occurred under particularly distressing circumstances. The method is now seldom used.

ARTIFICIAL VENTILATION BY INTERMITTENT POSITIVE PRESSURE

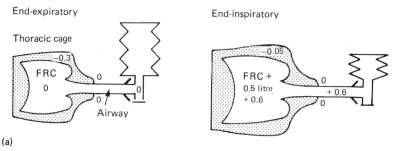

(a)

ARTIFICIAL VENTILATION BY CABINET RESPIRATOR

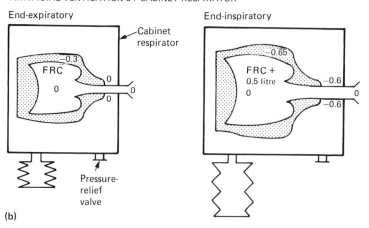

(b)

Figure 21.7 Comparison of artificial ventilation by (a) intermittent positive pressure (IPP) and (b) cabinet respirator (subatmospheric pressures only). The actual pressures differ in the two techniques, but the following pressure gradients are the same in both cases: mouth-to-ambient; alveolar-to-intrathoracic (transmural); intrathoracic-to-ambient. Ambient pressure refers to the pressure surrounding the trunk and is therefore cabinet pressure in the latter case. Static values for supine anaesthetized patient: lung compliance, 1.5 l/kPa (150 ml/cmH$_2$O); thoracic cage compliance, 2 l/kPa (200 ml/cmH$_2$O); total compliance. 0.85 l/kPa (85 ml/cmH$_2$O). (Intrathoracic space is shown stippled.) Figures indicate pressures relative to atmosphere in kilopascals.

Cuirass ventilators are a simplified form of cabinet ventilators in which the application of subatmospheric pressure is confined to the anterior abdominal wall. Function depends on a good airtight seal. They are less efficient than cabinet ventilators and suffer from the same disadvantages. However, they are much more convenient to use and may be useful to supplement inadequate spontaneous breathing. High frequency ventilation by chest wall compression is possible (Zidulka et al., 1983) and this may be favourable for clearance of secretions. It may find a role in combination with IPPV.

Intermittent mandatory ventilation (IMV)

IMV was introduced by Downs and his colleagues in Gainsville in 1973. The essential feature is provision of a parallel inspiratory gas circuit which allows the patient to take a spontaneous breath between artificial breaths. This confers three major advantages. Firstly, a spontaneous inspiration is not obstructed by a closed inspiratory valve and this helps to prevent the patient fighting the ventilator. It is very distressing for a conscious patient to attempt to inhale against the closed valves of a mechanical ventilator and it results in a large abdominal/thoracic pressure gradient which may cause gastric regurgitation. It has been claimed that the use of IMV reduces the demand for sedatives. The second advantage is the facilitation of weaning, which is considered further below. IMV permits a gradual resumption of spontaneous breathing, during which ventilator support is only gradually reduced. Excellent results have been claimed (Downs, Perkins and Modell, 1974). Thirdly, the patient is enabled to breathe spontaneously at any time during prolonged ventilation; this may prevent respiratory muscle atrophy and helps to reduce the mean intrathoracic pressure.

Some of these advantages of IMV are so obvious that it is hard to understand why its introduction was so long delayed. Most modern ventilators now provide IMV as a normal feature. The parallel circuit for spontaneous breathing should provide humidified inspired gas with the correct oxygen concentration. The pressure should also be appropriate to any expiratory pressure which is in use, and this is discussed below. Unfortunately, many ventilators using demand valves impose a substantial inspiratory load for spontaneous breaths. This increases the work of breathing (Gibney, Wilson and Pontoppidan, 1982).

A review by Weisman et al. (1983) challenges the concept that continuous spontaneous breathing is beneficial for a patient on IPPV. They point out that few of the advantages claimed for IMV have been demonstrated in controlled trials. Nevertheless, the conduct of a controlled trial in these circumstances is not easy, as it is extremely difficult to control the variables.

Interaction between patient and ventilator

The major weakness of all the ventilator systems mentioned above is that they lack feedback from the patient to the ventilator, which cannot, therefore, respond to any spontaneous respiratory activity by the patient. However, for many years there have been ventilators in which the inspiratory phase could be triggered with a spontaneous breath. More recently there has appeared a generation of ventilators in which the applied minute volume can be modified by the spontaneous minute volume which the patient is able to achieve.

Triggered and synchronized ventilators

The onset of the inspiratory phase of a ventilator may be brought forward by detection of the subatmospheric pressure generated by a spontaneous breath. This has three distinct applications. This was originally introduced as an aid to weaning for which it was rather disappointing (see below). Later it came to be used to assist an inadequate inspiration in a partially paralysed patient in whom it is desirable to preserve the spontaneous respiration rhythm. More recently it has been found to be a most effective method of synchronizing the ventilator to spontaneous respiration. In this application, it is an adjunct to IMV and is called synchronized IMV (SIMV). *Figure 21.8* shows the synchronization of artificial ventilation to a spontaneous respiratory rhythm with the CPU-1 ventilator (Nunn and Lyle, 1986).

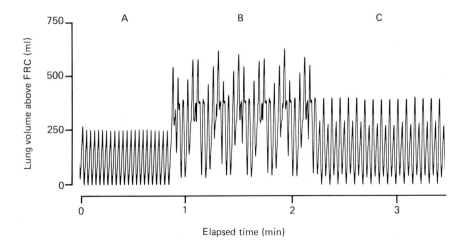

Figure 21.8 Synchronization of artificial ventilation with spontaneous breathing in a model patient using the Ohmeda CPU-1 ventilator. A: spontaneous breathing (tidal volume 250 ml at 26 b.p.m.). B: artificial ventilation superimposed (tidal volume 350 ml at 20 b.p.m.). C: synchronization mode used to obtain augmentation of alternate breaths at 13 b.p.m. (Reproduced from Nunn and Lyle (1986) by permission of the Editors of the British Journal of Anaesthesia)

Mandatory minute volume (MMV)

Hewlett, Platt and Terry (1977) described a simple technique for controlling the volume of artificial ventilation so that the total of spontaneous and artificial ventilation did not fall below a preset value. The principle is outlined in *Figure 21.9a*. If the patient is able to achieve the preset level of MMV, the ventilator remains inoperative. If the patient stops breathing, the ventilator then supplies the preset level of MMV. If the patient is able to achieve a part of the MMV, his contribution is subtracted from the total and the ventilator supplies the difference (*Figure 21.9b*). There is provision for the spontaneous ventilation to exceed the MMV.

This system was slow to be recognized but is now available commercially in the CPU-1 and Erica ventilators. It has a number of applications. Firstly, it can be an effective technique for weaning (see below). Secondly, spontaneous breaths by a ventilated patient do not necessarily increase the minute volume as would occur with IMV. Thus hypocapnia is avoided and the patient's respiratory efforts are not discouraged. Thirdly, for a patient who is breathing spontaneously, MMV provides an excellent safeguard against any reduction in spontaneous breathing which might result from such causes as sleep, administration of opiate, respiratory muscle fatigue or the fluctuations of a myasthenic crisis.

Positive end-expiratory pressure (PEEP)

A great variety of pathological conditions, as well as general anaesthesia, result in a decrease in FRC. The deleterious effect of this on gas exchange has been considered elsewhere (page 360) and it is reasonable to consider increasing the FRC by the application of PEEP, first described by Hill and his colleagues in 1965.

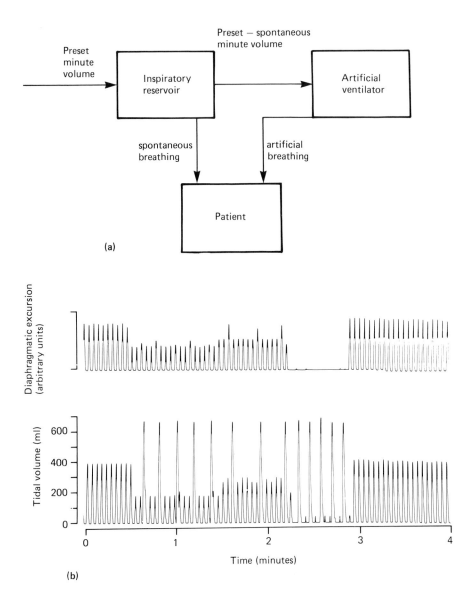

(a)

(b)

Figure 21.9 (a) The principle of mandatory minute volume (MMV). The mandatory minute volume is set on the rotameters and the patient breathes as much as he is able from the inspiratory reservoir. What is left is supplied as artificial ventilation (see text). (b) The upper trace shows the 'diaphragmatic excursion' of a model patient. The lower trace shows lung volume in the mandatory minute volume mode using the system of Hewlett, Platt and Terry (1977). For the first 30 seconds, the tidal volume of 400 ml at 18 b.p.m. (minute volume 7.2 l/min) is in excess of the mandatory minute volume setting (6.3 l/min). Thereafter, changes in spontaneous tidal volume result in intermittent breaths of artificial ventilation to preserve the required mandatory minute volume. Total apnoea supervenes at 2.3 minutes and ventilation is then totally artificial. (Reproduced from Nunn (1983) by courtesy of the Editors of the Japanese Journal of Clinical Anaesthesia*)*

Expiratory pressure can also be raised during spontaneous breathing and both forms are best considered together. The terminology is confusing and this chapter adheres to the definitions illustrated in *Figure 21.10*. Note in particular sPEEP in which a patient inhales spontaneously from ambient pressure but exhales against PEEP. This involves him in a considerable amount of additional work of breathing because he must raise his entire minute volume to the level of PEEP which is applied. This is undesirable and continuous positive airway pressure (CPAP) is much to be preferred to sPEEP. Unfortunately, true CPAP is difficult to achieve.

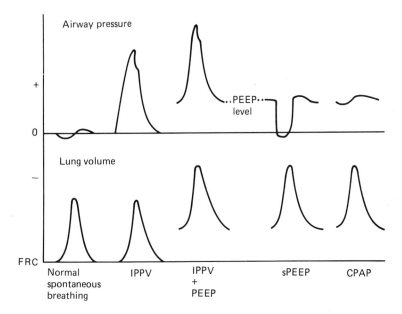

Figure 21.10 Definitions of nomenclature applied in this book to: IPPV, intermittent positive pressure ventilation; PEEP, positive end-expiratory pressure; sPEEP, true PEEP applied during spontaneous breathing; and CPAP, continuous positive airway pressure applied during spontaneous breathing. Note the unsatisfactory pressure swings during sPEEP. (Reproduced from Nunn (1984) by permission of the Editors of Anesthesiology Clinics)

Biased demand valves usually result in a pronounced dip in inspiratory pressure, increasing the total work of breathing. Loaded bellows are better but less convenient to manufacture. An exceptionally good circuit is the weighted bellows with balanced PEEP valve, described by Hewlett, Platt and Terry (1977), in which the inspiratory/expiratory pressure difference is only about 0.1 kPa (1 cmH$_2$O) during spontaneous breathing. The problem has been considered further by Hillman and Finucane (1985).

PEEP may be achieved by many techniques. The simplest is to exhale through a preset depth of water but more convenient methods are spring-loaded valves or diaphragms pressed down by gas or a column of water. It is also possible to use venturis and fans opposing the direction of expiratory gas flow.

Respiratory effects

Lung volume. End-expiratory alveolar pressure will equal the level of applied PEEP and this will reset the FRC in accord with the pressure/volume curve of the respiratory system (see *Figure 2.8*). For example, PEEP of 1 kPa (10 cmH$_2$O) will increase FRC by 500 ml in a patient with a compliance of 0.5 l/kPa (50 ml/cmH$_2$O). In many patients this may be expected to raise the tidal range above the closing capacity (page 41). It will also reduce airway resistance according to the inverse relationship between lung volume and airway resistance (see *Figure 3.10*). It may also change the relative compliance of the upper and lower parts of the lung (*Figure 21.11*), thereby improving the ventilation of the dependent overperfused parts of the lung.

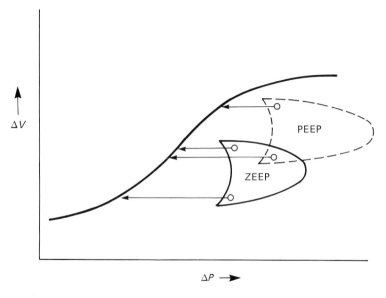

Figure 21.11 Effect of positive end-expiratory pressure (PEEP) on the relationship between regional pressure and volume in the lung (supine position). Note that compliance is greater in the upper part of the lung with zero end-expiratory pressure (ZEEP) and in the lower part of the lung with PEEP, which thus improves ventilation in the dependent zone of the lung. (Diagram kindly supplied by Professor J. Gareth Jones)

Dead space. Acute application of PEEP does not alter the dead space/tidal volume ratio (Lawler, 1987). However, there is indirect evidence that long-term application of PEEP causes an increase in the dead space, probably because of bronchiolar dilatation (Slavin et al., 1982).

Arterial Po_2. It is unlikely that PEEP improves arterial oxygenation in patients with healthy lungs but there is no doubt of the decrease in pulmonary shunting which is obtained in a wide range of pulmonary pathology, including oedema, collapse and the adult respiratory distress syndrome. This has resulted in PEEP being widely applied in the field of intensive care, and Kirby and his colleagues (1975) extended its use to levels in excess of 1.5 kPa (15 cmH$_2$O). During anaesthesia, it has been repeatedly observed that PEEP does little to improve arterial oxygenation in the patient with sound lungs. Nevertheless, it has now been shown that the level of pulmonary shunting is decreased (Bindslev et al., 1981). However, the accompanying decrease in cardiac output reduces the mixed venous oxygen saturation which counteracts the effect of a reduction in the shunt, resulting in a virtually unchanged arterial Po_2. Indeed, Dantzker, Lynch and Weg (1980) have suggested that shunt reduction in patients with adult respiratory distress syndrome is secondary to reduction in cardiac output (page 173).

Lung water. It was for many years believed that PEEP 'squeezed' oedema fluid out of the lung and that this was the cause of the dramatic improvement in arterial Po_2 which often followed the application of PEEP to patients with pulmonary oedema. However, there is now good evidence that lung water is not decreased by PEEP (Miller et al., 1981; Rizk and Murray, 1982). The improvement in arterial Po_2 is probably due to opening up of closed alveoli, transfer of oedema fluid to the interstitial compartment (page 433) and the reduction in cardiac output which reduces shunting in a wide range of circumstances (Cheney and Colley, 1980).

Intrapleural pressure. The intrapleural pressure is protected from the level of PEEP by the transmural pressure gradient of the lungs. Patients with diseased lungs tend to have an increased transmural pressure gradient which limits the rise in intrapleural pressure (*Figure 21.12*). Therefore their cardiovascular systems are better protected against the adverse effects of PEEP (see below).

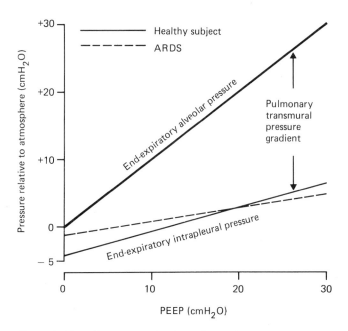

Figure 21.12 End-expiratory alveolar and intrapleural pressures as a function of positive end-expiratory pressure (PEEP). The lower continuous line shows intrapleural pressure in the relaxed healthy subject (Butler and Smith, 1957). The broken line shows values of intrapleural pressure in patients with adult respiratory distress syndrome (ARDS) taken from the work of Jardin et al. (1981). Absolute values of pressure probably reflect experimental technique and cannot be compared between the two studies. (Reproduced from Nunn (1984) by permission of the Editor of Anesthesiology Clinics)

Permeability. It has been found that PEEP increases the permeability of the lung to DTPA, a tracer molecule which does not readily cross the alveolar/capillary membrane (Rizk et al., 1984). However, it appears that this effect may be related to lung volume rather than to any damage to the membrane.

Barotrauma. A sustained increase in the transmural pressure gradient can damage the lung. The commonest forms of barotrauma attributable to artificial ventilation with or without PEEP are subcutaneous emphysema, pneumomediastinum and pneumothorax (Kumar et al., 1973). Tension lung cysts and hyperinflation of a lung or lobe have also been reported but the incidence of these complications is very variable. Pulmonary barotrauma probably starts as disruption of the alveolar membrane, with air entering the interstitial space and tracking back to the mediastinum along the bronchovascular bundles into the mediastinum from which it can reach the peritoneum, the pleural cavity or the subcutaneous tissues. Radiological demonstration of pulmonary interstitial gas may provide an early warning of barotrauma.

There is no agreement on the effect of PEEP on pulmonary barotrauma but Kumar et al. (1973) concluded that moderate levels of PEEP did not increase the level of barotrauma. However, Downs and Chapman (1976) found a very high incidence of barotrauma in patients exposed to PEEP in excess of 2 kPa (20 cmH$_2$O).

In patients who died following a prolonged period of exposure to PEEP, Slavin and his collegues (1982) demonstrated at autopsy a gross dilatation of terminal and respiratory bronchioles which they termed bronchiolectasis (*Figure 21.13*). Development of the condition was found to be related to the level of PEEP and

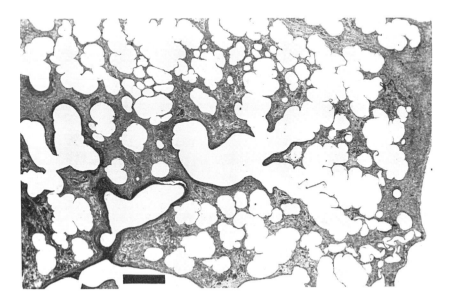

Figure 21.13 Histological appearances of bronchiolectasis in a patient who died after 16 days of artificial ventilation with positive end-expiratory pressure of 0.5 kPa (5 cmH$_2$O). Terminal and respiratory bronchioles are grossly dilated and surrounding alveoli are collapsed. Diameter of a normal terminal bronchiole is 0.5 mm. Scale bar is 1 mm. (Reproduced from Nunn (1984) by permission of the Editors of Anesthesiology Clinics)

the duration of its application. Indirect evidence suggested that it resulted in a large increase in dead space. Follow-up of a group of patients who had survived the use of PEEP indicated a return to normal pulmonary function with normal values for dead space (Navaratnarajah et al., 1984). The condition of bronchiolectasis appears to be analogous to bronchopulmonary dysplasia described in infants ventilated for respiratory distress syndrome (Taghizadeh and Reynolds, 1976).

Cardiovascular effects

Initially there was great reluctance to use PEEP because of the circulatory hazard which had been described in the classic paper of Cournand and his colleagues in 1948. Not too many papers in this field have two Nobel prize winners amongst their authors.

Cardiac output. There is general agreement that moderate levels of PEEP have relatively little effect on cardiac output. Suter, Fairley and Isenberg (1975) found in patients with acute pulmonary failure that PEEP had little effect on cardiac output up to 'best PEEP' (the level of PEEP which maximized oxygen flux). Bindslev et al. (1981) reported a 7 per cent decrease in cardiac output with 0.9 kPa (9 cmH$_2$O) of PEEP. Similar results were obtained by Jardin et al. (1981) in patients suffering from adult respiratory distress syndrome (*Figure 21.14*). Increased levels of PEEP caused substantial decreases in cardiac output in all three studies, and the response is clearly shown in *Figure 21.14*, which also shows the favourable effect of blood volume expansion.

There is general agreement that the main cause of the reduction in cardiac output is obstruction to filling of the right atrium, caused by the rise in intrathoracic pressure. The role of other factors has been hotly debated and consideration has been given to factors such as increased pulmonary capillary resistance (increased right ventricular afterload), decreased left ventricular compliance and decreased myocardial contractility. Furthermore, plasma from animals subjected to PEEP will depress contractility of isolated heart muscle preparations, suggesting the release of a negative inotrope (Grindlinger et al., 1979). This subject has been reviewed by the author (1984), and current views on the effect of PEEP on the circulation are summarized in *Figure 21.15*.

Oxygen flux. Increasing the level of PEEP tends to improve the arterial Po$_2$ while decreasing the cardiac output. As PEEP is increased the oxygen flux (the product of cardiac output and arterial oxygen content, page 256) tends to rise to a maximum and then falls (Suter, Fairley and Isenberg, 1975). Suter and his colleagues described their 'best PEEP' as the level which maximized oxygen flux. However, they did not optimize cardiac output with fluid replacement (see *Figure 21.14*) or with α-adrenergic stimulation or positive inotropes. It seems likely that they would have found optimal oxygen flux at higher levels of PEEP had they done so.

Arterial blood pressure. Figure 21.14 shows the decline in arterial pressure closely following the change in cardiac output. In Jardin's study the compensatory contraction of the peripheral vascular bed was only about half that required for maintenance of the arterial pressure in the face of the declining cardiac output. It has been suggested that this is due to PEEP causing inhibition of the cardiovascular regulatory centres (Cassidy, Gaffney and Johnson, 1981).

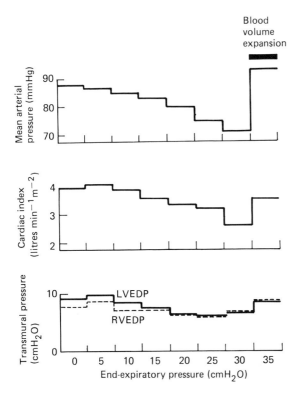

Figure 21.14 Cardiovascular responses as a function of positive end-expiratory pressure (PEEP) in patients with adult respiratory distress syndrome. Left and right ventricular end-diastolic pressure (LVEDP and RVEDP) were measured relative to intrapleural pressure. (Drawn from the data of Jardin et al. (1981) and reproduced from Nunn (1984) by permission of the Editors of Anesthesiology Clinics)

Interpretation of vascular pressures. Atrial pressures are normally measured relative to atmospheric pressure. When PEEP is applied, atrial pressures tend to be increased relative to atmospheric. However, relative to intrathoracic pressure, they are reduced at higher levels of PEEP (*Figure 21.14*). It is the transmural pressure gradient and not the level relative to atmosphere which is relevant to atrial filling.

An additional problem arises when the tip of a Swan–Ganz catheter lies in zone 1 of the lung where there is no pulmonary blood flow (page 131). It is presumed that the application of PEEP increases the extent of zone 1 and an artefact may thus be introduced into the measurement of pulmonary capillary wedge pressure (Roy et al., 1977).

Renal effects

Patients undergoing IPPV tend to become oedematous. Protein depletion and inappropriate fluid loading may be factors but there is now evidence that PEEP may itself reduce glomerular filtration (Marquez et al., 1979). Arterial pressure tends to be reduced as described above, while central venous pressure is raised. Therefore, the pressure gradient between renal artery and vein is reduced and this

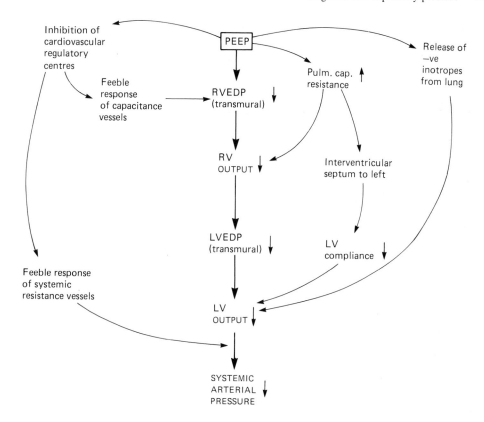

Figure 21.15 Summary of the cardiovascular effects of positive end-expiratory pressure (PEEP). See text for full explanation. RVEDP and LVEDP, right and left ventricular end-diastolic pressure; RV and LV, right and left ventricular

has a direct effect on renal blood flow. In addition, PEEP causes elevated levels of vasopressin, possibly due to activation of left atrial receptors. However, the change in vasopressin level is insufficient to explain the changes in urinary flow rate.

Negative (subatmospheric) end-expiratory pressure (NEEP)

The potentially deleterious effect of PEEP on the circulation not only delayed its introduction into clinical practice but also led to the use of NEEP, partly to facilitate expiration and partly for its supposedly beneficial effect on the circulation. NEEP was a fashionable extra on ventilators between about 1960 and 1970.

Respiratory effects

NEEP during expiration was seen as the counterpart of overpressure during inspiration, and *Figure 21.3b* shows how it might be used to obtain a reduction in the time required for expiration. However, expiration is fundamentally different from inspiration during IPPV. During inspiration there can be no question of airway collapse because the inflation pressure acts to distend the airways. During expiration, pressure gradients are acting to compress the airways as shown in *Figure 3.7*. Application of NEEP may then act directly to collapse the airways and so make matters worse. This is most likely to occur in patients with increased tendency to flow-related airway collapse, who are just the patients in whom some assistance to expiration might be required.

It might appear that the application of NEEP would increase the tidal volume by instituting a type of push–pull tidal exchange on either side of FRC. This, however, is unlikely to occur if FRC is close to residual volume, which tends to be the case during anaesthesia (page 357) and also in many patients who have severe respiratory problems. In such patients the inspiratory reserve remains the only practicable zone for increasing the tidal volume.

There has been no demonstration of any improvement of gas exchange with NEEP. In fact, Sykes et al. (1970) found the alveolar/arterial Po_2 gradient to be increased and Watson (1962b) found an increase in dead space.

Circulatory effects

If PEEP embarrasses the circulation, it appeared logical that NEEP would be beneficial. Unfortunately, this has not been borne out in practice. Scott, Stephen and Davie (1972), using NEEP of 0.5–0.7 kPa (5–7 cmH$_2$O), found no significant improvement in either cardiac output or arterial blood pressure in six patients undergoing artificial ventilation in an intensive care unit. Similar results were reported during anaesthesia (Prys-Roberts et al., 1967). Part of the difficulty probably lies in communicating the subatmospheric pressure to the intrathoracic space. *Figure 19.11* shows that below FRC in the anaesthetized patient, the pressure/volume curve is very flat and the pulmonary transmural pressure gradient becomes very large as the lung volume decreases below FRC. It is not possible to communicate a subatmospheric pressure from the inside of a collapsed balloon to the exterior. As in the case of the respiratory effects, the supposed circulatory benefits of NEEP have not stood the test of time and the technique is now virtually obsolete.

Weaning

Weaning depends upon obtained stable and satisfactory values for a range of respiratory variables, and typical criteria are listed in *Table 21.5*. The commonest technique of weaning is the abrupt cessation of artificial ventilation for periods of 2–3 minutes, with gradual prolongation of these periods depending upon the performance of the patient during the last period. Whereas this approach is satisfactory for an uncomplicated case and for healthy patients recovering from neuromuscular block, it may well be unsatisfactory for patients in whom ventilatory capacity and gas exchange function are marginal. Ventilatory capacity cannot, of course, be measured while the patient is still on a ventilator. Attempts to wean such patients often result in deterioration of minute volume and blood gases during short periods of spontaneous breathing but there may be late deterioration caused by factors such as fatigue of the respiratory muscles.

Table 21.5 Criteria for weaning

Tests of ventilatory capacity	
VC	$\geq$ 10–15 ml/kg
FEV$_1$	$\geq$ 10 ml/kg
Peak insp. pressure	-20 to -30 cmH$_2$O
Resting minute volume	> 10 l/min (doubled with max. effort)
Tests of blood oxygenation	< 40–47 kPa (300–350 mmHg)
(A–a) Po$_2$ difference	< 10–20%
Shunt	< 55–60%
Dead space/tidal volume	

(After Weisman et al., 1983)

No single variable is a reliable indicator of the success of a wean. Minute volume is probably the most useful but it is also necessary to take into account arterial Po$_2$ and Pco$_2$, bearing in mind that the latter will rise only slowly (page 226). In addition to these measurements, it is necessary to observe the patient for signs of fatigue, distress and dyscoordinated breathing.

In cases of difficulty, various alternative techniques of weaning may be tried.

Triggered ventilators (page 410) have been used to encourage the patient to re-establish spontaneous respiration. However, results were generally disappointing and the technique is now seldom used. It has even been suggested that the patient might come to realize that he need not make a full respiratory effort and so be discouraged.

Respiratory stimulants may be helpful, and doxapram is the best agent since it shows minimal tachyphylaxis. An intravenous infusion in the range 1–8 mg/min may be started just before disconnecting the ventilator. This may be continued for some days, with gradual reduction of the infusion rate.

Intermittent mandatory ventilation (page 409) is a very valuable aid to weaning, which is accomplished by progressive reduction of the mandatory ventilation. This approach avoids the abrupt transition between artificial and spontaneous ventilation and supplies the patient with a fall-back level of ventilation which is progressively reduced. Clearly a dangerous situation might arise if spontaneous ventilation suddenly deteriorated in the late phase of a wean when the mandatory ventilation had been reduced to a level insufficient to maintain life. However, monitoring of the patient should avoid this eventuality and the method has gained wide acceptance. Nevertheless, opinions differ on the value of IMV for weaning (Downs, Perkins and Modell, 1974; Weisman et al., 1983).

Mandatory minute volume (page 411) assists weaning from a completely different standpoint. The patient is left to resume spontaneous breathing if and when he is able. By whatever amount he is able to breathe, the artifical ventilation is reduced by the same amount so that arterial Pco$_2$ should remain approximately the same. No active intervention is required by staff and the ratio of spontaneous to artificial ventilation may fluctuate widely for a considerable period before spontaneous breathing becomes fully established. Essentially the patient is allowed to wean himself in his own time, with the guarantee that his minute volume will be protected whether he breathes or not.

It should, however, be stressed that although the minute volume is protected, there is no guarantee that the alveolar ventilation will remain constant. If the patient takes rapid and shallow breaths, this may be interpreted as an adequate minute volume while an increased dead space/tidal volume ratio may make the alveolar ventilation inadequate. In this connection it should be noted that the Erica ventilator in the MMV mode disregards low levels of spontaneous respiration. The efficacy of MMV for weaning has not yet been tested in a controlled trial.

Ventilation of the newborn

This subject is considered in Chapter 18.

Chapter 22

Extracorporeal gas exchange

The stimulus for the development of extracorporeal gas exchangers was cardiac surgery. Certain procedures were possible with stopped circulation, often prolonged by the induction of hypothermia. However, more intricate operations required an open heart for periods in excess of 20 minutes and this could not be achieved safely with simple cardiac arrest and hypothermia.

The design of extracorporeal gas exchangers has been based on the principles of the real lung. A large interface is required between blood and gas and this has been achieved both with and without a membrane at the interface which would correspond to the alveolar/capillary membrane.

Factors in design

The lungs of an adult have an interface between blood and gas of the order of 126 m^2 (page 16). It is not possible to achieve this in an artificial substitute and artificial lungs can be considered to have a very low 'diffusing capacity'. Nevertheless, they function satisfactorily within limits for the following reasons. Firstly, the real lung is adapted for maximal exercise, while patients on cardiopulmonary bypass are usually close to basal metabolic rate or less if hypothermia is used. Secondly, under resting conditions at sea level, there is an enormous reserve in the capacity of the lung to achieve equilibrium between pulmonary capillary blood and alveolar gas (see *Figure 8.2*). Therefore a subnormal diffusing capacity does not necessarily result in arterial hypoxaemia. Thirdly, it is possible to operate an artificial lung with an 'alveolar' oxygen concentration in excess of 90%, compared with 14% for real alveolar gas under normal circumstances. This greatly increases the gas transfer for a given 'diffusing capacity' of the artificial lung (page 189). Fourthly, there is no great difficulty in increasing the 'ventilation/perfusion ratio' of a membrane artificial lung above the value of about 0.8 in the normal lung at rest. Fifthly, the 'capillary transit time' of the artificial lung can be increased beyond the time of about 0.75 second in the real lung. This facilitates the approach of blood Po_2 to 'alveolar' Po_2 (see *Figure 8.2*). Finally, in certain types of gas-exchangers, it is possible to use countercurrent flow between gas and blood. This does not occur in the lungs of mammals. Carbon dioxide exchanges much more readily than oxygen because of its greater blood and lipid solubility. Therefore, in general, elimination of carbon dioxide does not present a major problem and the limiting factor of an artificial lung is oxygenation.

423

Against these favourable design considerations, there are certain advantages of the real lung, apart from its very large surface area, which are difficult to emulate. Firstly, the pulmonary capillaries have a diameter close to that of the erythrocyte. Therefore, each erythrocyte is brought into very close contact with the alveolar gas (see *Figure 1.7*). Streamline flow through much wider channels in a membrane artificial lung tends to result in a stream of erythrocytes remaining at a distance from the interface. Much thought has been devoted to the creation of turbulent flow to counteract this effect. In contrast, there is a very favourable diffusion distance in a bubble oxygenator when foaming occurs. Secondly, the vascular endothelium is specially adapted to prevent undesirable changes in the formed elements of blood, particularly neutrophils and platelets. Most artificial surfaces cause clotting of blood, and artificial lungs therefore require the use of anticoagulants. Further adverse changes result from denaturation of protein (see below). Thirdly, the lung has an extensive non-respiratory function in the uptake, synthesis and biotransformation of many constituents of the blood (see Chapter 11). This function is lost when the lungs are bypassed. Fourthly, the lung is an extremely efficient filter with an effective pore size of about 10 μm for flow rates of blood up to about 25 l/min. This is difficult to achieve with any man-made filter.

Types of extracorporeal gas exchangers

With blood/gas interface

Bubble oxygenators. The simplest design of extracorporeal oxygenator stems from the well-tried wash bottle of the chemist. By breaking up the gas stream into small bubbles, it is possible to achieve very large surface areas of interface. However, the smaller the bubbles, the greater the tendency for them to remain in suspension when the blood is returned to the patient. This is dangerous because of the direct access of the blood to the cerebral circulation. A compromise is to break the gas stream into bubbles ranging from 2 to 7 mm diameter, giving an effective area of interface of the order of 15 m². With a mean red cell transit time of 1–2 seconds and a 'ventilation/perfusion ratio' of unity or slightly more and an oxygen concentration of more than 90%, this gives an acceptable outflow blood Po_2 with blood flow rates up to about 6 l/min (Finlayson and Kaplan, 1979). The Pco_2 of the outflowing blood must be controlled by admixture of carbon dioxide with the inflowing oxygen in the gas phase. Priming volumes range from 400 to 900 ml. Gas is passed through the blood in a reservoir of about 1 litre capacity in which foaming takes place. Blood is then passed to a second reservoir for 'debubbling' to take place with the help of an antifoaming compound (e.g. Dow Corning Medical Antifoam-A).

Disc and vertical screen oxygenators. These devices have been used to film blood over a large surface area which is directly exposed to gas. This prevents the danger of bubbles remaining in the blood and there tends to be less damage to the blood. However, it is not practicable to obtain the large surface areas of a bubble oxygenator and the apparatus is troublesome to clean and maintain. These devices are now declining in popularity.

Membrane oxygenators

Two types of membrane are in use. Silicone rubber can be formed into a continuous thin uniform membrane. Rubber is a lipid and is freely permeable to oxygen, carbon dioxide and anaesthetic gases. An alternative approach is the use of membranes of polypropylene, Teflon or polyacrylamide which contain small pores ranging from 0.1 to 5 μm diameter (Finlayson and Kaplan, 1979). These pores tend to fill with protein which then forms a layer over the blood side of the membrane, the whole being freely permeable to the respiratory gases. However, performance declines over several hours which is not the case with a silicone rubber membrane. Microporous membranes can weep if the apparatus is primed with a protein-free solution, but in normal use can withstand a hydrostatic pressure gradient of the order of normal arterial blood pressure. Surface areas of the order of 10 m^2 can be achieved.

A major problem has been the mixing of blood as it flows across the membrane. The blood pathway is much thicker than the normal pulmonary capillary and a slow moving boundary layer impairs gas exchange. This has been avoided by designs which encourage mixing of the blood stream.

Blood pumps

Blood normally passes from the body to the oxygenator via a cannula in a major vein. After leaving the oxygenator, the pressure must be raised to permit re-entry into the patient's arterial circulation. Roller pumps are now universally used for this purpose and are adjusted to be not quite occlusive. This minimizes damage to the formed elements of the blood. There is no convincing evidence that performance is better with pulsatile blood flow.

Damage to blood

Damage due to non-occlusive roller pumps is almost negligible. Damage due to oxygenators is probably far less than that which results from surgical suction in removing blood from the operative site and, during cardiac surgery, this factor tends to obscure the differences attributable to the type of oxygenator. However, during prolonged extracorporeal oxygenation for respiratory failure, the influence of the type of oxygenator becomes important and membrane oxygenators are then superior to bubble oxygenators.

Protein denaturation

Contact between blood and either gas bubbles or plastic surfaces results in protein denaturation and plastic surfaces become coated with a layer of protein. With membrane oxygenators this tends to be self-limiting, but bubble oxygenators cause a continuous and progressive loss of protein. This is the main factor which limits their prolonged use.

Complement activation

Complement activation occurs when blood comes into contact with any artificial surface and complement C5a is known to be formed after cardiopulmonary bypass surgery (Chenoweth et al., 1981). This results in margination of neutrophils on vascular endothelium, possible consequences of which are considered on page 488.

Erythrocytes

Damage may amount to shortened survival or actual destruction of erythrocytes due to shear forces, turbulence, foaming or the use of occlusive pumps. Surgical suction is generally more damaging than the oxygenator. Without suction, the damage to erythrocytes with membrane oxygenators is within reasonable limits for many hours and they are superior in this respect to bubble oxygenators. Released haemoglobin is initially bound to proteins but eventually saturates the receptors and is excreted through the kidneys. Red cell ghosts are now believed to be more damaging than free haemoglobin and they may need to be removed by filtration.

Leucocytes and platelets

Counts of these elements are usually reduced by an amount which is in excess of the changes attributable to haemodilution. Platelets are lost by adhesion and aggregation, and postoperative counts are commonly about half the preoperative value (Finlayson and Kaplan, 1979).

Coagulation

No oxygenator can function without causing coagulation of the blood. Anti-coagulation is therefore a *sine qua non* of the technique and heparinization is universally employed for this purpose. This inevitably results in excess bleeding from any surgical incision.

Prolonged extracorporeal oxygenation for respiratory failure

It has long been known that extracorporeal oxygenation can be maintained for a few days in patients with respiratory failure. For reasons outlined above, membrane oxygenators are superior to bubble oxygenators for this application. It was hoped that the 'resting of the lung' might permit healing and recovery in patients with the adult respiratory distress syndrome (ARDS), considered in Chapter 26. This hypothesis led to the multi-centre randomized prospective trial of extracorporeal membrane oxygenation (ECMO) for patients with ARDS (Zapol et al., 1979).

Entry criteria were either:

1. Arterial Po_2 below 6.7 kPa (50 mmHg) for more than 2 hours, while breathing 100% oxygen, with positive end-expiratory pressure (PEEP) at least 0.5 kPa (5 cmH$_2$O).
    or
2. Arterial Po_2 below 6.7 kPa (50 mmHg) for more than 12 hours, while breathing 60% oxygen, with PEEP at least 0.5 kPa (5 cmH$_2$O) and a shunt fraction greater than 30 per cent.

Exclusion criteria included a pulmonary capillary wedge pressure of more than 3.3 kPa (25 mmHg), chronic pulmonary disease, malignancy, etc. Patients were then randomly allocated to conventional intermittent positive pressure ventilation (IPPV) or ECMO.

The study was terminated after treatment of the first 90 patients when it was found that mortality was more than 90 per cent in both groups with no statistically significant difference between the two forms of treatment. There has been much discussion on the reasons for the failure of the ECMO trial but Zapol pointed out that the use of venoarterial bypass would have reduced pulmonary perfusion and pulmonary arterial pressure by about 30 per cent. Possible adverse consequences of loss of pulmonary perfusion are outlined above.

Extracorporeal removal of carbon dioxide

A radically new approach to artificial gas exchange has been developed by Gattinoni and his colleagues in Milan. In essence, he has restricted extracorporeal gas exchange to removal of carbon dioxide and maintained oxygenation by a modification of apnoeic mass movement oxygenation. The lungs are either kept motionless or are ventilated two to three times per minute (low-frequency positive-pressure ventilation with extracorporeal CO_2 removal—LFPPV-ECCO$_2$R) (Gattinoni et al., 1980; Pesenti et al., 1981).

The technique depends on two important differences between the exchange of carbon dioxide and oxygen. Firstly, membrane oxygenators remove carbon dioxide some 10–20 times more effectively than they take up oxygen. Secondly, the normal arterial oxygen content (20 ml/100 ml) is very close to the maximum oxygen capacity, even with 100% oxygen in the gas phase (22 ml/100 ml). Therefore, there is little scope for superoxygenation of a fraction of the pulmonary circulation to compensate for a larger fraction of the pulmonary circulation in which oxygenation does not take place. In contrast, the normal mixed venous carbon dioxide content is 52 ml/100 ml compared with an arterial carbon dioxide content of 48 ml/100 ml and there is therefore ample scope for removing a larger than normal fraction of carbon dioxide from a part of the pulmonary circulation to compensate for a remaining fraction which does not undergo any removal of carbon dioxide (*Figure 22.1*). I believe it is true to say that, although the underlying physiology is self-evident, this difference between carbon dioxide and oxygen has escaped attention in recent years.

It is therefore possible to maintain carbon dioxide homoeostasis by diversion of only a small fraction of the cardiac output through an extracorporeal membrane oxygenator (Gattinoni et al., 1980). This is best illustrated by means of the Fick equation for carbon dioxide:

$$\begin{array}{c}\text{carbon}\\\text{dioxide}\\\text{removal}\end{array} = \begin{array}{c}\text{pulmonary}\\\text{blood flow}\end{array} \left(\begin{array}{c}\text{mixed venous}\\\text{CO}_2\text{ content}\end{array} - \text{arterial CO}_2\text{ content}\right)$$

Under normal circumstances, typical values might be:

$$240 = 6000 \ (52/100 - 48/100)$$
(values in ml and ml/min)

Using Gattinoni's technique with a flow through the membrane oxygenator of 1.3 l/min, typical values might be:

$$240 = 1300 \ (52/100 - 33.5/100)$$

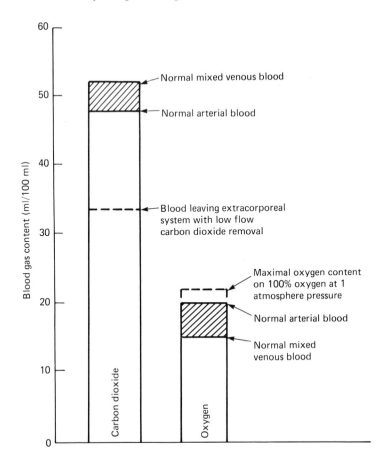

Figure 22.1 Comparison of absolute contents of carbon dioxide and oxygen in blood at 1 atmosphere pressure. Note that there is ample reserve potential for removing carbon dioxide below the level attained in normal arterial blood. In contrast, the maximal possible oxygen content of blood at 1 atmosphere is not greatly in excess of the level in normal arterial blood. This difference makes possible the extracorporeal removal of carbon dioxide (but not the supply of oxygen) by passing a small fraction of the cardiac output through an extracorporeal gas exchanger.

The outflow from the membrane oxygenator would thus be 1.3 l/min with a carbon dioxide content of 33.5 ml/100 ml, corresponding to a P_{CO_2} of about 2 kPa (15 mmHg). This would account for removal of the whole of the normal metabolic production of carbon dioxide. Furthermore, there is no necessity for the bypass to be venoarterial and the far simpler venovenous bypass has been used by Gattinoni. As a result there is no reduction in pulmonary blood flow or pressure.

With P_{CO_2} held constant by extracorporeal removal of carbon dioxide, there is no obstacle to the continued uptake of oxygen by mass movement apnoeic oxygenation, a process which is normally terminated after about 30 minutes by progressive increase in P_{CO_2} (see page 228). All that is necessary is to replace the alveolar gas with oxygen and connect the trachea to a supply of oxygen, which is then drawn into the lungs at a rate equal to the metabolic consumption of oxygen, and this should continue indefinitely. In fact, Gattinoni recommends ventilation of the lungs two to three times a minute with long end-expiratory pauses and PEEP of about 1.5 kPa (15 cmH$_2$O). This is clearly beneficial for preservation of compliance and airway patency but imposes minimal danger of barotrauma.

The technique would seem to expose the lungs to very high concentrations of oxygen and the possibility of oxygen toxicity (Chapter 29). In practice this does not appear to have been a problem, possibly due to induction of superoxide dismutase during an earlier stage of therapy (page 490). Furthermore, the air which flows through the membrane exchanger maintains the nitrogen tension of the body and this does not appear to interfere with the uptake of oxygen. Alternatively, the oxygen concentration of the gas passing through the membrane exchanger can be increased to make a contribution to oxygenation of the arterial blood.

Gattinoni et al. (1980) described the reversal of respiratory failure in three patients who fulfilled the entry criteria of the ECMO trial and might therefore have been expected to have a 90 per cent mortality. Since then, Gattinoni has described a series of 18 patients, all fulfilling the ECMO entry criteria, of whom 11 survived (Gattinoni et al., 1983). LFPPV-ECCO$_2$R was maintained for an average of 6 days. Reports of use of this technique in other centres are still sparse at the time of writing (Hickling, 1986; Hickling et al., 1986).

Chapter 23

Pulmonary oedema

Pulmonary oedema is defined as an increase in pulmonary extravascular water, which occurs when transudation or exudation exceeds the capacity of the lymphatic drainage.

Anatomical factors
(see Chapter 1)

The pulmonary capillary endothelial cells abut against one another at fairly loose junctions which are of the order of 5 nm (50 Å) wide (DeFouw, 1983). These junctions permit the passage of quite large molecules and the pulmonary lymph contains albumin at about half the concentration in plasma.

Epithelial cells meet at tight junctions with a gap of only about 1 nm (DeFouw, 1983). The tightness of these junctions is crucial for prevention of the escape of large molecules, such as albumin, from the interstitial fluid into the alveoli.

The lung has a well developed lymphatic system draining the interstitial tissue through a network of channels around the bronchi and pulmonary vessels towards the hilum. Lymphatic vessels cannot be identified at alveolar level but may be seen in association with bronchioles. Down to airway generation 11 (see *Table 1.1*), the lymphatics lie in a potential space around the air passages and vessels, separating them from the lung parenchyma.

In the hilum of the lung, the lymphatic drainage passes through several groups of tracheobronchial lymph glands, where they receive tributaries from the superficial subpleural plexus. Most of the lymph from the left lung usually enters the thoracic duct where it can be conveniently sampled in the sheep. The right side drains into the right lymphatic duct. However, the pulmonary lymphatics often cross the midline and pass independently into the junction of internal jugular and subclavian veins on the corresponding sides of the body. Studies in dogs have indicated that approximately 15 per cent of the flow in the thoracic duct derives from the lungs (Meyer and Ottaviano, 1972).

The normal lymphatic drainage from human lungs is only about 10 ml/h. Lymphatic flow can increase greatly when transudation into the interstitial spaces is increased. This presumably occurs when pulmonary oedema is threatened but it cannot be conveniently measured in man.

Stages of pulmonary oedema

Whatever the aetiology of pulmonary oedema, it is possible to recognize at least four stages. With gradual onset of the condition, pulmonary oedema passes progressively through the four stages. However, in fulminating cases, it may first appear as the fourth stage. There will usually be a prodromal stage in which pulmonary lymphatic drainage is increased but there is no detectable increase in extravascular water.

Stage I. Interstitial pulmonary oedema

In its mildest form, there is an increase in interstitial fluid but without passage of oedema fluid into the alveoli. With the light microscope this is first detected as cuffs of distended lymphatics, typically '8'-shaped around the adjacent branches of the bronchi and pulmonary artery (*Plate 2* and *Figure 23.1*). When well developed, the cuffing accounts for the butterfly shadow in the chest radiograph. Electron microscopy shows fluid accumulation in the alveolar septa but this is charac-

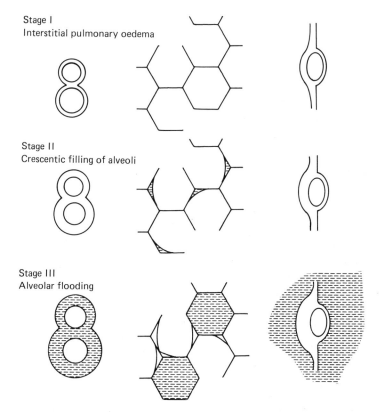

Figure 23.1 Stages in the development of pulmonary oedema. On the left is shown the development of the cuff of distended lymphatics around the branches of the bronchi and pulmonary arteries. In the middle is the appearance of the alveoli by light microscopy (fixed in inflation). On the right is the appearance of the pulmonary capillaries by electron microscopy. The active side of the capillary is to the right. For an explanation of the stages, see text.

teristically confined to the 'service' side of the pulmonary capillary which contains the stroma, leaving the geometry of the 'active' side unchanged (see *Figure 1.9*). Thus, gas exchange is better preserved than might be expected from the overall increase in lung water.

Physical signs are generally absent in stage I and the alveolar/arterial Po_2 gradient is normal or only slightly increased. Diagnosis rests on the chest radiograph and the demonstration of causative factors such as an increased wedge pressure.

Stage II. Crescentic filling of the alveoli

With further increase in extravascular lung water, interstitial oedema of the alveolar septa is increased and fluid begins to pass into the alveolar lumina. It first appears as crescents in the angles between adjacent septa, at least in lungs which have been fixed in inflation (*Figure 23.1*). The centre of the alveoli and most of the alveolar walls remain clear, and gas exchange is not grossly abnormal.

Stage III. Alveolar flooding

In the third stage, there is quantal alveolar flooding. Some alveoli are totally flooded while others, frequently adjacent, have only the crescentic filling or else no fluid at all in their lumina. It appears that fluid accumulates up to a point at which there is a critical radius of curvature when surface tension sharply increases the transudation pressure gradient. This would produce flooding on an all-or-none basis for each individual alveolus.

Clearly there can be no effective gas exchange in the capillaries of an alveolar septum which is flooded on both sides and the overall defect of gas exchange may be considered as venous admixture or shunt. It is not helpful to consider the condition as an impaired diffusing capacity. Rales can be heard during inspiration and the lung fields show an overall opacity superimposed on the butterfly shadow. Due to the difference in pulmonary vascular pressures (page 122), alveolar flooding tends to occur in the dependent parts of the lungs.

Stage IV. Froth in the air passages

When alveolar flooding is extreme, the air passages become blocked with froth which moves to and fro with breathing. This effectively stops all gas exchange and is rapidly fatal unless treated.

The mechanism of pulmonary oedema

The Starling equation and fluid exchange across the endothelium

Transudation of intravascular fluid must be considered in two stages, the first from the microcirculation into interstitial space (i.e. across the endothelium) and the second from the interstitial space into the alveoli (i.e. across the epithelium) (*Figure 23.2*). Passage of fluid across the endothelium is promoted by the hydrostatic pressure differential but counteracted by the osmotic pressure of the plasma proteins. The balance of pressures is normally sufficient to prevent any appreciable transudation but it may be upset in a wide variety of pathological circumstances.

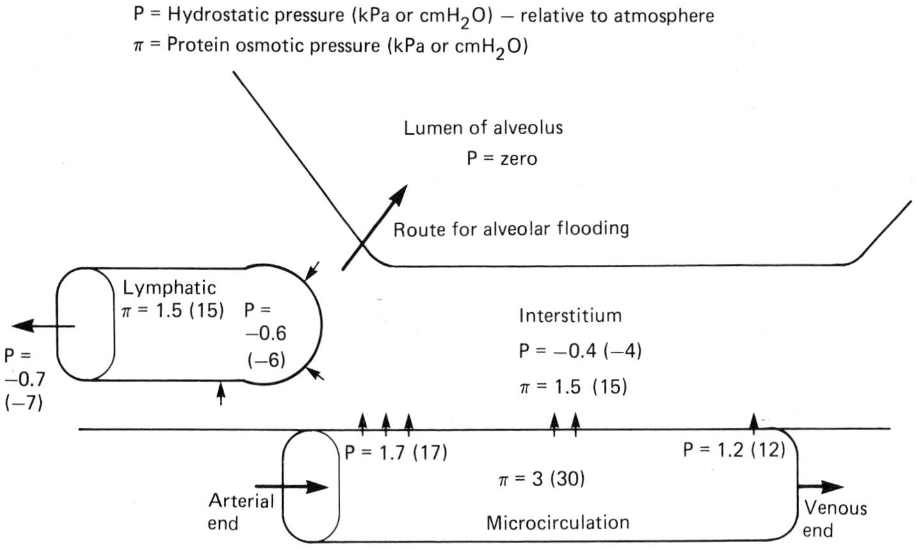

P = Hydrostatic pressure (kPa or cmH$_2$O) — relative to atmosphere

π = Protein osmotic pressure (kPa or cmH$_2$O)

Lumen of alveolus
P = zero

Route for alveolar flooding

Lymphatic
π = 1.5 (15)   P = −0.6 (−6)

P = −0.7 (−7)

Interstitium
P = −0.4 (−4)
π = 1.5 (15)

P = 1.7 (17)

π = 3 (30)

P = 1.2 (12)

Arterial end

Microcirculation

Venous end

Figure 23.2 Normal values for hydrostatic and plasma protein osmotic pressures in the pulmonary microcirculation and interstitium. Values are taken from Staub (1984).

It is customary to display the relationship between fluid flow and the balance of pressures in the form of the Starling equation. For the endothelial barrier this is as follows:

$$\dot{Q} = K[(Pmv - Ppmv) - \Sigma(\Pi mv - \Pi pmv)]$$

$\dot{Q}$ is the flow rate of transudated fluid which, in equilibrium, will be equal to the lymphatic drainage.

K   is the hydraulic conductance (i.e. flow rate of fluid per unit pressure gradient across the endothelium.

Pmv   is the hydrostatic pressure in the microvasculature.

Ppmv   is the hydrostatic pressure in the perimicrovascular tissue (i.e. the interstitium).

Σ is the reflection coefficient, in this case applying to albumin. It is an expression of the permeability of the endothelium to the solute (albumin). A value of unity indicates total reflection corresponding to zero concentration of the solute in the interstitial fluid. A value of zero indicates free passage of the solute across the membrane and, with equal concentrations on both sides of the membrane, such a solute could exert no osmotic pressure across the membrane. This normally applies to the crystalloids in plasma.

Πmv is the osmotic pressure the solute exerts within the microvasculature.

Πpmv is the osmotic pressure the solute exerts in the perimicrovascular tissue.

Under normal circumstances in man, the pulmonary lymph flow ($\dot{Q}$) is about 10 ml/hour with a protein content about half that of plasma. The pulmonary microvascular pressure (Pmv) is in the range 0–2 kPa (0–15 mmHg), relative to atmosphere, depending on the vertical height within the lung field (see *Figure 6.4*). Furthermore, there is a progressive decrease in capillary pressure from its arterial to its venous end, since approximately one-half of the pulmonary vascular resistance is across the capillary bed (see *Figures 6.3* and *23.2*). It is meaningless to talk about the mean pulmonary capillary pressure.

The hydrostatic pressure in the perimicrovascular tissue is not easy to measure. However, using implanted pressure-measuring capsules, Meyer, Meyer and Guyton (1968) found an average pressure of 1.3 kPa (10 mmHg) below atmospheric. Bhattacharya, Gropper and Staub (1984), studying the excised dog lung held at an inflation pressure of 0.5 kPa (5 cmH$_2$O), found interstitial pressures at the alveolar junctions some 0.4 kPa (4 cmH$_2$O) less than the alveolar pressure (*Figure 23.2*). There was a gradient in interstitial pressure from alveoli to hilum where the pressure was about 0.7 kPa (7 cmH$_2$O) less than alveolar pressure. There was no vertical gradient in interstitial pressures such as might have been expected from gravity.

With increasing pulmonary oedema, the interstitial space can accommodate large volumes of water with only small increases in pressure, the interstitial compliance being high. Some 500 ml can be accommodated in the interstitium and lymphatics of the human lungs with a rise of pressure of only about 0.2 kPa (2 cmH$_2$O) (Staub, 1984). However, above a certain critical level of pressure, fluid in the interstitial space floods into the alveoli through a high conductance pathway which has not yet been defined. Staub (1983) has compared this with an overflowing bath tub.

The capacity and compliance of the interstitium for water are increased at larger lung volumes (Gee and Williams, 1979) and this is considered to be one of the mechanisms by which positive end-expiratory pressure (PEEP) improves gas exchange although it does not decrease the total amount of lung water (page 415).

The reflection coefficient for albumin (Σ) in the healthy lung is about 0.5. The overall osmotic pressure gradient between blood and interstitial fluid is about 1.5 kPa (11.5 mmHg). Thus there is a small balance favouring transudation. There is a considerable safety margin in the upper part of the lung where the microvascular hydrostatic pressure is lowest. However, in the dependent part of the lung, where the hydrostatic pressure is highest, the safety margin is relatively slender.

Gram-for-gram, albumin exerts about twice the osmotic pressure of the globulins which have a higher molecular weight. However, the total osmotic pressure of the plasma proteins is not simply the summation of the albumin and globulin fractions because of protein–protein interaction (Staub, 1984).

Fluid exchange across the alveolar epithelium

The permeability of this membrane is considered in Chapter 8 (page 203). It is freely permeable to gases, water and hydrophobic substances. However, it is virtually impermeable to albumin and small solutes.

It is possible to construct a Starling equation for the epithelium (Staub, 1983) but there are considerable uncertainties about the osmotic pressure of the alveolar lining fluid. It has even been suggested that the alveolar lining is largely dry (Hills, 1982), which would make the concept meaningless. However, it does appear that transudation across the alveolar epithelium is virtualy zero unless the integrity of the barrier is compromised or the interstitial pressure increases above a critical level.

Aetiology

On the basis of the Starling equations, it is possible to make a rational approach to the aetiology of pulmonary oedema. There are four groups of aetiological factors, classified according to their effect on factors in the Starling equation.

Increased capillary pressure (haemodynamic pulmonary oedema)

This group comprises the commonest causes of pulmonary oedema. Basically the mechanism is an elevation of the hydrostatic pressure gradient across the pulmonary capillary wall, until it exceeds the osmotic pressure of the plasma proteins. Interstitial fluid accumulates until its pressure exceeds a critical value which then results in alveolar flooding. The oedema fluid has a protein content which is less than that of normal pulmonary lymph (Staub, 1984).

Absolute hypervolaemia may result from overtransfusion, from excessive and rapid administration of other blood volume expanders or from accidental access of irrigation fluids through open venous channels in hollow organs, as for example during prostatectomy.

Relative pulmonary hypervolaemia may result from redistribution of the circulating blood volume into the lungs. This may result from use of the Trendelenburg position or occlusive limb tourniquets. Vasopressor mechanisms and drugs act on the systemic circulation to a greater extent than the pulmonary circulation and so redirect blood into the pulmonary circulation.

Raised pulmonary venous pressure will inevitably result in an increase in pulmonary capillary pressure. This may occur from any form of left heart failure, including left ventricular failure, dysrhythmias, mitral valve lesions and rare conditions such as atrial myxoma. It is also possible that there may be vasoconstriction in the pulmonary veins and this apears to be caused by histamine (page 129) and perhaps also in Gram-negative septicaemia (Kuida et al., 1958).

Increased pulmonary blood flow may raise the pulmonary capillary pressure sufficiently to precipitate pulmonary oedema. This may result from a left-to-right cardiac shunt, anaemia or, rarely, as a result of exercise.

Subatmospheric airway pressure was once popular in an attempt to improve cardiac output (page 419). It is uncertain whether this could increase the transmural hydrostatic pressure gradient or whether the capillary pressure would change with the alveolar pressure.

Increased permeability of the alveolar/capillary membrane (permeability oedema)

This group comprises the next commonest causes of pulmonary oedema. The mechanism is the loss of integrity of the alveolar/capillary membrane, allowing albumin and other macromolecules to enter the alveoli. The osmotic pressure gradient which opposes transudation is then lost. The oedema fluid has a protein content which approaches that of plasma (Staub, 1984).

The alveolar/capillary membrane can be damaged either directly or indirectly by many agents which are reviewed in Chapter 26. Apart from the possibility of the condition progressing to the adult respiratory distress syndrome, permeability pulmonary oedema is always potentially very dangerous. The presence of protein in the alveoli tends to make the oedema refractory and the protein may become organized into a so-called hyaline membrane.

Decreased osmotic pressure of the plasma proteins

As in the previous category, the mechanism here is a reduction in the osmotic pressure gradient opposing transudation. Although seldom the primary cause of pulmonary oedema, a reduced plasma albumin concentration is very common in the seriously ill patient and it must decrease the microvascular pressure threshold at which transudation commences.

Lymphatic obstruction

As in other tissues, obstruction of the pulmonary lymphatic drainage is a potential cause of pulmonary oedema. There can be no lymphatic drainage immediately after transplantation of a lung and there is a tendency towards oedema until the lymphatics are re-formed.

Miscellaneous causes

'Neurogenic' pulmonary oedema may follow head injuries or other cerebral lesions. It has been demonstrated that it does not occur in the denervated lung but the mechanism remains a mystery at the time of writing.

Sudden expansion of a collapsed lung may result in pulmonary oedema confined to the one side and probably caused by increased permeability (Pavlin, Nessly and Cheney, 1981). The problem may arise after aspiration of a pneumothorax or a pleural effusion. Lungs which have been collapsed for some time should be re-expanded slowly and by not more than 1 litre at one time.

Pulmonary oedema occurring at high altitude is well documented although the mechanism is still open to speculation. It is considered in Chapter 14 (page 315). Also within the miscellaneous category is pulmonary oedema following diamorphine overdosage.

Pathophysiology

The most important physiological abnormality of pulmonary oedema is venous admixture or shunt. Pulmonary arterial blood mingles with pulmonary venous blood without having undergone gaseous exchange. This results in an increased alveolar/arterial P_{O_2} gradient and hypoxaemia which may be life threatening.

Hypercapnia is not generally a problem. In severe pulmonary oedema, the hypoxaemia is the more pressing disorder. In less severe pulmonary oedema, there is usually an increased respiratory drive due partly to hypoxaemia and partly to stimulation of J receptors (page 94). As a result the P_{CO_2} is usually normal or somewhat decreased. If a patient with severe pulmonary oedema is treated with a high concentration of inspired oxygen there may be hypercapnia due to the interference with gas exchange.

Physiological principles of treatment

Symptomatic treatment

The highest priority is to restore the arterial P_{O_2}. The inspired oxygen concentration should be increased, up to 100% if necessary. Sitting the patient up is a simple means of reducing the central blood volume. Morphine may exert its beneficial effect by peripheral vasodilatation.

If there is froth in the airway, it will be necessary to pass a tracheal tube and aspirate the froth. Artificial ventilation is necessary if the oedema is severe, and the results are often spectacular. Artificial ventilation is often combined with positive end-expiratory pressure (PEEP). It was originally thought that this drove the fluid back into the circulation but there is no evidence that extravascular lung water is reduced by PEEP (page 415). The success of PEEP probably depends on forcing airway liquid down the tracheobronchial tree and opening up of alveoli which were previously not ventilated. By increasing the lung volume, the capacity of the interstitium to hold liquid is increased (Gee and Williams, 1979). Pare et al. (1983), studying dogs with haemodynamic pulmonary oedema, found that PEEP did not alter the total amount of lung water but a greater proportion was in the extra-alveolar interstitial space.

Treatment of the cause

Treatment of the underlying cause of pulmonary oedema follows directly from the Starling equation and an understanding of the aetiology.

In *haemodynamic pulmonary oedema*, the essential feature of treatment is reduction of the wedge pressure. Depending on the precise aetiology, treatment is directed towards improvement of left ventricular function and/or reduction of blood volume. Venous occlusive cuffs on the limbs are a valuable emergency method of reduction of circulating blood volume. Diuretics act more slowly. Essentially the patient is titrated to the left along his Frank–Starling curve (*Figure 23.3*). In addition the curve is moved upwards and to the left, if this is possible, using positive inotropes as an adjunct to correction of left ventricular malfunction.

In *permeability pulmonary oedema*, treatment should be directed towards restoration of the integrity of the alveolar/capillary membrane. Unfortunately, no particularly successful measures are available towards this end (see Chapter 26). It is, however, important to minimize the wedge pressure even though this is not the primary cause of the oedema. Attempts may be made to increase the plasma albumin concentration if it is reduced.

Clinical measurement

As an indication of impending or actual haemodynamic pulmonary oedema, the most useful measurement is the left atrial or wedge pressure. The Swan–Ganz catheter has revolutionized management in such patients.

Measurement of the integrity of the alveolar/capillary membrane is more difficult (see page 203). Laboratory methods are available for animals, but the only practical approach for clinical use is measurement of the rate of loss of a gamma-emitting tracer molecule from the lung into the circulation. The most sensitive

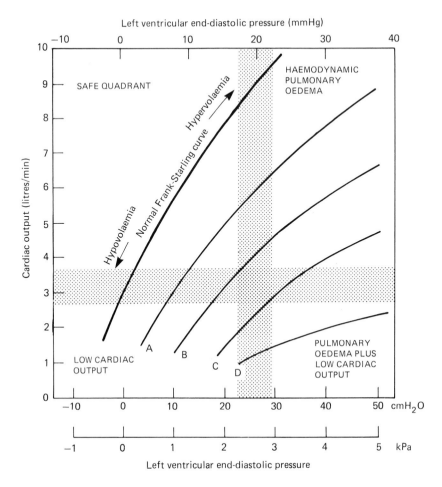

Figure 23.3 Quadrant diagram relating cardiac output to left ventricular end-diastolic pressure. The thick curve is a typical normal Frank–Starling curve. To the right are shown curves representing progressive left ventricular failure. Top left is the safe quadrant which contains a substantial part of the normal Frank–Starling curve but progressively less of the curves representing ventricular failure. Top right is the quadrant representing normal cardiac output but raised left atrial pressure, attained at the upper end of relatively normal Frank–Starling curves (e.g. hypervolaemia). There is a danger of haemodynamic pulmonary oedema. Bottom left is the quadrant representing normal or low left atrial pressure but low cardiac output, attained at the lower end of all Frank–Starling curves (e.g. hypovolaemia). The patient is in shock. Bottom right is the quadrant representing both low cardiac output and raised left atrial pressure. There is simultaneous danger of pulmonary oedema and shock, and the worst Frank–Starling curves hardly leave this quadrant.

tracer is ^{99m}TcDTPA (metastable technetium-99-labelled diethylene triamine penta-acetate, molecular weight 492 daltons) (Jones, Royston and Minty, 1983). The half-time of clearance from the lung fields is usually in the range 40–100 minutes in the healthy non-smoker. The half-time is reduced below 40 minutes following a variety of lung insults. However, it is within the range 10–40 minutes in apparently healthy smokers (page 340) and this limits its scope for the early detection of a damaged alveolar/capillary membrane.

Measurement of lung water would be an extremely valuable diagnostic and prognostic aid to the management of pulmonary oedema. It is easy enough to measure lung water gravimetrically at postmortem and there is usually sufficient protein in alveolar fluid for it to stain and be clearly visible by light microscopy.

Measurement of lung water during life has proved elusive. A great deal of effort has been devoted to the double indicator method. This uses the techniques for the measurement of pulmonary or central blood volume by dye dilution (page 137) but with two indicators. One indicator is chosen to remain within the circulation while the other (usually 'coolth' or tritiated water) diffuses into the interstitial fluid. Extravascular lung water is then derived as the difference between the volumes as measured with the two indicators. Staub (1974) discussed the limitations of these methods and there is still widespread agreement that the method is technically very difficult since a high level of accuracy is required to demonstrate small changes in lung water. Thoracic electrical impedance is an alternative approach but is also beset with difficulties. Only rarely will control measurements be available before the onset of pulmonary oedema.

Chapter 24

Pulmonary collapse and atelectasis

Pulmonary collapse may be defined as an acquired state in which the lungs or a part of the lungs become airless due to approximation of alveolar walls. Atelectasis is strictly defined as a state in which the lungs of a newborn have never been expanded but the term is often used as a synonym for collapse.

The lungs themselves have an elastic recoil which, if unopposed, causes a decrease in lung volume to the point at which airways are closed. Trapped gas must eventually be absorbed by the pulmonary blood flow since the total partial pressure of gases in mixed venous blood is always less than atmospheric. Thus, collapse may be caused by two entirely different mechanisms. Firstly, there may, in the first instance, be loss of the forces opposing the retraction of the lung which is followed by absorption of trapped gas. Secondly, there may be absorption of gas trapped behind an obstructed airway which can easily overcome any force tending to hold the lung expanded.

Loss of forces opposing retraction of the lung

The equilibrium state of the isolated lung is total collapse (see *Figure 2.3*). When the lung volume is decreased to closing capacity, airway closure commences, particularly in the dependent parts of the lung (page 62). At residual volume, at least in older subjects, all airways are closed and all alveolar gas is trapped. Trapped gas will then be removed by the pulmonary circulation as described below. In due course the lung will become completely airless.

The lungs are normally prevented from collapse by the outward elastic recoil of the rib cage and the tone of the diaphragm (page 34). The pleural cavity normally contains no gas but, if a small bubble of gas is introduced, its pressure is subatmospheric (see *Figure 2.4*). Pulmonary collapse due to loss of forces opposing lung retraction may be considered under five headings as follows.

Voluntary reduction of lung volume

It seems unlikely that voluntary reduction of lung volume below closing capacity will cause overt collapse of lung in a subject breathing air. However, in older subjects, there is an increase in the alveolar/arterial P_{O_2} gradient, suggesting trapping of alveolar gas (see *Figure 19.8*). If the subject has been breathing 100% oxygen, collapse may easily follow reduction of lung volume (see below).

Excessive external pressure

Ventilatory failure is the more prominent aspect of an external pressure in excess of about 6 kPa (60 cmH$_2$O) which is not communicated to the airways. However, some degree of pulmonary collapse could also occur and this is a normal consequence of the great depths attained by diving mammals while breath holding. An approximately normal lung volume is maintained during conventional diving operations when respired gas is maintained at the surrounding water pressure.

It is theoretically possible to induce collapse by the application of a subatmospheric pressure to the airways. Velasquez and Farhi (1964) demonstrated increased shunting in dogs under these circumstances.

Loss of integrity of the rib cage

Multiple rib fractures or the old operation of thoracoplasty may impair the elastic recoil of the rib cage to the point at which partial lung collapse results. This depends entirely on the extent of the injury to the rib cage but six or more ribs fractured in two places will usually result in collapse. However, extensive trauma to the rib cage also causes interference with the mechanics of breathing which is generally more serious than collapse.

Intrusion of abdominal contents into the chest

Extensive atelectasis results from a congenital defect of the diaphragm. Abdominal contents may completely fill one-half of the chest with total atelectasis of that lung. Paralysis of one side of the diaphragm causes the diaphragm to lie higher in the chest with a tendency to basal collapse on that side. An extensive abdominal mass (e.g. tumour or ascites) may force the diaphragm into the chest.

Space occupation of the pleural cavity

Air introduced into the pleural cavity reduces the forces opposing retraction of the lung and this is a potent cause of collapse. A *closed pneumothorax* is a fixed volume of air which may cause collapse in relation to the volume of air introduced. The intrapleural pressure rises in proportion to the volume of air in the cavity and is above atmospheric in a *tension pneumothorax*. The affected lung is then totally collapsed and the mediastinum is displaced towards the opposite side. This is a life-threatening condition requiring immediate relief of the pressure. An *open pneumothorax* communicates with the atmosphere and results in pendulum breathing in addition to collapse. It occurs at thoracotomy, where pendulum breathing is prevented by artificial ventilation but collapse may still occur and indeed is often induced to improve surgical access. In 'one-lung anaesthesia', a divided airway is used to ventilate the non-exposed lung while the exposed lung is allowed to collapse.

The pleural cavity may also be occupied by an effusion, empyema or a haemothorax. All of these may result in collapse. Less commonly there may be a significant intrusion in the thoracic cavity by tumour, cardiomegaly or haemopericardium.

Absorption of trapped gas

Absorption of alveolar gas trapped beyond obstructed airways may be the consequence of reduction in lung volume by the mechanisms described above. However, it is the primary cause of collapse when there is total or partial airway obstruction at normal lung volume. Obstruction is commonly due to secretions, pus, blood or tumour but may be due to intense local bronchospasm or mucosal oedema. Bronchial blockers have been used for the deliberate production of collapse.

Gas trapped beyond the point of airway closure is absorbed by the pulmonary blood flow. The total of the partial pressures of the gases in mixed venous blood is always less than atmospheric (see *Table 29.2*), although pressure gradients for the individual component gases between alveolar gas and mixed venous blood may be quite different.

The effect of respired gases

If the patient has been breathing 100% oxygen prior to obstruction, the alveoli will contain only oxygen, carbon dioxide and water vapour. Since the last two together normally amount to less than 13.3 kPa (100 mmHg), the alveolar P_{O_2} will usually be in excess of 88 kPa (660 mmHg). However, the P_{O_2} of the mixed venous blood is unlikely to exceed about 6.7 kPa (50 mmHg) so the alveolar/mixed venous P_{O_2} gradient will be of the order of 80 per cent of an atmosphere. Absorption collapse will thus be rapid and there will be no nitrogen in the alveolar gas to maintain inflation.

The situation is much more favourable in a patient who has been breathing air since most of the alveolar gas is then nitrogen which is at a tension of only about 0.5 kPa (4 mmHg) below that of mixed venous blood (Klocke and Rahn, 1961). Alveolar nitrogen tension rises above that of mixed venous blood as oxygen is absorbed and eventually the nitrogen will be fully absorbed. Collapse must eventually occur but the process is much slower than in the patient who has been breathing oxygen. *Figure 24.1* shows a computer simulation of the time required for collapse with various gas mixtures (Webb and Nunn, 1967). Nitrous oxide/oxygen mixtures may be expected to be absorbed almost as rapidly as 100% oxygen. This is partly because nitrous oxide is much more soluble in blood than nitrogen, and partly because the mixed venous tension of nitrous oxide is usually much less than the alveolar tension, except after a long period of inhalation.

When the inspired gas composition is changed *after* obstruction and trapping occur, complex patterns of absorption may ensue. The inhalation of nitrous oxide after airway occlusion has occurred while breathing air results in temporary expansion of the trapped volume (*Figure 24.1*). This is caused by large volumes of the more soluble nitrous oxide passing from blood to alveolus in exchange for smaller volumes of the less soluble nitrogen passing in the reverse direction. This phenomenon also applies to air embolus, pneumothorax, residual air from a pneumoencephalogram and, indeed, any air space in the body. It is potentially dangerous and may contraindicate the use of nitrous oxide as an anaesthetic (Munson and Merrick, 1967).

Magnitude of the pressure gradients

It needs to be stressed that the forces generated by the absorption of trapped gases are not trivial. The total partial pressure of gases in mixed venous blood is normally

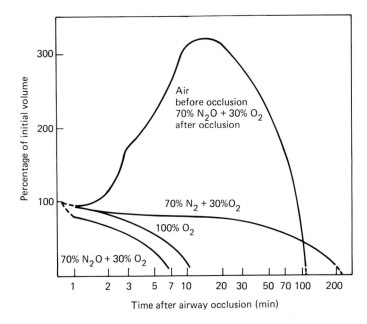

Figure 24.1 The lower curves show the rate of absorption of the contents of sections of the lung whose air passages are obstructed, resulting in sequestration of the contents. The upper curve shows the expansion of the sequestered gas when nitrous oxide is breathed by a patient who has recently suffered regional airway obstruction while breathing air. In all other cases, it is assumed that the inspired gas is not changed after obstruction has occurred. Similar considerations apply to gas sequestered in other parts of the body, and the data apply to pneumothorax, gas emboli and air introduced during pneumoencephalography. (Reproduced from Webb and Nunn (1967) by permission of the authors and the Editor of Anaesthesia*)*

87.4 kPa (656 mmHg). The corresponding pressure of the alveolar gases is 95.1 kPa (713 mmHg), allowing for water vapour pressure at 37°C. The difference, 7.7 kPa (57 mmHg or 77 cmH$_2$O), is sufficient to overcome any forces opposing recoil of the lung. Absorption collapse after breathing air may therefore result in drawing the diaphragm up into the chest, reducing rib cage volume or displacing the mediastinum. If the patient has been breathing oxygen, the total partial pressure of gases in the mixed venous blood is barely a tenth of an atmosphere (see *Table 29.2*) and absorption of trapped alveolar gas generates enormous forces.

Effect of reduced ventilation/perfusion ratio

Absorption collapse may still occur in the absence of total airway obstruction provided that the ventilation/perfusion ($\dot{V}/\dot{Q}$) ratio is sufficiently reduced. It is now well established that older subjects as well as those with a pathological increase in scatter of $\dot{V}/\dot{Q}$ ratios may have substantial perfusion of areas of lung with $\dot{V}/\dot{Q}$ ratios in the range 0.01–0.1. This shows as a characteristic 'shelf' in the plot of perfusion against $\dot{V}/\dot{Q}$ (*Figure 24.2*). These grossly hypoventilated areas are liable to collapse if the patient breathes oxygen (*Figure 24.2b*). If the $\dot{V}/\dot{Q}$ ratio is less than 0.05, ventilation even with 100% oxygen cannot supply the oxygen which is removed (assuming the normal arterial/mixed venous oxygen content difference of 0.05 ml/ml). As the $\dot{V}/\dot{Q}$ ratio decreases below 0.05, so the critical inspired oxygen con-

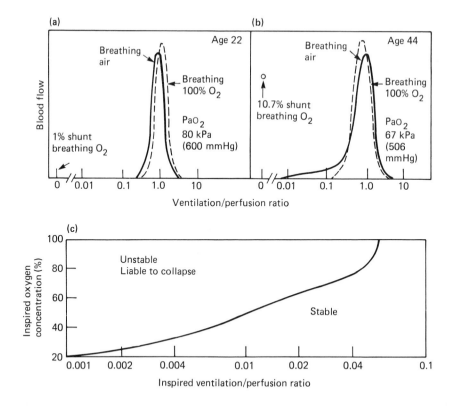

Figure 24.2 Inspiration of 100% oxygen causes collapse of alveoli with very low ventilation/perfusion ratios. (a) The minor change in the distribution of blood flow (in relation to V̇/Q̇ ratio) when a young subject breathes oxygen. Collapse is minimal and a shunt of 1 per cent develops. (b) The changes in an older subject with a 'shelf' of blood flow distributed to alveoli with very low V̇/Q̇ ratios. Breathing oxygen causes collapse of these alveoli and this is manifested by disappearance of the shelf and appearance of an intrapulmonary shunt of 10.7 per cent. (c) The inspired oxygen concentration relative to the inspired V̇/Q̇ ratio which is critical for absorption collapse. (Redrawn from Wagner et al. (1974) by permission of the authors and the Editor of the Journal of Clinical Investigation, *and from Dantzker, Wagner and West (1975) by permission of the authors and the Editor of the* Journal of Applied Physiology)

centration necessary for collapse also decreases (*Figure 24.2c*). There is no difficulty in demonstrating that pulmonary collapse may be induced in healthy middle-aged subjects by breathing oxygen at close to residual volume (Nunn et al., 1965b, 1978).

The effect of collapse

Perfusion through a collapsed lung or part of lung is one of the most important causes of intrapulmonary shunting (page 167). At least in the short term, some perfusion continues through the collapsed area and this is regulated mainly by hypoxic pulmonary vasoconstriction (page 127). In the absence of alveolar gas, the P_{O_2} which governs pulmonary vascular resistance is the mixed venous P_{O_2} (Marshall and Marshall, 1983). It has been observed that, in the presence of collapse, the shunt fraction of the pulmonary blood flow is directly proportional to the cardiact ouput (page 173), and this has been attributed to the effect of cardiac output on the mixed venous P_{O_2} (Marshall and Marshall, 1985). Thus, with a reduced cardiac output, the mixed venous P_{O_2} will be reduced (according to the Fick principle) and hypoxic pulmonary vasoconstriction in the area of the collapse will be increased. Therefore the shunt fraction will be decreased. However, the blood flowing through the shunt is more desaturated and these two effects counteract each other so that the arterial P_{O_2} is little changed. This complex problem is further discussed on pages 249 et seq.

Sudden re-expansion of an area of collapsed lung may result in pulmonary oedema (page 436).

Diagnosis of pulmonary collapse

The diagnosis may be made on physical signs but reliance is usually placed on chest radiography. In the upright position, collapse is commonest in the basal segments, often concealed behind the cardiac shadow unless the exposure is appropriate. Collapse in the supine position may well occur in the dorsal parts of the lung which are then dependent. This is not easy to detect radiologically since it may form a thin sheet parallel to the plate in an anteroposterior exposure. In the lateral view it may be obscured by the vertebral column. Computerized tomography has been successfully used to detect what appears to be dorsal collapse during anaesthesia, after conventional means had failed (Brismar et al., 1985).

Collapse results in a reduction in pulmonary compliance, which has been suggested as a diagnostic aid (Butler and Smith, 1957; Bendixen, Hedley-Whyte and Laver, 1963; Velasquez and Farhi, 1964). Its value in diagnosis is limited by the wide scatter in normal values. However, a sudden reduction may give an indication of collapse provided, of course, that control measurements were available before collapse.

Collapse also reduces the functional residual capacity and arterial P_{O_2}. However, in a study of absorption collapse, there was little to choose between these measurements and changes in the chest radiograph for the detection of minimal collapse (Nunn et al., 1978). When present, it was detected by all three methods. In patients undergoing intensive care, a reduction in arterial P_{O_2} cannot distinguish between the three very common conditions of pulmonary collapse, consolidation and oedema.

Treatment

This should be directed at the cause. Factors opposing the elastic recoil of the lung should be removed wherever possible. For example, pneumothorax, pleural effusion and ascites should be drained as necessary. In other cases, particularly impaired integrity of the chest wall, it may be preferable to treat the patient with intermittent positive pressure ventilation. It is usually possible to restore normal lung volume by appropriate control of airway pressures.

When collapse is caused by regional airway obstruction, the most useful methods in both treatment and prevention are by chest physiotherapy, combined when necessary with tracheobronchial toilet, through either a tracheal tube or a bronchoscope. Fibreoptic bronchoscopy alone will often clear an obstructed airway and permit re-expansion.

A logical approach is hyperinflation of the chest or an artificial 'sigh'. Many ventilators are equipped to provide an intermittent 'sigh' but evidence of its efficacy is elusive. It does nothing to reduce the alveolar/arterial P_{O_2} gradient during anaesthesia (Panday and Nunn, 1968). However, voluntary maximal inspirations have been effective in clearing areas of absorption collapse in subjects who had been breathing oxygen near residual volume (Nunn et al., 1978). The process imparted a distinctive tearing sensation in the chest but rapidly restored to normal both chest radiograph and arterial P_{O_2}. Mention has been made above of the possibility of pulmonary oedema following sudden re-expansion of collapsed lung.

Chapter 25

Pulmonary embolism

The pulmonary circulation may be blocked by embolism, which may be gas, thrombus, fat, tumour or foreign body. The architecture of the microvasculature is well adapted to minimize the resultant infarct. Large numbers of pulmonary capillaries tend to arise from metarterioles at right angles and there are abundant anatomoses throughout the microcirculation (see *Plate 5*). This tends to preserve circulation distal to the impaction of a small embolus.

Air embolism

An embolus may arise from pneumothorax and pulmonary barotrauma but is most commonly iatrogenic during either neurosurgery or cardiac surgery. Compressed air was formerly used to increase the speed of a blood transfusion and this was associated with some disastrous cases of embolism if the blood was exhausted before the pressure was released. Some small degree of air embolism is almost inevitable in all types of intravenous therapy.

In neurosurgery, the usual source of air embolism is the use of the sitting position for posterior fossa surgery. This results in a subatmospheric venous pressure at the operative site and air may enter dural veins which are held open by their structure. In open cardiac surgery, it is almost impossible to remove all traces of air from the ventricles before closing the heart.

Detection of air embolism

Early diagnosis of air embolism is essential in neurosurgery, and there are three principal methods in routine use. Bubbles in circulating blood give a very characteristic sound with a precordial Doppler probe. The method is, if anything, too sensitive, since a shower of small bubbles produces a particularly large signal. The second method is based on the appearance of nitrogen in the expired air. There should be no significant exhaled nitrogen after the first 15 minutes of an anaesthetic in which the patient breathes a mixture of oxygen and nitrous oxide. The appearance of nitrogen is easily detected with a mass spectrometer and is diagnostic of air entering the circulation. The third and simplest method is based on the end-expired CO_2 concentration which is easily measured with an infrared analyser. Many factors influence the end-expiratory concentration but a sudden decrease is likely to be either cardiac arrest or air embolism. More recently it has been shown that transoesophageal echocardiography is an efficient method of detecting air embolism and, furthermore, it is the only practicable method of detecting paradoxical air embolism (see below) (Cucchiara et al., 1984; Furuya and Okumura, 1984).

Effects of air embolus

Provided there is no major intracardiac right-to-left shunt, small quantities of air are filtered out by the lungs where they are gradually absorbed and no harm results. However, massive air embolism (probably in excess of 100 ml) may cause cardiac arrest either by frothing in the right ventricle or by massive occlusion of the pulmonary circulation. Treatment then requires aspiration of air through a cardiac catheter, which is difficult.

Paradoxical air embolism. Rarely, there may be passage of air emboli from the right to left heart without there being an overt right-to-left shunt. This is important because air then enters the systemic arterial circulation where there may be embolism and infarction, particularly of the brain. The cause is failure of complete closure of the foramen ovale. It is possible to pass a probe through such a foramen ovale in 20–35 per cent of the adult population (Edward, 1960) but paradoxical embolism does not usually occur because pressure is slightly higher in the left atrium than the right. However, Perkins-Pearson, Marshall and Bedford (1982) demonstrated that in anaesthetized patients in the sitting position, right atrial pressure exceeded the pulmonary capillary wedge pressure in about half of their patients. Furthermore, right atrial pressure increased further in relation to wedge pressure when positive end-expiratory pressure was applied, presumably due to inceased pulmonary vascular resistance (Perkins and Bedford, 1984). Clearly, under these circumstances there is an increased chance of paradoxical air embolism.

Apart from intracardiac passage of an air embolus, it is possible that air bubbles may pass through the pulmonary circulation, although surface forces in the microvasculature render this unlikely. In small vessels, the radii of curvature of the air bubbles is so small that the interfaces are able to support very large pressure differences. This effect may be demonstrated *in vitro* by noting the very high pressures which can be maintained across a series of bubbles in water lying in a glass capillary tube (Jamin's tube). Neverthless, one clinical report suggests that paradoxical pulmonary air embolism through the pulmonary circulation is possible (Marquez et al., 1981).

Pulmonary arterial pressure is increased by a large embolus due to the right ventricle working against an increased pulmonary vascular resistance.

Alveolar dead space is increased according to the proportion of the pulmonary circulation which is occluded (Severinghaus and Stupfel, 1957). The resultant increase in arterial/end-tidal P_{CO_2} gradient is the basis of detection of air embolism by infrared CO_2 as described above.

Thromboembolism

The commonest pulmonary embolus consists of detached venous thromboses, particularly from veins in the thigh and the pelvic venous plexuses. Smaller thrombi are filtered in the lungs without causing symptoms but larger emboli may impact in major vessels, typically at a bifurcation forming a saddle embolus. This may cause a catastrophic increase in pulmonary vascular resistance with acute right heart failure or cardiac arrest. The only effective treatment is then embolectomy. In less severe cases, dispersal of the thrombus may be accelerated with streptokinase which can be infused though a pulmonary artery catheter lying in the blocked branch.

The primary physiological lesion is an increase in alveolar dead space with an increased arterial/end-tidal P_{CO_2} gradient. However, this does not usually cause hypercapnia since hyperventilation is almost always present and arterial P_{CO_2} is usually below the normal range. Arterial P_{O_2} is also decreased and, in dogs, this has been shown to be due to increased intrapulmonary shunting (Stein et al., 1961).

Other deleterious effects result from breakdown and removal of the thrombus, a process for which the lung is well adapted. Many proteins and particularly fibrin monomers are known to counteract the effect of surfactant, so decreasing compliance (Seeger et al., 1985). Bronchospasm is a well recognized complication (Windebank, Boyd and Moran, 1973) and has been attributed to local release of serotonin (5-hydroxytryptamine) from the platelets in the clot and also to local hypocapnia in the part of the lung without effective pulmonary circulation.

Diagnosis of embolus due to thrombus

In massive pulmonary embolus due to thrombus, the diagnosis is only too obvious. In less severe cases, the diagnosis may be made by pulmonary angiography or a perfusion scan. However, the methods based on gas analysis described above for air embolism are not applicable.

Measurement of physiological dead space may help in the diagnosis but the wide scatter of normal values reduces the discrimination of the test.

Fat embolism

Fracture of long bones may be associated with fat embolism which stains characteristically with osmic acid. It has been thought that blood lipids might coalesce and form the emboli. However, fragments of bone marrow with the normal architecture have been found embedded in the lung fields at postmortem after fat embolism.

Lipid appears to pass through the pulmonary circulation to invade the systemic circulation. Surface forces between blood and lipid are much less than between blood and air and so would not offer the same hindrance to passage through the lungs. In the systemic circulation, fat emboli cause the characteristic petechiae in the anterior axillary folds. In addition, fat may be found in the urine and there is often evidence of cerebral involvement.

There is initially an increase in physiological dead space (Greenbaum et al., 1965) but this is soon accompanied by an increase in shunt (Prys-Roberts et al., 1970) which is probably caused by the release of substances in the lung which cause spasm of the airways and open up anastomotic channels between pulmonary artery and vein. The position is often further complicated by superadded infection.

Chapter 26

Adult respiratory distress syndrome

Ashbaugh and his colleagues (1967) described a condition in adults which was similar to the respiratory distress sydrome in infants and later Petty and Ashbaugh (1971) introduced the term 'adult respiratory distress syndrome' (ARDS). It is a characteristic form of parenchymal lung failure, often terminal, which may follow any one or more of a wide range of predisposing conditions. There are a great many synonyms for ARDS, including shock lung, respirator lung, pump lung and Da Nang lung. Many of these names prejudge the aetiology in a quite unjustifiable manner.

Definition

There is no universal agreement on the criteria for the diagnosis of ARDS. Neither is there any single diagnostic test which distinguishes the condition. However, the essential features are as follows:

1. Acute respiratory failure requiring artificial ventilation.
2. Severe hypoxaemia with a large increase in the alveolar/arterial Po_2 gradient. There is no agreement on the precise degree of hypoxaemia for the definition of ARDS, and proposals range from an arterial Po_2 of 6.7 to 10 kPa (50–75 mmHg) while breathing an inspired oxygen concentration variously cited within the range 50–100%. Alternatively, the critical level of hypoxaemia has been defined as an arterial Po_2 which is less than 20 per cent of the inspired Po_2.
3. Bilateral diffuse infiltration on the chest radiograph.
4. Stiff lungs with a total compliance of the respiratory system which is less than 5 ml/kPa (50 ml/cmH$_2$O). It should, however, be noted that this is within the normal range for an anaesthetized patient who has healthy lungs.
5. Pulmonary oedema should not be cardiogenic and the pulmonary wedge pressure should not be elevated. Different definitions of ARDS require the wedge pressure to be less than various values ranging from 1.6 to 2.4 kPa (12–18 mmHg). Objections have been raised to inclusion of this criterion. Lloyd, Newman and Brigham (1984) pointed out that this would exclude the diagnosis of ARDS where it coexisted with a condition which caused an increased left atrial pressure.

In addition to the criteria listed above, various authors suggest that one or more of the known predisposing conditions should have been present and that the clinical course has followed the recognized pattern (see below). In addition, it is noted that the histology is usually diagnostic but it is seldom indicated or advisable to take a lung biopsy. There is no reliable laboratory test to confirm the diagnosis.

In part, the diagnosis of ARDS depends on exclusion of other conditions. Sometimes it is not easy to separate it from other conditions such as pulmonary embolus, fibrosing alveolitis, bronchopneumonia and virus pneumonia, which may present many similar features. There has been much debate on whether ARDS exists as a discrete entity or whether it is more profitable to regard the conditions following the various predisposing factors as separate disorders.

It would be helpful if there could be a standardized definition of ARDS. Differences in the criteria greatly complicate comparisons of incidence, mortality, aetiology and efficacy of therapy in different centres. Diagnostic criteria have been presented and discussed by Pepe et al. (1982), Fein et al. (1983), Fowler et al., (1983), Lloyd, Newman and Brigham (1984) and Stevens and Raffin (1984).

Clinical course

Four phases may be recognized in the development of ARDS. In the first the patient is dyspnoeic and tachypnoeic but there are no other abnormalities. The chest radiograph is normal at this stage, which lasts for about 24 hours. In the next phase there is hypoxaemia but the arterial Pco_2 remains normal or subnormal. There are minor abnormalities of the chest radiograph. This phase may last for 1 or 2 days. Diagnosis is easily missed in these prodromal stages and is very dependent on the history of one or more predisposing conditions.

It is only in phase three that the diagnostic criteria of true ARDS become established. There is severe arterial hypoxaemia due to an increased alveolar/ arterial Po_2 gradient, and the Pco_2 may be slightly elevated. The lungs become stiff and the chest radiograph shows the characteristic bilateral diffuse infiltrates. Artificial ventilation is usually instituted at this stage.

The fourth phase is terminal and comprises massive bilateral consolidation with unremitting hypoxaemia, the arterial Po_2 characteristically being less than 7 kPa (52.5 mmHg) when the inspired oxygen concentration is 100%. Dead space is substantially increased and the arterial Pco_2 is only with difficulty kept in the normal range by the use of a large minute volume (10–20 l/min).

Not every patient progresses through all these phases and the condition may resolve at any stage. It is difficult to predict whether the condition will progress and there is no useful laboratory test. Serial observations of the chest radiograph and the alveolar/arterial Po_2 gradient are the best guides to progress.

Predisposing conditions and risk factors

Although the clinical and histopathological picture of ARDS is remarkably consistent, it has been described as the sequel to a very large range of predisposing conditions (*Table 26.1*)). Recognition of the predisposing factors is important for predicting which patients are at risk.

By no means are all the conditions in *Table 26.1* equally likely to proceed to ARDS. Analysis of some of the more important risk factors has been undertaken by Pepe et al. (1982), Fein et al. (1983) and Fowler et al. (1983). Pepe's group found the highest single risk factor was the sepsis syndrome: 38 per cent of patients

Table 26.1 Some predisposing conditions for ARDS

Direct injury	Indirect injury
Pulmonary contusion	Septicaemia
Gastric aspiration	Shock or prolonged hypotension
Near-drowning	Non-thoracic trauma
Inhalation of toxic gases and vapours	Cardiopulmonary bypass
Some infections	Head injury
Fat embolus	Pancreatitis
Amniotic fluid embolus	Diabetic coma
Radiation	Multiple blood transfusions
Bleomycin	

in this category developed ARDS. The incidence was 30 per cent in patients who aspirated gastric contents, 24 per cent in patients with multiple emergency transfusions (more than 22 units in 12 hours) and 17 per cent in patients with pulmonary contusions. Multiple minor fractures produced an incidence of only 8 per cent, and numbers were too small to evaluate near-drowning, pancreatitis and prolonged hypotension. Over all, 25 per cent of patients with a single risk factor developed ARDS but this rose to 42 per cent with two factors and 85 per cent with three. Sepsis was, however, seldom associated with the other factors, and in most of the patients with sepsis who developed ARDS it was the only risk factor. The number and nature of the risk factors was a better predictor than the injury severity score or measurements of initial oxygenation.

Fein's group followed 116 patients with septicaemia and found an 18 per cent incidence of ARDS but this was greatly increased if the patient also had thrombocytopenia (46 per cent incidence) or a period of 60 minutes with a systolic blood pressure less than 8 kPa (60 mmHg) (64 per cent incidence). No patient without hypotension proceeded to develop ARDS. Most infections were Gram negative but some were Gram positive and a few were fungal. Age and sex did not affect the likelihood of development of ARDS.

Fowler's group followed 993 patients considered to be at risk as a result of cardiopulmonary bypass surgery, burns, bacteraemia, transfusions of 10 or more units of blood, major fractures, disseminated intravascular coagulation (DIC), aspiration of gastric contents or pneumonia. As a single factor, aspiration had the highest incidence of ARDS (35.6 per cent) followed by DIC (22.2 per cent) and pneumonia (11.9 per cent). Other factors, including bacteraemia, all showed an incidence of less than 6 per cent. Patients with multiple risk factors had an incidence of 24.6 per cent compared with 5.8 per cent for a single risk factor.

These studies clearly show major differences in the incidence and causation of ARDS in particular patient populations. Others in this field have encountered many cases attributable to multiple trauma and also to treatment with bleomycin. Difficult though it may be to extrapolate from a particular study to one's own practice, the major predisposing conditions are now agreed to be septicaemia (particularly Gram negative), aspiration of gastric contents, DIC, multiple trauma (particularly with pulmonary contusion) and multiple transfusions. It is now rare to see the condition following evacuation and resuscitation of exsanguinated casualties from the battlefield. This was commonplace in Vietnam where overenthusiastic replacement of circulatory volume may have been a factor. No case of ARDS occurred in the Falklands campaign (J.M. Beeley, personal communication).

It is extremely difficult, if not impossible, to separate the toxic effects of high concentrations of oxygen from the pathological condition which required their use. This problem is considered on page 492 but it seems unlikely that high concentrations of oxygen *per se* are a major aetiological factor in the causation of ARDS.

Incidence and mortality

The much-quoted American Lung Program of 1972 estimated the incidence in the USA to be 150 000 cases a year, which would correspond to 130 per year in a typical British health district of 200 000 people. The incidence in the UK is probably much less than this and, although no reliable statistics exist, it seems unlikely that there are more than about 20 cases a year in the average British health district.

The reasons for this discrepancy are not clear. Possibly the diagnostic criteria tend to be different and the definition cited above has considerable latitude in the precise degree of arterial hypoxaemia. It would be helpful if there were an internationally standardized definition of ARDS.

There is, however, considerable agreement that the overall mortality of ARDS is of the order of 50 per cent whatever the criteria of diagnosis. It tends to be higher in cases which follow septicaemia, and was reported as 81 per cent by Fein et al. (1983) and 78 per cent by Fowler et al. (1983).

Histopathology

Although of diverse aetiology, the histological appearances of ARDS are remark-ably consistent and give it the distinction of being considered a discrete clinical entity. Bachofen and Weibel (1982), after extensive study of autopsy material, have divided the histological changes into two stages: acute and subacute or chronic.

The acute stage

The acute stage is characterized by damaged integrity of the blood/gas barrier. The changes are primarily in the interalveolar septa and cannot be satisfactorily seen with light microscopy. Electron microscopy shows extensive damage to the type I alveolar epithelial cells (page 17), which may be totally destroyed (*Figure 26.1*). Meanwhile the basement membrane is usually preserved and the endothelial cells still tend to form a continuous layer with apparently intact cell junctions. Endothelial permeability is nevertheless increased although the morphological basis for the change is not evident. Interstitial oedema is found, predominantly on the 'service' side of the capillary where endothelium and epithelium are separated by a tissue space (see *Figure 1.7*). Fortunately, the oedema tends to spare the 'active' side of the capillary where endothelium and epithelium are in close apposition. This differentiation between the two sides of the pulmonary capillary is also seen in cardiogenic oedema.

Protein-containing fluid leaks into the alveoli, which also contain erythrocytes and leucocytes in addition to amorphous material comprising strands of fibrin (*Figure 26.1*). The exudate may form into sheets which line the alveoli as the so-

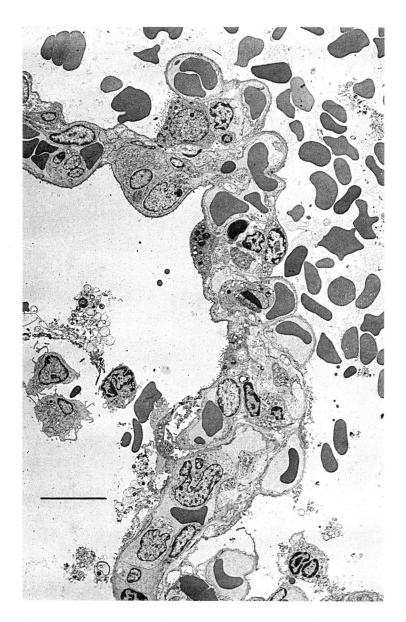

Figure 26.1 Electron micrograph of an alveolar septum in the early stages of adult respiratory distress syndrome. On the right-hand side of the septum there are many examples of damage to alveolar epithelium but the endothelium tends to remain intact. The alveolar gas spaces to left and right contain many erythrocytes, leucocytes, cell debris and fibrin strands. No hyaline membrane has yet formed. The scale bar (bottom left) is 10 μm.(Reproduced from Bachofen and Weibel (1982) by permission of the authors and the Editors of Chest Medicine*)*

called hyaline membrane. Intravascular coagulation is common at this stage and, in patients with septicaemia, capillaries may be completely plugged with leucocytes, and the underlying endothelium may then be damaged.

The subacute or chronic stage

Attempted repair and proliferation predominate in the chronic stage of ARDS. Within a few days of the onset of the condition, there is a thickening of endothelium, epithelium and the interstitial space. The type I epithelial cells are destroyed and replaced by type II cells (page 18) which proliferate but do not differentiate into type I cells as normal. They remain cuboidal and about ten times the thickness of the type I cells which they have replaced. This appears to be a non-specific response to damaged type I cells and is similar to that which results from exposure to high concentrations of oxygen (page 492). Type I cells are end-cells and cannot divide. They are derived from type II cells which appear to be much more robust.

The interstitial space is greatly expanded by oedema fluid, fibres and a variety of proliferating cells. Fibrosis commences after the first week and ultimately fibrocytes predominate: extensive fibrosis is seen in resolving cases. Within the alveoli, the protein-rich exudate may organize to produce the characteristic 'hyaline membrane' which effectively destroys the structure of the alveoli. This is clearly visible with light microscopy.

Pathophysiology

In established ARDS, lung compliance is greatly reduced and this seems to be adequately explained by the histological changes described above. It is also very likely that there is impaired production and function of surfactant (Fein et al., 1982). Functional residual capacity is reduced by collapse, tissue proliferation and increased elastic recoil.

Alveolar/capillary permeability is increased in the early stages and this may be demonstrated by the enhanced transit of various tracer molecules across the alveolar/capillary membrane (page 203).

Dantzker and his colleagues (1979) have applied the technique of multiple inert gas wash-out (page 181) to patients with ARDS to determine the pattern of distribution of ventilation and perfusion. They found a bimodal distribution of circulation, one part to areas of normal ventilation/perfusion ($\dot{V}/\dot{Q}$) ratio and another to areas of zero or very low $\dot{V}/\dot{Q}$ ratio. This was sufficient to explain the alveolar/arterial P_{O_2} gradient without the need to invoke changes in diffusion capacity. In the clinical situation, this state of affairs is easily characterized in terms of physiological dead space (page 156) and shunt (page 174). Further characterization of the defect is of little practical benefit in the management of the patient.

The shunt is usually so large (i.e. more than 40 per cent) that increasing the inspired oxygen concentration will not produce a normal arterial P_{O_2} (see the iso-shunt chart, *Figure 7.11*). The increased dead space, which may exceed 70 per cent of tidal volume, requires a large increase in minute volume in an attempt to preserve a normal arterial P_{O_2}. Gaseous homoeostasis is further compromised by the fact that the oxygen consumption of the patient is usually increased even though he is paralysed and ventilated artificially (Sibbald and Dredger, 1983).

Mechanisms of causation of ARDS

The diversity of predisposing conditions suggests that there may be several possible mechanisms, at least in the early stages of development of ARDS. Nevertheless, the end-result is remarkably similar (Stevens and Raffin, 1984). In all cases initiation of the syndrome seems to be damage to the alveolar/capillary membrane with transudation often increased by pulmonary venoconstriction (Malik, Selig and Burhop, 1985). Thereafter, development of the condition is accelerated by a series of positive feedback mechanisms. The initial insult to the alveolar/capillary membrane may be direct or indirect by one of several postulated mechanisms.

Direct injury to the lung

Direct injury to the lung seems to be sufficient to explain the initiation of ARDS in certain situations. These include gastric aspiration, near-drowning, inhalation of toxic gases, pulmonary contusion and, possibly, pulmonary oxygen toxicity. Certain bacterial toxins may act directly on pulmonary endothelium.

Indirect injury to the lung

Much attention has recently been given to cellular and humoral mechanisms which may damage the alveolar/capillary membrane. The cells which appear capable of damaging the membrane include neutrophils, basophils and macrophages. In addition, platelets also have the possibility of releasing arachidonic acid metabolites. Damage may be inflicted by a large number of substances, including bacterial endotoxin, oxygen-derived free radicals, proteases, thrombin, fibrin, fibrin degradation products, histamine, bradykinin, 5-hydroxytryptamine (serotonin), platelet-activating factor (PAF) and some arachidonic acid metabolites. Various chemotactic agents, especially complement C5a, probably play a major role in directing formed elements onto the pulmonary endothelium. It seems improbable that any one mechanism is responsible for all cases of ARDS. It is more likely that different mechanisms operate in different predisposing conditions and in different animal models of ARDS.

Malik, Selig and Burhop (1985) have drawn attention to the fact that many of the humoral mediators, including histamine and some arachidonic acid metabolites, cause pulmonary venoconstriction. This raises pulmonary capillary pressure and compounds the effect of increased permeability. It has also been noted that many proteins, including albumin but particularly fibrin monomer, can antagonize the action of surfactant (Seeger et al., 1985).

Neutrophil-mediated injury has been extensively considered as a possible mechanism (see reviews by Fantone and Ward, 1982; Rinaldo and Rogers, 1982, Tate and Repine, 1982; Brigham and Meyrick, 1984; Glausner and Fairman, 1985). The postulated sequence of events begins with activation of complement C5a which is known to cause margination of neutrophils on the vascular endothelium. Complement C5a is known to be activated in sepsis (Hammerschmidt et al., 1983), after cardiopulmonary bypass surgery (Chenoweth et al., 1981) and in many other conditions which may lead to ARDS. Neutrophils have been seen packed in the pulmonary capillaries of lung specimens from patients with ARDS (see below).

However, there is no doubt that margination of very large numbers of neutrophils in the pulmonary circulation may occur without any resultant pulmonary damage (Glausner and Fairman, 1985). This occurs, for example, during haemodialysis with a cellophane membrane.

Under other circumstances it seems very likely that neutrophils marginated in the pulmonary circulation may damage the endothelium. The postulated sequence of events is that the neutrophils are first primed with the bactericidal contents of their lysosomes. This may occur in response to endotoxin which will also cause neutrophils to adhere firmly to the pulmonary capillary endothelium. In addition, complement C5a results in temporary adherence to endothelium but its most important effect is to trigger the neutrophil into inappropriate release of its lysosomal contents. Instead of being released into phagocytic vesicles, they come into direct contact with the endothelium which is thereby damaged.

Four groups of substances released from neutrophils have been considered as potentially damaging to the endothelium. Firstly, there are oxygen-derived free radicals, considered in detail in Chapter 29. These are powerful and important bactericidal agents which also have the capacity to damage the endothelium by lipid peroxidation and other means. In addition, they inactivate α_1-antitrypsin. The second group comprises proteolytic enzymes, which not only damage the endothelium directly but also produce elastin fragments which are chemotactic for monocytes and macrophages (Senior, Griffen and Mecham, 1980). Of the proteases, elastase is particularly damaging. The third group comprises the arachidonic metabolites, prostaglandins, thromboxanes and leukotrienes, various members of which cause vasoconstriction, increase vascular permeability and are chemotactic for neutrophils. They are discussed further in Chapter 11. The fourth group comprises platelet-activating factors resulting in intravascular coagulation. Fibrin and fibrin degradation products may themselves contribute to the tissue damage. It will be seen that numerous positive feedback loops amplify the tissue damage once it is started.

Proof of the role of neutrophils has been sought by studies of neutrophil-depleted animals, but with contradictory results. While neutrophils certainly possess the potential for endothelial damage, it seems very unlikely that they are the sole cause of ARDS. Their role in the causation of increased alveolar/capillary permeability has been critically reviewed by Glausner and Fairman (1985).

Macrophages and basophils may also produce substances which damage the endothelium. For various reasons, research has concentrated on the neutrophil. However, this does not exclude the possibility that macrophages and basophils may play an important role. Macrophages contain a wide range of bactericidal agents similar to those of the neutrophil and they are already present in the normal alveolus (page 19). Their numbers increase greatly in ARDS. Basophils share many of the properties of neutrophils described above. Their potential role has not been excluded.

Platelets are present in the pulmonary capillaries in large number in ARDS. Aggregation in that site is associated with increased capillary hydrostatic pressure, possibly due to release of arachidonic acid metabolites. They may also play a role in maintenance of the integrity of the endothelium (Malik, Selig and Burhop, 1985).

Principles of management

Management is essentially supportive since there is no specific therapy yet shown to be effective in arresting the development of ARDS. Indeed, specific therapy may well depend upon the particular predisposing condition. The main objectives of supportive therapy are fourfold:

1. To maintain a safe arterial Po_2.
2. To minimize pulmonary transudation.
3. To prevent complications, particularly sepsis.
4. To maintain the circulation.

Patients are always ventilated and often with positive end-expiratory pressure (PEEP) to improve arterial Po_2. At one time it seemed that the early use of PEEP might prevent the development of ARDS (Schmidt et al., 1976). However, it now seems unlikely that there is any such effect (Fein et al., 1982; Pepe, Hudson and Carrico, 1984). Inspired oxygen concentration should be carefully controlled to avoid dangerous hypoxia, on the one hand, and the possibility of pulmonary oxygen toxicity on the other hand. Satisfactory gaseous exchange may be impossible by conventional means and thought has been given to the use of high frequency ventilation and extracorporeal techniques (Chapters 21 and 22). To discourage oedema formation attempts may be made to raise the serum albumin which is commonly reduced. Also the fluid balance should be adjusted to keep the wedge pressure rather low (0.7–1.3 kPa or 5–10 mmHg) (Fein et al., 1982).

There has been some evidence in favour of the use of massive doses of steroids in the prodromal stages of ARDS, at least in patients with sepsis (Sibbald et al., 1981). However, more recently, Weigelt et al. (1985) failed to show any benefit and both Weigelt and DeMaria et al. (1985) found an increased incidence of sepsis in patients receiving high-dose steroids.

Certain specific drugs have been used in an attempt to block the processes believed to be responsible for the development of the condition. Steroids have been extensively tried with a view to stabilization of lysosomal membranes but no clear conclusions have yet been forthcoming (Fein et al., 1982). There are many drugs which can retard the formation of fibrous tissue and their role in ARDS has been considered by Rinaldo and Rogers (1982).

Therapy for ARDS remains disappointing, with a very high mortality in spite of great expenditure of resources in both therapy and research. The major shortcoming is specific therapy, which must await an understanding of the mechanism of development of the condition.

Problems of research into ARDS

Research into ARDS is notoriously difficult. Human studies are bedevilled by the difficulty of predicting which patients will develop the condition, and this is compounded by the relatively small and decreasing number of cases which are seen in some research centres. When the condition has developed, the patient is clearly not in any condition to give informed consent for research and there are evident difficulties in approaching the relatives of a patient with a condition carrying a 50 per cent mortality.

The obvious solution to these difficulties would appear to be the use an animal model. There have, however, been great difficulties in establishing an animal model which mimics the disease in man. Various substances have been used to mimic ARDS, including oleic acid, paraquat, phorbol myristate acetate, α-naphthyl-thiourea (ANTU) and high concentrations of oxygen. Although severe lung damage can be produced in certain species, there is no certainty that the condition is a true model of ARDS. Furthermore, effective therapy may be confined to the particular model. The problem is compounded by marked species differences in response.

Chapter 27

The effects of changes in the carbon dioxide tension

A number of special difficulties hinder an understanding of the effects of changes in P_{CO_2}. Firstly, there is the problem of species difference, which is a formidable obstacle to the interpretation of animal studies in this as in other fields. The second difficulty arises from the fact that carbon dioxide can exert its effect in a number of ways. For example, the so-called 'inert gas' narcotic effect would presumably be produced by carbon dioxide in accord with its physical properties, although it is more likely to exert its effects upon the central nervous system by means of its unique ability to alter the intracellular pH (page 219). This is quite apart from the fact that a change in P_{CO_2} usually alters the pH of the circulating blood. In addition, it remains possible that carbon dioxide can exert specific effects unrelated to the mechanisms listed above, although this would be difficult to prove. The third difficulty in the understanding of the effects of carbon dioxide arises from the fact that the gas seems to act at many different sites in the body. Sometimes the action of carbon dioxide at different sites produces opposite effects upon a particular function, and the action of carbon dioxide upon blood pressure (*Figure 27.1*) is an example of the complexity of the manner in which its effects may be produced. The subject has been reviewed by Foëx (1980), Prys-Roberts (1980) and Utting (1980).

Effects upon the nervous system

Carbon dioxide has at least five major effects upon the brain:

1. It is the major factor governing cerebral blood flow.
2. It may be presumed to exert the inert gas narcotic effect in accord with its physical properties which are similar to those of nitrous oxide.
3. It influences the excitability of the neurones, particularly relevant in the case of the reticuloactivating system.
4. It is the main factor influencing the intracellular pH, which is known to have important effects upon the metabolism of the cell.
5. It influences the CSF pressure through changes in cerebral blood flow.

The interplay of these effects is difficult to understand, although the gross changes produced are well established.

Effects on consciousness. Carbon dioxide was used as an anaesthetic by Henry Hill Hickman in 1824, later by Ozanam (1862), and finally by Leake and Waters (1928).

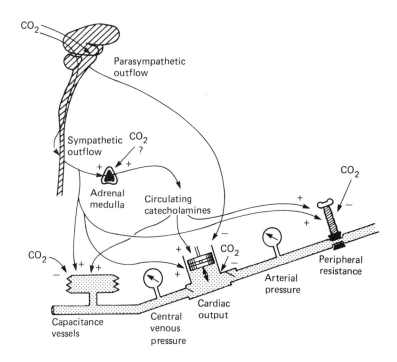

27.1 The complexity of the mechanisms by which carbon dioxide may influence the circulatory system. The overall effect in the anaesthetized patient is an increase in cardiac output which is roughly proportional to the arterial Pco_2. The rise in cardiac output exceeds the rise in blood pressure and this may be described as a fall in peripheral resistance (total). In spite of the rise of cardiac output, there is an increase in central venous pressure. This implies that capacitance vessels are contracted to cause a rise in filling pressure with which the increased cardiac output does not keep pace. In the absence of sympathetic nervous system activity, the direct effect of carbon dioxide upon the myocardium causes a fall of cardiac output and a profound fall in peripheral resistance is also seen. A fall in arterial blood pressure is then inevitable.

Thirty per cent carbon dioxide is sufficient for the production of anaesthesia, and this concentration results in an isoelectric electroencephalogram (Clowes, Hopkins and Simeone, 1955). However, use of carbon dioxide as an anaesthetic in man is complicated by the frequent occurrence of convulsions at about the concentration required for anaesthesia (Leake and Waters, 1928). Higher concentrations have been shown to be tolerated in dogs, in whom the tendency to convulsions disappears when the Pco_2 rises above about 33.3 kPa (250 mmHg). Carbon dioxide has been widely used as a routine anaesthetic agent for small laboratory animals.

The effect of varying levels of Pco_2 on the susceptibility of a patient to anaesthesia has been widely debated. It has been claimed that hyperventilation and hypocapnia enhance the actions of agents used to produce general anaesthesia (Gray and Rees, 1952) and this is supported by the demonstration of a reduced threshold to the pain of tibial pressure (Clutton-Brock, 1957). These effects have been variously attributed to decreased excitation of the reticuloactivating system or to cerebral hypoxia resulting from the combined effects of cerebral vasoconstriction and shift of the oxyhaemoglobin dissociation curve. However, Eisele, Eger and Muallem (1967) found that, in dogs, the minimal alveolar concentration (MAC) of halothane required for anaesthesia was unaltered by changes of P_{CO_2} within the range 2–12.7 kPa (15–95 mmHg). Above 12.7 kPa the narcotic effect of carbon dioxide was apparent and the halothane requirement was progressively reduced until, at P_{CO_2} 32.7 kPa (245 mmHg), anaesthesia was achieved with carbon dioxide alone. In patients with ventilatory failure, carbon dioxide narcosis occurs when the P_{CO_2} rises above 12–16 kPa (90–120 mmHg) (Westlake, Simpson and Kaye, 1955; Refsum, 1963).

Narcosis by carbon dioxide is not due primarily to its inert gas narcotic effects, because its oil solubility predicts a very much weaker narcotic than it appears to be. It seems likely that the major effect on the central nervous system is by alteration of the intracellular pH with consequent derangements of metabolic processes (Woodbury and Karler, 1960). Eisele's results (Eisele, Eger and Muallem, 1967) showed that the narcotic effect correlated better with cerebrospinal fluid pH than with arterial P_{CO_2}.

Cerebral blood flow rises with P_{CO_2} within the range 3–13 kPa (approximately 20–100 mmHg). The effect is exerted on the cerebral vascular resistance by means of changes in the extracellular pH in the region of the arterioles. The full response curve is S-shaped (*Figure 27.2*). The response at very low P_{CO_2} is probably limited by the vasodilator effect of tissue hypoxia, and the response above 16 kPa (120 mmHg) seems to represent maximal vasodilation, since there is little further increase in cerebral blood flow when the P_{CO_2} is raised as high as 59 kPa (440 mmHg)

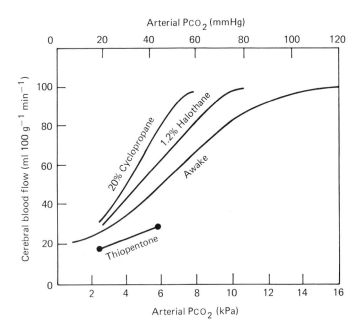

Figure 27.2 Relationship of cerebral blood flow to arterial P_{CO_2} in awake and anaesthetized patients. Lower concentrations of cyclopropane (5% and 13%) appear to reduce cerebral blood flow (Alexander et al., 1968). Data are drawn from various sources, including Reivich (1964), Lassen (1959), Pierce et al. (1962), Smith and Wollman (1972) and Alexander et al. (1968)

(Reivich, 1964). The changes shown in *Figure 27.2* represent the brain as a whole and it is not possible to generalize about regional changes. It should also be remembered that sensitivity to carbon dioxide may be lost in the region of tumours, infarctions or trauma. There is commonly a fixed vasodilatation in these areas giving rise to so-called luxury perfusions (Lassen, 1966). Far from being luxurious, this may cause dangerous increases in intracranial pressure. Conversely, some areas of the brain may develop focal ischaemia without the ability to respond to increased P_{CO_2}.

Areas with either luxury perfusion or focal ischaemia may respond to altered P_{CO_2} in the opposite direction to the normal, as is shown in *Figure 27.2*. Thus a high P_{CO_2} may increase blood flow through normal brain tissue and actually decrease perfusion through ischaemic areas which have lost their response to carbon dioxide. This has been termed the intracerebral steal (Hoedt-Rasmussen et al., 1967). The reverse phenomenon may occur when P_{CO_2} is lowered in patients with an area of luxury perfusion. Vasoconstriction in the surrounding normal tissue may divert blood flow towards the abnormal area of luxury perfusion which has no ability to respond to lowered P_{CO_2}. This has been termed the inverse steal or Robin Hood syndrome (Lassen and Palvalgyi, 1968).

Since hyperventilation is commonly practised during anaesthesia (Gray and Rees, 1952), while other patients are allowed to become severely hypercapnic (Birt and Cole, 1965), it is important to know the extent to which anaesthesia may modify the effect of P_{CO_2} on the cerebral blood flow. Pierce et al. (1962) studied the effect of hyperventilation on human volunteers anaesthetized with thiopentone at normal levels of P_{CO_2}: cerebral blood flow was reduced in accord with the reduced cerebral oxygen consumption (*Table 27.1*), but further vasoconstriction occurred with hyperventilation (*Figure 27.2*), resulting in a substantial fall in jugular venous P_{O_2}. Brain tissue P_{O_2} would undoubtedly have been reduced but there is no convincing biochemical or psychometric evidence that the practice of hyperventilation during anaesthesia results in any significant level of cerebral damage. Inhalational anaesthetics have a direct cerebral vasodilator effect and accentuate the response to P_{CO_2}.

Intracranial pressure tends to rise with increasing P_{CO_2}, probably as a result of cerebral vasodilatation. This has important implications in the management of patients with head injuries and in those undergoing neurosurgery. Hyperventilation is now one of the standard methods of reducing intracranial pressure after head injury (Shenkin and Bouzarth, 1970) but some patients react in the opposite direction. A valuable approach is to monitor intracranial pressure and so determine the optimal P_{CO_2} for individual patients with head injuries.

Hyperventilation has long been a standard method for controlling brain tension during neurosurgical operations (Marrubini, Rossanda and Tretola, 1964). Halothane and other inhalational anaesthetics may cause a dangerous rise in intracranial pressure in patients with intracranial tumours (Jennett, McDowall and Barker, 1967) but this effect may be partly mitigated by prior induction of hypocapnia, as suggested by Jennett and his co-workers and later confirmed by Adams et al. (1972).

Effects upon the autonomic and endocrine systems

Survival in severe hypercapnia is, to a large extent, dependent on the autonomic response. A great many of the effects of carbon dioxide on other systems are due wholly or in part to the autonomic response to carbon dioxide.

Table 27.1 Effects of hyperventilation and anaesthesia on cerebral blood flow and oxygenation in man

State of patient or subject	Cerebral oxygen consumption $(ml\ 100\ g^{-1}\ min^{-1})$	Cerebral blood flow $(ml\ 100\ g^{-1}\ min^{-1})$	Internal jugular venous P_{O_2} kPa	mmHg
Conscious				
Arterial P_{CO_2}				
5.3 kPa (40 mmHg)	3.0	44.0	4.7–5.3	35–40
Arterial P_{CO_2}				
2.7 kPa (20 mmHg)	3.0	22.0	—	—
Anaesthetized:				
thiopentone				
Arterial P_{CO_2}				
5.9 kPa (44 mmHg)	1.5	27.6	4.7	35
Arterial P_{CO_2}				
2.4 kPa (18 mmHg)	1.7	16.4	2.4	18
halothane 1.0%				
Arterial P_{CO_2}				
5.5 kPa (41 mmHg)	2.2*	54.4*	5.3†	40†

Data on the conscious subject from Smith and Wollman (1972).
Data on patients anaesthetized with thiopentone from Pierce et al. (1962).
*Data on patients anaesthetized with halothane from Christensen, Hoedt-Rasmussen and Lassen (1967).
†Data on blood from superior sagittal sinus of dogs breathing 2% halothane (derived from oxygen saturation) (McDowall, 1967).

Nahas, Ligou and Mehlman (1960) and Millar (1960) have clearly shown the increase in plasma levels of both adrenaline and noradrenaline caused by an elevation of P_{CO_2} during apnoeic mass-movement oxygenation (*Figure 27.3*). In moderate hypercapnia there is a proportionate rise of adrenaline and noradrenaline, but in gross hypercapnia (P_{CO_2} more than 27 kPa or 200 mmHg) there is an abrupt rise of adrenaline. Similar, though very variable, changes have been obtained over a lower range of P_{CO_2} in human volunteers inhaling carbon dioxide mixtures (Sechzer et al., 1960).

The relationship between P_{CO_2} and plasma catecholamine levels is considerably influenced by the administration of inhalational anaesthetic agents. Higher levels of adrenaline and noradrenaline are obtained during cyclopropane anaesthesia than in the unanaesthetized subject. Price et al. (1960) reported levels of 10 µg/l with a P_{CO_2} increase to only 10.7 kPa (80 mmHg) during cyclopropane administration. However, the same group found that plasma catecholamine levels of patients under halothane anaesthesia rose in much the same way as in conscious subjects.

The effect of an increased level of circulating catecholamines is, to a certain extent, offset by a decreased sensitivity of target organs when the pH is reduced (Tenney, 1956). This is additional to the general depressant direct effect of carbon dioxide on target organs. There is also evidence that the anterior pituitary is stimulated by carbon dioxide, resulting in increased secretion of ACTH (Tenney, 1960). Acetylcholine hydrolysis is reduced at low pH and therefore certain parasympathetic effects may be enhanced during hypercapnia.

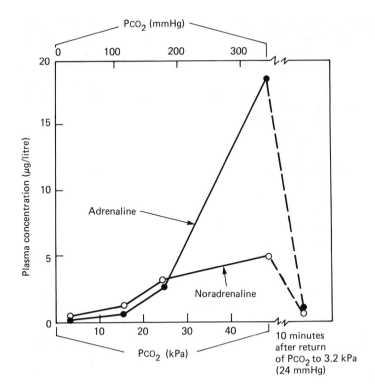

Figure 27.3 This graph shows the changes in plasma catecholamine levels in the dog during the rise of P_{CO_2} from 2.9 to 45 kPa (22 to 338 mmHg)in the course of 1 hour of apnoeic oxygenation. After 10 minutes of ventilation with oxygen, P_{CO_2} returned to 3.2 kPa (24 mmHg). Catecholamines were almost back to control values but the adrenaline remained higher than the noradrenaline. (Prepared from Table 4 of Millar, 1960)

It has been suggested that sudden reduction of P_{CO_2} after a period of hypercapnia results in a further elevation of the plasma catecholamine level (see review by Tenney and Lamb, 1965). However, it is difficult to find experimental evidence for this view and there is, in fact, quite a lot of evidence to suggest the contrary. Millar (1960) showed a rapid fall of both adrenaline and noradrenaline within minutes of reduction of a gross elevation of P_{CO_2} (*Figure 27.3*). Some support for the theory of posthypercapnic elevation of plasma catecholamine levels has been derived from the cardiovascular response to reduction of an elevated P_{CO_2}. This is considered below.

Effects upon the respiratory system

Chapter 4 discusses the role of carbon dioxide in the control of ventilation. In general the maximal stimulant effect is attained within the P_{CO_2} range 13.3–20 kPa (100–150 mmHg) (Graham, Hill and Nunn, 1960). At higher levels of P_{CO_2} the stimulation is reduced, while at very high levels respiration is depressed and later ceases altogether. Graham, Hill and Nunn (1960) made the curious observation that dogs maintained at a very high tension of carbon dioxide (above 46.7 kPa or 350 mmHg) eventually started breathing again. The breathing was of a gasping character but was sufficient to maintain life for at least an hour without any artificial assistance to ventilation. The breathing in this state (termed 'supercarbia') is uninfluenced by changes in P_{CO_2} or by vagal section. The P_{CO_2}/ventilation response curve is generally displaced to the right and its slope reduced by the action of anaesthetic agents and other depressant drugs (see Chapter 19). In profound anaesthesia the response curve may be flat, or even sloping downwards, and carbon dioxide then acts as a respiratory depressant.

Reduction of P_{CO_2} does not always lead to apnoea in the naive subject, who is unaware of Haldane's classic work (page 76). However, during anaesthesia, reduction of P_{CO_2} below the threshold value usually results in apnoea (Fink, 1961). Therefore, to restore spontaneous respiration at the end of an operation in which artificial hyperventilation has been employed, it is necessary either to raise the P_{CO_2} above the apnoeic threshold value (Ivanov and Nunn, 1969) or to awaken the patient. References to the effects of carbon dioxide on the control of breathing are given in Chapter 4.

A raised P_{CO_2} causes vasoconstriction in the pulmonary circulation (page 128) but the effect is less marked than that of hypoxia (Barer, Howard and McCurrie, 1967).

Effects upon oxygenation of the blood

Quite apart from the effect of carbon dioxide upon ventilation, it exerts two other important effects which influence the oxygenation of the blood. Firstly, if the concentration of nitrogen (or other 'inert' gas) remains constant, the concentration of carbon dioxide in the alveolar gas can increase only at the expense of oxygen which must be displaced. Secondly, an increase in P_{CO_2} causes a displacement of the oxygen dissociation curve to the right (page 263). In a patient with gross hypercapnia, Prys-Roberts, Smith and Nunn (1967) reported visibly desaturated arterial blood although the P_{O_2} was 14 kPa (105 mmHg). Unfortunately, the saturation was not measured but subsequent studies suggested that a value of the order of 90% would be expected.

Effects upon the circulatory system
(see review by Foëx, 1980)

The effects of carbon dioxide upon the circulation are complicated by the alternative modes of action upon the different components of the system (see *Figure 27.1*). Many actions are in opposition to each other and, under different circumstances, the overall effect of carbon dioxide upon certain circulatory functions can be entirely reversed.

Myocardial contractility and heart rate are diminished by elevated P_{CO_2} in the isolated preparation (Jerusalem and Starling, 1910), probably as a result of change in pH. However, in the intact subject the depressant direct action of carbon dioxide is overshadowed by the stimulant effect mediated through the sympathetic system. Blackburn et al. (1972) clearly showed a positive inotropic effect with increasing

Pco$_2$ in the dog and demonstrated that this is prevented by β-adrenergic blockade. Cullen and Eger (1974) agreed with Prys-Roberts et al. (1967) that, in artificially ventilated man, increased Pco$_2$ raises cardiac output and slightly reduces total peripheral resistance. As a result, blood pressure tends to be increased. Cullen and Eger obtained similar results during spontaneous breathing.

At very high levels of Pco$_2$ it is likely that cardiac output falls. Study of a single dog by Severinghaus, Mitchell and Nunn (unpublished) showed a progressive decline of cardiac output with increasing Pco$_2$ in supercarbia (*Table 27.2*). The response of cardiac output to increased Pco$_2$ is diminished by most anaesthetics and by spinal analgesia (Gregory et al., 1974; and a survey of other studies by Cullen and Eger, 1974).

Table 27.2 Circulatory changes at very high Pco$_2$ observed in a single dog by Severinghaus, Mitchell and Nunn (unpublished)

Time	Arterial blood					Cardiac output (l/min)	Blood pressure syst/diast	
	Pco$_2$		pH	Po$_2$				
	kPa	mmHg		kPa	mmHg		kPa	mmHg
11:51	6.8	51	7.32	39.2	294	3.14	22.0/15.3	165/115
12:35	52.4	393	6.50	27.2	204	2.34	22.0/14.7	165/110
13:00	62.4	468	6.42	20.3	152	0.98	12.0/ 8.0	90/60
13:15	72.0	540	6.41	16.0	120	0.64	11.3/ 6.0	85/45
14:33	6.4	48	7.28	39.1	293	1.29	15.3/12.7	115/95

The dog breathed spontaneously in the state of 'supercarbia' above a Pco$_2$ of 44.9 kPa (337 mmHg) which was attained at 12:25

Pco$_2$ was gradually reduced from 13:16 until 14:33

Cyclopropane anaesthesia was used when the Pco$_2$ was low.

Anaesthesia was terminated at 14:40 and the dog regained consciousness at 14:55. Recovery was uneventful.

Arrhythmias have been reported in unanaesthetized man during acute hypercapnia but have seldom been of serious import (cases reviewed by Nunn, 1962b). The position is, however, more dangerous under anaesthesia with cyclopropane (Lurie et al., 1958) and with halothane (Black et al., 1959), and possibly with other agents which have not yet been adequately studied in man. With these anaesthetic agents it appears that arrhythmias will always occur above a 'Pco$_2$ arrhythmic threshold', which is reported to be surprisingly constant for a particular patient under particular conditions. The mean value is 9.9 kPa (74 mmHg) for cyclopropane and 12.3 kPa (92 mmHg) for halothane. Multifocal ventricular extrasystoles have been reported and the danger of ventricular fibrillation cannot be discounted. Most investigators have found that arrhythmias (short of ventricular fibrillation) have little effect upon the blood pressure and appear to do the patient no obvious harm.

It should be noted that Graham, Hill and Nunn (1960) raised the Pco$_2$ of a series of dogs to 73.3 kPa (550 mmHg) and found no arrhythmias regardless of whether the dogs were receiving cyclopropane or halothane. This is a good example of the importance of species difference and illustrates the error which may arise from extrapolation of evidence from animal experiments to man.

Arrhythmias caused by elevated P_{CO_2} in anaesthetized patients occur at catecholamine levels which are above normal, but which are not *per se* high enough to cause arrhythmias. It therefore seems that arrhythmias are caused, at least in part, by a direct action of carbon dioxide on the heart (Price et al., 1958).

Brown and Miller (1952) reported that ventricular fibrillation may follow the sudden reduction of a high P_{CO_2} in dogs. Graham, Hill and Nunn (1960) were unable to confirm these observations after precipitous falls of P_{CO_2} caused by ventilation with oxygen. They suggested that, in the study of Brown and Miller, the dogs may have suffered hypoxia caused by ventilation with air in the presence of a high P_{CO_2}. It now seems unlikely that this is a serious problem in the clinical context.

Blood pressure

Blood pressure is generally raised as P_{CO_2} increases in both conscious and anaesthetized patients (see above). However, the response is variable and certainly cannot be relied upon as an infallible diagnostic sign of hypercapnia. At very high levels of P_{CO_2}, the blood pressure declines and appears to be the cause of death if the condition of supercarbia persists for much more than an hour (Graham, Hill and Nunn, 1960). Hypotension accompanies an elevation of P_{CO_2} if there is blockade of the sympathetic system by ganglioplegic drugs or spinal blockade (Payne, 1958). There is general agreement that hypotension follows a sudden fall of an elevated P_{CO_2}.

Regional blood flow appears to be influenced by the P_{CO_2} in different ways for different organs (Tenney and Lamb, 1965). Brain (Kety and Schmidt, 1948; Lassen, 1959), heart and skin blood flow increases with rising P_{CO_2}, while skeletal muscle blood flow is reduced by hypercapnia, although this effect is much diminished by general anaesthesia (McArdle and Roddie, 1958). Vance, Brown and Smith (1973) showed that hypocapnia (P_{CO_2} 3.3 kPa or 25 mmHg) in anaesthetized dogs caused a highly significant reduction in myocardial blood flow. However, oxygen extraction was increased and myocardial oxygen consumption was unchanged.

Effect upon the kidney

Renal blood flow and glomerular filtration rate are little influenced by minor changes of P_{CO_2}. However, at high levels of P_{CO_2} there is constriction of the glomerular afferent arterioles, leading to anuria. This effect is abolished in the denervated kidney (Irwin, Draper and Whitehead, 1957).

Chronic hypercapnia results in increased resorption of bicarbonate by the kidneys, further raising the plasma bicarbonate level, and constituting a secondary or compensatory 'metabolic alkalosis'. Chronic hypocapnia decreases renal bicarbonate resorption, resulting in a further fall of plasma bicarbonate and producing a secondary or compensatory 'metabolic acidosis'. In each case the arterial pH returns towards the normal value but the bicarbonate ion concentration departs even further from normality.

Although acute changes of P_{CO_2} do not produce a true metabolic acid-base change, the interpolation technique of Siggaard-Andersen et al. (1960) indicates an apparent base deficit of about 2 mmol/l when the P_{CO_2} of a normal patient is acutely raised from 5.3 to 10.7 kPa (40 to 80 mmHg). Similarly, a base excess of about 2 mmol/l appears when the P_{CO_2} is acutely lowered to 2.7 kPa (20 mmHg). The explanation of this artefact is to be found above (page 216).

Effect upon blood electrolyte levels

Hypercapnia is accompanied by a leakage of potassium ions from the cells into the plasma (Clowes, Hopkins and Simeone, 1955). Hepatectomy has demonstrated that most of the potassium comes from the liver, probably in association with glucose which is mobilized in response to the rise in plasma catecholamine levels (Fenn and Asano, 1956). Since it takes an appreciable time for the potassium ions to be transported back into the intracellular compartment, repeated bouts of hypercapnia at short intervals result in a stepwise rise in plasma potassium.

A reduction in the ionized fraction of the total calcium has, in the past, been thought to be the cause of the tetany which accompanies severe hypocapnia. However, the changes which occur are too small to account for tetany, which only occurs in parathyroid disease when there has been a fairly gross reduction of ionized calcium (Tenney and Lamb, 1965). Hyperexcitability affects all nerves and spontaneous activity ultimately occurs. The spasms probably result from activity in proprioceptive fibres causing reflex muscle contraction.

Effect upon drug action

Changes in P_{CO_2} may affect drug action as a result of a great number of different mechanisms. Firstly, the distribution of the drug may be influenced by changes in perfusion of organs. Secondly, the ionization of drugs may be altered by the change in blood pH. Thirdly, the solubility of the drug in body fluids and the protein binding may be influenced. The effects of changes in P_{CO_2} and pH on the older neuromuscular blockers have been studied by Hughes (1970), who also reviewed the earlier literature. Dann (1971) reported no effect of changes in P_{CO_2} on the duration of action of the steroid neuromuscular blocker pancuronium.

Bedside recognition of hypercapnia

Hyperventilation is the cardinal sign of a hypercapnia due to an increased concentration of carbon dioxide in the inspired gas, whether it be endogenous or exogenous. However, this sign will be absent in the paralysed patient and also in those in whom hypercapnia is the result of hypoventilation. Such patients, including those with chronic obstructive airway disease, constitute the great majority of those with hypercapnia; dyspnoea may or may not be present. In patients with central failure of respiratory drive (including 'blue bloaters'), dyspnoea may be entirely absent. On the other hand, when hypoventilation results from mechanical failure in the respiratory system (airway obstruction, pneumothorax, pulmonary fibrosis, etc.), dyspnoea is usually obvious. This problem is discussed further on page 381 in relation to *Figure 20.2*.

In patients with chronic bronchitis, hypercapnia is usually associated with a flushed skin and a full and bounding pulse with occasional extrasystoles. The blood pressure is often raised but this is not a reliable sign. Muscle twitchings and a characteristic flap of the hands may be observed when coma is imminent. Convulsions may occur. The patient will become comatose when the P_{CO_2} reaches a level in the range 12–16 kPa (90–120 mmHg) (see above). Hypercapnia should always be considered in cases of unexplained coma.

It would be wrong to believe that hypercapnia can always be reliably diagnosed on clinical examination. This is particularly true when there is a neurological basis for hypoventilation. Now that it has become so simple to measure the arterial P_{CO_2}, an arterial sample should be taken in all cases of doubt.

Chapter 28

Hypoxia

Biochemical changes in hypoxia

The essential feature of hypoxia is the cessation of oxidative phosphorylation when the mitochondrial P_{O_2} falls below the critical level. Anaerobic pathways, in particular the glycolytic pathway (see *Figure 10.3*), then come into play. Glycolysis is initiated under hypoxic conditions by the accumulation of adenosine diphosphate (ADP) which acts on rate-limiting steps in the metabolic pathway.

Anaerobic metabolism produces only one-nineteenth of the yield of adenosine triphosphate (ATP) per mole of glucose, when compared with aerobic metabolism (page 236). Therefore, during hypoxia, the ATP/ADP ratio of the brain falls and there is a decline in the level of high energy compounds, including phosphocreatine (*Figure 28.1*). The changes are very rapid in an organ with a high metabolic rate and, in the rat brain, respiratory arrest results in a precipitous fall of all high energy compounds within a few minutes (Kaasik, Nilsson and Siesjö, 1970b). Very similar changes occur in response to arterial hypotension. These changes will rapidly block cerebral function but organs with a lower energy requirement will continue to function for a longer time. Relative resistance to hypoxia is discussed below in relation to survival times.

The end-products of aerobic metabolism are carbon dioxide and water, both of which are easily diffusible and lost from the body. The main anaerobic pathway produces hydrogen and lactate ions which are retained within the brain, since the blood/brain barrier is relatively impermeable to charged ions. In the rest of the body hydrogen and lactate ions escape into the circulation where they may be conveniently quantified in terms of the base deficit, excess lactate or lactate/pyruvate ratio.

In severe cerebral hypoxia, it seems likely that a major part of the dysfunction and damage is due to intracellular acidosis. In particular, pH falls below the optimum for certain enzymes and intracellular acidosis may be the main cause of the development of postanoxic cerebral oedema. When anoxia follows chronic hypoxia, there is, surprisingly, less evidence of cell damage than in acute anoxia. It has been suggested that this is due to the reduction in lactic acid formation, owing to glucose depletion during the period of chronic hypoxaemia (Lindenberg, 1963; Geddes, 1967), since a 19-fold increase in glucose consumption is required to maintain ATP production during anoxia. This quantity of glucose is beyond the capacity of the transport mechanism of the neurones, which therefore suffer energy

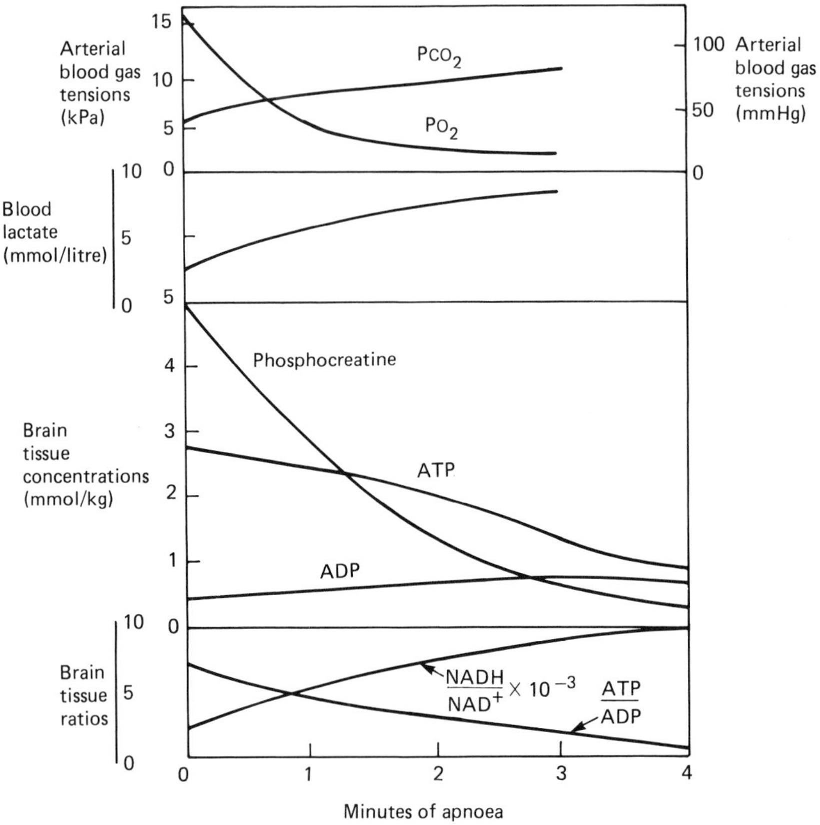

Figure 28.1 Time course of changes during 4 minutes of respiratory arrest in anaesthetized and curarized rats previously breathing 30% oxygen. Recovery of all values, except blood lactate, was complete within 5 minutes of restarting pulmonary ventilation after 3 minutes' apnoea. Effects of sustained levels of hypoxaemia were reported by Siesjö and Nilsson (1971). (Drawn from the data of Kaasik, Nilsson and Siesjö, 1970a)

depletion and reduction of intracellular glucose concentration as well as intracellular acidosis during anoxia.

It has been mentioned in Chapter 10 (page 239) that acidosis inhibits the rate-limiting enzyme 6-phosphofructokinase (see *Figure 10.3*). This limits the production of ATP and may also result in hyperglycaemia. Fructose-1,6-diphosphate enters the pathway below the stage which is rate-limited by lactacidosis and also avoids the expenditure of two molecules of ATP in its derivation from glucose. Therefore four molecules of ATP are produced from one of fructose-1,6-diphosphate in comparison with two from one molecule of glucose:

Fructose-1,6-diphosphate + 2Pi + 4ADP → 2 lactic acid + 4ATP + 2H$_2$O

(compare with equation on page 239)

Furthermore there is no subsequent stage in the pathway which is significantly rate-limited by acidosis. Additional benefits from fructose-1,6-diphosphate are that it activates pyruvic acid kinase (see *Figure 10.3*) and increases production of 2,3-diphosphoglycerate (2,3-DPG) (see *Figure 10.16*), and it is also suggested that it has a positive inotropic effect on the myocardium. Initial results suggest that it may have a very promising role in the treatment of various types of hypoxia (Webb, 1984).

Quantification of cerebral hypoxia presents considerable difficulty since the usual indicators (hydrogen and lactate ions) are not released into the jugular venous blood. It is possible to detect rapid changes of CSF pH and lactate during arterial hypotension (Kaasik, Nilsson and Siesjö, 1970a) since the CSF is on the same side of the blood/brain barrier as the neurones. However, an index of hypoxia available from the jugular venous blood is more elusive. Venous P_{O_2} is perhaps the best of the simple measurements. Arterial/venous differences offer further possibilities but, again, lactate and base deficit are not helpful. A better index is the ratio of arterial/venous differences of oxygen and glucose. With full aerobic metabolism the theoretical ratio is 6:1 (moles). A decrease indicates anaerobic consumption of glucose (usually in increased quantity) and the validity of this index is not affected by the blood/brain barrier.

P_{O_2} levels and hypoxia

Cellular P_{O_2}

The cellular P_{O_2} is the starting point for quantitative consideration of hypoxia. Oxidative phosphorylation to form ATP occurs in the mitochondria and will continue down to P_{O_2} of about 0.13 kPa, or 1 mmHg (page 241). P_{O_2} gradients within the cell are considered on page 201, and there is reason to believe that neurones will no longer function when the P_{O_2} at their surface is reduced below about 2.7 kPa (20 mmHg). P_{O_2} varies from one cell to another and is also different in different parts of the same cell. There are therefore insuperable difficulties in defining or measuring 'the tissue P_{O_2}'.

Venous P_{O_2}

Venous P_{O_2} is a more feasible measurement than cellular P_{O_2}, and the venous P_{O_2} approximates to the mean P_{O_2} at the surface of the cells in the region drained by the venous blood. Some cells close to the arterial end of the capillaries will have a higher P_{O_2} while others lying between the venous end of two or more capillaries will have a lower P_{O_2} (see *Figure 8.3*). Nevertheless, the venous P_{O_2} is a useful and practicable measure of the state of oxygenation of an organ, and conciousness is usually lost when the internal jugular venous P_{O_2} falls below about 2.7 kPa (20 mmHg) whatever the cause (McDowell, personal communication). The significance of the venous P_{O_2} is lost when there are shunts which permit arterial blood to mix with blood draining the tissue, but significant shunts do not occur in the organs which are most vulnerable to hypoxia.

The lowest tolerable level of arterial P_{O_2}

We may now extend this argument and consider in what circumstances the venous P_{O_2} may fall below the critical level of 2.7 kPa (20 mmHg), which in normal blood corresponds to 32% saturation and about 6.4 ml/100 ml oxygen content. If the brain has a mean oxygen consumption of 46 ml/min and a blood flow of 620 ml/min, it follows that the arterial/venous oxygen content difference is about 7.4 ml/100 ml. Thus, *under these conditions*, an arterial oxygen content of 13.8 ml/100 ml is the minimum which will avoid cerebral hypoxia. With normal haemoglobin concentration, pH, etc., this would correspond to a saturation of 68% and an arterial P_{O_2} of 4.8 kPa (36 mmHg). This calculation and others under various different conditions are set out in *Table 28.1*.

This calculation leads to the conclusion that an arterial P_{O_2} of less than 4.8 kPa (36 mmHg) would result in cerebral hypoxia, *if all other factors remained normal*. However, other factors may not be normal. They may be unfavourable as a result of multiple disability in the patient (e.g. anaemia or a decreased cerebral blood flow). Alternatively, there may be favourable factors, including the powerful homoeostatic mechanisms which exist to protect the brain from hypoxia. These include the polycythaemia of chronic arterial hypoxaemia, increased cerebral blood flow in anaemia and the vasopressor response to cerebral hypoxia. Cerebral vascular resistance is diminished by reduced arterial blood pressure and arterial hypoxaemia. Cerebral oxygen requirements are reduced by hypothermia or anaesthesia (see *Table 27.1*). The possible combinations of conditions are so great that it is not feasible to discuss every possible situation. Instead, certain important examples have been selected which illustrate the fundamentals of the problem, and these are set out in *Table 28.1*.

A twofold increase of cerebral blood flow would permit a further fall of arterial P_{O_2} from 4.8 to 3.6 kPa (36 to 27 mmHg) before the cerebral venous P_{O_2} reached 2.7 kPa (20 mmHg). This is important, as an increase in cerebral blood flow may be expected to follow severe hypoxia. Polycythaemia (e.g. a haemoglobin concentration of 18 g/dl) does not confer the same degree of benefit and the lower limit of arterial P_{O_2} would then be 4.3 kPa (32 mmHg). Alkalosis, which may be expected to result from the hypoxic drive to respiration, confers no advantage at all. Considerable advantage derives from hypothermia, but this is all due to the reduction in cerebral metabolism and not at all to the shift of the dissociation curve.

Uncompensated ischaemia is dangerous and, with a 45 per cent reduction in cerebral blood flow, any reduction of arterial P_{O_2} exposes the brain to risk of hypoxia. Uncompensated anaemia is almost equally dangerous, although an increase in cerebral blood flow restores a satisfactory safety margin. In the example in *Table 28.1*, a 40 per cent reduction of blood oxygen capacity and a 40 per cent increase of cerebral blood flow permits the arterial P_{O_2} to fall to 5.3 kPa (40 mmHg) without the cerebral venous P_{O_2} falling below 2.7 kPa (20 mmHg), a situation which is close to that in uncomplicated arterial hypoxaemia. The last line in *Table 28.1* shows the very dangerous combination of anaemia and ischaemia. In this example the haemoglobin concentration is reduced to about 11 g/dl and the cerebral blood flow to three-quarters of the normal value. Neither abnormality is very serious considered separately, but in combination the arterial P_{O_2} cannot be reduced below its normal value without the risk of cerebral hypoxia.

Table 28.1 must not be taken too literally, since there are many minor factors which have not been considered. However, it is a general rule that maximal cerebral

Table 28.1 Lowest arterial oxygen levels compatible with a cerebral venous Po$_2$ of 2.7 kPa (20 mmHg) under various conditions

	Blood O$_2$ capacity (ml/100 ml)	Brain O$_2$ consump. (ml/min)	Cerebral blood flow (ml/min)	Cerebral venous blood				Art./ven. O$_2$ content difference (ml/100 ml)	Arterial blood			
				Po$_2$ (kPa)	Po$_2$ (mmHg)	Sat (%)	O$_2$ content (ml/100 ml)		O$_2$ content (ml/100 ml)	Sat. (%)	Po$_2$ (kPa)	Po$_2$ (mmHg)
Normal values	20	46	620	4.4	33	63	12.6	7.4	20.0	97.5	13.3	100
Uncompensated arterial hypoxaemia	20	46	620	2.7	20	32	6.4	7.4	13.8	68	4.8	36
Arterial hypoxaemia with increased cer. blood flow	20	46	1240	2.7	20	32	6.4	3.7	10.1	50	3.6	27
Arterial hypoxaemia with polycythaemia	25	46	620	2.7	20	32	8.0	7.4	15.4	61	4.3	32
Arterial hypoxaemia with alkalosis*	20	46	620	2.7	20	46	9.2	7.4	16.6	82	4.9	37
Arterial hypoxaemia with hypothermia†	20	23	620	2.7	20	57	11.4	3.7	15.1	75	3.6	27
Uncompensated cerebral ischaemia	20	46	340	2.7	20	32	6.4	13.5	19.9	98	14.9	112
Uncompensated anaemia	12	46	620	2.7	20	32	3.8	7.4	11.2	93	8.9	67
Anaemia with increased cer. blood flow	12	46	870	2.7	20	32	3.8	5.3	9.1	75	5.3	40
Combined anaemia and ischaemia	15	46	460	2.7	20	32	4.8	10.0	14.8	97	12.3	92

*pH 7.6   †temp. 30°C; cerebral O$_2$ consumption reduced to half normal

vasodilatation may be expected to occur in any condition (other than cerebral ischaemia) which threatens cerebral oxygenation. We must also bear in mind that there may be circumstances in which the critical organ is not the brain but the heart, liver or kidney.

The most important message of this discussion is that there is no simple answer to the question 'What is the safe lower limit of arterial P_{O_2}?'. Acclimatized mountaineers have remained conscious during exercise at high altitude with arterial P_{O_2} values as low as 2.7 kPa (20 mmHg) (page 319). Patients presenting with severe respiratory disease tend to remain conscious down to the same level of arterial P_{O_2} (Refsum, 1963; McNicol and Campbell, 1965). However, both acclimatized mountaineers and patients with chronic respiratory disease have compensatory polycythaemia and maximal cerebral vasodilatation. Uncompensated subjects who are acutely exposed to hypoxia are unlikely to remain conscious with an arterial P_{O_2} of less than about 3.6 kPa (27 mmHg) but considerable individual variation must be expected.

The question of fitness for surgery and anaesthesia in the presence of a disorder of a factor which influences oxygen flux cannot be decided in isolation but must be answered after considering the other relevant factors and the patient as a whole. It is particularly important to consider the additional disturbances which may be expected to result from the proposed intervention.

Compensatory mechanisms in hypoxia

Hypoxia presents a serious threat to the body, and compensatory mechanisms usually take priority over other changes. Thus, for example, in hypoxia with concomitant hypocapnia, hyperventilation and increase in cerebral blood flow occur in spite of the decreased P_{CO_2} (Turner et al., 1957). Certain compensatory mechanisms will come into play whatever the reason for the hypoxia, although their effectiveness will depend to a large extent on the cause. For example, hyperventilation will be largely ineffective in stagnant hypoxia since hyperventilation while breathing air can do little to increase the oxygen content of arterial blood, and usually nothing to increase perfusion.

Hyperventilation results from a decreased arterial P_{O_2} but the response is non-linear (*Figure 4.6*). There is little effect until arterial P_{O_2} is reduced to about 7 kPa (52.5 mmHg): maximal response is at 4 kPa (30 mmHg). The interrelationship between hypoxia and other factors in the control of breathing is discussed in Chapter 4.

Pulmonary distribution of blood flow is improved by hypoxia as a result of increase in pulmonary arterial pressure (page 127).

Cardiac output is increased by hypoxia, together with the regional blood flow to almost every major organ, particularly the brain.

Haemoglobin concentration is not increased in acute hypoxia in man but it is increased in chronic hypoxia due to residence at altitude and chronic respiratory disease.

The dissociation curve is displaced to the right by an increase in 2,3-DPG and by acidosis which may also be present. This tends to increase tissue Po_2 (see *Figure 10.15*).

The sympathetic system is concerned in many of the responses to hypoxia. The immediate response is reflex and is initiated by chemoreceptor stimulation: it occurs before there is any measurable increase in circulating catecholamines although this does occur in due course. Reduction of cerebral and probably myocardial vascular resistance is not dependent on the autonomic system but depends on local responses in the vicinity of the vessels themselves.

Anaerobic metabolism is increased in severe hypoxia in an attempt to maintain the level of ATP (page 239).

Organ survival times

Lack of oxygen stops the machine and then wrecks the machinery. The time of circulatory arrest up to the first event (survival time) must be distinguished from the duration of anoxia which results in the second event (revival time), the latter being defined as the time beyond which no recovery of function is possible. Anoxia lasting more than the survival time but less than the revival time may result in prolonged impairment of function during recovery which may not be complete.

Survival times depend on many factors. There is a very large difference between different organs, ranging from less than 1 minute for the cerebral cortex to about 2 hours for skeletal muscle. Heart is intermediate with a survival time of about 5 minutes, liver and kidney probably being about 10 minutes. Revival times tend to be about four times as long as survival times, but the ratio is greater in the case of the brain, which has a revival time of the order of 5 minutes.

Apart from the inherent differences in sensitivity of organs, survival time is influenced by oxygen consumption and oxygen stores in the tissue. An inactive organ (such as a heart in asystole or the brain in hypothermia) has increased resistance to hypoxia, and there is a small but definite increase in survival time when tissue Po_2 has been increased by hyperbaric oxygenation. Hypothermia both decreases oxygen demand and increases the solubility of oxygen in the tissue.

Survival of an organ after anoxia depends on many secondary factors which influence oxygen transport during the recovery phase. If the heart has been severely affected by generalized hypoxaemia, there may be a reduced perfusion of other organs during recovery. Tissue oedema, particularly of the brain, may decrease the local perfusion and oxygen transport for a considerable time during recovery.

Chapter 29

Hyperoxia and oxygen toxicity

Hyperoxia

Extreme hyperventilation, while breathing air, may raise the arterial P_{O_2} to about 16 kPa (120 mmHg). Higher levels can be obtained only by oxygen enrichment of the inspired gas or by elevation of the ambient pressure. Although by this means the arterial P_{O_2} can be raised to very high levels, the increase in arterial oxygen content is relatively small in the normal subject, since the arterial oxygen saturation is normally close to 95% (*Table 29.1*). Apart from raising this to 100%, additional oxygen can be carried only in physical solution. Provided that the arterial/mixed venous oxygen content difference remains constant, it follows that venous oxygen content will rise by the the same value as the arterial oxygen content. The consequences in terms of venous P_{O_2} are shown in *Table 29.1* and are important because tissue P_{O_2} apaproximates more closely to venous P_{O_2} than to arterial P_{O_2}. Note particularly the trivial rise in venous P_{O_2} when breathing oxygen at normal barometric pressure. It is necessary to breathe oxygen at 3 atmospheres absolute (ATA) pressure before there is an appreciable rise in venous P_{O_2}. The same applies to tissue P_{O_2}.

It is convenient to consider two degrees of hyperoxia. The first applies to the inhalation of oxygen-enriched gas at normal pressure, while the second involves inhaling oxygen at raised pressure and is termed hyperbaric oxygenation. Nevertheless, it is important to remember that the inhalation of air at raised pressures results in hyperoxia. An air-breathing diver at a depth of 50 metres of sea water would have an arterial P_{O_2} comparable to that of a man breathing oxygen at sea level.

Hyperoxia resulting from breathing oxygen-enriched gas at normal pressure

The commonest indications for oxygen enrichment of the inspired gas are the prevention of arterial hypoxaemia ('anoxic anoxia') caused either by hypoventilation (page 388) or by venous admixture (page 171. Oxygen enrichment of the inspired gas may also be used to mitigate the effects of hypoperfusion ('stagnant hypoxia') but the data in *Table 29.1* show that there will be only a marginal improvement in oxygen flux (page 256). Although the improvement may be marginal, it may also be critical in certain situations. Thus Freeman (1962) demonstrated reduction in mortality in critically bled dogs following the administration of

Table 29.1 Oxygen levels attained in the normal subject by changes in the oxygen tension of the inspired gas

	At normal barometric pressure		At 2 ATA	At 3 ATA
Inspired gas	Air	Oxygen	Oxygen	Oxygen
Inspired gas P_{O_2} (humidified)				
(kPa)	20	95	190	285
(mmHg)	150	713	1425	2138
Arterial P_{O_2}*				
(kPa)	13	80	175	270
(mmHg)	98	600	1313	2025
Arterial oxygen content†				
(ml/100 ml)	19.3	21.3	23.4	25.5
Arterial/venous oxygen content				
difference (ml/100 ml)	5.0	5.0	5.0	5.0
Venous oxygen content				
(ml/100 ml)	14.3	16.3	18.4	20.5
Venous P_{O_2}				
(kPa)	5.2	6.4	9.1	48.0
(mmHg)	39	48	68	360

Tissue perfusion may be reduced by elevation of P_{O_2}. This tends to increase the arterial/venous oxygen content difference which will limit the rise in venous P_{O_2}. The increases in venous P_{O_2} shown in this Table will therefore be too great in certain circumstances.

*Reasonable values have been assumed for P_{CO_2} and alveolar/arterial P_{O_2} difference.

†Normal values are assumed for Hb, pH, etc.

oxygen but, in hypoperfusion, improvement of perfusion is generally more important than raising the arterial P_{O_2}.

'Anaemic anoxia' will be only partially relieved by oxygen therapy but, since the combined oxygen is less than in a subject with normal haemoglobin concentration, the effect of additional oxygen carried in solution will be relatively more important.

Clearance of gas loculi in the body may be greatly accelerated by the inhalation of oxygen which may also be considered as denitrogenation. The principle of this form of therapy depends on the reduction of the total tension of the dissolved gases in the venous blood. This results in the capillary blood having additional capacity to carry away gas dissolved from the loculi. Total gas tensions in venous blood are always slightly less than atmospheric (*Table 29.2*) and this is of critical importance in prevention of the accumulation of air in potential spaces such as the pleural cavity, in which the pressure is subatmospheric (page 27). When breathing 100% oxygen the total pressure of gases in the venous blood is little more than one-tenth of an atmosphere (*Table 29.2*). Oxygen is therefore useful in the treatment of air embolus and pneumothorax, and has also been used to relieve intestinal distension (Down and Castleden, 1975).

Carbon monoxide poisoning has long been recognized as an indication for oxygen therapy. Not only is the oxygen content of the arterial blood improved but also the rate of dissociation of carboxyhaemoglobin is increased (Sharp, Ledingham and Norman, 1962).

Table 29.2 Normal arterial and mixed venous blood gas tensions

	kPa		mmHg	
	Arterial blood	Venous blood	Arterial blood	Venous blood
Breathing air				
P_{O_2}	13.3	5.3	100	40
P_{CO_2}	5.3	6.1	40	46
P_{N_2}	76.0	76.0	570	570
Total gas tensions	94.6	87.4	710	656
Breathing oxygen				
P_{O_2}	80.0	6.7	600	50*
P_{CO_2}	5.3	6.1	40	46
P_{N_2}	0	0	0	0
Total gas tensions	85.3	12.8	640	96

*See Table 29.1

Hyperbaric oxygenation

Hyperbaric oxygenation may be regarded as an extension of normal therapy and it is the only means by which arterial P_{O_2} values in excess of 90 kPa (675 mmHg) may be obtained.

In hyperbaric oxygen therapy, it is easy to be deluded into thinking that the tissues will be exposed to much the same P_{O_2} as applies in the chamber. Terms such as 'drenching the tissues with oxygen' have been used but are really meaningless. In fact, the simple calculations shown in *Table 29.1*, supported by experimental observations, show that large increases in venous and presumably tissue P_{O_2} do not occur until the P_{O_2} of the arterial blood is of the order of 270 kPa (2025 mmHg), when the whole of the tissue oxygen requirements can be met from the dissolved oxygen. The relationship between arterial and tissue P_{O_2} varies from one tissue to another, and oxygen-induced vasoconstriction (in the brain for example) limits the rise in venous and tissue P_{O_2}.

When the dissolved oxygen in the arterial blood is sufficient for tissue oxygen requirements there will be only a small quantity of reduced haemoglobin in the venous blood. Since this reduces the buffering power and carbamino carriage of carbon dioxide in the blood, it was suggested that carbon dioxide retention might result (Gessel, 1923). In fact, the increase in tissue P_{CO_2} from this cause is unlikely to exceed 1 kPa (7.5 mmHg). However, in the brain this might result in a significant increase in cerebral blood flow, causing a secondary rise in tissue P_{O_2}.

Clinical applications of hyperbaric oxygenation

Around 1960 it appeared that hyperbaric oxygenation would become a most important and widespread form of therapy. In fact, enthusiasm has waned and it has never passed into universal use. However, it is still practised in a few centres where it is claimed that the advantages are substantial. Clear answers to its value have been slow to emerge from controlled trials, which are admittedly very difficult to conduct in the conditions for which benefit is claimed.

Prolongation of the safe period of circulatory arrest would seem at first sight to be an obvious application. However, consideration of the realities shown in *Table 29.1* suggests it may be less promising than was hoped. Results have proved to be disappointing at normal temperatures although somewhat better during hypothermia (Ledingham and Norman, 1965) when oxygen consumption is reduced and the solubility of oxygen in tissue fluids is increased.

Hyperbaric oxygen has a minor theoretical role in the management of severe pulmonary shunting. The iso-shunt diagram (page 171) shows that even 100% oxygen can do little to improve arterial Po_2 when the shunt is greater than about 40 per cent. However, hyperbaric oxygenation will restore a normal arterial Po_2 in the presence of a shunt up to 50 per cent (*Table 29.3*).

Table 29.3 Oxygen levels with 50 per cent shunt

	Pulmonary end-capillary blood			Arterial blood			Mixed venous blood		
	Po_2		O_2 content (ml/100 ml)	Po_2		O_2 content (ml/100 ml)	Po_2		O_2 content (ml/100 ml)
Oxygen at:	(kPa)	(mmHg)		(kPa)	(mmHg)		(kPa)	(mmHg)	
1 ATA*	80	600	21	6.3	47	16	4.0	30	11
2 ATA*	173	1 300	23	8.3	62	18	4.7	35	13
3 ATA*	267	2 000	25	26.7	200	20	5.6	42	15

*The pressure in atmospheres absolute (ATA) is equal to the sum of the barometric pressure and the gauge pressure (which shows the difference between the chamber pressure and the atmosphere). It is very important to distinguish clearly between absolute' and gauge pressure since both scales are in routine use in different laboratories.

Hypoxia due to hypoperfusion can be relieved by hyperbaric oxygenation when the perfusion is only marginally inadequate. The small increase in oxygen content of the arterial blood clearly cannot compensate for a gross failure of perfusion. Satisfactory results have been obtained in experimental ligation of the left circumflex coronary artery in dogs (Smith and Lawson, 1958). However, evidence of satisfactory results in clinical myocardial infarction has remained elusive (Cameron et al., 1965). There have been isolated case reports of patients with severe cerebral ischaemia who have regained consciousness during hyperbaric oxygenation (Ingvar, 1965).

It has been suggested that preservation of partially severed limbs may be improved with hyperbaric oxygenation (Smith et al., 1961). It has also been claimed that mortality from haemorrhagic shock has been reduced by hyperbaric oxygenation (Attar, Scanlan and Cowley, 1966). There are also reports that varicose and senile ulcers heal more rapidly with intermittent exposure to hyperbaric oxygen.

Infection seems to be the most enduring field of application of hyperbaric oxygenation following good results which were obtained with anaerobic infections (Brummelkamp, 1965). High partial pressures of oxygen will increase the production of oxygen-derived free radicals which are cidal not only to anaerobes but also to aerobes (page 487).

Radiotherapy has been employed under conditions of hyperbaric oxygenation since 1955, the rationale being based on the synergistic effect of radiation and oxygen which tends to spare hypoxic areas of tumours. The subject was reviewed by Foster (1965) but results have been disappointing and the technique is seldom used today.

Carbon monoxide remains a strong indication for hyperbaric oxygenation (Sharp, Ledingham and Norman, 1962). However, its clinical value is maximal at the very early stages when hyperbaric facilities are least likely to be available. This consideration led to interest in the possibility of mounting small pressure chambers in ambulances (Williams and Hopkinson, 1965). However, the exploitation of natural gas has resulted in a great decrease in the incidence of carbon monoxide poisoning.

At the time of writing, there has been great interest in the therapeutic value of hyperbaric oxygenation in multiple sclerosis. Fischer, Marks and Reich (1983) reported a favourable response after 12 months in a double-blind controlled clinical trial of 40 patients in which the treated group received oxygen at 2 atmospheres total pressure while the placebo group inhaled 10% oxygen in nitrogen, also at 2 atmospheres. However, these findings were not confirmed in a larger study by Wiles et al. (1986). Neither were they confirmed in other studies cited by these authors, who concluded that there is no basis for recommending hyperbaric oxygen in the treatment of multiple sclerosis. However, there are reports of a beneficial effect in patients with cerebral infarction secondary to occlusion of a carotid or middle cerebral artery (Kapp, 1981).

Techniques for the administration of oxygen under orthobaric and hyperbaric conditions are described on pages 273 et seq.

Oxygen toxicity

The oxygen molecule and derived species

Although ground state oxygen (dioxygen) is a powerful oxidizing agent, the molecule is stable and with an indefinite half-life. However, the oxygen molecule is capable of subtle modifications which transform it into a range of free radicals and other highly toxic substances, most of which are far more reactive than oxygen itself. A comprehensive account may be found in the excellent book by Halliwell and Gutteridge (1985).

The dioxygen molecule (*Figure 29.1*) is unusual in having two unpaired electrons in the outer (2P) shell. Thus dioxygen itself qualifies as a free radical but stability is conferred by the fact that the orbits of the two unpaired electrons are parallel. Furthermore, the two unpaired electrons also confer the property of paramagnetism which has been exploited as a method of gas analysis that is almost specific for oxygen.

Under a wide range of circumstances, considered below, the oxygen molecule may be partially reduced by receiving a single electron which pairs with one of the unpaired electrons to form a very reactive unstable free radical known by various names such as the superoxide anion or the superoxide free radical (O^- in *Figure 29.1*). This species is both an anion and a free radical. It is the first and crucial stage

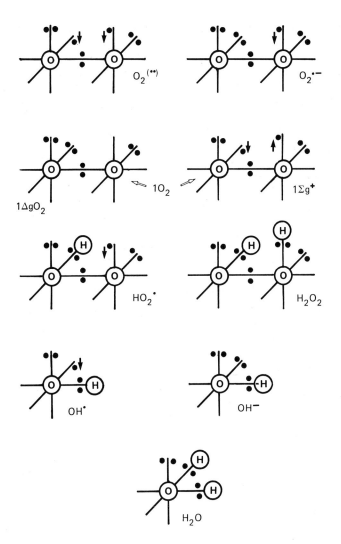

Figure 29.1 Outer orbital ring of electrons in (from the top left): ground state oxygen or dioxygen (O_2); superoxide anion ($O_2^{\cdot-}$); two forms of singlet oxygen ($1o_2$); peroxy free radical ($HO_2^{\cdot}$); hydrogen peroxide (H_2O_2); hydroxyl free radical ($HO^{\cdot}$); hydroxyl ion (OH^-); and water H_2O. The arrows indicate unpaired electrons. See text for properties and interrelationships.

in the production of a series of toxic oxygen-derived free radicals and other compounds. It is relatively stable in aqueous solution at body pH but has a rapid biological decay due to the ubiquitous presence of superoxide dismutase (see below). Being charged, superoxide anion does not readily cross cell membranes.

Other possible modifications of the oxygen molecule are internal rearrangements of one of the unpaired electrons to form two possible species, both known as singlet oxygen ($1o_2$). In $1\Delta gO_2$, one unpaired electron is transferred to the orbit of the other (*Figure 29.1*), imparting an energy level 22.4 kcal/mol above the ground state. There being no remaining unpaired electron, $1\Delta gO_2$ is not a free radical. In $1\Sigma g^+$, the rotation of one unpaired electron is reversed, which imparts an energy level 37.5 kcal/mol above the ground state and this species is still a free radical. $1\Sigma g^+$ is extremely reactive and rapidly decays to the $1\Delta gO_2$ form which is particularly relevant in biological systems and especially to lipid peroxidation (see below).

Superoxide anion may acquire a hydrogen ion to form the hydroperoxyl radical thus:

$$O_2^{\cdot-} + H^+ = HO_2^{\cdot}$$

The reaction is pH dependent with a pK of 4.8 so the equilibrium is far to the left in biological systems.

Acquisition of two hydrogen ions and two electrons results in the formation of hydrogen peroxide (*Figure 29.1*) which, though not a free radical, is a powerful and toxic oxidizing agent, that plays an important role in oxygen toxicity. It is continuously generated by various reactions in the body and is destroyed in the liver by catalase and peroxidases.

Figure 29.2 shows the three-stage reduction of oxygen through the superoxide anion and hydrogen peroxide to water which is the fully reduced and stable state. This contrasts with the more familiar single-stage reduction of oxygen to water which occurs in the terminal cytochrome (page 237). The first step in *Figure 29.2* is the acquisition of a single electron by molecular oxygen to form the superoxide anion which then undergoes a dismutation. In this reaction, two molecules of

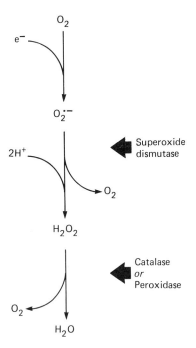

Figure 29.2 Three-stage reduction of oxygen to water. The first reaction is a single electron reduction to form the superoxide anion free radical. In the second reaction the first products of the dismutation reaction are dioxygen and a short-lived intermediate which then receives two protons to form hydrogen peroxide.

superoxide anion exchange an electron whereby one reverts to molecular oxygen and the other is converted into a short-lived intermediate which acquires two hydrogen ions to become hydrogen peroxide. This dismutation reaction proceeds spontaneously but is greatly accelerated by the intracellular enzyme superoxide dismutase (SOD) which is present in most living tissue and is an important defence against oxygen toxicity.

Hydrogen peroxide breaks down slowly into water and molecular oxygen. This reaction is also greatly accelerated by a number of intracellular enzymes, catalase (CAT) or one of various peroxidases. These enzymes also constitute an important defence against oxygen toxicity and both SOD and CAT can be induced. Unlike the single-stage reduction of oxygen, the three-stage reaction shown in *Figure 29.2* is not inhibited by cyanide.

Although it is likely that both the superoxide anion and hydrogen peroxide have direct toxic effects, they interact to produce even more dangerous species. To the right of *Figure 29.3* is shown the Fenton or Haber–Weiss reaction which results in the formation of the harmless hydroxyl ion together with two extremely reactive species, the hydroxyl free radical (OH·) and singlet oxygen (1_2). It seems likely that they are mainly responsible for the toxic effects of oxygen. The Fenton reaction is more likely to take place under biological circumstances and it is catalysed by metals, particularly ferrous iron. To the left of *Figure 29.3* is shown the reaction of hydrogen peroxide with chloride ion to form hypochlorous acid. This occurs in the

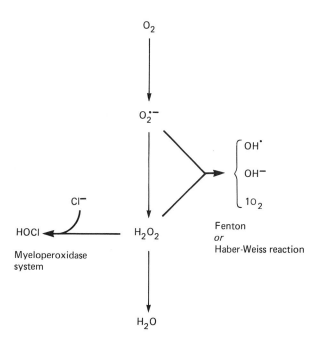

Figure 29.3 Interaction of superoxide anion and hydrogen peroxide in the Fenton or Haber–Weiss reaction to form hydroxyl free radical, hydroxyl ion and singlet oxygen. Hypochlorous acid is formed from hydrogen peroxide by the myeloperoxidase system. (Reproduced from Nunn (1985b) by courtesy of the Editor of the Journal of the Royal Society of Medicine)

phagocytic vesicle of the neutrophil and plays a major role in bacterial killing. Lucid accounts of these changes and their clinical relevance have been written by Del Maestro (1980) and Fantone and Ward (1982).

In many respects, the changes described above are similar to those caused by ionizing radiation, with the hydroxyl free radical (OH$^-$) being a major product in both cases. It is therefore hardly surprising that the effect of radiation is increased by high partial pressures of oxygen, to which reference was made above. As tissue P_{O_2} is reduced below about 2 kPa (15 mmHg), there is progressively increased resistance to radiation damage until, at zero P_{O_2}, resistance is increased threefold (Gray et al., 1953).

Sources of electrons for the reduction of oxygen to superoxide anion

The existence of the superoxide anion was first deduced by McCord and Fridovich in 1968 from a reaction in which the electron was donated by the conversion of xanthine to uric acid by the enzyme xanthine oxidase (*Figure 29.4*). This long remained a laboratory technique for the production of oxygen-derived free radicals in cell cultures and organ perfusion techniques. However, hypoxanthine may be formed from ATP under hypoxic or ischaemic conditions, and, especially during reperfusion, reaction with oxygen and xanthine oxidase may result in liberation of oxygen-derived free radicals. Xanthine oxidase catalyses the conversion of both hypoxanthine to xanthine and xanthine to uric acid. It seems probable that, under certain circumstances, this mechanism may play a role in reperfusion tissue damage or postischaemic shock (McCord and Roy, 1982; Parks, Bulkley and Granger, 1983). Its relevance would seem to be limited by the rather sparse distribution of xanthine oxidase within the body. In man the enzyme is largely confined to liver and the mucosa of small bowel but also seems to be present in the capillary endothelium of many organs, including the lung (Jarasch et al., 1981). Rat lungs

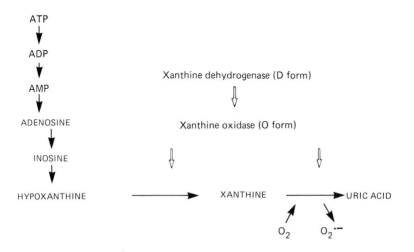

Figure 29.4 Generation of superoxide anion from oxygen by the reaction of xanthine and xanthine oxidase. Also shown are the pathways from ATP to hypoxanthine and the conversion of xanthine dehydrogenase to xanthine oxidase, both of which changes occur in hypoxia.

contain appreciable quantities of xanthine oxidase and it has been demonstrated in this species that pulmonary hyperoxic damage can be increased by perfusion of the organ with hypoxanthine (Saugstad et al., 1984). The relevance of these observations to human pulmonary hyperoxic damage is not yet established. In common with other enzymes, xanthine oxidase is released from the damaged liver (Shammea, Nasrallah and Al-Khalidi, 1973). The naturally occurring enzyme is actually in the form of xanthine dehydrogenase (type D) which does not produce superoxide anion unless it has been converted to xanthine oxidase itself (type O).

A major source of electrons for the reduction of oxygen to superoxide anion is ferrous iron which loses an electron during conversion to the ferric state. This is an important aspect of the toxicity of ferrous iron and has been proposed as a mechanism of rheumatoid arthritis (Blake et al., 1981). A similar reaction also occurs during the spontaneous oxidation of haemoglobin to methaemoglobin (page 262). It is for this reason that large quantities of SOD, CAT and other protective agents are present in the young erythrocyte. They become depleted during ageing of the erythrocyte and their exhaustion may well determine the life of the cell. In addition to the role of ferrous iron acting as an electron source in generating superoxide anion, reference was made above to its catalytic role in the Fenton reaction, which generates the hydroxyl free radical and singlet oxygen.

Of great biological importance is the production of oxygen-derived free radicals as bactericidal agents by neutrophils and macrophages, a major discovery by Babior, Kipnes and Curnutte (1973). The electron is donated from NADPH by the enzyme NADPH oxidase which is located within the membrane of the phagocytic vesicle (*Figure 29.5*). NADPH is generated by the hexose monophosphate shunt. This mechanism is activated by phagocytosis and is accompanied by an enormous increase in the oxygen consumption of the cells. This is the so-called respiratory burst, which is probably responsible for most of the oxygen consumption by shed blood (page 280), a process which is known to be cyanide resistant. Superoxide anion is released into the phagocytic vesicle, where it is reduced to hydrogen peroxide which then reacts with chloride ions to form hypochlorous acid in the myeloperoxidase reaction (see *Figure 29.3*). NAPDH oxidase is absent in chronic granulomatous disease which results in a serious disability to contend with infection. Absence of myeloperoxidase is less serious. Oxygen-derived free radicals are also involved in the killing of malarial parasites (Clark and Hunt, 1983).

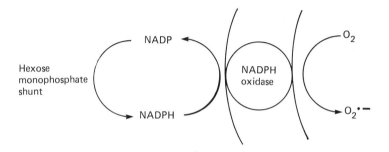

Figure 29.5 Single-stage reduction of oxygen by NADPH oxidase located in the membrane of the phagocytic vesicle of a neutrophil.

Although the NADPH oxidase system has extremely important biological advantages, it can also act in an inappropriate manner to the disadvantage of the organism. There seems little doubt that it can damage the endothelium of the lung and it may well play a part in the production of the adult respiratory distress syndrome (ARDS) (Chapter 26). The suggested sequence of events starts with margination of neutrophils in the pulmonary capillary circulation. This is normally harmless but, under certain circumstances, may result in the discharge of oxygen-derived free radicals, not only into phagocytic vesicles but also onto the surface of the endothelium. The endothelium is damaged by lipid peroxidation and other mechanisms (see below), and increased permeability to macromolecules then initiates the full syndrome of ARDS (Fantone and Ward, 1982; Rinaldo and Rogers, 1982; Tate and Repine, 1983).

Various drugs and toxic substances can act as an analogue of NADPH oxidase and transfer an electron from NADPH to molecular oxygen. The best example of this is paraquat which can, in effect, insert itself into an electron transport chain, alternating between its singly and doubly ionized form (*Figure 29.6*). This process is accelerated at high levels of P_{O_2} and so there is a synergistic effect between paraquat and oxygen. Paraquat is concentrated in the alveolar epithelial type II cell where the P_{O_2} is as high as anywhere in the body. Due to the very short half-life of the oxygen-derived free radicals, damage is confined to the lung. Bleomycin and various antibiotics can act in a similar manner but usually at high dose levels.

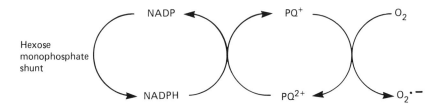

Hexose monophosphate shunt

Figure 29.6 Role of paraquat (PQ) in the reduction of oxygen to superoxide anion. Compare with Figure 29.5.

There is also evidence that generation of oxygen-derived free radicals is increased when normal oxygen usage is increased. Thus during severe exercise, lipid peroxidation occurs which can be reversed by pretreatment with vitamin E (Clark, Cowden and Hunt, 1985).

Whatever other factors may apply, the production of oxygen-derived free radicals is increased at high levels of P_{O_2} (Freeman and Crapo, 1981; Freeman, Topolsky and Crapo, 1982). It would appear that the normal tissue defences against free radicals (discussed below) are effective against free radicals produced in the absence of any abnormal electron donor up to a tissue P_{O_2} of the order of 60 kPa (450 mmHg). This level is not reached in any tissue under natural conditions. It can, however, be reached in the lungs during the inhalation of more than 70% oxgen at normal pressures but in other tissues only under hyperbaric conditions. This accords with the development of clinical oxygen toxicity as discussed below.

Factors promoting the production of oxygen-derived free radicals include:

High partial pressures of oxygen
Increased oxygen consumption

Ferrous iron and haemoglobin
Paraquat
NADPH oxidase and phagocytosis
Complement activation
Xanthine oxidase
Glucose oxidase
Ionizing radiation

Biological targets of oxygen-derived free radicals

The three main targets are deoxyribonucleic acid (DNA), lipids and sulphydryl-containing proteins. All three are also sensitive to ionizing radiation. The mechanisms of both forms of damage have much in common and synergism occurs.

Breakage of chromosomes in cultures of Chinese hamster lung fibroblasts by high concentrations of oxygen was demonstrated by Sturrock and Nunn (1978) (*Figure 29.7*). The same authors showed that 48 hours' exposure to 95% oxygen increased the rate of mutations by a factor of 25. It is not yet clear to what extent damage to DNA is responsible for pulmonary oxygen toxicity.

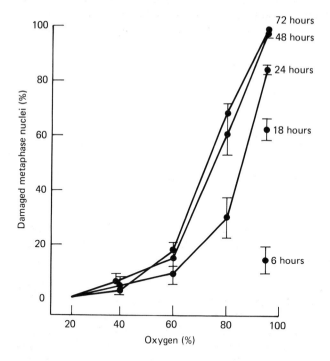

Figure 29.7 Breakage of chromosomes in a culture of Chinese hamster lung fibroblasts by oxygen at various concentrations and for varying durations of exposure. (Reproduced from Sturrock and Nunn (1978) by courtesy of the Editors of Mutation Research*)*

There is little doubt that lipid peroxidation is a major mechanism of tissue damage by oxygen-derived free radicals. The interaction of a free radical with an unsaturated fatty acid not only disrupts that particular lipid molecule but also generates another free radical so that a chain reaction ensues until stopped by a free radical scavenger. Lipid peroxidation disrupts cell membranes and accounts for the loss of integrity of the alveolar/capillary barrier in pulmonary oxygen toxicity.

Damage to sulphydryl-containing proteins is less fully understood but includes the inactivation of a range of enzymes including some which may be involved in oxygen convulsions (see below).

Defences against oxygen-derived free radicals

It will be clear from the foregoing account that life as we know it would not be possible without extensive mechanisms for protection of the living organism from the ravages of oxygen-derived free radicals. It is likely that such mechanisms commenced to evolve as soon as the first photosynthetic organisms began discharging oxygen into the primite atmosphere, an event which can be dated to about 2000 million years ago (Nunn, 1968).

The defensive system operates in depth. Of special importance are the enzymes superoxide dismutase (SOD) and catalase (CAT), the actions of which are described above. These are widely distributed in all aerobic organisms and can be induced, particularly in the young. Thus, 7 days' exposure of rats to 85% oxygen increased tissue levels of SOD and also increased tolerance to subsequent exposure to 100% oxygen (Crapo and Tierney, 1974). SOD may also be induced by injection of endotoxin (Frank, Summerville and Massaro, 1980). However, this effect is blocked by acetylsalicylic acid (Klein, Trouwborst and Salt, 1985) which would interfere with prostaglandin metabolism (see *Figure 11.3*). No less important is the glutathione/glutathione peroxidase system which scavenges not only the oxygen-derived free radicals themselves but also free radicals formed during lipid peroxidation as described above. Two molecules of the tripeptide (glycine–cysteine–glutamic acid) glutathione (GSH) are oxidized to one molecule of reduced glutathione (GSSG) by the formation of a disulphide bridge linking the cysteine residues. GSH is re-formed from GSSG by the enzyme glutatione reductase, hydrogen being supplied by NADPH and hydrogen ions. NADPH is formed by the pentose phosphate pathway which can be rate-limiting in the maintenance of the GSH/GSSG ratio. Other antioxidants and free radical scavengers include ascorbic acid (important for the hydroxyl free radical), vitamin E (α-tocopherol), dimethylthiourea and dimethylsulphoxide. Their therapeutic role is by no means clear at the time of writing.

Two other drugs require special mention. Desferrioxamine is not a free radical scavenger but is an iron-chelating agent. Since ferrous iron is both a potent source of electrons for conversion of oxygen to the superoxide anion and a catalyst in the Fenton reaction, it may well prove to have a therapeutic role which is likely to extend beyond the haemachromatoses and acute iron poisoning (Gutteridge et al., 1985).

The role of steroids is not yet clarified. Sturrock and Hulands (1980) have shown that maximal doses of methylprednisolone give considerable protection from the chromosome-breaking effect of oxygen described above (Sturrock and Nunn, 1978). Dexamethasone in high dosage has been found to have therapeutic value in the late stage of pulmonary oxygen toxicity in rats but to decrease survival when used in the early stages of exposure (Koizumi, Frank and Massaro, 1985). It will be difficult if not impossible to confirm the value of steroids in the treatment of pulmonary oxygen toxicity in man.

There are difficulties in the therapeutic use of SOD and CAT because they are intracellular enzymes with very short half-lives in plasma. There is therefore little scope for their use by direct intravenous injection. In certain circumstances, induction may be feasible as a prophylactic measure and this must often have occurred during the early stages of treatment of ARDS, when the inspired oxygen concentration has been gradually increased to counter progressive failure of gas exchange. It is possible for these enzymes to enter cells if they are administered in liposomes and their plasma half-life may also be extended by conjugation with polyethylene glycol. Experimental use of SOD and CAT in these forms has been described by Turrens, Crapo and Freeman (1984), Padmanabhan et al. (1985) and McDonald et al. (1985).

Factors protecting from oxygen-derived free radical attack include:

Superoxide dismutase
Catalase
Glutatione/glutathione peroxidase system
Other peroxidases
Induction of above enzymes
Inhibition of xanthine oxidase
Iron chelation
Antioxidants:
   vitamin C (ascorbate)
   vitamin E (α-tocopherol
   dimethylsulphoxide
   dimethylthiourea
   n-acetylcysteine
Steroids (possibly)

Clinical oxygen toxicity

The most important clinical conditions in which oxygen has been identified as the sole precipitating cause are oxygen convulsions, pulmonary oxygen toxicity and retrolental fibroplasia. In addition, it is believed that the therapeutic use of high oxygen concentrations may contribute to lung damage in certain conditions for which it is required because of the defect in gas exchange.

Oxygen convulsions (the Paul Bert effect)

It is well established that exposure to oxygen at a partial pressure in excess of 2 atmospheres absolute (2 ATA) may result in convulsions, which are usually lethal to divers and so limit the depth to which closed circuit oxygen apparatus can be used. It is interesting that the threshold for oxygen convulsions is close to that at which brain tissue P_{O_2} is likely to be sharply increased (see *Table 29.1*). The relationship to cerebral tissue P_{O_2} is supported by the observation that an elevation of P_{CO_2} lowers the threshold for convulsions (Lambertsen, 1965). High P_{CO_2} increases cerebral blood flow and therefore raises the tissue P_{O_2} relative to the arterial P_{O_2}. Hyperventilation and anaesthesia each provide limited protection.

The mechanism of causation of oxygen convulsions is not yet clear. It is, however, established that brain gamma-aminobutyric acid (GABA) levels decrease prior to convulsion and the change correlates with the severity of the convulsion (Wood and Watson, 1963). Furthermore, the threshold for change in GABA levels is similar to the threshold for convulsions (Wood, Watson and Murray, 1969). Association of two phenomena does not necessarily prove that the relationship is causal but GABA is an inhibitory neurotransmitter and it is not unreasonable to suggest that a reduced level might result in convulsions. The change in GABA levels may be due to inactivation of sulphydryl-containing enzymes which are one of the targets for free radical attack. Both convulsions and depression of GABA levels occur when the brain tissue P_{O_2} level is sufficiently high for the increased production of free radicals to overwhelm the natural defences.

Pulmonary oxygen toxicity

Pulmonary tissue P_{O_2} is the highest in the body and the lung is therefore the organ most vulnerable to oxygen toxicity. However, there are formidable obstacles to clinical investigation. There are obvious difficulties in the way of direct experimentation in man, and interpretation of animal studies is complicated by species differences. Study of oxygen toxicity in the clinical environment is complicated by the presence of the pulmonary pathology which necessitated the use of oxygen.

Cellular changes. Weibel reviewed the classic studies of his group in 1971. Electron microscopy has shown that, in rats exposed to 1 atmosphere of oxygen, the primary change is in the capillary endothelium, which becomes vacuolated and thin. Permeability is increased and fluid accumulates in the interstitial space. At a later stage, in monkeys, the epithelial lining is lost over large areas of the alveoli. This process affects the type I cell (page 17) and is accompanied by proliferation of the type II cell which is relatively resistant to oxygen. Massaro and Massaro (1978) suggested that this was an essential defence mechanism to re-establish the integrity of the blood/gas interface. Weibel postulated that the cytological differentiation of the type I cell decreases its resistance to oxygen-induced damage. Over all, the alveolar/capillary membrane is greatly thickened, partly because of the substitution of type II cells for type I and partly because of interstitial accumulation of fluid.

Limits of survival. Pulmonary effects of oxygen vary greatly between different species, probably because of different levels of provision of defences against free radicals as outlined above. Most strains of rats will not survive for much more than 3 days in 1 atmosphere of oxygen. Monkeys generally survive oxygen breathing for about 2 weeks, and man is probably even more resistant. Pulmonary oxygen tolerance curves for normal man have been prepared by Clark and Lambertsen (1971), but these are based on reduction in vital capacity which is a very early stage of oxygen toxicity. There is an approximately inverse relationship between P_{O_2} and duration of tolerable exposure. Thus 20 hours of 1 atmosphere had a similar effect to 10 hours of 2 atmospheres or 5 hours of 4 atmospheres. There is also general agreement that man can withstand 10 hours' exposure to 1 atmosphere of oxygen, with nothing more than substernal distress and a measurable reduction in vital capacity.

American astronauts breathed 100% oxygen at a pressure of one-third of an atmosphere until the Apollo fire of 1967 (see below). There is abundant evidence that prolonged exposure to this environment does not result in demonstrable pulmonary oxygen toxicity, thus establishing a P_{O_2} of 34 kPa (255 mmHg) as a safe level. It also shows that the significant factor is partial pressure and not concentration. In contrast, the concentration of oxygen rather than its partial pressure is the important factor in absorption collapse of the lung (page 442).

Oxygen toxicity in the presence of pre-existing pulmonary pathology. Some limited information on human pulmonary oxygen toxicity has been obtained in the course of therapeutic administration of oxygen.

Nash, Blennerhassett and Pontoppidan (1967) reviewed 70 patients who died after prolonged artificial ventilation. Pulmonary abnormalities (particularly fibrin membranes, oedema and fibrosis) were greater in those patients who had received more than 90% oxygen. However, the higher concentrations of oxygen would probably have been used in those patients with the more severe defects in gas exchange and it is, therefore, difficult to distinguish between the effects of oxygen itself and the conditions which required its use. The same problem was tackled by Gilbe, Salt and Branthwaite (1980) who, in an extensive review of patients ventilated for long periods with high concentrations of oxygen, concluded that adverse effects of oxygen on the alveolar epithelium were rarely of practical importance in hypoxaemic patients.

An elegant attempt to avoid the complicating factor of pre-existing pulmonary disease was made by Singer and his colleagues (1970), who ventilated a group of patients with 100% oxygen for 24 hours after cardiac surgery. Two further patients received oxygen for 5 and 7 days respectively. Various indices of pulmonary function (V_D/V_T ratio, shunt and compliance) were not significantly different from a control group receiving less than 42% oxygen.

Barber, Lee and Hamilton (1970) studied patients with irreversible head injuries and compared a group receiving 100% oxygen for 31–72 hours with a control group ventilated with air. There were no differences in lung histology between the two groups.

Pulmonary absorption collapse. Whatever the uncertainties about the susceptibility of man to pulmonary oxygen toxicity, there is no doubt that high concentrations of oxygen in zones of the lung with low ventilation/perfusion ratios will result in collapse (page 444). This may be demonstrated in the healthy but middle-aged volunteer. A few minutes of breathing oxygen at residual lung volume results in radiological evidence of collapse, a reduced arterial P_{O_2} and substernal pain on attempting a maximal inspiration (Nunn et al., 1965b, 1978).

Ventilatory depression. Perhaps the greatest danger of oxygen therapy is the production of ventilatory depression in patients who have lost their sensitivity to carbon dioxide and rely upon the hypoxic drive to breathing (page 382). This is particularly dangerous in the patient with chronic bronchitis (the 'blue bloater'). *Figure 20.3* shows the alarmingly rapid onset of respiratory depression when a patient with chronic hypercapnia resulting from long-standing poliomyelitis breathed oxygen.

Balancing the risks. Prevention of dangerous hypoxia is always the first priority and must be treated in spite of the various hazards associated with the use of oxygen. This point was firmly stressed by Gilbe, Salt and Branthwaite (1980). A reasonably safe arterial P_{O_2} is 10 kPa (75 mmHg) but, if this cannot be maintained without resorting to dangerous levels of inspired oxygen concentrations (in excess of 60%), it may be necessary to settle for a lower arterial Po_2 and 6.7 kPa (50 mmHg) has been suggested by Hutchison, Flenley and Donald (1964). In fact, the safe lower level of arterial Po_2 for an individual patient depends on many factors (page 474) and no general rule can be formulated. Levels of the order of 3 kPa (23 mmHg) have been tolerated by Himalayan mountaineers.

Administration of high inspired concentrations of oxygen can usually be avoided by attention to various aspects of patient care, including bronchodilatation, clearance of secretions, artificial ventilation and positive end-expiratory airway pressure. Inspired oxygen concentrations should never be higher than necessary and a process of titration is necessary. It is particularly important that staff be aware of the danger of precipitating ventilatory depression or apnoea by the use of oxygen. It should be noted that even very severe respiratory depression while breathing 100% oxygen will probably not result in immediate hypoxia because of apnoeic mass-movement oxygenation (page 228). However, Pco_2 will rapidly increase (page 230).

Other hazards of oxygen

Retrolental fibroplasia (RLF)

Shortly after RLF was first described in 1942, it became established that hyperoxia was the major aetiological factor. This led to the use of oxygen being strictly curtailed in the management of neonates. This resulted in an increase in morbidity and mortality attributable to hypoxia and thereafter oxygen was carefully monitored and titrated in the hope of steering the narrow course between the Scylla and Charybdis of hypoxia and RLF (see review by Lucey and Dangman, 1984). This policy has not eradicated the condition and there is now overwhelming evidence that RLF may occur in infants who have never received additional oxygen. Vitamin E has been used in the attempt to prevent RLF but it is currently believed that hyperoxia is but one of a variety of factors which may cause RLF by changes in the retinal oxygen supply. There is a well established inverse relationship between birth weight and the incidence of RLF, but Flynn (1984) presents the case against major surgery (with administration of anaesthetic gases and oxygen) being a significant risk factor.

The fire hazard

Fire risk is enormously increased by the use of high concentrations of oxygen, even at reduced barometric pressure. The problem had been reviewed by Denison, Ernsting and Cresswell (1966) but was tragically highlighted by the death of the three American astronauts breathing 100% oxygen at one-third of an atmosphere, in 1967, to which reference was made above. Cabin atmospheres for the American space programme are now 64% oxygen and 36% nitrogen at a total pressure of 34.5 kPa (259 mmHg). This substantially reduces the fire hazard.

Techniques for orthobaric and hyperbaric oxygen therapy are considered on pages 273 et seq.

Appendix A

Physical quantities and units of measurement

SI units

As with the previous edition, we are still in a state of transition from old to new metric units. The old system was based on the centimetre–gram–second (CGS) and was supplemented with many non-coherent derived units such as the millimetre of mercury for pressure and the calorie for work which could not be related to the basic units by factors which were powers of ten. The new system, the Système Internationale or SI, is based on the metre–kilogram–second (MKS) and comprises base and derived units which are obtained simply by multiplication or division without the introduction of numbers, not even powers of ten.

Base units are metre (length), kilogram (mass), second (time), ampere (electric current), kelvin (thermodynamic temperature), ·mole (amount of substance) and candela (luminous intensity).

Derived units include newton (force: kilograms metre second^{-2}), pascal (pressure: newton metre^{-2}), joule (work: newton metre) and hertz (periodic frequency: second^{-1}).

Special non-SI units are recognized as having sufficient practical importance to warrant retention for general or specialized use. These include litre, day, hour, minute and the standard atmosphere.

Non-recommended units include the dyne, bar and calorie and gravity-dependent units such as the kilogram-force, centimetre of water and millimetre of mercury, which are expected to disappear within a few years.

The introduction of SI units into anaesthesia and respiratory physiology was reviewed by Padmore and Nunn (1974). While it is still too early to define the full extent of the change of units, it is clear that the kilopascal will replace the millimetre of mercury for blood gas tensions. The change is complete in many countries and has now started in the USA, where mmHg had been replaced by the almost identical torr. The introduction of the kilopascal for fluid pressures in the medical field is being delayed for, what appears to the author, an entirely specious attachment to the mercury or water manometer. The scale on a sphygmo-manometer or central venous pressure manometer can easily be engraved to read kilopascals and we appear to be condemned to a further period during which we record arterial pressure in mmHg, venous pressure in cmH$_2$O, cerebrospinal fluid pressure in mmH$_2$O and, in the author's intensive therapy unit, a suction pump calibrated in cmHg. The existing situation would be less dangerous if all staff knew the relationship between a millimetre of mercury and a centimetre of water.

The replacement of the calorie by the joule should end the confusion between the calorie and the Calorie (kilocalorie). It is not yet clear whether the 'amount of substance' (mol) will replace the gas volume in expressions of, for example, oxygen consumption. This transition would be fairly inconvenient. It is likely that the litre will replace the '100 ml' as the reference quantity of a liquid.

In this book, both SI and old units are given in situations in which the change is likely to be made in the life of this edition. It is hoped that text and figures can be read with equal facility by those accustomed to each system. Conversion factors are listed in *Table A.1*). For the physical quantities listed below, the dimensions are

Table A.1 Conversion factors for units of measurement

Force	
1 N (newton)	= 10^5 dyn
Pressure	
1 kPa (kilopascal)	= 7.50 mmHg
	= 10.2 cmH$_2$O
	= 0.009 87 standard atmospheres
	= 10 000 dyn/cm^2 (microbars)
1 standard atmosphere	= 101.3 kPa
	= 760 mmHg
	= 1033 cmH$_2$O
	= 10 m of sea water (specific gravity 1.033)
1 mm Hg(almost equal to the torr)	= 1.36 cmH$_2$O
Compliance	
1 l kPa^{-1}	= 0.098 l/cmH$_2$O
Flow resistance	
1 kPa l^{-1} s	= 10.2 cmH$_2$O/l/sec
Work	
1 J (joule)	= 0.102 kilopond metres
	= 0.239 calories
Power	
1 W (watt)	= 1 J s^{-1}
	= 6.12 kp m min^{-1}
Surface tension	
1 N m^{-1} (newton/metre or pascal metre)	= 1000 dyn/cm
Note: 1mN m^{-1}	= 1 dyn/cm
Amount of substance	
1 mmol of oxygen	= 22.39 ml (STPD)
1 mmol of carbon dioxide	= 22.26 ml (STPD)

In the figures and text of this book 1 kPa has been taken to equal 7.5 mmHg or 10 cmH$_2$O

given in mass/length/time (MLT) units. These units provide a most useful check of the validity of equations and other expressions which are derived in the course of studies of respiratory function. Only quantities with identical MLT units can be added or subtracted and the units must be the same on the two sides of an equation.

Volume (dimensions: L^3)

In this book we are concerned with volumes of blood and gas. Strict SI units would be cubic metres and submultiples. However, the litre (1) and millilitre (ml) are recognized as special non-SI units and will remain in use. For practical purposes, we may ignore changes in the volume of liquids which are caused by changes of temperature. However, the changes in volume of gases caused by changes of temperature or pressure are by no means negligible and constitute an important source of error if they are ignored. Gas volumes are usually measured at ambient (or environmental) temperature and pressure, either dry (as from a cylinder passing through a rotameter) or saturated with water vapour at ambient temperature (e.g. an expired gas sample). Customary abbreviations are ATPD (ambient temperature and pressure, dry) and ATPS (ambient temperature and pressure, saturated).

It is not good practice to report gas volumes under the conditions prevailing during their measurement. In the case of oxygen uptake, carbon dioxide output and the exchange of 'inert' gases, we need to know the actual quantity (i.e. number of molecules) of gas exchanged and this is most conveniently expressed by stating the gas volume as it would be under standard conditions; i.e. 0°C, 101.3 kPa (760 mmHg) pressure and dry (STPD). Conversion from ATPS to STPD is by application of Charles' and Boyle's laws (see Appendix B). A table of conversion factors is given in Appendix C. In the case of volumes which relate to anatomical measurements (e.g. vital capacity, tidal volume and dead space) it is necessary to express gas volumes as they would be at body temperature and pressure, saturated with water vapour (BTPS). Conversion from ATPS to BTPS is also based on Charles' and Boyle's laws, and factors are listed in Appendix C.

Amount of substance (dimensionless)

In clinical chemistry there is a progressive move towards reporting concentrations in terms of 'amount of substance' concentration (mmol l^{-1}) in place of mass concentration (mg/100 ml). In the respiratory field this may be extended to gases and vapours. For an ideal gas, 1 mmol corresponds to 22.4 ml, and this figure applies to oxygen and nitrogen. For non-ideal gases such as nitrous oxide and carbon dioxide the figure is reduced to 22.25.

Gas concentrations may be expressed as mmol/l, and for a mixture of ideal gases the sum of the concentrations of the components would be 44.6 mmol/l at standard temperature and pressure (dry). The advantages and disadvantages of expressing gas concentrations in terms of millimoles were reviewed by Piiper et al. (1971). If haemoglobin is expressed as millimoles of the monomer, then 1 mmol of haemoglobin combines with 1 mmol of oxygen.

Fluid flow rate (dimensions: L^3/T, or L^3T^{-1})

In the case of liquids, flow rate is the physical quantity of cardiac output, regional blood flow, etc. The strict SI units would be metre^3 second^{-1}, but litres per minute (l/min) and millilitres per minute (ml/min) are special non-SI units which may be retained. For gases, the dimension is applied to the delivery rate of fresh gases in anaesthetic gas circuits, minute volume of respiration, oxygen consumption, etc. The units are the same as those for liquids except that litres per second are used for the high instantaneous flow rates which occur during the course of inspiration and expiration.

In the case of gas flow rates, just as much attention should be paid to the matter of temperature and pressure as when volumes are being measured. Measurement is usually made at ambient temperature, but gas exchange rates are reported after correction to STPD, while ventilatory gas flow rates should be corrected to BTPS. As a very rough rule, gas volumes at STPD are about 10 per cent less than at ATPS, while volumes at BTPS are about 10 per cent more.

Force (dimensions: MLT^{-2}) (LT^{-2} or L/T^2 are the units of acceleration)

In respiratory physiology we are chiefly concerned with force in relation to pressure, which is force per unit area. An understanding of the units of force is essential to an understanding of the units of pressure. Force, when applied to a free body, causes it to change either the magnitude or the direction of its velocity.

The units of force are of two types. The first is the force resulting from the action of gravity on a mass and is synonymous with weight. It includes the kilogram-force and the pound-force (as in the pound per square inch). All such units are non-recommended under the SI and will disappear. The second type of unit of force is absolute and does not depend on the magnitude of the gravitational field. In the CGS system, the absolute unit of force was the dyne and this has been replaced under the MKS system and the SI by the newton (N) which is defined as the force which will give a mass of 1 kilogram an acceleration 1 metre per second per second.

$$1 \text{ N} = 1 \text{ kg m s}^{-2}$$

Pressure (dimensions: MLT^{-2}/L^2, or $ML^{-1}T^{-2}$)

Pressure is defined as force per unit area. The SI unit is the pascal (Pa) which is 1 newton per square metre.

$$1 \text{ Pa} = 1 \text{ N m}^{-2}$$

The pascal is inconveniently small (one hundred-thousandth of an atmosphere) and the kilopascal (kPa) has been adopted for general use in the medical field. Its introduction is simplified by the fact that the kPa is very close to 1 per cent of an atmosphere. Thus a standard atmosphere is 101.3 kPa and the Po_2 of dry air is very close to 21 kPa: 1 kPa is also approximately equal to 10 cmH$_2$O. The kilopascal will replace the millimetre of mercury and the centimetre of water, both of which are gravity based. The centimetre of water can be considered as the pressure at the bottom of a centimetre cube of water which would be one gram-force acting on a square centimetre.

The standard atmosphere may continue to be used under SI. It is defined as $1.013\,25 \times 10^5$ pascals.

The torr came into use only shortly before the move towards SI units. This is unfortunate for the memory of Torricelli, as the torr will disappear from use. The torr is defined as exactly equal to 1/760 of a standard atmosphere and it is therefore very close to the millimetre of mercury, the two units being considered identical for practical purposes. The only distinction is that the torr is absolute, while the millimetre of mercury is gravity based.

The bar is the absolute unit of pressure in the old CGS system and is defined as 10^6 dyn/cm^2. The unit was convenient because the bar is close to 1 atmosphere (1.013 bars) and a millibar is close to 1 centimetre of water (0.9806 millibars).

Compliance (dimensions: $M^{-1}L^4T^2$)

The term 'compliance' is used in respiratory physiology to denote the volume change of the lungs in response to a change of pressure. The dimensions are therefore volume divided by pressure, and the commonest units have been litres (or millilitres) per centimetre of water. It is likely that this will change to litres per kilopascal (l/kPa). Elastance is the reciprocal of compliance.

Resistance to fluid flow (dimensions: $ML^{-4}T^{-1}$)

Under conditions of laminar flow (see *Figure 3.2*) it is possible to express resistance to gas flow as the ratio of pressure difference to gas flow rate. This is analogous to electrical resistance which is expressed as the ratio of potential difference to current flow. The dimensions of resistance to gas flow are pressure difference divided by gas flow rate, and typical units in the respiratory field have been cmH$_2$O/litre/ second or dynes sec cm^{-5} in absolute units. Appropriate SI units will probably be kilopascals litre^{-1} second (kPa l^{-1} s).

Work (dimensions: ML^2T^{-2}, derived from $MLT^{-2} \times L$ or $ML^{-1}T^{-2} \times L^3$)

Work is done when a force moves its point of application or gas is moved in response to a pressure gradient. the dimensions are therefore either force times distance or pressure times volume, in each case simplifying to ML^2T^{-2}. The multiplicity of units of work has caused confusion in the past. Under SI, the erg, calorie and kilopond-metre will disappear in favour of the joule, which is defined as the work done when a force of 1 newton moves its point of application 1 metre. It is also the work done when a litre of gas moves in response to a pressure gradient of 1 kilopascal. This represents a welcome simplification.

$$1\ J = 1\ N\ m = 1\ l\ kPa$$

The kilojoule will replace the kilocalorie in metabolism.

Power (dimensions: ML^2T^{-2}/T or ML^2T^{-3})

Power is the rate at which work is done and so has the dimensions of work divided by time. The SI unit is the watt, which equals 1 joule per second. Power is the correct dimension for the rate of continuous expenditure of biological energy, although one talks loosely about the 'work of breathing', for example (page 104). This is incorrect and 'power of breathing' is the correct term.

Surface tension (dimensions: MLT^{-2}/L or MT^{-2})

Surface tension has become important to the respiratory physiologist since the realization of the part it plays in the 'elastic' recoil of the lungs (page 24). The CGS units of surface tension are dynes per centimetre (of interface). The appropriate SI unit would be the newton per metre. This has the following rather curious relationships:

$$1 \text{ N/m} = 1 \text{ Pa m} = 1 \text{ kg/s}^2$$

The unit for surface tension is likely to be called the pascal metre (Pa m) which is identical to the newton per metre. A millinewton per metre (or a millipascal metre) is identical in value to the familiar CGS unit, the dyn/cm.

General notes

The symbol for second is now changed from sec to s. In the case of temperature, the symbol °C now represents degrees Celsius and not degrees Centigrade. The values are identical.

Division may be indicated by a solidus (/) provided that only one is used. For example, m/s and m s^{-1} are equally correct for metres per second. In expressions with more than two terms, confusion may be avoided by the exclusive use of negative indices (see Padmore and Nunn, 1974).

Appendix B

The gas laws

A knowledge of physics is more important to the understanding of the respiratory system than of any other system of the body. Not only gas transfer but also ventilation and perfusion of the lungs occur largely in response to physical forces, with vital processes playing a less conspicuous role than is the case, for example, in brain, heart or kidney. Much of this book is concerned with physics, and it may be helpful to review those aspects which are most relevant to the behaviour of gases in the respiratory system.

Physical quantities and units of measurement are perennial sources of confusion in respiratory physiology. Apart from any inherent difficulty, we suffer from an unnecessary duplication of units, particularly those of pressure. Appendices A and C are intended to resolve some of these difficulties but they need not be read by those readers who have already obtained a grasp of the subject.

Certain physical attributes of gases are customarily presented under the general heading of the gas laws. These are of fundamental importance in respiratory physiology.

Boyle's law describes the inverse relationship between the volume and absolute pressure of a perfect gas at constant temperature:

$$PV = K \qquad \qquad ...(1)$$

where P represents pressure and V represents volume. At temperatures near their boiling point, gases deviate from Boyle's law. At room temperature, the deviation is negligible for oxygen and nitrogen and is of little practical importance for carbon dioxide or nitrous oxide. Anaesthetic vapours show substantial deviations.

Charles' law describes the direct relationship between the volume and absolute temperature of a perfect gas at constant pressure:

$$V = KT \qquad \qquad ...(2)$$

where T represents the absolute temperature. There are appreciable deviations at temperatures immediately above the boiling point of gases. Equations (1) and (2) may be combined as follows:

$$PV = RT \qquad \qquad ...(3)$$

where R is the universal gas constant, which is the same for all perfect gases and has the value of 8.1314 joules/degree kelvin/mole. From this it may be derived that the mole volume of all perfect gases is 22.4 litres at STPD. Carbon dioxide and nitrous oxide deviate from the behaviour of perfect gases to the extent of having mole volumes of 22.2 litres at STPD.

Van der Waals' equation is an attempt to improve the accuracy of equation (3) in the case of non-perfect gases. It makes allowance for the finite space occupied by gas molecules and the forces which exist between them. The Van der Waals equation includes two additional constants:

$$(P + a/V^2)\,(V - b) = RT \qquad \qquad ...(4)$$

where a corrects for the attraction between molecules and b corrects for the volume occupied by molecules. This expression is of particular interest to anaesthetists since the constants for anaesthetic gases are related to their anaesthetic potency (Wulf and Featherstone, 1957).

An alternative method of correction for non-ideality is to express equation (3) in the following form:

$$PV/RT = Z \qquad \qquad ...(5)$$

For a perfect gas, Z equals unity. For a particular gas at a particular temperature and pressure, the non-ideality may be expressed as the special value for Z (usually less than unity) which may be obtained from tables.

Since Z has a special value for each gas at each temperature and pressure, useful tables of Z values are necessarily very cumbersome. It is therefore much more convenient to replace Z with a power series as follows:

$$PV/RT = 1 + B/V + C/V^2 + ... \qquad \qquad ...(6)$$

The constants B, C, etc., are known as virial coefficients and vary only with temperature for a particular gas. Compilations are therefore simplified and the serious student is referred to Dymond and Smith (1969) or to Kaye and Laby (1966) which is more generally available but less complete. Values for B may be positive or negative and it is seldom necessary to use more than the one coefficient.

Adiabatic heating. A great deal of respiratory physiology can fortunately be understood without much knowledge of thermodynamics. However, a recurrent problem is the heating which occurs when a gas is compressed. This effect is sufficiently large to be a readily detectable source of error in such techniques as the body plethysmograph (page 45), and the use of a large rigid container as a simulator for the paralysed thorax.

Henry's law describes the solution of gases in liquids with which they do not react. It does not apply to vapours which, in the liquid state, are infinitely miscible with the solvent (e.g. ether in olive oil) (Nunn, 1960b). The general principle of Henry's law is simple enough. The number of molecules of gas dissolving in the solvent is directly proportional to the partial pressure of the gas at the surface of the liquid, and the constant of proportionality is an expression of the solubility of the gas in the liquid. This is a constant for a particular gas and a particular liquid at a particular temperature but usually falls with rising temperature.

For many people, confusion arises from the multiplicity of units which are used. For example, when considering oxygen dissolved in blood, it has been customary to consider the amount of gas dissolved in units of vols per cent (ml of gas (STPD) per 100 ml blood) and the pressure in mmHg. Solubility is then expressed as vols per cent/mmHg, the value for oxygen in blood at 37°C being 0.003. However, for carbon dioxide in blood, we tend to use units of mmol/l of carbon dioxide per mmHg. The units are then mmol l^{-1} mmHg^{-1}, the value for carbon dioxide in blood at 37°C being 0.03. Both vols per cent and mmol/l are valid measurements of the quantity (mass or number of molecules) of the gas in solution and are interchangeable with the appropriate conversion factor.

Physicists are more inclined to express solubility in terms of the *Bunsen coefficient*. For this, the amount of gas in solution is expressed in terms of volume of gas (STPD) per unit volume of solvent (i.e. one-hundredth of the amount expressed as vols per cent) and the pressure is expressed in atmospheres.

Biologists, on the other hand, prefer to use a related term—the *Ostwald coefficient*. This is the volume of gas dissolved, expressed as its volume under the conditions of temperature and pressure at which solution took place. It might be thought that this would vary with the pressure in the gas phase, but this is not so. If the pressure is doubled, according to Henry's law, twice as many molecules of gas dissolve. However, according to Boyle's law, they would occupy half the volume at double the pressure. Therefore, if Henry's and Boyle's laws are obeyed, the Ostwald coefficient will be independent of changes in pressure at which solution occurs. It will differ from the Bunsen coefficient only because the gas volume is expressed as the volume it would occupy at the temperature of the experiment rather than at 0°C. Conversion is thus in accord with Charles' law and the two coefficients will be identical at 0°C. This should not be confused with the fact that, like the Bunsen coefficient, the Ostwald coefficient falls with rising temperature.

The partition coefficient is the ratio of the number of molecules of gas in one phase to the number of molecules of gas in another phase when equilibrium between the two has been attained. If one phase is gas and another a liquid, the liquid/gas partition coefficient will be identical to the Ostwald coefficient. Partition coefficients are also used to describe partitioning between two media (e.g. oil/water, brain/blood, etc.). At the time of writing, it is still too early to say when SI units will come into general use for expression of solubility (see Appendix A). The coherent unit is millimole litre^{-1} kilopascal^{-1}.

Graham's law of diffusion governs the influence of molecular weight on the diffusion of a gas through a gas mixture. Diffusion rates through orifices or through porous plates are inversely proportional to the square root of the molecular weight. This factor is only of importance in the gaseous part of the pathway between ambient air and the tissues, and is of limited importance in the whole process of 'diffusion' as understood by the respiratory physiologist.

Dalton's law of partial pressure states that, in a mixture of gases, each gas exerts the pressure which it would exert if it occupied the volume alone. This pressure is known as the partial pressure (or tension) and the sum of the partial pressures equals the total pressure of the mixture. Thus, in a mixture of 5% carbon dioxide in oxygen at a total pressure of 101 kPa (760 mmHg), the carbon dioxide exerts a partial pressure of $5/100 \times 101 = 5.05$ kPa (38 mmHg). In general terms:

$$P_{CO_2} = F_{CO_2} \times P_B$$

(Note that fractional concentration is expressed as a fraction and not as a percentage: per cent concentration $= F \times 100$.)

In the alveolar gas at sea level, there is about 6.2% water vapour, which exerts a partial pressure of 6.3 kPa (47 mmHg). The available pressure for other gases is therefore $(P_B - 6.3)$ kPa or $(P_B - 47)$ mmHg.

Tension is synonymous with partial pressure and is applied particularly to gases dissolved in a liquid such as blood. Molecules of gases dissolved in liquids have a tendency to escape, but net loss may be prevented by exposing the liquid to a gas mixture in which the tension of the gas exactly balances the escape tendency. The two phases are then said to be in equilibrium and the tension of the gas in the liquid is considered equal to that of the tension of the gas in the gas mixture with which it is in equilibrium. Thus a blood P_{CO_2} of 5.3 kPa (40 mmHg) means that there would be no net exchange of carbon dioxide if the blood were exposed to a gas mixture which had a P_{CO_2} of 5.3 kPa (40 mmHg).

Appendix C

Conversion factors for gas volumes

Conversion factors for gas volumes—ATPS to BTPS

Gas volumes measured by spirometry and other methods usually indicate the volume at ambient temperature and pressure, saturated (ATPS). Tidal volume, minute volume, dead space, lung volumes, etc., should be converted to the volumes as they would be in the lungs of the patient at body temperature and pressure, saturated (BTPS).

Table C.1 Factors for conversion of gas volumes measured under conditions of ambient temperature and pressure, saturated (ATPS) to the volumes which would be occupied under conditions of body temperature and pressure, saturated (BTPS)

Ambient temperature (°C)	Conversion factor	Saturated water vapour pressure	
		kPa	mmHg
15	1.129	1.71	12.8
16	1.124	1.81	13.6
17	1.119	1.93	14.5
18	1.113	2.07	15.5
19	1.108	2.20	16.5
20	1.103	2.33	17.5
21	1.097	2.48	18.6
22	1.092	2.64	19.8
23	1.086	2.80	21.0
24	1.081	2.99	22.4
25	1.075	3.16	23.7
26	1.069	3.66	25.2

Derivation of correction factors:

$$\text{volume}_{(\text{BTPS})} = \text{volume}_{(\text{ATPS})} \left(\frac{273 + 37}{273 + t} \right) \left(\frac{P_B - P_{H_2O}}{P_B - 6.3} \right)$$

P_B is barometric pressure and the Table has been prepared for a barometric pressure of 100 kPa (750 mmHg): variations within the range 99–101 kPa (740–760 mmHg) have a negligible effect upon the factors.

t is ambient temperature (°C). The Table has been prepared for a body temperature of 37°C: variations within the range 35–39°C are of small importance.

P_{H_2O} is the water vapour presure of the sample (kPa).

Conversion factors for gas volumes—ATPS to STPD

Measurement of absolute amounts of gases (e.g. oxygen consumption) requires conversion of measured gas volumes to standard conditions (0°C, 101.3 kPa (760 mmHg), dry). Under these conditions, one mole of an ideal gas occupies 22.4 litres.

Table C.2 Factors for conversion of gas volumes measured under conditions of ambient temperature and pressure, saturated (ATPS) to the volumes which would be occupied under conditions of standard temperature and pressure, dry (STPD)−0°C, 101.3 kPa (760 mmHg)

Ambient temperature (°C)	Barometric pressure, kPa (mmHg)			
	97.3 (730)	98.7 (740)	100 (750)	101.3 (760)
15	0.895	0.907	0.919	0.932
16	0.890	0.903	0.915	0.928
17	0.886	0.899	0.911	0.923
18	0.882	0.894	0.907	0.919
19	0.878	0.890	0.902	0.915
20	0.873	0.886	0.898	0.910
21	0.869	0.881	0.893	0.906
22	0.865	0.877	0.889	0.901
23	0.860	0.872	0.885	0.897
24	0.856	0.868	0.880	0.892
25	0.851	0.863	0.875	0.887
26	0.847	0.859	0.871	0.883

Derivation of correction factors:

$$\text{volume}_{(STPD)} = \text{volume}_{(ATPS)} \left(\frac{273}{273 + t} \right) \left(\frac{P_B - P_{H_2O}}{101} \right)$$

P   is barometric pressure (kPa).

t is ambient temperature.

P_{H_2O} is the saturated vapour pressure of water at ambient temperature (see *Table C.1.*

Appendix D

Symbols, abbreviations and definitions

Symbols

Symbols used in this book are in accord with the recommendations of the committee for standardization of definitions and symbols in respiratory physiology (Pappenheimer et al., 1950). The use of these symbols is very helpful for an understanding of the quantitative relationships which are so important in respiratory physiology.

Primary symbols (large capitals) denoting physical quantities.

        F fractional concentration of gas
        P pressure, tension or partial pressure of a gas
        V volume of a gas
        Q volume of blood
        C content of a gas in blood
        S saturation of haemoglobin with oxygen
        R respiratory exchange ratio (RQ)
        D diffusing capacity

   · denotes a time derivative; e.g. $\dot{V}$ ventilation
                      $\dot{Q}$ blood flow

Secondary symbols denoting location of quantity.

in gas phase (small capitals)	*in blood* (lower case)
I inspired gas	a arterial blood
E expired gas	v venous blood
A alveolar gas	c capillary
D dead space	t total
T tidal	s shunt
B barometric (usually pressure)	

  ⁻ denotes mixed or mean; e.g. $\bar{v}$ mixed venous blood
                             $\bar{E}$ mixed expired gas
   ′ denotes end; e.g. E′ end-expiratory gas
                     c′ end-capillary blood

Tertiary symbols indicating particular gases.

> O_2 oxygen
> CO_2 carbon dioxide
> N_2O nitrous oxide
> etc.

f denotes the respiratory frequency

BTPS, ATPS and STPD: see *Appendix C*

Examples of respiratory symbols

> $P_{A_{O_2}}$ alveolar oxygen tension
> $C\bar{v}_{O_2}$ oxygen content of mixed venous blood
> $\dot{V}_{O_2}$ oxygen consumption

The system is well adapted to the expression of quantitative relationships.

$$\dot{Q}\,(Ca_{O_2} - C\bar{v}_{O_2}) = \dot{V}_{O_2} \qquad \text{(Fick equation)}$$

$$V_D = V_E \left(\frac{Pa_{CO_2} - P\bar{E}_{CO_2}}{Pa_{CO_2}} \right) \text{(Bohr equation)}$$

$$R = \frac{\dot{V}_{CO_2}}{\dot{V}_{O_2}}$$

Definitions of words used in a special sense or which have little general use

Ambient: surrounding or environmental (e.g. room air).

Parameter: a quantity which is a constant in a particular relationship, but which varies from one relationship to another; e.g. *a* and *b* in the equation $y = a + bx$ (*x* and *y* are variables).

Variable: any quantity of which the value is likely to change; e.g. haemoglobin concentration might be considered as a variable over a number of days but as a parameter when a series of blood samples are drawn in rapid succession without there being a change of haemoglobin concentration. P_{O_2} would probably be a variable in both situations.

Phase: a continuous fluid medium. The lungs contain a gas phase and a blood phase, separated by the alveolar/capillary membrane.

Appendix E

Nomograms and correction charts

Blood gas correction nomograms for time

This nomogram (*Figure E.1*) is designed for the application of corrections for metabolism occurring between sampling and analysis when blood at 37°C is drawn into a 5 ml glass or 2 ml plastic syringe at room temperature, followed by storage at room temperature. Elapsed time between sampling and analysis is shown on the ordinate. Line charts indicate the change in P_{CO_2} (which rises), pH (which falls) and base excess (which falls). A graph is required for the change in P_{O_2} (which falls) because the rate of fall depends upon the P_{O_2}. For details, see Kelman and Nunn (1966b).

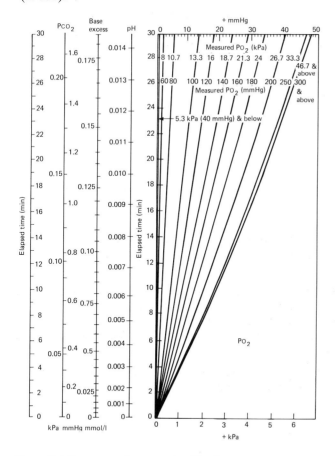

Figure E.1 Nomogram for correcting blood P_{CO_2}, P_{O_2}, pH and base excess for metabolic changes occurring between sampling and analysis. (Reproduced from Kelman and Nunn (1966b) by permission of the Editors of the Journal of Applied Physiology*)*

Blood gas correction nomogram for temperature (*Figure E.2*)

Enter with the patient's temperature on the abscissa. *Multiply* the measured gas tension by the factor shown on the ordinate, using the appropriate curve for P_{O_2} based on the saturation of the sample. The broken line should be used for P_{CO_2}, whatever the level of P_{CO_2}. The line chart at the top of the graph may be used for the pH correction which should be *added*. For details, see Kelman and Nunn (1966b).

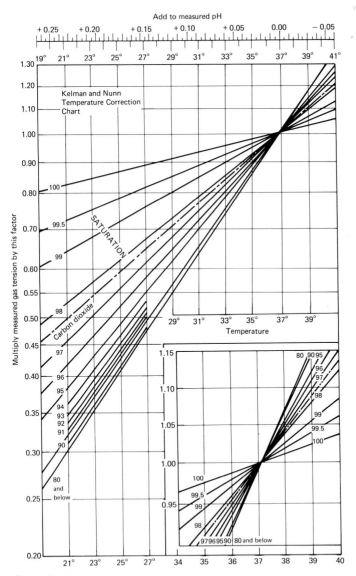

Figure E.2 Nomogram for correction of blood P_{CO_2}, P_{O_2} and pH for differences between temperature of patient and electrode system (assumed to be 37°C). (Reproduced from Kelman and Nunn (1966b) by permission of the Editors of the Journal of Applied Physiology)

Nomogram for haemoglobin dissociation curve

The right-hand line charts of *Figure E.3* give corresponding values for Po_2 and saturation under standard conditions (temperature 37°C; pH, 7.40; base excess, zero). The remaining lines indicate the factors by which the actual measured Po_2 should be multiplied to give the 'virtual Po_2' with which to enter the standard dissociation curve for determination of saturation. When more than one factor is required, they should be multiplied together (page 263).

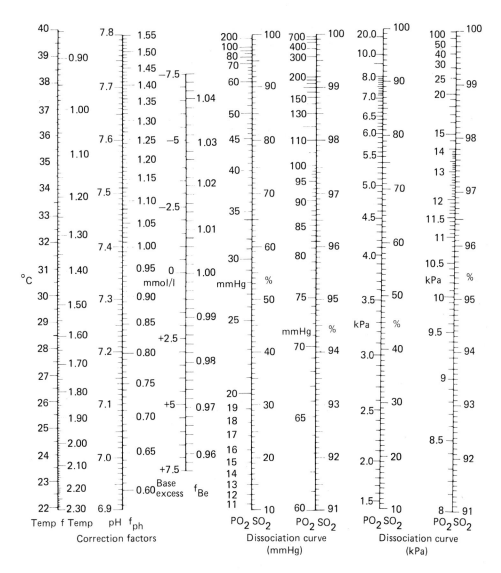

Figure E.3 Line charts representing the oxyhaemoglobin dissociation curve. (Reproduced after Kelman and Nunn (1966b) by permission of the Editors of the Journal of Applied Physiology*)*

The Siggaard-Andersen curve nomogram

The *in vitro* relationship between pH and P_{CO_2} of oxygenated blood is indicated either by a line joining two points obtained after *in vitro* equilibration or by a line passing through the actual arterial values and with a slope indicated by the haemoglobin concentration. The slope is that of a line joining the normal arterial point (indicated by a small circle in the diagram) and the appropriate point on the haemoglobin scale (i.e. 15 g/dl in the example). Intersections of the buffer line indicate three indices of metabolic acid–base state: buffer base, standard bicarbonate and base excess which is currently in vogue. Interpolation of P_{CO_2} indicates corresponding (*in vitro*) pH values and *vice versa*.

The example in *Figure E.4* is normal arterial blood (*in vitro* changes); other equilibration curves are shown in *Figure 9.5*.

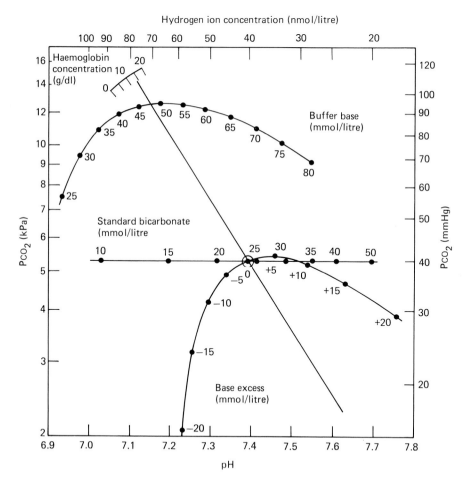

Figure E.4 The Siggaard-Andersen curve nomogram relating pH and P_{CO_2} for oxygenated blood in vitro.
(Adapted from Siggaard-Andersen (1982) with permission of the author and Editors of the Scandinavian Journal of Clinical and Laboratory Investigation*)*

Nomogram for RQ and oxygen consumption

The respiratory exchange ratio of a patient breathing air may be determined from the concentrations of oxygen and carbon dioxide in the expired gas by using the left-hand section of *Figure E.5*. Oxygen consumption may be determined from the mixed expired oxygen concentration and the volume of gas expired in 2 or 3 minutes, by using the right-hand section of *Figure E.5*. The nomogram for calculation of the respiratory exchange ratio has only a very small error. The nomogram for calculating the oxygen consumption has an error of less than 10 ml/min if the respiratory exchange ratio is within the limits 0.7–0.9. For details, see Nunn (1972).

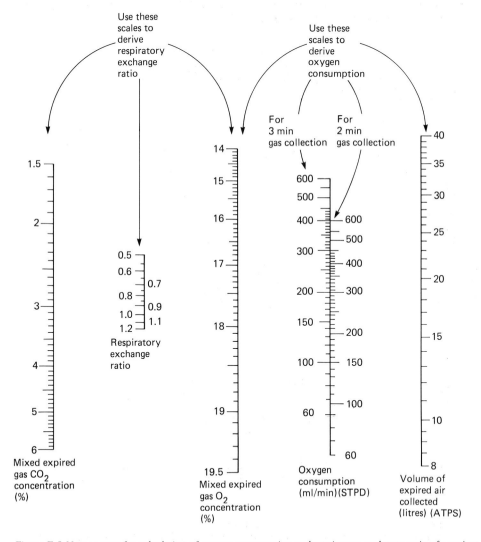

Figure E.5 Nomograms for calculation of oxygen consumption and respiratory exchange ratio of a patient breathing air. (Reproduced from Nunn (1972) by permission of the Editor of the British Medical Journal*)*

The iso-shunt chart

Figure E.6 is a diagram of the theoretical relationship between arterial P_{O_2} and inspired oxygen concentration for different values of virtual shunt. The shaded areas enclose all relationships within the limits of haemoglobin concentration 10–14 g/dl and arterial P_{CO_2} 3.3–5.3 kPa (25–40 mmHg). Virtual shunt is defined as the shunt which gives the relationships depicted when the arterial/mixed venous oxygen content difference is 5 ml/100ml. For further details, *see* page 170 and Benatar, Hewlett and Nunn (1973).

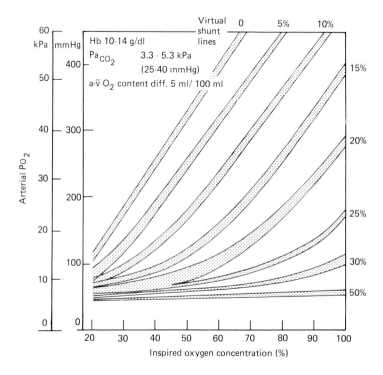

Figure E.6 Iso-shunt lines for control of oxygen therapy. (Reproduced from Benatar, Hewlett and Nunn (1973) by permission of the Editor of the British Journal of Anaesthesia*)*

Air–oxygen mixing chart

The chart shown in *Figure E.7* is used for determining air and oxygen flow rates required to give various total gas flow rates at various oxygen concentrations. (Chart prepared by Dr A.M. Hewlett.)

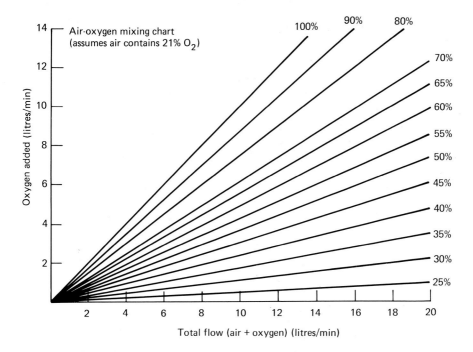

Figure E.7 Air–oxygen mixing chart for oxygen therapy. (Reproduced from Richardson, Chinn and Nunn (1976) by permission of the Editor of the British Journal of Anaesthesia)

Appendix F

The exponential function

The field of applied respiratory physiology contains many examples of exponential functions. Appreciation of some of the mathematical intricacies is helpful to understanding the practical implications of certain aspects of the basic physiology. Apart from the author, there may well be others in the biomedical sphere who did not have the benefit of formal instruction in this aspect of mathematics. Appendix F has therefore been included to provide a simple account of those aspects of exponential functions which are relevant to applied respiratory physiology. Readers who are not versed in advanced mathematics may find the less orthodox books are helpful, particularly *Mathematics for the Million* by Lancelot Hogben (1951) and *Calculus Made Easy* by Silvanus P. Thompson (1965).

General statement

An exponential function describes a change in which the rate of change of one variable, in relation to the other, is proportional to the magnitude of the first variable. Thus, if y varies with respect to x, the rate of change of y with respect to x (i.e. dy/dx)* varies in proportion to the value of y at that instant. That is to say:

$$\frac{dy}{dx} = ky$$

where k is a constant.

This general equation appears with minor modifications in three main forms. To the biological worker they may be conveniently described as the tear-away, the wash-out and the wash-in.

The tear-away exponential function

This must be described first, as it is the simplest form of the exponential function. It is, however, the least important of the three in relation to respiratory function.

---

*dy/dx is the mathematical shorthand for rate of change of y with respect to x. The 'd' means a very small bit of'; dy/dx thus means a very small bit of y divided by a very small bit of x. This is equal to the slope of the graph of y against x at that point. In the case of a curve, it is the slope of a tangent drawn to the curve at that point.

Simple statement

In a tear-away exponential function, the quantity under consideration increases at a rate which is in direct proportion to its actual value—the richer one is, the faster one makes money.

Examples

Classic examples are compound interest, and the mythical water-lily which doubles its diameter every day (*Figure F.1*). A typical biological example is the free spread of a bacterial colony in which (for example) each bacterium divides every 20 minutes. The doubling time of this example would be 20 minutes.

Mathematical statement

By convention we consider y as the quantity which is changing in relation to x. However, in relation to respiratory function, x almost invariably represents time and so we shall take the liberty of replacing x with t throughout. The tear-away function may thus be represented as follows:

$$\frac{dy}{dt} = ky$$

A little mathematical processing will convert this equation into a more useful form, which will indicate the instantaneous value of y at any time, t.
  First multiply both sides by dt/y:

$$\frac{1}{y}\, dy = k\, dt$$

Next integrate both sides with respect to t:

$$\log_e y + C_1 = kt + C_2$$

(C_1 and C_2 are constants of integration and may be collected on the right-hand side.)

$$\log_e y = (C_2 - C_1) + kt$$

Finally, take antilogs of each side to the base e:

$$y = e^{(C_2 - C_1)} \times e^{kt}$$

At zero time, $t = 0$ and $e^{kt} = 1$. Therefore the constant $e^{(C_2 - C_1)}$ equals the initial value of y which we may call y_0. Our final equation is thus:

$$y = y_0\, e^{kt}$$

y_0 is the initial value of the variable y at zero time.
e is the base of natural or napierian logarithms (discovered in 1619 before the circulation of the blood was known). This constant (2.718 28...) possesses many remarkable properties which are lucidly expounded for the non-specialist by Hogben (1951).

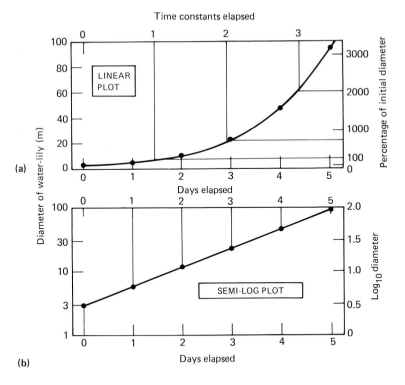

Figure F.1 The growth of a water-lily which doubles its diameter every day—a typical tear-away exponential function. Initial diameter, 3 metres; size doubled every day (i.e. doubling time = 1 day). Compare the figures in the table below with those in Table F.1.

Diameter of water-lily $= 3e^{t/1.44}$
(t is measured in days, diameter in metres)

Elapsed time (days)	Diameter of water-lily	
	metres	percentage of initial diameter
0	3	100
1	6	200
1.44	8.2	272
2	12	400
2.88	22.2	739
3	24	800
4	48	1 600
4.32	60.3	2 009
5	96	3 200

k is a constant which defines the speed of the particular function. For example, it will differ by a factor of two if our mythical water-lily doubles its size every 12 hours instead of every day. In the case of the wash-out and wash-in, we shall see that k is directly related to certain important physiological quantities, from which we may predict the speed of certain biological changes.

To many of us, e is unfamiliar and fairly alarming. We may, if we wish, avoid it by using the more familiar base 10:

$$y = y_0 10^{k_1 t}$$

This is a perfectly valid way of expressing a tear-away exponential function, but you will notice that the constant k has changed to k_1. This new constant does *not* have the simple relationships of physiological variables mentioned above. It does, however, bear a constant relationship to k, as follows:

$$k_1 = 0.4343k \text{ (approx.)}$$

When an exponential function is considered to proceed by steps of whole numbers, it is known as a geometrical progression.

Graphical representation

On linear graph paper, a tear-away exponential functional rapidly disappears off the top of the paper (*Figure F.1*). If plotted on semi-logarithmic paper (time on a linear axis and y on a logarithmic axis), the plot becomes a straight line and this is a most convenient method of presenting such a function. The logarithmic plots in *Figures F.1–F.3* are all plotted on semi-log paper.

The wash-out or die-away exponential function

The account of the tear-away exponential function has really been a curtain-raiser for the wash-out or die-away exponential function, which is of great importance to the biologist in general, and the respiratory physiologist in particular.

Simple statement

In a wash-out exponential function, the quantity under consideration falls at a rate which decreases progressively in proportion to the distance it still has to fall. It approaches but, in theory, never reaches zero.

Examples

Classic examples are cooling curves, radioactive decay and (nearer home) water running out of the bath. In the last example the rate of flow down the plug-hole is proportional to the pressure of water, which is proportional to the depth of water in the bath, which in turn is proportional to the quantity of water in the bath (assuming that the sides are vertical). Therefore, the flow rate of water down the plug-hole is proportional to the amount of water left in the bath, and decreases as the bath empties. The last molecule of bath water takes an infinitely long time to drain away. A similar example is the mountaineer who each day ate half of the food which he carried. In this way he made his food last indefinitely.

Biological examples include:

1. Passive expiration (*Figure F.2*).
2. The elimination of inhalational anaesthetics.
3. The fall of arterial P_{CO_2} to its new level after a step increase in ventilation.

4. The fall of arterial P_{O_2} to its new level after a step decrease in ventilation.
5. The fall of blood P_{CO_2} towards the alveolar level as it progresses along the pulmonary capillary.
6. The fall of blood P_{O_2} towards the tissue level as blood progresses through the tissue capillaries.

Mathematical statement

When a quantity *decreases* with time, the rate of change is *negative*. Therefore, the wash-out exponential function is written thus:

$$\frac{dy}{dt} = -ky$$

from which we may derive the following equations, which give the value of y at any time t:

$$y = y_0 e^{-kt}$$

which is simply another way of saying:

$$y = \frac{y_0}{e^{kt}}$$

y_0 is again the initial value of y at zero time. In *Figure F.2*, y_0 is the initial value of (lung volume−FRC) at the start of expiration; that is to say, the tidal volume inspired.
e is again the base of natural logarithms (2.718 28...).
k is the constant which defines the rate of decay, and really comes into its own in the wash-out exponential function. It is the reciprocal of a most important quantity known as the *time constant*. There are three things which should be known about the time constant:

1. *Figure F.2* shows a tangent drawn to the first part of the curve. This shows the course events would take if the initial rate were maintained instead of slowing down in the manner characteristic of the wash-out curve. The time which would then be required for completion would be $1/k$ which is called the *time constant* and designated by the Greek letter tau (τ). The wash-out exponential function may thus be written:

$$y = y_0 e^{-t/\tau}$$

2. After 1 time constant, y will have fallen to $1/e$ of its initial value, or approximately 37 per cent of its initial value.
   After 2 time constants, y will have fallen to $1/e^2$ of its initial value, or approximately 13.5 per cent of its initial value.
   After 3 time constants, y will have fallen to $1/e^3$ of its initial value, or approximately 5 per cent of its initial value.
   After 5 time constants, y will have fallen to $1/e^5$ of its initial value, or approximately 1 per cent of its initial value.
   (More precise values are indicated in *Table F.1*).

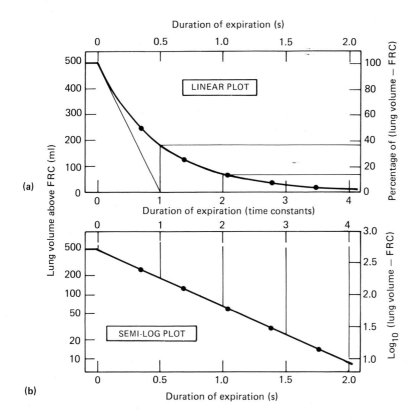

Figure F.2 Passive espiration—a typical wash-out exponential function. Tidal volume, 500 ml; compliance, 0.5 l/kPa (50 ml/cmH₂O); airway resistance 1 kPa l⁻¹ s (10 cmH₂O/1000 ml/sec); time constant, 0.5 s; half-life, 0.35 s. The points on the curves indicate the passage of successive half-lives.

	Elapsed time (constants)	Lung volume remaining above FRC	
		ml	percentage of tidal volume
Lung volume above FRC = $500e^{-(t/0.5)}$	0	500	100
	0.69	250	50
	1	184	36.8
	2	67.5	13.5
	3	25	5.0
	4	9	1.8

Note that the logarithmic co-ordinate has no zero. This accords with the lung volume approaching, but never actually equalling, the FRC.

3. The time constant is often determined by physiological factors. When air escapes passively from a distended lung, the time constant is governed by two variables, compliance and resistance(Chapters 2, 3 and 21).

Let V represent the lung volume (above FRC), then $-(dV/dt)$ is the instantaneous expiratory gas flow rate. Assuming Poiseuille's law is obeyed (page 47):

$$-\frac{dV}{dt} = \frac{P}{R}$$

when P is the instantaneous alveolar-to-mouth pressure gradient and R is the airway resistance.

But

$$\text{compliance } C = \frac{V}{P}$$

therefore

$$-\frac{dV}{dt} = \frac{1}{CR}V$$

or

$$\frac{dV}{dt} = -\frac{1}{CR}V$$

Then by integration and the taking of antilogs as described above:

$$V = V_0 e^{-(t/CR)}$$

By analogy with the general equation of the wash-out exponential function, it is clear that $CR = 1/k = \tau$ (the time constant). Thus the *time constant equals the product of compliance and resistance.*[*] This is analogous to the discharge of an electrical capacitor through a resistance, when the time constant of discharge equals the product of the capacitance and the resistance. Analysis of the passive expiration has been considered in greater detail on page 42 and by Bergman (1969).

Rather similar is the wash-out of anaesthetic from a body or organ. Here the 'capacitance' equals the product of the mass of the body or organ and the solubility in it of the agent. The agent's 'resistance' to escape is inversely related to ventilation, diffusion, blood flow, renal function, etc. In the more complex situations, wash-out curves remain exponential in form but are compounded of a number of individual wash-out curves. Each has its own time constant which equals the product of capacitance (for the anaesthetic) and resistance (to wash-out) for

---

[*] It is strange at first sight that two quantities as complex as compliance and resistance should have a product as simple as time. In fact, the mass/length/time units check perfectly well (*see* Appendix A).

$$\text{compliance} \times \text{resistance} = \text{time}$$
$$M^{-1}L^4T^2 \times ML^{-4}T^{-1} = T$$

each part. An example of the technique for separation of individual components from an overall wash-out curve is the analysis of nitrogen clearance curves (Comroe et al., 1962).

Wash-out of a substance from an organ by perfusion with blood which is free of the substance is another example of a wash-out exponential function where the time constant may be stated in terms of certain physiological factors.

Let Q represent the volume of an organ and C be the concentration in the organ of a substance whose solubility in the organ equals its solubility in blood.

Imagine a small quantity of blood (dQ) to enter the organ. The concentration is then reduced by dC:

$$\frac{C - dC}{C} = \frac{Q + dQ}{Q}$$

Subtracting 1 from each side:

$$-\frac{dC}{C} = \frac{dQ}{Q}$$

If blood enters the organ at a constant rate, dQ/dt may be represented by $\dot{Q}$ (the usual symbol for blood flow rate). It then follows that:

$$-\frac{dC}{C} = \frac{\dot{Q}.dt}{Q}$$

and so

$$-\frac{dC}{dt} = \frac{\dot{Q}}{Q} C$$

from which if follows that:

$$C = C_0 e^{-(\dot{Q}/Q)t}$$

Again, by analogy, it is clear that $Q/\dot{Q} = 1/k = \tau$ (the time constant). Thus the *time constant equals the tissue volume divided by its blood flow.*

Similarly, the time constant of wash-out of a substance from the alveolar gas equals the FRC divided by the alveolar ventilation (assuming that none of the substance crosses the alveolar/capillary membrane during the process, as is nearly true with helium, for example).

This important relationship is used in the nitrogen wash-out test of uniformity of intrapulmonary gas mixing, in which gas is considered as being washed out of two compartments, one fast and one slow. A compound wash-out curve is obtained and is subsequently analysed for different components (Comroe et al., 1962). It is also the basis of the Lassen and Ingvar (1961) technique for measurement of organ blood flow. The theory is delightfully simple. The time constant is determined for the wash-out of a freely diffusible radioactive substance from the organ. Since the reciprocal of the time constant equals the organ blood flow divided by the organ volume, the answer is immediately available in blood flow per unit volume of tissue (usually expressed as ml min^{-1} 100 ml of tissue). This again makes the assumption that the solubility of the substance is the same for blood and tissue. If it is not, a correction factor can easily be applied.

Half-life. It is often convenient to use the half-life instead of the time constant. This is the time required for *y* to change by a factor of two (or a half). The special attraction of the half-life is its ease of measurement. The half-life of a radioactive element may be determined quite simply. First of all the degree of activity is measured and the time noted. Its activity is then followed and the time noted at which its activity is exactly half the initial value. The difference between the two times is the half-life and is constant at all levels of activity. Half-lives are shown in *Figures F.1–F.3* as dots on the curves. For a particular exponential function there is a constant relationship between the time constant and the half-life.

Half-life = 0.69 times the *time constant*
Time constant = 1.44 times the *half-life*

(For practical purposes, the time constant is 1.5 times the half-life.)

Graphical representation

Plotting a wash-out exponential function is similar to the tear-away function (*Figure F.2*). Semi-log paper may be used in the same way and is of considerable practical importance as the curve (being straight) may then be defined by far fewer observations. It is also easy to extrapolate backwards to zero time if the initial value is required but could not be measured directly for some reason. It is, for example, an essential step in the measurement of cardiac output with a dye which is rapidly lost from the circulation (page 137).

The wash-in exponential function

The wash-in function is also of special importance to the respiratory physiologist and is the mirror image of the wash-out function.

Simple statement

In a wash-in exponential function, the quantity under consideration rises towards a limiting value, at a rate which decreases progressively in proportion to the distance it still has to rise.

Examples

A typical example would be a mountaineer who each day manages to climb half the remaining distance between his overnight camp and the summit of the mountain. His rate of ascent declines exponentially and he will never reach the summit. A graph of his altitude plotted against time would resemble a 'wash-in' curve.

Biological examples include the reverse of those listed for the wash-out function:

1. Inflation of the lungs of a paralysed patient by a sustained increase of mouth pressure (*Figure F.3*).
2. The uptake of inhalational anaesthetics.
3. The rise of arterial P_{CO_2} to its new level after a step decrease of ventilation.
4. The rise of arterial P_{O_2} to its new level after a step increase of ventilation.

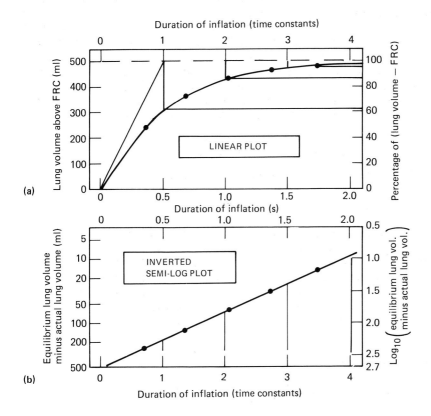

Figure F.3 Passive inflation of the lungs with a sustained mouth pressure—a typical wash-in exponential function. Eventual tidal volume, 500 ml; compliance, 0.5 l/kPa (50 ml/cmH₂O); airway resistance, 1 kPa l⁻¹ s (10 cm H₂O/1000 ml/sec); time constant, 0.5 s; half-life, 0.35 s. The points on the curves indicate the passage of successive half-lives.

	Elapsed time (constants)	Lung volume attained above FRC	
		ml	percentage of tidal volume
Lung volume above FRC = $500\,(1 - e^{-(t/0.5)})$	0	0	0
	0.69	250	50
	1	316	63.2
	2	433	86.5
	3	475	95.0
	4	491	98.2

Note that, for the semi-log plot, the log scale (ordinate) is from above downwards and indicates the difference between the equilibrium lung volume (inflation pressure maintained indefinitely) and the actual lung volume. Use log graph paper upside down.

5. The rise of blood P_{O_2} to the alveolar level as it progresses along the pulmonary capillary.
6. The rise of blood P_{CO_2} to the venous level as blood progresses through the tissue capillaries.

Mathematical statement

With a wash-in exponential function, y increases with time and therefore the rate of change is positive. As time advances, the rate of change falls towards zero. The initial value of y is often zero but y approaches a final limiting value which we may designate y_∞, that is the value of y when time is infinity (∞). A change of this type is indicated thus:

$$\frac{dy}{dt} = k(y_\infty - y)$$

As y approaches y_∞ so the quantity within the parentheses approaches zero, and the rate of change slows down. The corresponding equation which indicates the instantaneous value of y is:

$$y = y_\infty (1 - e^{-kt})$$

y_∞ is the limiting value of y (attained only at infinite time).
e is again the base of natural logarithms.
k is a constant defining the rate of build-up and, as is the case of the wash-out function, it is the reciprocal of the *time constant* the significance of which is described above. It is the time which would be required to reach completion, if the initial rate were maintained without slowing down.

After 1 time constant, y will have risen to approximately $100 - 37 = 63$ per cent of its final value.
After 2 time constants, y will have risen to approximately $100 - 13.5 = 86.5$ per cent of its final value.
After 3 time constants, y will have risen to approximately $100 - 5 = 95$ per cent of its final value.
After 5 time constants, y will have risen to approximately $100 - 1 = 99$ per cent of its final value.
(More precise values are indicated in *Table F.1*.)

Finally, the time constant for a wash-in exponential function equals the product of compliance and resistance, tissue volume divided by blood flow, or FRC divided by alveolar ventilation as the case may be. As above, the time constant is approximately 1.5 times the half-life.

There are many examples of both a wash-in and a wash-out in a single system with fixed parameters. The time constant for each function will then be the same. A classic example is the charging of an electrical capacitor through a resistance, and then allowing it to discharge to earth through the same resistor. The time constant to the same for each process and equals the product of capacitance and resistance. *Figure F.3* shows inflation of the lung by a sustained pressure applied to the mouth. Assuming that compliance and airway resistance are the same for inflation and expiration, the inflation curve in *Figure F.3* will be the mirror image of the

Table F.1 Percentage change of y after lapse of different numbers of time constants

Time elapsed in time constants	Tear-away function $y = y_0 e^{kt}$ (expressed as % of y_0)	Wash-out function $y = y_0 e^{-kt}$ (expressed as % of y_0)	Wash-in function $y = y_\infty(1 - e^{-kt})$ (expressed as % of y_∞)
0	100	100	0
0.693*	200	50	50
1	272	36.8	63.2
2	739	13.5	86.5
3	2 009	4.98	95.02
4	5 460	1.83	98.17
5	14 841	0.67	99.33
10	2 202 650	0.004 5	99.995 5
∞	∞	0	100

*Half-life or doubling time.

Note. $272 = 100 \times e$
   $739 = 100 \times e^2$
   $2\ 009 = 100 \times e^3$
   etc.

expiration curve in *Figure F.2,* and each will have the same time constant (equal to compliance times resistance).

Graphical representation

The wash-in function may be represented on linear paper as for the other types of exponential function. However, for the semi-log plot, the paper must be turned upside down and the plot made as indicated in *Figure F.3*. The curve will then be a straight line.

References and further reading

Abraham, A.S., Cole, R.B. and Bishop, J.M. (1968) Reversal of pulmonary hypertension by prolonged oxygen administration to patients with chronic bronchitis. *Circulation Res.* **23**, 147

Abraham, A.S., Cole, R.B., Green, I.D., Hedworth-Whitty, R.B., Clarke, S.W. and Bishop, J.M. (1969) Factors contributing to the reversible pulmonary hypertension of patients with acute respiratory failure studied by serial observations during recovery. *Circulation Res.* **24**, 51

Abreu e Silva, F.A., MacFadyen, U.M., Williams, A. and Simpson, H. (1985) Sleep apnoea in infancy. *Jl R. Soc. Med* **78**, 1005

Adair, G.S. (1925) The hemoglobin system. VI. The oxygen dissociation curve of hemoglobin. *J. biol. Chem.* **63**, 529

Adams, R.W., Gronert, G.A., Sundt, T.M. and Michenfelder, J.D. (1972) Halothane, hypocapnia, and cerebrospinal fluid pressure in neurosurgery. *Anesthesiology* **37**, 510

Agostoni, E. (1962) Diaphragm activity and thoraco-abdominal mechanics during positive pressure breathing. *J. appl. Physiol.* **17**, 215

Agostoni, E. (1963) Diaphragm activity during breath-holding: factors related to its onset. *J. appl. Physiol.* **18**, 30

Agostoni, E., Sant' Ambrogio, G. and Carrasco, H.D.P. (1960) Electromyography of the diaphragm in man and transdiaphragmatic pressure. *J. appl. Physiol.* **15**, 1093

Aitken, R.S. and Clarke-Kennedy, A.E. (1928) On the fluctuations in the composition of the alveolar air during the respiratory cycle in muscular exercise. *J. Physiol.* **65**, 389

Alabaster, V.A. (1980) Inactivation of endogenous amines in the lungs. In: *Metabolic Activities of the Lung*, Ciba Foundation Symposium, no. 78. Amsterdam: Excerpta Medica

Alexander, J.I., Spence, A.A., Parikh, R.K. and Stuart, B. (1973) The role of airway closure in postoperative hypoxaemia. *Br. J. Anaesth.* **45**, 34

Alexander, S.C., James, F.M. Colton, E.T., Gleaton, H.R. and Wollman, H. (1968) Effects of cyclopropane on cerebral blood flow and carbohydrate metabolism in man. *Anesthesiology* **29**, 170

Anderson, D.O. and Ferris, B.G. (1962) Role of tobacco smoking in the causation of chronic respiratory disease. *New Engl. J. Med.* **267**, 787

Angus, G.E. and Thurlbeck, W.M. (1972) Number of alveoli in the human lung. *J. appl. Physiol.* **32**, 483

Anthonisen, N.R., Danson, J., Robertson, P.C. and Ross, W.R.D. (1969) Airway closure as a function of age. *Resp. Physiol.* **8**, 58

Armitage, G.H. and Taylor, A.B. (1956) Non-bronchospirometric measurement of differential lung function. *Thorax* **11**, 281

Arndt, H., King, T.K.C. and Briscoe, W.A. (1970) Diffusing capacities and ventilation:perfusion ratios in patients with the clinical syndrome of alveolar capillary block. *J. clin. Invest.* **49**, 408

Arnone, A. (1972) X-ray diffraction study of binding of 2,3-diphosphoglycerate to human deoxyhaemoglobin. *Nature* **237**, 146

Ashbaugh, D.G., Bigelow, D.B., Petty, T.L. and Levine, B.E. (1967) Acute respiratory distress in adults. *Lancet* **2**, 319

Ashton, H., Stepney, R. and Thompson, P.W. (1979) Self-titration by cigarette smokers. *Br. med. J.* **2**, 357

Asmussen, E. (1965) Muscular exercise. *Handbk Physiol., section 3*, **2**, 939

Asmussen, E. and Neilsen, M. (1946) Studies on the regulation of respiration in heavy work. *Acta physiol. scand.* **12**, 171

Asmussen, E. and Nielsen, M. (1960) Aveolar–arterial gas exchange at rest and during work at different oxygen tensions. *Acta physiol. scand.* **50**, 153

Astrup, P. and Severinghaus, J.W. (1986) *The History of Blood Gases, Acids and Bases*. Copenhagen: Munksgaard

Attar, S., Scanlan, E. and Cowley, R.A. (1966) Further evaluation of hyperbaric oxygen in haemorrhagic shock. In *Proceedings of the Third International Conference on Hyperbaric Medicine*, edited by I.W. Brown and B.G. Cox. Washington DC: National Academy of Sciences

Aub, J.C. and DuBois, E.F. (1917) The basal metabolism of old men. *Archs intern. Med.* **19**, 823

Austrian, R., McClement, J.H., Renzetti, A.D., Donald, K.W., Riley, R.L. and Cournand, A. (1951) Clinical and physiological features of some types of pulmonary diseases with impairment of alveolar–capillary diffusion. *Am. J. Med.* **11**, 667

Avery, M.E. and Mead, J. (1959) Surface properties in relation to atelectasis and hyaline membrane disease. *Archs Dis. Childh.* **97**, 517

Babior, B.M., Kipnes, R.S. and Curnutte, J.T. (1973) The production by leukocytes of superoxide, a potential bactericidal agent. *J. clin. Invest.* **52**, 741

Bachofen, M. and Weibel, E.R. (1982) Structural alterations of lung parenchyma in the adult respiratory distress syndrome. *Clins chest Med.* **3**, 35

Bachrach, A.J. (1982) A short history of man in the sea. In: *The Physiology and Medicine of Diving*, edited by P.B. Bennett and D.H. Elliott. London: Baillière Tindall

Bainton, C.R. and Mitchell, R.A. (1965) Posthyperventilation apnea in awake man. *Fedn Proc.* **24**, 273

Bake, B., Wood, L., Murphy, B., Macklem, P.T. and Milic-Emili, J. (1974) Effect of inspiratory flow rate on regional distribution of inspired gas. *J. appl. Physiol.* **37**, 8

Bakhle, Y.S. (1968) Conversion of angiotensin I to angiotensin II by cell-free extracts of dog lung. *Nature* **220**, 919

Bakhle, Y.S. (1980) Pulmonary angiotensin-converting enzyme and its inhibition. In: *Metabolic Activities of the Lung*. Ciba Foundation Symposium, no. 78. Amsterdam: Excerpta Medica

Bakhle, Y.S. and Block, A.J. (1976) Effects of halothane on pulmonary inactivation of noradrenalin and prostaglandin E_2 in anaesthetized dogs. *Clin. Sci.* **50**, 87

Bakhle, Y.S. and Ferreira, S.H. (1985) Lung metabolism of eicosanoids: prostaglandins, prostacyclin, thromboxane and leukotrienes. *Handbk Physiol. section 3*, **1**, 365

Bakhle, Y.S. and Vane, J.R. (1977) (eds) *Metabolic Functions of the Lung*. New York: Marcel Dekker

Banner, N.R. and Govan, J.R. (1986) Long term transtracheal oxygen delivery through microcatheter in patients with hypoxaemia due to chronic obstructive airway disease. *Br. med. J.* **293**, 111

Barber, R.E., Lee, J. and Hamilton, W.K. (1970) Oxygen toxicity in man. A prospective study in patients with irreversible brain damage. *New Engl. J. Med.* **283**, 1478

Barcroft, J. (1920) Physiological effects of insufficient oxygen supply. *Nature* **106**, 125

Barer, G.R., Howard, P. and McCurrie, J.R. (1967) The effect of carbon dioxide and changes in blood pH on pulmonary vascular resistance in cats. *Clin. Sci.* **32**, 361

Barer, G.R., Howard, P., McCurrie, J.R. and Shaw, J.W. (1969) Changes in the pulmonary circulation after bronchial occlusion in anaesthetized dogs and cats. *Circulation Res.* **25**, 747

Barnes, P.J. (1984) The third nervous system in the lung: physiology and clinical perspectives. *Thorax* **39**, 561

Barth, L. (1954) Untersuchungen über die Diffusionsatmung des Menschen. In *Anaesthesieprobleme. Abh. dt. Akad. Wiss. Berl., Klasse für med.*

Bates, D.V., Macklem, P.T. and Christie, R.V. (1971) *Respiratory Function in Disease*, 2nd edn. Philadelphia, Pa. and London: W.B. Saunders

Bay, J., Nunn, J.F. and Prys-Roberts, C. (1968) Factors influencing arterial PO_2 during recovery from anaesthesia. *Br. J. Anaesth.* **40**, 398

Beamer, W.C., Prough, D.S., Royster, R.L., Johnston, W.E. and Johnson, J.C. (1984) High frequency ventilation produces auto-PEEP. *Crit. Care Med.* **12,** 734

Bellville, J.W. and Seed, J.C. (1960) The effect of drugs on the respiratory response to carbon dioxide. *Anesthesiology* **21,** 727

Benatar, S.R. Hewlett, A.M. and Nunn, J.F. (1973) The use of iso-shunt lines for control of oxygen therapy. *Br. J. Anaesth.* **45,** 711

Bend, J.R., Serabjit-Singh, C.J. and Philpot, R.M. (1985) The pulmonary uptake, accumulation and metabolism of xenobiotics. *A. Rev. Pharmacol. Toxiocol.* **25,** 97

Bendixen, H.H. and Bunker, J.P. (1962) Measurement of inspiratory force in anesthetized dogs. *Anesthesiology* **23,** 315

Bendixen, H.H., Hedley-Whyte, J. and Laver, M.B. (1963) Impaired oxygenation in surgical patients during general anesthesia with controlled ventilation. *New Engl. J. Med.* **269,** 991

Bendixen, H.H., Smith, G.M. and Mead, J. (1964) Pattern of ventilation in young adults. *J. appl. Physiol.* **19,** 195

Benesch, R. and Benesch, R.E. (1967) Effects of organic phosphates from human erythrocytes on the allosteric properties of haemoglobin. *Biochem. Biophys. Res. Commun.* **26,** 162

Bennett, E.D., Jayson, M.I.V., Rubinstein, D. and Campbell, E.J.M. (1962) The ability of man to detect added non-elastic loads to breathing. *Clin. Sci.* **23,** 155

Bennett, P.B. (1982a) Inert gas narcosis. In: *The Physiology and Medicine of Diving,* edited by P.G. Bennett and D.H. Elliott. London: Baillière Tindall

Bennett, P.B. (1982b) The high pressure nervous syndrome in man. In: *The Physiology and Medicine of Diving,* edited by P.B. Bennett and D.H. Elliott. London: Ballière Tindall.

Benumof, J.L. (1982) One-lung ventilation: which lung should be PEEPed? *Anesthesiology* **56,** 161

Benzinger, T. (1937) Untersuchungen über die Atmung und den Gasstoffwechsel insbesondere bei Sauerstoffmangel und Unterdruck, mit fortlaufend unmittelbar aufzeichnenden Methoden. *Ergebn. Physiol.* **40,** 1

Berger, A.J. and Hornbein, T.F. (1987) Control of respiration. In: *Physiology and Biophysics,* vol. 2, 21st edn, edited by H.D. Patton, A.F. Fuchs, B. Hille and A.M. Scher. Philadelphia, Pa: W.B. Saunders

Bergman, N.A. (1963) Distribution of inspired gas during anesthesia and artificial ventilation. *J. appl. Physiol.* **18,** 1085

Bergman, N.A. (1966) Measurement of respiratory resistance in anesthetized subjects. *J. appl. Physiol.* **21,** 1913

Bergman, N.A. (1967) Effects of varying waveforms on gas exchange. *Anesthesiology* **28,** 390

Bergman, N.A. (1969) Properties of passive exhalations in anesthetized subjects. *Anesthesiology* **30,** 379

Bergman, N.A. and Tien, Y.K. (1983) Contribution of the closure of pulmonary units to impaired oxygenation during anesthesia. *Anesthesiology* **59,** 395

Bergman, N.A. and Waltemath, C.L. (1974) A comparison of some methods for measuring total respiratory resistance. *J. appl. Physiol.* **36,** 131

Bernstein, L. and Mendel, D. (1951) Accuracy of spirographic tracings at high rates. *Thorax* **6,** 297

Bernstein, L., D'Silva, J.L. and Mendel, D. (1952) The effect of rate on MBC determination with a new spirometer. *Thorax* **7,** 225

Bertrand, F., Hugelin, A. and Vibert, J.F. (1974) A stereologic model of pneumotaxic oscillator based on spatial and temporal distributions of neuronal bursts. *J. Neurophysiol.* **37,** 91

Bhattacharya, J., Gropper, M.A. and Staub, N.A. (1984) Interstitial fluid pressure gradient measured by micropuncture in excised dog lung. *J. appl. Physiol.* **56,** 271

Bindslev, L.G., Hedenstierna, G., Santesson, J., Gottlieb, I. and Carvallhas, A. (1981) Ventilation–perfusion distribution during inhalation anaesthesia. *Acta anaesth. scand.* **25,** 360

Birt, C. and Cole, P.V. (1965) Some physiological effects of closed circuit halothane anaesthesia. *Anaesthesia* **30,** 258

Biscoe, T.J. (1971) Carotid body structure and function. *Physiol. Rev.* **5,** 437

Biscoe, T.J. and Millar, R.A. (1964) The effect of halothane on carotid sinus baroreceptor activity. *J. Physiol.* **173,** 24

Biscoe, T.J. and Willshaw, P. (1981) Stimulus–response relationships of the peripheral arterial chemoreceptors. In: *Regulation of Breathing,* Part I, edited by T.F. Hornbein. New York: Marcel Dekker

Bitter, H.S. and Rahn, H. (1956) Redistribution of alveolar blood flow with passive lung distension. *Wright Air Dev. Ctr. Tech. Rep.* 56–466, 1

Bjertnaes, L.J. (1977) Hypoxia induced vasoconstriction in isolated perfused lungs exposed to injectable or inhalation anaesthetics. *Acta anaesth. scand.* **21,** 133

Black, A.M.S. and Torrance, R.W. (1971) Respiratory oscillations in chemoreceptor discharge in the control of breathing. *Resp. Physiol.* **13,** 221

Black, G.W., Linde, H.W., Dripps, R.D. and Price, H.L. (1959) Circulatory changes accompanying respiratory acidosis during halothane (Fluothane) anaesthesia in man. *Br. J. Anaesth.* **31,** 238

Blackburn, J.P., Conway, C.M., Leigh, J.M., Lindop, M.J. and Reitan, J.A. (1972) $PaCO_2$ and the pre-ejection period. *Anesthesiology* **37,** 268

Blake, D.R., Hall, N.D., Bacon, P.A., Dieppe, P.A., Halliwell, B. and Gutteridge, J.M.C. (1981) The importance of iron in rheumatoid disease. *Lancet* **2,** 1142

Bledsoe, S.W. and Hornbein, T.F. (1981) Central chemosensors and the regulation of their chemical environment. In: *Regulation of Breathing,* Part I, edited by T.F. Hornbein. New York: Marcel Dekker

Blitt, C.D., Brown, B.R., Wright, B.J., Gandolfi, A.J. and Sipes, G. (1979) Pulmonary biotransformation of methoxyflurane. *Anesthesiology* **51,** 528

Bodman, R.I. (1963) Clinical applications of pulmonary function tests. *Anaesthesia* **18,** 355

Bohr, C. (1891) Über die Lungenathmung. *Skand. Arch. Physiol.* **2,** 236

Bohr, C. (1909) Über die spezifische Tätigkeit der Lungen bei der respiratorischen Gasaufnahme. *Skand. Arch. Physiol.* **22,** 221

Boidin, M.P. (1985) Airway patency in the unconscious patient. *Br. J. Anaesth.* **57,** 306

Bookallil, M. and Smith, W.D.A. (1964) A proportional respiratory sampling apparatus. *Br. J. Anaesth.* **36,** 527

Boothby, W.M. and Sandiford, I. (1924) Basal metabolism. *Physiol. Rev.* **18,** 1085

Borland, C., Chamberlain, A., Higenbottam, T., Shipley, M. and Rose, G. (1983) Carbon monoxide yield of cigarettes and its relation to cardiorespiratory disease. *Br. med. J.* **287,** 1583

Boushey, H.A., Holtzman, M.J., Sheller, J.R. and Nadel, J.A. (1980) Bronchial hyperreactivity. *Am. Rev. resp. Dis.* **121,** 389

Bowes, G. and Phillipson, E.A. (1984) Arousal responses to respiratory stimuli during sleep. In: *Sleep and Breathing,* edited by N.A. Saunders and C.E. Sullivan. New York: Marcel Dekker

Brady, J.P., Cotton, E.C. and Tooley, W.H. (1964) Chemoreflexes in the newborn infant: effects of 100% oxygen on heart rate and ventilation. *J. Physiol.* **172,** 332

Braunitzer, G. (1963) Molekulare struktur der Hämoglobine. *Nova Acta Acad. Caesar. Leop. Carol.* **26,** 471

Breuer, J. (1868) Die Selbsteurung der Athmung durch den Nervus Vagus. *Sber. Akad. Wiss. Wien* **58,** 909

Brigham, K.L. and Meyrick, B. (1984) Interactions of granulocytes with the lungs. *Circulation Res.* **54,** 623

Briscoe, W.A., Forster, R.E. and Comroe, J.H. (1954) Alveolar ventilation at very low tidal volumes. *J. apply. Physiol.* **7,** 27

Brismar, B., Hedenstierna, G., Lundquist, H., Strandberg, A., Svensson, L. and Tokics, L. (1985) Pulmonary densities during anesthesia with muscular relaxation — a proposal of atelectasis. *Anesthesiology* **62,** 422

Brown, E.B. and Miller, F. (1952) Ventricular fibrillation following a rapid fall in alveolar carbon dioxide concentration. *Am. J. Physiol.* **169,** 56

Brown, E.S., Johnson, R.P. and Clements, J.A. (1959) Pulmonary surface tension. *J. appl. Physiol.* **14,** 717

Brummelkamp, W.H. (1965) Reflections on hyperbaric oxygen therapy at 2 atmospheres absolute for *Clostridium welchii* infections. In: *Hyperbaric Oxygenation,* edited by I. Ledingham. Edinburgh and London: Churchill Livingstone

Brusasco, V., Knopp, T.J., Schmid, E.R. and Rehder, K. (1984) Ventilation–perfusion relationship during high-frequency ventilation. *J. appl. Physiol.* **56,** 454

Burton, A.C. (1951) On the physical equilibrium of small blood vessels. *Am. J. Physiol.* **164,** 319

Butler, J. (1960) The work of breathing through the nose. *Clin. Sci.* **19,** 55

Butler, J. and Smith, B.H. (1957) Pressure–volume relationships of the chest in the completely relaxed anaesthetised patient. *Clin. Sci.* **16,** 125

Butler, J., White, H.C. and Arnott, W.M. (1957) The pulmonary compliance in normal subjects. *Clin. Sci.* **16,** 709

Butler, W.J., Bohn, D.J., Bryan, A.C. and Froese, A.B. (1980) Ventilation by high frequency oscillation in humans. *Anesth. Analg.* **59,** 577

Butt, M.P., Jalowayski, A., Modell, J.H. and Giammona, S.T. (1970) Pulmonary function after resuscitation from near drowning. *Anesthesiology* **32,** 275

Cain, C.C. and Otis, A.B. (1949) Some physiological effects resulting from added resistance to respiration. *J. Aviat. Med.* **20,** 149

Cain, S.M. and Otis, A.B. (1961) Carbon dioxide transport in anesthetized dogs during inhibition of carbonic anhydrase. *J. appl. Physiol.* **16,** 1023

Cameron, A.J.V., Gibb, B.H., Ledingham, I. McA. and McGuinness, J.B. (1965) A controlled clinical trial of hyperbaric oxygen in the treatment of acute myocardial infarction. In: *Hyperbaric Oxygenation,* edited by I. Ledingham. Edinburgh and London: Churchill Livingstone

Campbell, E.J.M. (1952) An electromyographic study of the role of the abdominal muscles in breathing. *J. Physiol.* **117,** 222

Campbell, E.J.M. (1955) An electromyographic examination of the role of the intercostal muscles in breathing in man. *J. Physiol.* **129,** 12

Campbell, E.J.M. (1957) The effects of increased resistance to expiration on the respiratory behaviour of the abdominal muscles and intra-abdominal pressure. *J. Physiol.* **136,** 556

Campbell, E.J.M. (1958) *The Respiratory Muscles and the Mechanics of Breathing.* London: Lloyd-Luke

Campbell, E.J.M. (1960a) Simplification of Haldane's apparatus for measuring CO_2 concentration in respired gases in clinical practice. *Br. med. J.* **1,** 457

Campbell, E.J.M. (1960b) A method of controlled oxygen administration which reduces the risk of carbon-dioxide retention. *Lancet* **2,** 12

Campbell, E.J.M. (1962) RIpH. *Lancet* **1,** 681

Campbell, E.J.M. and Guz, A. (1981) Breathlessness. In: *Regulation of Breathing,* Part II, edited by T.F. Hornbein. New York: Marcel Dekker

Campbell, E.J.M. and Howell, J.B.L. (1960) Simple rapid methods of estimating arterial and mixed venous PCO_2. *Br. med J.* **1,** 458

Campbell, E.J.M. and Howell, J.B.L. (1962) Proprioceptive control of breathing. In: Ciba Foundation Symposium on *Pulmonary Structure and Function*, edited by A.V.S. de Rueck and M. O'Connor. Edinburgh and London: Churchill Livingstone

Campbell, E.J.M. and Howell, J.B.L. (1963) The sensation of breathlessness. *Br. med. Bull.* **19,** 36

Campbell, E.J.M., Howell, J.B.L. and Peckett, B.W. (1957) The pressure–volume relationships of the thorax of anaesthetized human subjects. *J. Physiol.* **136,** 563

Campbell, E.J.M., Nunn, J.F. and Peckett, B.W. (1958) A comparison of artificial ventilation and spontaneous respiration with particular reference to ventilation–blood-flow relationships. *Br. J. Anaesth.* **30,** 166

Campbell, E.J.M., Westlake, E.K. and Cherniack, R.M. (1957) Simple methods of estimating oxygen consumption and efficiency of the muscles of breathing. *J. appl. Physiol.* **11,** 303

Campbell, E.J.M., Freedman, S., Smith, P.S. and Taylor, ME. (1961) The ability of man to detect added elastic loads to breathing. *Clin. Sci.* **20,** 223

Campbell, E.J.M., Freedman, S., Clark, T.J.H., Robson, J.G. and Norman, J. (1967) The effect of muscular paralysis induced by tubocurarine on the duration and sensation of breath-holding. *Clin. Sci.* **32,** 425

Campbell, E.J.M., Godfrey, S., Clark, T.H.J., Freedman, S. and Norman, J. (1969) The effect of muscular paralysis induced by tubocurarine on the duration and sensation of breath holding during hypercapnia. *Clin. Sci.* **36,** 323

Carlens, E., Hanson, H.E. and Nordenström, B. (1951) Temporary occlusion of the pulmonary artery. *J. thorac. Surg.* **22,** 527

Caro, C.G., Butler, J. and DuBois, A.B. (1960) Some effects of restriction of chest cage expansion on pulmonary function in man. *J. clin. Invest.* **39,** 573

Cascorbi, H.F. and Singh-Amaranath, A.V. (1972) Fluroxene toxicity in mice. *Anesthesiology* **37,** 480

Cassidy, S.S., Gaffney, F.A. and Johnson, R.L. (1981) A perspective in PEEP. *New Engl. J. Med.* **304,** 421

Castleden, C.M. and Cole, P.V. (1974) Variations in carboxyhaemoglobin levels in smokers. *Br. med. J.* **4,** 736

de Castro, F. (1926) Sur la structure et l'innervation de la glande intercarotidienne. *Trab. Lab. Invest. biol. Univ. Madrid* **24,** 365

Cater, D.B., Garatini, S., Marina, F. and Silver, I.A. (1961) Changes of oxygen tension in brain and somatic tissues induced by vasodilator and vasoconstrictor drugs. *Proc. R. Soc. B* **155,** 136

Cater, D.B., Hill, D.W., Lindop, P.J., Nunn, J.F. and Silver, I.A. (1963) Oxygen washout studies in the anesthetized dog. *J. appl. Physiol.* **18,** 888

Catley, D.M., Thornton, C., Jordan, C., Lehane, J.R., Royston, D. and Jones, J.G. (1985) Pronounced, episodic oxygen desaturation in the postoperative period. *Anesthesiology* **63,** 20

Cerretelli, P., Cruz, J.C., Farhi, L.E. and Rahn, H. (1966) Determination of mixed venous O_2 and CO_2 tensions and cardiac output by a rebreathing method. *Resp. Physiol.* **1,** 258

Ceruti, E. (1966) Chemoreceptor reflexes in the newborn infant: effect of cooling on the response to hypoxia. *Pediatrics* **37,** 556

Chakrabarti, M.K., Gordon, G. and Whitwam, J.G. (1986) Relationship between tidal volume and deadspace during high frequency ventilation. *Br. J. Anaesth.* **58,** 11

Channin, E. and Tyler, J. (1962) Effect of increased breathing frequency on inspiratory resistance in emphysema. *J. appl. Physiol.* **17,** 605

Chanutin, A. and Curnish, R. (1967) Effect of organic and inorganic phosphates on the oxygen equilibrium of human erythrocytes. *Arch. Biochem. Biophys.* **121,** 96

Cheney, F.W. and Colley, P.S. (1980) The effect of cardiac output on arterial blood oxygenation. *Anesthesiology* **52,** 496

Chenoweth, D.E., Cooper, S.W., Hugli, T.E., Stewart, R.W., Blackstone, E.H. and Kirlin, J.W. (1981) Complement activation during cardiopulmonary bypass. *New Engl. J. Med.* **304,** 497

Chernick, V. (1981) The fetus and the newborn. In: *Regulation of Breathing,* Part II, edited by T.F. Hornbein. New York: Marcel Dekker

Christensen, M.S. (1974) Acid–base changes in cerebrospinal fluid and blood, and blood volume changes following prolonged hyperventilation in man. *Br. J. Anaesth.* **46,** 348

Christensen, M.S., Hoedt-Rasmussen, K. and Lassen, N.A. (1967) Cerebral vasodilatation by halothane anaesthesia in man and its potentiation by hypotension and hypercapnia. *Br. J. Anaesth.* **39,** 927

Christiansen, J., Douglas, C.G. and Haldane, J.S. (1914) The adsorption and dissociation of carbon dioxide by human blood. *J. Physiol.* **48,** 244

Clark, I.A. and Hunt, N.H. (1983) Evidence for reactive oxygen intermediates causing hemolysis and parasite death in malaria. *Infec. Immun.* **39,** 1

Clark, I.A., Cowden, W.B. and Hunt, N.H. (1985) Free radical-induced pathology. *Med. Res. Rev.* **5,** 297

Clark, J.M. and Lambertsen, C.J. (1971) Pulmonary toxicity — a review. *Pharmac. Rev.* **23,** 37

Clark, J.M., Hagerman, F.C. and Gelfand, R. (1983) Breathing patterns during submaximal and maximal exercise in elite oarsmen, *J. appl. Physiol.* **55,** 440

Clark, T.J.H. (1968) The ventilatory response to CO_2 in chronic airways obstruction measured by a rebreathing method. *Clin. Sci.* **34,** 559

Clark, T.J.H., Clarke, B.G. and Hughes, J.M.B. (1966) A simple technique for measuring changes in ventilatory response to carbon dioxide. *Lancet,* **2,** 368

Clarke, S.W., Jones, J.G. and Oliver, D.R. (1970) Resistance to two-phase gas–liquid flow in airways. *J. appl. Physiol.* **29,** 464

Clements, J.A. (1970) Pulmonary surfactant. *Am. Rev. resp. Dis.* **101,** 984

Clergue, F., Ecoffey, C., Derenne, J.P. and Viars, P. (1984) Oxygen drive to breathing during halothane anesthesia: effects of almitrine bismesilate. *Anesthesiology* **60**, 125

Clowes, G.H.A., Hopkins, A.L. and Simeone, F.A. (1955) A comparison of physiological effects of hypercapnia and hypoxia in the production of cardiac arrest. *Ann. Surg.* **142**, 446

Clutton-Brock, J. (1957) The cerebral effects of overventilation. *Br. J. Anaesth.* **29**, 111

Cockett, F.B. and Vass, C.C.N. (1951) A comparison of the role of the bronchial arteries in the bronchiectasis. *Thorax* **6**, 268

Cohen, J.J., Brackett, N.C. and Schwartz, W.B. (1964) The nature of the carbon dioxide titration curve in the normal dog. *J. clin. Invest.* **43**, 777

Cohen, P.J. and Behar, M.G. (1970) The in vitro effect of anesthesia on the oxyhemoglobin dissociation curve. *Fedn Proc.* **29**, 329

Cole, A.G.H., Weller, S.F. and Sykes, M.K. (1984) Inverse ratio ventilation compared with PEEP in adult respiratory failure. *Intens. Care Med.* **10**, 227

Cole, R.B. and Bishop, J. M. (1963) Effects of varying inspired oxygen tension on alveolar–arterial O_2 tension difference in man. *J. appl. Physiol.* **18**, 1043

Coleridge, J.C.G. and Coleridge, H.M. (1984) Afferent vagal C fibre innervation of the lungs and airways and its functional significance. *Rev. Physiol. Biochem. Pharmac.* **99**, 1

Colgan, F.J., Barrow, R.E. and Fanning, G. (1971) Constant positive-pressure breathing and cardio-respiratory function. *Anesthesiology* **34**, 145

Comroe, J.H. (1939) The location and function of the chemoreceptors of the aorta. *Am. J. Physiol.* **127**, 176

Comroe, J.H. and Botelho, S. (1947) The unreliability of cyanosis in the recognition of arterial anoxemia. *Am. J. med. Sci.* **214**, 1

Comroe, J.H. and Dripps, R.D. (1946) Artificial respiration *J. Am. med. Ass.* **130**, 381

Comroe, J.H. and Schmidt, C.F. (1938) The part played by reflexes from the carotid body in the chemical regulation of respiration in the dog. *Am. J. Physiol.* **121**, 75

Comroe, J.H., Nisell, O.I. and Nims, R.G. (1954) A simple method of concurrent measurement of compliance and resistance to breathing in anesthetized animals and man. *J. appl. Physiol.* **7**, 225

Comroe, J.H., Forster, R.E., DuBois, A.B., Briscoe, W.A. and Carlsen, E. (1962) *The Lung,* 2nd edn. Chicago: Year Book Medical; London: Lloyd-Luke

Conn, A.W. and Barker, G.A. (1984) Fresh water drowning and near drowning. *Can. Anaesth. Soc. J.* **31**, S38

Conn, A.W., Edmonds, J.F. and Barker, G.A. (1978) Near-drowning in cold fresh water: current treatment regimen. *Can. Anaesth. Soc. J.* **25**, 259

Connaughton, J.J., Douglas, N.J., Morgan, A.D., Shapiro, C.M., Critchley, J.A.J.H., Pauly, N. and Flenley, D.C. (1985) Almitrine improves oxygenation when both awake and asleep in patients with hypoxia and carbon dioxide retention caused by chronic bronchitis and emphysema. *Am. Rev. resp. Dis.* **132**, 206

Cooper, E.A. (1957) Infra-red analysis for the estimation of carbon dioxide in the presence of nitrous oxide. *Br. J. Anaesth* **30**, 486

Cooper, E.A. (1959) The estimation of minute volume. *Anaesthesia* **14**, 373

Cooper, E.A. (1961) Behaviour of respiratory apparatus. *Med. Res. Memo. Natn. Coal Bd med. Serv.* **2**

Cooper, E.A. and Smith, H. (1961) Indirect estimation of arterial pCO_2. *Anaesthesia* **16**, 445

Corda, M., von Euler, C. and Lennerstrand, G. (1965) Proprioceptive innervation of the diaphragm. *J. Physiol.* **178**, 161

Cormack, R.S. (1972) Eliminating two sources of error in the Lloyd–Haldane apparatus. *Resp. Physiol.* **14**, 382

Cormack, R.S. and Powell, J.N. (1972) Improving the performance of the infra-red carbon dioxide meter. *Br. J. Anaesth.* **44**, 131

Cormack, R.S., Cunningham, D.J.C. and Gee, J.B.L. (1957) The effect of carbon dioxide on the respiratory response to want of oxygen in man. *Q. Jl exp. Physiol.* **42**, 303

Cotes, J.E. (1975) *Lung Function,* 3rd edn. Oxford: Blackwell

Cotev, S., Lee, J. and Severinghaus, J.W. (1968) The effects of acetazolamide on cerebral blood flow and cerebral tissue P_{O_2}. *Anesthesiology* **29**, 471

Cournand, A., Motley, H.L., Werko, L. and Richards, D.W. (1948) Physiological studies of the effects of intermittent positive pressure breathing on cardiac output in man. *Am. J. Physiol.* **152**, 162

Cox, J., Woolmer, R.W. and Thomas, V. (1960) Expired air resuscitation. *Lancet* **1**, 727

Craig, A.B. (1961) Causes of loss of consciousness during underwater swimming. *J. appl. Physiol.* **16**, 583

Craig, D.B., Wahba, W.M., Don, H.F., Couture, J.G. and Becklake, M.R. (1971) 'Closing volume' and its relationship to gas exchange in seated and supine positions. *J. appl. Physiol.* **31**, 717

Crandall, E.D., Bidani, A. and Forster, R.E. (1977) Postcapillary changes in blood pH *in vivo* during carbonic anhydrase inhibition. *J. appl. Physiol.* **43**, 582

Crapo, J.D. and Tierney, D.F. (1974) Superoxide dismutase and pulmonary oxygen toxicity. *Am. J. Physiol.* **226**, 1401

Crawford, M. and Rehder, K. (1985) High-frequency small-volume ventilation in anesthetized humans. *Anesthesiology* **62**, 298

Cross, K.W., Klaus, M., Tooley, W.H. and Weisser, K. (1960) The response of the new-born baby to inflation of the lungs. *J. Physiol.* **151**, 551

Cucchiara, R.F., Nugent, M., Seward, J.B. and Messick, J.M. (1984) Air embolism in upright neurosurgical patients; detection and localization by two-dimensional transesophageal echocardiography. *Anesthesiology* **60**, 353

Cullen, D.J. and Eger, E.I. (1974) Cardiovascular effects of carbon dioxide in man. *Anesthesiology* **41**, 345

Cunningham, D.J.C. (1974) The control system regulating breathing in man. *Q. Rev. Biophys.* **6**, 433

Cunningham, D.J.C. and Ward, S.A. (1975a) The form of the respiratory interaction between an alternate-breath oscillation of $PACO_2$ and hypoxia in man. *J. Physiol.* **251**, 37P

Cunningham, D.J.C. and Ward, S.A. (1975b) The separate effects of alternate-breath oscillations of $PACO_2$ during hypoxia on inspiration and expiration. *J. Physiol.* **252**, 33P

Cunningham, D.J.C., Howson, M.G. and Pearson, S.B. (1973) The respiratory effects in man of altering the time profile of alveolar CO_2 and O_2 within each respiratory cycle. *J. Physiol.* **234**, 1

Cunningham, D.J.C., Kay, R.H. and Young, J.M. (1965) A fast response paramagnetic oxygen analyser. *J. Physiol.* **181**, 15P

Cunningham, D.J.C., Hey, E.N., Patrick, J.M. and Lloyd, B.B. (1963) The effect of noradrenalin infusion on the relation between pulmonary ventilation and the alveolar PO_2 and PCO_2 in man. *Ann. N.Y. Acad. Sci.* **109**, 756

Cushley, M.J., Tattersfield, A.E. and Holgate, S.T. (1984) Adenosine-induced bronchoconstriction in asthma. *Am. Rev. resp. Dis.* **129**, 380

Dail, C.W., Affeldt, J.E. and Collier, C.R. (1955) Clinical aspects of glossopharyngeal breathing. *J. Am. med. Ass.* **158**, 445

Dalhamn, T. and Rylander, R. (1965) Ciliastatic action of cigarette smoke. *Archs Otolaryngol.* **81**, 379

Daly, I. de B. and Daly, M. de B. (1959) The effects of stimulation of the carotid body chemoreceptors on the pulmonary vascular bed in the dog. *J. Physiol.* **148**, 201

Daly, N.J., Ross, J.C. and Behnke, R.H. (1963) The effect of changes in the pulmonary vascular bed produced by atropine, pulmonary engorgement and positive pressure breathing on diffusing and mechanical capacity of the lung. *J. clin. Invest.* **42**, 1083

Dann, W.L. (1971) The effects of different levels of ventilation in the action of pancuronium in man. *Br. J. Anaesth.* **43**, 959

Dantzker, D.R., Lynch, J.P. and Weg, J.G. (1980) Depression of cardiac output is a mechanism of shunt reduction in the therapy of acute respiratory failure. *Chest* **77**, 636

Dantzker, D.R., Wagner, P.D. and West, J.G. (1975) Instability of lung units with low V̇A/Q̇ ratios during O_2 breathing. *J. appl. Physiol.* **38**, 886

Dantzker, D.R., Brock, C.J., Dehart, P., Lynch, J.P. and Weg, J.G. (1979) Ventilation–perfusion distributions in adult respiratory distress syndrome. *Am. Rev. resp. Dis.* **120**, 1039

Datta, H., Stubbs, W.A. and Alberti, K.G.M.M. (1980) Substrate utilization by the lung. In: *Metabolic Activities of the Lung*, Ciba Foundation Symposium, no. 78. Amsterdam: Excerpta Medica

Davenport, H.T. and Valman, H.B. (1980) Resuscitation of the newborn. In: *General Anaesthesia*, 4th edn, vol. 2, edited by T.C. Gray, J.F. Nunn and J.E. Utting. London: Butterworths

Davidson, J.T., Whipp, B.J., Wasserman, K., Koyal, S.N. and Lugliani, R. (1974) Role of carotid bodies in breath-holding. *New Engl. J. Med.* **290**, 819

Davies, R.O., Edwards, M.W. and Lahiri, S. (1982) Halothane depresses the response of carotid body chemoreceptors to hypoxia and hypercapnia in the cat. *Anesthesiology* **57**, 153

Dawes, G.S. (1968) *Fetal and Neonatal Physiology*. Chicago: Year Book Publishers

Dawes, G.S., Fox, H.E., Leduc, B.M., Liggins, G.C. and Richards, R.T. (1972) Respiratory movements and rapid eye movement sleep in the foetal lamb. *J. Physiol.* **220**, 119

Defares, J.G., Lundin, G., Arborelius, M., Stromblad, R. and Svanberg, L. (1960) Effect of 'unilateral hypoxia' on pulmonary blood flow distribution in normal subjects. *J. appl. Physiol.* **15**, 169

DeFouw, D.O. (1983) Ultrastructural features of alveolar epithelial transport. *Am. Rev. resp. Dis.* **127**, S9

Dejours, P. (1962) Chemoreflexes in breathing. *Physiol. Rev.* **42**, 335

Dejours, P. (1964) Control of respiration in muscular exercise. *Handbk Physiol., section* 3, **1**, 631

Del Maestro, R.F. (1980) An approach to free radicals in medicine and biology. *Acta physiol. scand.* suppl. 492, 153

Delivoria-Papadopoulos, M., Roncevic, N.P. and Oski, F.A. (1971) Postnatal changes in oxygen transport of term, premature, and sick infants. *Pediat. Res.* **5**, 235

DeMaria, E.J., Reichman, W., Kenney, P.R., Armitage, J.M. and Gann, D.S. (1985) Septic complications of corticosteroid administration after central nervous system trauma. *Ann. Surg.* **202**, 248

Dempsey, J.A., Forster, H.V. and doPico, G.A. (1974) Ventilatory acclimatization to moderate hypoxemia in man. *J. clin. Invest.* **53**, 1091

Denison, D.M. (1984) Geometric estimates of lung and chest wall function. In: *Techniques in Respiratory Physiology,* Part II, edited by A.B. Otis. Amsterdam: Elsevier

Denison, D.M., Ernsting, J. and Cresswell, A.W. (1966) Fire and hyperbaric oxygen. *Lancet* **2**, 1404

Denison, D., Edwards, R.H.T., Jones, G. and Pope, H. (1971) Estimates of the CO_2 pressures in systemic arterial blood during rebreathing on exercise. *Resp. Physiol.* **11**, 186

Dickinson, J.G. (1985) Terminology and classification of acute mountain sickness. *Br. med. J.* **285**, 720

Dickinson, J., Heath, D., Gosney, J. and Williams, D. (1983) Altitude-related deaths in seven trekkers in the Himalayas. *Thorax* **38**, 646

Doll, R. and Hill, A.B. (1950) Smoking and carcinoma of the lung. *Br. med. J.* **2**, 739

Doll, R. and Peto, M. (1976) Mortality in relation to smoking: 20 years' observations on male British doctors. *Br. med. J.* **2**, 1525

Dollfuss, R.E., Milic-Emili, J. and Bates, D.V. (1967) Regional ventilation of the lung studied with boluses of ^{133}xenon. *Resp. Physiol.* **2**, 234

Don, H.F., Wahba, W.M. and Craig, D.B. (1972) Airway closure, gas trapping, and the functional residual capacity during anesthesia. *Anesthesiology* **36**, 533

Don, H.F., Wahba, M., Cuadrado, L. and Kelkar, K. (1970) The effects of anesthesia and 100 per cent oxygen on the functional residual capacity of the lungs. *Anesthesiology* **32**, 521

Donald, K.W. (1947) Oxygen poisoning in man. *Br. med. J.* **1**, 667 and 712

Donald, K.W. and Christie, R.V. (1949) A new method of clinical spirometry. *Clin. Sci.* **8**, 21

Donald, K.W., Renzetti, A., Riley, R.L. and Cournand, A. (1952) Analysis of factors affecting the concentrations of oxygen and carbon dioxide in gas and blood of lungs: results. *J. appl. Physiol.* **4**, 497

Donald, K.W., Bishop, J.M., Cumming, G. and Wade, O.L. (1953) Effect of nursing positions on cardiac output in man. *Clin. Sci.* **12**, 199

Douglas, C.G. and Haldane, J.S. (1909) The causes of periodic or Cheyne–Stokes breathing. *J. Physiol.* **38**, 401

Douglas, N.J., White, D.P., Pickett, C.K., Weil, J.V. and Zwillich, C.W. (1982) Respiration during sleep in normal man. *Thorax* **37**, 840

Dowman, C.E. (1927) Relief of diaphragmatic tic, following encephalitis, by section of phrenic nerves. *J. Am. med. Ass.* **88**, 95

Down, R.H.L. and Castleden, W.M. (1975) Oxygen therapy for pneumatosis coli. *Br. med. J.* **1**, 493

Downs, J.B. and Chapman, R.L. (1976) Treatment of bronchopleural fistula during continuous positive pressure ventilation. *Chest* **69**, 363

Downs, J.B., Perkins, H.M. and Modell, J.H. (1974) IMV — an evaluation. *Archs Surg.* **109**, 519

Draper, W.B. and Whitehead, R.W. (1944) Diffusion respiration in the dog anesthetized by pentothal sodium. *Anesthesiology* **5**, 262

DuBois, A.B., Botelho, S.Y. and Comroe, J.H. (1956) A new method of measuring airway resistance in man using a body plethysmograph. *J. clin. Invest.* **35**, 327

DuBois, A.B., Botelho, S.Y., Bedell, G.N., Marshall, R. and Comroe, J.H. (1956) A rapid plethysmographic method for measuring thoracic gas volume. *J. clin. Invest.* **35**, 322

Dueck, R., Young, I., Clausen, J. and Wagner, P.D. (1980) Altered distribution of pulmonary ventilation and blood flow following induction of inhalational anesthesia. *Anesthesiology* **52**, 113

Duffin, J., Triscott, A. and Whitwam, J.G. (1976) The effect of halothane and thiopentone on ventilatory responses mediated by the peripheral chemoreceptors in man. *Br. J. Anaesth.* **48**, 975

Duke, H.N. (1954) The site of action of anoxia on the pulmonary blood vessels of the cat. *J. Physiol.* **125**, 373

Dunbar, B.S., Ovassapian, A. and Smith, T.C. (1967) The effects of methoxyflurane on ventilation in man. *Anesthesiology* **28**, 1020

Dutton, R.E., Fitzgerald, R.S. and Gross, N. (1968) Ventilatory response to square-wave forcing of carbon dioxide at the carotid bodies. *Resp. Physiol.* **4**, 101

Dymond, J.H. and Smith, E.B. (1969) *The Virial Coefficients of Gases: a critical compilation.* Oxford: Oxford University Press

Eckenhoff, J.E., Enderby, G.E.H., Larson, A., Edridge, A. and Judevine, D.E. (1963) Pulmonary gas exchange during deliberate hypotension. *Br. J. Anaesth.* **35**, 750

Edlund, A., Bonfim, W., Kaijser, L., Olin, C., Patrono, C., Pinca, E. and Wennmalm, W. (1981) Pulmonary formation of prostacyclin in man. *Prostaglandins* **22**, 323

Edward, J.F. (1960) Inter-atrial communication. In: *Pathology of the Heart,* edited by J.E. Gould Springfield, Ill: Charles C Thomas

Effros, R.M. and Mason, G.R. (1983) Measurements of pulmonary epithelial permeability in vivo. *Am. Rev. resp. Dis.* **127**, S59

Eger, E.I. (1981) Isoflurane: a review. *Anesthesiology* **55**, 559

Eger, E.I., Dolan, W.M., Stevens, W.C., Miller, R.D. and Way, W.L. (1972) Surgical stimulation antagonizes the respiratory depression produced by forane. *Anesthesiology* **36**, 544

Eisele, J.H., Eger, E.I. and Muallem, M. (1967) Narcotic properties of carbon dioxide in the dog. *Anesthesiology* **28**, 856

Eisele, J.H., Trenchard, D., Burki, N. and Guz, A. (1968) The effect of chest wall block on respiratory sensation and control in man. *Clin. Sci.* **35**, 23

Eisele, J.H., Noble, M.I.M., Katz, J., Fung, D.L. and Hickey, R.F. (1972) Bilateral phrenic-nerve block in man. *Anesthesiology* **37**, 64

Elam, J.O. (1962) In: *Artificial Respiration,* edited by J.L. Whittenberger. New York and London: Harper and Row

Elam, J.O. and Greene, D.G. (1962) In: *Artificial Respiration,* edited by J.L. Whittenberger. New York and London: Harper and Row

Elliott, S.E., Segger, F.J. and Osborn, J.J. (1966) A modified oxygen gauge for the rapid measurement of Po_2 in respiratory gases. *J. appl. Physiol.* **21**, 1672

Ellis, F.R. and Nunn, J.F. (1968) The measurement of gaseous oxygen tension utilising paramagnetism: an evaluation of the Servomex OA 150 analyser. *Br. J. Anaesth.* **40**, 569

Ellis, H. and Feldman, S. (1983) *Anatomy for Anaesthetists,* 4th edn. Oxford: Blackwell Scientific

Ellison, R.G., Ellison, L.T. and Hamilton, W.F. (1955) Analysis of respiratory acidosis during anaesthesia. *Ann. Surg.* **141**, 375

Enghoff, H. (1931) Zur Frage des schädlichen Raumes bei der Atmung. *Skand. Arch. Physiol.* **63**, 15

Enghoff, H. (1938) Volumen inefficax. Bemerkungen zur Frage des schädlichen Raumes. *Uppsala Läk För Förh.* **44**, 191

Enghoff, H., Holmdahl, M. H:son and Risholm, L. (1951) Diffusion respiration in man. *Nature* **168**, 830

Ernsting, J. (1963) The effect of brief profound hypoxia upon the arterial and venous oxygen tensions in man. *J. Physiol.* **169**, 292

Ernsting, J. and McHardy, G.J.R. (1960) Brief anoxia following rapid decompression from 560 to 150 mmHg. *J. Physiol.* **153**, 73P

Eve, F.C. (1932) Actuation of the inert diaphragm by a gravity method. *Lancet* **2**, 995

Ezi-Ashi, T.I., Papworth, D.P. and Nunn, J.F. (1983) Inhalational anaesthesia in developing countries. *Anaesthesia* **38**, 736

Fairley, H.B. and Blenkarn, G.D. (1966) Effect on pulmonary gas exchange of variations in inspiratory flow rate during intermittent positive pressure ventilation. *Br. J. Anaesth.* **38**, 320

Fairweather, L.J., Walker, J. and Flenley, D.C. (1974) 2,3-Diphosphoglycerate concentrations and the dissociation of oxyhaemoglobin in ventilatory failure. *Clin. Sci.* **47**, 577

Faithfull, N. S. (1987) Fluorocarbons — current status and future applications. *Anaesthesia* **42**, 234

Fanta, C.H. and Drazen, J.M. (1983) Calcium blockers and bronchoconstriction. *Am. Rev. resp. Dis.* **127**, 673

Fantone, J.C. and Ward, P.A. (1982) Role of oxygen-derived free radicals and metabolites in leukocyte-dependent inflammatory reactions. *Am. J. Pathol.* **107**, 397

Farhi, L.I. (1964) Gas stores of the body. *Handbk Physiol., section 3*, **1**, 873

Featherstone, R.M., Muehlbaecher, C.A., DeBon, F.L. and Forsaith, J.A. (1961) Interactions of inert gases with proteins. *Anesthesiology* **22**, 6

Fein, A.M., Goldberg, S.K., Lippmann, M.L., Fischer, R. and Morgan, L. (1982) Adult respiratory distress syndrome. *Br. J. Anaesth.* **54**, 723

Fein, A.M., Lippmann, M., Holtzman, H., Eliraz, A. and Goldberg, S.K. (1983) The risk factors, incidence, and prognosis of ARDS following septicemia. *Chest* **83**, 40

Femi-Pearse, D., Afonja, A.O., Elegbeleye, O.O. and Odusote, K.A. (1976) Value of determination of oxygen consumption in tetanus. *Br. med. J.* **1**, 74

Fencl, V., Miller, T.B. and Pappenheimer, J.R. (1966) Studies of the respiratory response to disturbances of acid–base balance, with deductions concerning the ionic composition of cerebral interstitial fluid. *Am. J. Physiol.* **210**, 459

Fenn, W.O. and Asano, T. (1956) Effects of carbon dioxide inhalation on potassium liberation from the liver. *Am. J. Physiol.* **185**, 567

Fenn, W.O., Otis, A.B., Rahn, H., Chadwick, L.E. and Hegnauer, A.H. (1947) Displacement of blood from the lungs by pressure breathing. *Am. J. Physiol.* **151**, 258

Ferguson, J.K.W. (1936) Carbamino compounds of CO_2 with human haemoglobin and their role in the transport of CO_2. *J. Physiol.* **88**, 40

Ferguson, J.K.W. and Roughton, F.J.W. (1934) The direct chemical estimation of carbamino compounds of CO_2 with haemoglobin. *J. Physiol.* **83**, 68

Ferris, B.G., Mead, J., Whittenberger, J.L. and Saxton, G.A. (1952) Pulmonary function in convalescent poliomyelitis patients. 3. Compliance of the lungs and thorax. *New Engl. J. Med.* **40**, 664

Ferris, E.B., Engel, G.L., Stevens, C.D. and Webb, J. (1946) Voluntary breath holding. *J. clin. Invest.* **25**, 734

Filley, G.F., MacIntosh, D.J. and Wright, G.W. (1954) Carbon monoxide uptake and pulmonary diffusing capacity in normal subject at rest and during exercise. *J. clin. Invest.* **33**, 530

Fink, B.R. (1961) Influence of cerebral activity in wakefulness on regulation of breathing. *J. appl. Physiol.* **16**, 15

Fink, B.R. and Demarest, R.J. (1978) *Laryngeal Mechanics*. Cambridge, Mass: Harvard University Press

Fink, B.R., Ngai, S.H. and Holaday, D.A. (1958) Effect of air flow resistance on ventilation and respiratory muscle activity. *J. Am. med. Ass.* **168**, 2245

Finlayson, D.C. and Kaplan, J.A. (1979) Cardiopulmonary bypass. In: *Cardiac Anesthesia*, edited by J.A. Kaplan. London: Grune & Stratton

Finley, T.N., Swenson, E.W. and Comroe, J.H. (1962) The cause of arterial hypoxemia at rest in patients with 'alveolar–capillary block syndrome'. *J. clin. Invest.* **41**, 618

Finucane, K.E. and Colebatch, H.J.H. (1969) Elastic behavior of the lung in patients with airway obstruction. *J. appl. Physiol.* **26**, 330

Fischer, B.H., Marks, M. and Reich, T. (1983) Hyperbaric-oxygen treatment of multiple sclerosis. A randomized, placebo-controlled, double-blind study. *New Engl. J. Med.* **308,** 181

Fisher, A.B. and Forman, H.J. (1985) Oxygen utilization and toxicity in the lungs. *Handbook Physiol. section 3,* **1,** 231

Fishman, A.P. (1972) Pulmonary oedema. The water exchanging function of the lung. *Circulation* **46,** 390

Fishman, A.P. (1980) Vasomotor regulation of the pulmonary circulation. *A. Rev. Physiol.* **42,** 211

Fishman, A.P. (1985) Pulmonary circulation. *Handbk Physiol. section 3,* **1,** 93

Fleming, P.J. and Ponte, J. (1983) Control of respiration in the fetus and newborn. In: *Control of Respiration,* edited by D.J. Pallot. London: Croom Helm

Flenley, D.C. (1985a) Long-term home oxygen therapy. *Chest* **87,** 99

Flenley, D.C. (1985b) Disordered breathing during sleep. *Jl R. Soc. Med.* **78,** 1031

Flenley, D.C. (1985c) In: *Asthma and Bronchial Hyper-reactivity. Progress in Respiration Research 19,* edited by H. Herzog and A. Perruchoud. Basel: Karger

Flenley, D.C., Fairweather, L.J., Cooke, N.J. and Kirby, B.J. (1975) Changes in haemoglobin binding curve and oxygen transport in chronic hypoxic lung disease. *Br. med. J.* **1,** 602

Fletcher, R. (1984) Airway dead space, end-tidal CO_2 and Christian Bohr. *Acta anaesth. scand.* **28,** 408

Flynn, J.T. (1984) Oxygen and retrolental fibroplasia: update and challenge. *Anesthesiology* **60,** 397

Foëx, P. (1980) Effects of carbon dioxide on the systemic circulation. In: *The Circulation in Anaesthesia,* edited by C. Prys-Roberts. Oxford: Blackwell Scientific

Folkow, B. and Pappenheimer, J.R. (1955) Components of the respiratory dead space and their variation with pressure breathing and with broncho-active drugs. *J. appl. Physiol.* **8,** 102

Forrest, J.B. (1972) The effect of hyperventilation on pulmonary surface activity. *Br. J. Anaesth.* **44,** 313

Forster, H.V., Dempsey, J.A. and Chosy, L.W. (1975) Incomplete compensation of CSF $[H^+]$ in man during acclimatization to high altitude (4,300 m). *J. appl. Physiol.* **38,** 1067

Forster, H.V., Dempsey, J.A., Thomson, J., Vidruk, E. and doPico, G.A. (1972) Estimation of arterial P_{O_2}, P_{CO_2}, pH and lactate from arterialized venous blood. *J. appl. Physiol.* **32,** 134

Forster, R.E. (1964a) Rate of gas uptake by red cells. *Handbk Physiol., section 3,* **1,** 827

Forster, R.E. (1964b) Diffusion of gases. *Handbk Physiol., section 3,* **1,** 839

Foster, C.A. (1965) Hyperbaric oxygen and radiotherapy. In: *Hyperbaric Oxygenation,* edited by I. Ledingham. Edinburgh and London: Churchill Livingstone

Fourcade, H.E., Larson, C.P., Hickey, R.F., Bahlman, S.H. and Eger, E.I. (1972) Effects of time on ventilation during halothane and cyclopropane anesthesia. *Anesthesiology* **36,** 83

Fowler, A.A., Hamman, R.F., Good, J.T. et al (1983) Adult respiratory distress syndrome: risk with common predispositions. *Ann. intern. Med.* **98,** 593

Fowler, K.T. and Hugh-Jones, P. (1957) Mass spectrometry applied to clinical practice and research. *Br. med. J.* **1,** 1205

Fowler, W.S. (1948) Lung function studies. II. The respiratory dead space. *Am. J. Physiol.* **154,** 405

Fowler, W.S. (1950a) Lung function studies. IV. Postural changes in respiratory dead space and functional residual capacity *J. clin. Invest.* **29,** 1437

Fowler, W.S. (1950b) Lung function studies. V. Respiratory dead space in old age and in pulmonary emphysema. *J. clin. Invest.* **29,** 1439

Fowler, W.S. (1954) Breaking point of breath-holding. *J. appl. Physiol* **6,** 539

Fowler, W.S. and Blakemore, W.S. (1951) Lung function studies. VII. The effect of pneumonectomy on respiratory dead space. *J. thorac. Surg.* **21,** 433

Frank, L., Summerville, J. and Massaro, D. (1980) Protection from oxygen toxicity with endotoxin: role of the endogenous antioxidant enzymes of the lung. *J. clin. Invest.* **65,** 1104

Frayser, R., Rennie, I.D., Gray, G.W. and Houston, C.S. (1975) Hormonal and electrolyte response to exposure to 17,500 ft. *J. appl. Physiol.* **38,** 636

Freeman, B.A. and Crapo, J.D., (1981) Hyperoxia increases oxygen radical production in rat lungs and lung mitochondria. *J. biol. Chem.* **256,** 10986

Freeman, B.A., Topolsky, M.K. and Crapo, J.D. (1982) Hyperoxia increases oxygen radical production in rat lung homogenates. *Archs Biochem. Biophys.* **216,** 477

Freeman, J. (1962) Survival of bled dogs after halothane and ether anaesthesia. *Br. J. Anaesth.* **34,** 832

Freeman, J. and Nunn, J.F. (1963) Ventilation–perfusion relationships after haemorrhage. *Clin. Sci.* **24,** 135

Freund, F., Roos, A. and Dodd, R.B. (1964) Expiratory activity of the abdominal muscles in man during general anesthesia. *J. appl. Physiol.* **19,** 693

Froese, A.B. (1985) Effects of anesthesia and paralysis on the chest wall. In: *Effects of Anesthesia,* edited by B.G. Covino, H.A. Fozzard, K. Rehder and G. Strichartz. Bethesda, Md: American Physiological Society

Froese, A.B. and Bryan, A.C. (1974) Effects of anesthesia and paralysis on diaphragmatic mechanics in man. *Anesthesiology* **41,** 242

Froman, C. (1966) Correction of cerebrospinal fluid metabolic acidosis by intrathecal injection of bicarbonate. *Br. J. Anaesth.* **39,** 90

Froman, C. and Crampton-Smith. A. (1966) Hyperventilation associated with low pH of cerebrospinal fluid after intracranial haemorrhage. *Lancet* **1,** 780

Frumin, M.J., Epstein, R.M. and Cohen, G. (1959) Apneic oxygenation in man. *Anesthesiology* **20,** 789

Fujita, S., Zorick, F., Conway, W., Roth, T., Hartse, K.M. and Piccone, P. (1980) Uvulo-palato-pharyngoplasty: a new surgical treatment for upper airway sleep apnea. *Sleep Res.* **9,** 197

Fuleihan, S., Wilson, R.S. and Pontoppidan, H. (1976) Effect of mechanical ventilation with end-inspiratory pause on blood-gas exchange. *Anesth. Analg.* **55,** 122

Furuya, H. and Okumura, F. (1984) Detection of paradoxical air embolism by transeophageal echocardiography. *Anesthesiology* **60,** 374

Gail, D.B. and Lenfant, C.J.M. (1983) Cells of the lung: biology and clinical implications. *Am. Rev. resp. Dis.* **127,** 366

Gattinoni, L., Pesenti, A., Rossi, G.P. et al. (1980) Treatment of acute respiratory failure with low-frequency positive-pressure ventilation and extracorporeal removal of CO_2. *Lancet* **2,** 292

Gattinoni, L., Pesenti, A., Kolobow, T. and Damia, G. (1983) A new look at therapy of the adult respiratory distress syndrome: motionless lungs. *Int. Anesth. Clins* **21,** 97

Gautier, H. and Bertrand, F. (1975) Respiratory effects of pneumotaxic center lesions and subsequent vagotomy in chronic cats. *Resp. Physiol.* **23,** 71

Geddes, I.C. (1967) Recent studies in metabolic aspects of anaesthesia. In: *Modern Trends in Anesthesia—3,* edited by F.T. Evans and T.C. Gray. London: Butterworths

Geddes, D.M., Nesbitt, K., Traill, T. and Blackburn, J.P. (1979) First pass uptake of ^{14}C-propranolol by the lung. *Thorax* **34,** 810

Gee, M.H. and Williams, D.O. (1979) Effect of lung inflation on perivascular cuff fluid volume in isolated dog lung lobes. *Microvasc. Res.* **17,** 192

Gehr, P., Bachofen, M. and Weibel, E.R. (1978) The normal lung: ultrastructure and morphometric estimation of diffusion capacity. *Resp. Physiol.* **32,** 121

Georg, G., Lassen, N.A., Mellemgaard, K. and Vinther, A. (1965) Diffusion in the gas phase of the lungs in normal and emphysematous subjects. *Clin. Sci.* **29,** 525

Gerrard, J.W., Cockcroft, D.W., Mink, J.T., Cotton, D.J., Poonawala, R. and Dosman, J.A. (1980) Increased nonspecific bronchial reactivity in cigarette smokers with normal lung function. *Am. Rev. resp. Dis.* **122,** 577

Gersh, B.J. (1980) Measurement of intravascular pressures. In: *The Circulation in Anesthesia,* edited by C. Prys-Roberts. Oxford: Blackwell Scientific

Gerst, P.H., Rattenborg, C. and Holaday, D.A. (1959) The effects of hemorrhage on pulmonary circulation and respiratory gas exchange. *J. clin. Invest.* **38,** 524

Gessell, R. (1923) On the chemical regulation of respiration. *Am. J. Physiol.* **66,** 5

Giammona, S.T. and Modell, J.H. (1967) Drowning by total immersion. Effects on pulmonary surfactant of distilled water, isotonic saline and sea water. *Am. J. Dis. Child.* **114,** 612

Gibney, R.T., Wilson, R.S. and Pontoppidan, H. (1982) Comparison of work of breathing on high gas flow and demand valve continuous positive airway pressure systems. *Chest* **82,** 692

Gilbe, C.E., Salt, J.C. and Branthwaite, M.A. (1980) Pulmonary function after prolonged mechanical ventilation with high concentrations of oxygen. *Thorax* **35,** 907

Gillis, C.N. (1973) Metabolism of vasoactive hormones by lung. *Anesthesiology* **39**, 626

Gillis, C.N. and Pitt, B.R. (1982) The fate of circulating amines with the pulmonary circulation. *A. Rev. Physiol.* **44**, 269

Ginn, R. and Vane, J.R. (1968) Disappearance of catecholamines from the circulation. *Nature* **219**, 740

Glauser, F.L. and Fairman, R.P. (1985) The uncertain role of the neutrophil in increased permeability pulmonary edema. *Chest* **88**, 601

Glazier, J.B., Hughes, J.M.B., Maloney, J.E. and West, J.B. (1967) Vertical gradient of alveolar size in lungs of dogs frozen intact. *J. appl. Physiol.* **23**, 694

Glazier, J.B., Hughes, J.M.B., Maloney, J.E. and West, J.B. (1969) Measurements of capillary dimensions and blood volume in rapidly frozen lungs. *J. appl. Physiol.* **26**, 65

Glossop, M.W. (1963) A simple method for the estimation of carbon dioxide concentration in the presence of nitrous oxide. *Br. J. Anaesth.* **35**, 17

Gluck, L. (1971) Biochemical development of the lung. *Clin. Obstet. Gynec.* **14**, 710

Gluck, L., Kulovich, M.V., Borer, R.C., Brenner, P.H., Anderson, G.G. and Spellacy, W.N. (1971) Diagnosis of the respiratory distress syndrome by amniocentesis. *Am. J. Obstet. Gynec.* **109**, 440

Godfrey, S. and Wolf. E. (1972) An evaluation of rebreathing methods for measuring mixed venous P_{CO_2} during exercise. *Clin. Sci.* **42**, 345

Gold, M.I. and Helrich, M. (1967) Ventilation and blood gases in anaesthetized patients. *Can. Anaesth. Soc. J.* **14**, 424

Goldman, M., Knudson, R.J., Mead, J., Paterson, N., Schwaber, J.R. and Wohl, M.E. (1970) A simplified measurement of respiratory resistance by forced oscillation. *J. apply. Physiol.* **28**, 113

Gooden, B.A. (1982) The diving response in clinical medicine. *Aviat. Space Environ. Med.* **53**, 273

Gordh, T. (1945) Postural circulatory and respiratory changes during ether and intravenous anesthesia. *Acta chir. scand.* **92**, suppl. 102, 26

Gothard, J.W.W. and Branthwaite, M.A. (1984) The effects of thoracic surgery. In: *Effects of anesthesia and surgery on pulmonary mechanisms and gas exchange. International Anesthesiology Clinics,* vol. 22, no. 4, edited by J.G. Jones. Boston, Mass: Little, Brown

Gracey, D.R., Divertie, M.B. and Brown, A.L. (1968) Alveolar–capillary membrane in idiopathic interstitial pulmonary fibrosis. *Am. Rev. resp. Dis.* **98**, 16

Graham, G.R., Hill, D.W. and Nunn, J.F. (1960) Die Wirkung hoher CO_2 -Konzentrationen auf Kreislauf und Atmung. *Anaesthesist* **9**, 70

Granit, R. (1955) *Receptors and Sensory Perception.* New Haven, Ct, and London: Yale University Press

Gray, L.H., Conger, A.D., Ebert, M., Hornsey, S. and Scott, O.C.A. (1953) The concentration of oxygen dissolved in tissues at the time of irradiation as a factor in radiotherapy. *Br. J. Radiol.* **26**, 638

Gray, T.C. and Rees, G.J. (1952) The role of apnoea in anaesthesia for major surgery. *Br. med. J.* **2**, 891

Greenbaum, R., Nunn, J.F., Prys-Roberts, C., Kelman, G.R. and Silk, F.F. (1965) Cardio-pulmonary function after fat embolism. *Br. J. Anaesth.* **37**, 554

Greenbaum, R., Bay, J., Hargreaves, M.D., Kain, M.L., Kelman, G.R., Nunn, J.F., Prys-Roberts, C. and Siebold, K. (1967a) Effects of higher oxides of nitrogen on the anaesthetized dog. *Br. J. Anaesth.* **39**, 393

Greenbaum, R., Nunn, J.F., Prys-Roberts, C. and Kelman, G.R. (1967b) Metabolic changes in whole human blood (*in vitro*) at 37°C. *Resp. Physiol.* **2**, 274

Green, D.G., Bauer, R.O., Janney, C.D. and Elam, J.O. (1957) Oxygen and carbon dioxide exchange and energy cost of expired air resuscitation. *J. Am. med. Ass.* **167**, 328

Gregory, G.A. (1981) Resuscitation of the newborn. In: *Anesthesia,* vol. 2, edited by R.D. Miller. London: Churchill Livingstone

Gregory, G.A., Kitterman, J.A., Phibbs, P.H., Tooley, W.H. and Hamilton, W.K. (1971) Treatment of the idiopathic respiratory-distress syndrome with continuous positive airway pressure. *New Engl. J. Med.* **284**, 1333

Gregory, G.A., Eger, E.I., Smith, N.T. and Cullen, B.F. (1974) The cardiovascular effects of carbon dioxide in man awake and during diethyl ether anesthesia. *Anesthesiology* **40**, 301

Gregory, I.C. (1973) Assessment of Van Slyke manometric measurements of oxygen content. *J. appl. Physiol.* **34**, 715

Gregory, I.C. (1974) The oxygen and carbon monoxide capacities of foetal and adult blood. *J. Physiol.* **236**, 625

Grindlinger, G.A., Manny, J., Justice, R., Dunham, B., Shepro, D. and Hechtman, H.B. (1979) Presence of negative inotropic agents in canine plasma during positive end-expiratory pressure. *Circulation Res.* **45**, 460

Grollman, A. (1929) The determination of the cardiac output of man by the use of acetylene. *Am. J. Physiol.* **88**, 285

Guilleminault, C., van den Hoed, J. and Mitler, M.M. (1978) Clinical overview of the sleep apnea syndromes. In: *Sleep Apnea Syndromes,* edited by C. Guilleminault and W.C. Dement. New York: Alan R. Liss

Gurtner, G. and Burns, B. (1975) Physiological evidence consistent with the presence of a specific O_2 carrier in the placenta. *J. appl. Physiol.* **39**, 728

Gurtner, G.H. and Fowler, W.S. (1971) Interrelationships of factors affecting the pulmonary diffusing capacity. *J. appl. Physiol.* **30**, 619

Gutteridge, J.M.C., Rowley, D.A., Griffiths, E. and Halliwell, B. (1985) Low molecular weight iron complexes and oxygen radical reactions in idiopathic haemochromatosis. *Clin. Sci.* **68**, 463

Guz. A., Nobel, M.I.M., Trenchard, D., Cochrane, H.L. and Makey, A.R. (1964) Studies on the vagus nerves in man: their role in respiratory and circulatory control. *Clin. Sci.* **27**, 293

Guz, A., Noble, M.I.M., Widdicombe, J.G., Trenchard, D. and Mushin, W.W. (1966a) Peripheral chemoreceptor block in man. *Resp. Physiol.* **1**, 38

Guz, A., Noble, M.I.M., Widdicombe, J.G., Trenchard, D., Mushin, W.W. and Makey, A.R. (1966b) The role of the vagal and glossopharyngeal afferent nerves in respiratory sensation, control of breathing and arterial pressure regulation in conscious man. *Clin. Sci.* **30**, 161

Guz, A., Noble, M.I.M., Eisele, J.H. and Trenchard, D. (1971) The effect of lung deflation on breathing in man. *Clin. Sci.* **40**, 451

Hagberg, J.M., Mullin, J.P. and Nagle, F.J. (1978) Oxygen consumption during constant-load exercise. *J. appl. Physiol.* **45**, 381

Haldane, J.S. (1920) A new apparatus for accurate blood-gas analysis. *J. Path. Bact.* **23**, 443

Haldane, J.S. and Priestley, J.G. (1905) The regulation of the lung ventilation. *J. Physiol.* **32**, 225

Hales, S. (1731) *Vegetable Staticks: analysis of the air,* p. 240. London

Halliwell, B. and Gutteridge, J.M.C. (1985) *Free Radicals in Biology and Medicine.* Oxford: Clarendon Press

Halsey, M.J. (1982) The effects of high pressure on the central nervous system. *Physiol. Rev.* **62**, 1341

Halsey, M.J., Wardley-Smith, B. and Green, C.J. (1978) Pressure reversal of general anaesthesia — a multi-site expansion hypothesis. *Br. J. Anaesth.* **50**, 1091

Hamburger, H.J. (1918) Anionenwanderungen in serum und Blut unter dem Einfluss von CO_2. Säure und Alkali. *Biochem. Z.* **86**, 309

Hammerschmidt, D.E. (1983) Activation of the complement system and of granulocytes in lung injury: the adult respiratory distress syndrome. *Adv. Inflamm. Res.* **5**, 147

Hanks, E.C., Ngai, S.H. and Fink, B.R. (1961) The respiratory threshold for carbon dioxide in anesthetized man. *Anesthesiology* **22**, 393

Haponik, E.F., Smith, P.L., Bohlman, M.E., Allen, R.P., Goldman, S.M. and Bleecker, E.R. (1983) Computerized tomography in obstructive sleep apnea. *Am. Rev. resp. Dis.* **127**, 221

Hardy, C., Robinson, C., Lewis, R.A., Tattersfield, A.E. and Holgate, S.T. (1985) Airway and cardiovascular responses to inhaled prostacyclin in normal and asthmatic subjects. *Am. Rev. resp. Dis.* **131**, 18

Harlan, W.R. and Said, S.I. (1969) Selected aspects of lung metabolism. Chapter 12 in: *The Biological Basis of Medicine,* edited by E.E. Bittar and N. Bittar. New York and London: Academic Press

Harper, R.M. and Sauerland, E.K. (1978) The role of the tongue in sleep apnea. In: *Sleep Apnea Syndromes,* edited by C. Guilleminault and W.C. Dement. New York: Alan R. Liss

Harries, M.G. (1981) Drowning in man. *Crit. Care Med.* **9**, 407

Harris, E.A., Hunter, M.E., Seelye, E.R., Vedder, M. and Whitlock, R.M.L. (1973) Prediction of the physiological dead-space in resting normal subjects. *Clin. Sci.* **45,** 375

Harris, P. and Heath, D. (1962) *The Human Pulmonary Circulation.* Edinburgh and London: Churchill Livingstone

Hasselbalch, K.A. (1916) Berechnung der Wasserstoffzahl des Blutes usw. *Biochem. Z.* **78,** 112

von Hayek, H. (1960) *The Human Lung.* Translated from *Die Menschliche Lunge* by V.E. Krahl. New York and London: Hafner

Head, H. (1889) On the regulation of respiration. *J. Physiol.* **10,** 1

Heaton, R.W., Henderson, A.F. and Costello, J.F. (1984) Cold air as a bronchial provocation technique. *Chest* **86,** 810

Hedenstierna, G. (1985) Differential ventilation in bilateral lung disease. *Europ. J. Anaesthesiol.* **2,** 1

Hedenstierna, G. and McCarthy, G. (1975) Mechanics of breathing, gas distribution and functional residual capacity at different frequencies of respiration during spontaneous and artificial ventilations. *Br. J. Anaesth,* **47,** 706

Hedenstierna, G., Baehrendtz, S., Klingstedt, C., Santesson, J. Soderborg, B., Dhalborn, M. and Bindslev, L. (1984) Ventilation and perfusion of each lung during differential ventilation with selective PEEP. *Anesthesiology* **61,** 369

Hendenstierna, G., Standberg, A., Brismar, B., Lundquist, H., Svensson, L. and Tokics, L. (1985) Functional residual capacity, thoracoabdominal dimensions and central blood volume during general anesthesia with muscle paralysis and mechanical ventilation. *Anesthesiology* **62,** 247

Heijman, K., Heijman, L., Jonzon, A., Sedin, G., Sjostrand, U. and Widman, B. (1972) High frequency positive pressure ventilation during anesthesia and routine surgery in man. *Acta anesth. scand.* **16,** 176

Heller, M.L. and Watson, T.R. (1961) Polarographic study of arterial oxygenation during apnea in man. *New Engl. J. Med.* **264,** 326

Hemmingsen, A. and Scholander, P.E. (1960) Specific transport of oxygen through hemoglobin solutions. *Science* **132,** 1379

Hempleman, H.V. and Lockwood, A.P.M. (1978) *The Physiology of Diving in Man and Other Animals.* London: Edward Arnold

Henderson, L.J. (1909) Das Gleichgewicht zwischen Basen und Säuren im tierischen Organismus. *Ergebn. Physiol.* **8,** 254

Henderson, Y., Chillingworth, F.P. and Whitney, J.L. (1915) The respiratory dead space. *Am. J. Physiol.* **38,** 1

Heneghan, C.P.H., Bergman, N.A. and Jones, J.G. (1984) Changes in lung volume and $(PA_{O_2} - Pa_{O_2})$ during anaesthesia. *Br. J. Anaesth.* **56,** 437

Heneghan, C.P.H., Bergman, N.A., Jordan, C., Lehane, J.R. and Catley, D.M. (1986) Effect of isoflurane on bronchomotor tone in man. *Br. J. Anaesth.* **58,** 24

Herholdt, J.D. and Rafn, C.G. (1796) *Life-saving Methods for Drowning Persons.* Copenhagen: T. Tikiob. Reprinted in 1960; Aarhuus, Denmark: Stiftsbogtrykkerie

Hering, E. (1868) Die Selbsteuerung der Athmung durch den Nervus Vagus. *Sber. Akad. Wiss. Wien* **57,** 672

Hewlett, A.M., Platt, A.S. and Terry, V.G. (1977) Mandatory minute volume. *Anaesthesia* **32,** 163

Hewlett, A.M., Hulands, G.H., Nunn, J.F. and Minty, K.B. (1974a) Functional residual capacity during anaesthesia. I: Methodology. *Br. J. Anaesth.* **46,** 479

Hewlett, A.M., Hulands, G.H., Nunn, J.F. and Heath, J.R. (1974b) Functional residual capacity. II: Spontaneous respiration. *Br. J. Anaesth.* **46,** 486

Hewlett, A.M., Hulands, G.H., Nunn, J.F. and Milledge, J.S. (1974c) Functional residual capacity during anaesthesia. III: Artificial ventilation. *Br. J. Anaesth.* **46,** 495

Heymans, C. and Neil, E. (1958) *Reflexogenic Areas of the Cardiovascular System.* Boston, Mass: Little Brown; London: Churchill

Heymans, C., Bouckaert, J.J. and Dautrebande, L. (1930) Sinus carotidien et réflexes respiratoire. *Archs int. Pharmacodyn Thér.* **39,** 400

Heymans, J.F. and Heymans, C. (1927) Sur les modifications directes et sur la régulation reflexe de l'activité du centre respiratoire de la tête isolée du chien. *Archs int. Pharmacodyn. Thér.* **33,** 272

Hickey, R.F., Visick, W., Fairley, H.B. and Fourcade, H.E. (1973) Effects of halothane anesthesia on functional residual capacity and alveolar–arterial oxygen tension difference. *Anesthesiology* **38,** 20

Hickling, K.G. (1986) Extracorporeal CO_2 removal in severe adult respiratory distress syndrome. *Anaesth. intens. Care* **14,** 46

Hickling, K.G., Downward, G., Davis, F.M. and A'Court, G. (1986) Management of severe ARDS with low frequency positive pressure ventilation and extracorporeal CO_2 removal. *Anaesth. intens. Care* **14,** 79

Hickman, H.H. (1824). A letter on suspended animation. Ironbridge, W. Smith (addressed to T.A. Knight of Downton Castle)

Higgins, H.L. and Means, J.H. (1915) The effect of certain drugs on the respiration and gaseous metabolism in normal human subjects. *J. Pharmac. exp. Ther.* **7,** 1

Hill, J.D., Main, F.B., Osborn, J.J. and Gerbode, F. (1965) Correct use of respirator on cardiac patient after operation. *Archs Surg.* **91,** 775

Hillman, D.R. and Finucane, K.E. (1985) Continuous positive airway pressure: a breathing system to minimize work. *Crit. Care Med.* **13,** 38

Hills, B.A. (1982) What forces keep the air spaces of the lung dry? *Thorax* **37,** 713

Hoedt-Rasmussen, K., Skinhoj, E., Paulson, O., Ewald, J., Bjerrum, J.K., Fahrenkrug, A. and Lassen, N.A. (1967) Regional cerebral blood flow in acute apoplexy. The 'luxury perfusion syndrome' of brain tissue. *Archs Neurol.* **17,** 271

Hoff, H.E. and Breckenridge, C.G. (1949) The medullary origin of respiratory periodicity in the dog. *Am. J. Physiol.* **158,** 157

Hogben, L. (1951). *Mathematics for the Million,* 3rd edn. London: Allen and Unwin

Holmdahl, M. H:son. (1953) Apnoeic diffusion oxygenation in electroconvulsion therapy. *Acta Soc. Med. uppsal.* **58,** 269

Holmdahl, M. H:son (1956) Pulmonary uptake of oxygen acid–base metabolism and circulation during prolonged apnoea. *Acta chir. scand.* suppl. 212

Hornbein, T.F. and Pavlin, E.G. (1975) Distribution of H^+ and HCO_3^- between CSF and blood during respiratory alkalosis in dogs. *J. Physiol,* **228,** 1149

Hornbein, T.F. and Roos, A. (1963) Specificity of H ion concentration as a carotid chemoreceptor stimulus. *J. appl. Physiol.* **18,** 580

Hornbein, T.F., Griffo, Z.J. and Roos, A. (1961) Quantitation of chemoreceptor activity: interrelation of hypoxia and hypercapnia. *J. Neurophysiol.* **24,** 561

Howell, J.B.L., Permutt, S., Proctor, D.F. and Riley, R.L. (1961) Effect of inflation of the lung on different parts of pulmonary vascular bed. *J. appl. Physiol.* **16,** 71

Hughes, J.M.B., Glazier, J.B., Maloney, J.E. and West, J.B. (1968) Effect of lung volume on the distribution of pulmonary blood flow in man. *Resp. Physiol.* **4,** 58

Hughes, J.M.B., Grant, B.J.B., Greene, R.E., Iliff, L.D. and Milic-Emili, J. (1972) Inspiratory flow rate and ventilation distribution in normal subjects and in patients with simple chronic bronchitis. *Clin. Sci.* **43,** 583

Hughes, R. (1970) The influence of changes in acid–base balance on neuromuscular blockade in cats. *Br. J. Anaesth.* **42,** 658

Hugh-Jones, P. and West, J.B. (1960) Detection of bronchial and arterial obstruction by continuous gas analysis from individual lobes and segments of the lung. *Thorax* **15,** 154

Hulands, G.H., Green, R., Iliff, L.D. and Nunn, J.F. (1970) Influence of anaesthesia on the regional distribution of perfusion and ventilation in the lung. *Clin. Sci.* **38,** 451

Hultgren, H.N. (1978) High altitude pulmonary edema. In: *Lung Water and Solute Exchange,* edited by N. Staub. New York: Marcel Dekker

Hunninghake, G.W. and Crystal, R.G. (1983) Cigarette smoking and lung destruction. Accumulation of neutrophils in the lungs of cigarette smokers. *Am. Rev. resp. Dis.* **128,** 833

Hussain, S.N.A., Simkus, G. and Roussos, C. (1985) Respiratory muscle fatigue: a cause of ventilatory failure in septic shock. *J. appl. Physiol.* **58,** 2033

Hutchison, D.C.S., Flenley, D.C. and Donald, K.W. (1964) Controlled oxygen therapy in respiratory failure. *Br. med. J.* **2,** 1159

Hutchison, D.C.S., Cook, P.J.L., Barter, C.E., Harris, H. and Hugh-Jones, P. (1971) Pulmonary emphysema and α_1-antitrypsin deficiency. *Br. med. j.* **1**, 689

Hyatt, R.E., Zimmerman, I.R., Peters, G.M. and Sullivan, W.J. (1970) Direct write out of total respiratory resistance. *J. appl. Physiol.* **28**, 675

Ingvar, D.H. (1965) In: *Hyperbaric Oxygenation,* discussion page 199, edited by I. Ledingham. Edinburgh and London: Churchill Livingstone

Irwin, R.L., Draper, W.B. and Whitehead, R.W. (1957) Urine secretion during diffusion respiration after apnea from neuromuscular block. *Anesthesiology* **18**, 594

Ivanov, S.D. and Nunn, J.F. (1968) Influence of duration of hyperventilation on rise time of P_{CO_2} after step reduction of ventilation. *Resp. Physiol.* **4**, 243

Ivanov, S.D. and Nunn, J.F. (1969) Methods of elevation of P_{CO_2} for restoration of spontaneous breathing after artificial ventilation of anaesthetised patients. *Br. J. Anaesth.* **41**, 28

Jain, S.K., Trenchard, D., Reynolds, F., Noble, M.I.M. and Guz, A. (1973) The effect of local anaesthesia of the airway on respiratory reflexes in the rabbit. *Clin. Sci.* **44**, 519

Jarasch, E.-D., Grund, C., Bruder, G., Heid, H.W., Keenan, T.W. and Franke, W.W. (1981) Localization of xanthine oxidase in mammary-gland epithelium and capillary endothelium. *Cell* **25**, 67

Jardin, F., Farcot, J.-C., Boisante, L., Curien, N., Margairaz, A. and Bourdarias, J.-P. (1981) Influence of positive end-expiratory pressure on left ventricular performance. *New Engl. J. Med.* **304**, 387

Jennett, S. (1984) Snoring and its treatment. *Br. med. J.* **289**, 335

Jennett, W.B., McDowall, D.G. and Barker, J. (1967) The effect of halothane on intracranial pressure in cerebral tumours: report of two cases. *J. Neurosurg.* **26**, 270

Jerusalem, E. and Starling, E.H. (1910) On the significance of carbon dioxide for the heart beat. *J. Physiol.* **40**, 279

Johnson, S.R. (1951) The effect of some anesthetic agents on the circulation in man. *Acta chir. scand.* **102**, suppl. 158

Jones, J.G., Royston, D. and Minty, B.D. (1983) Changes in alveolar–capillary barrier function in animals and humans. *Am. Rev. resp. Dis.* **127**, S51

Jones, J.G., Faithfull, D., Jordan, C. and Minty, B. (1979) Rib cage movement during halothane anaesthesia in man. *Br. J. Anaesth.* **51**, 399

Jones, J.G., Minty, B.D., Lawler, P., Hulands, G., Crawley, J.C.W. and Veall, N. (1980) Increased alveolar epithelial permeability in cigarette smokers. *Lancet* **1**, 66

Jones, J.G., Minty, B.D., Royston, D. and Royston, J.P. (1983) Carboxyhaemoglobin and pulmonary epithelial permeability in man. *Thorax* **38**, 129

Jones, R.D., Commins, B.T. and Cernik, A.A. (1972) Blood lead and carboxyhaemoglobin levels in London taxi drivers. *Lancet* **2**, 302

Jorfeldt, L., Lewis, D.H., Löfström, J.B. and Post, C. (1979) Lung uptake of lidocaine in healthy volunteers. *Acta anaesth. scand.* **23**, 567

Juno, P., Marsh, M., Knopp, T.J. and Rehder, K. (1978) Closing capacity in awake and anesthetized–paralyzed man. *J. appl. Physiol.* **44**, 238

Junod, A.F. (1985) 5-Hydroxytryptamine and other amines in the lung. *Handbk Physiol. section 3,* **1**, 337

Kaasik, A.E., Nilsson, L. and Siesjö, B.K. (1970a) The effect of asphyxia upon the lactate, pyruvate and bicarbonate concentrations of brain tissue and cisternal CSF, and upon the tissue concentrations of phosphocreatine and adenine nucleotides in anesthetized rats. *Acta physiol. scand.* **78**, 433

Kaasik, A.E., Nilsson, L. and Siesjö, B.K. (1970b) The effect of arterial hypotension upon the lactate, pyruvate and bicarbonate concentrations of brain tissue and cisternal CSF, and upon the tissue concentrations of phosocreatine and adenine nucleotides in anesthetized rats. *Acta physiol. scand.* **78**, 448

Kain, M.L., Panday, J. and Nunn, J.F. (1969) The effect of intubation on the dead space during halothane anaesthesia. *Br. J. Anaesth.* **41**, 94

Kalia, M., Senapati, J.M., Parida, B. and Panda, A. (1972) Reflex increase in ventilation by muscle receptors with nonmedullated fibers (C fibers). *J. appl. Physiol.* **32**, 189

Kaneko, K., Milic-Emili, M.E., Dolovich, M.B., Dawson, A. and Bates, D.V. (1966) Regional distribution of ventilation and perfusion as a function of body position. *J. appl. Physiol.* **21**, 767

Kao, F.F. (1963) An experimental study of the pathways involved in exercise hyperpnoea employing cross-circulation techniques. In: *The Regulation of Human Respiration,* edited by D.J.C. Cunningham and B.B. Lloyd. Oxford: Blackwell Scientific

Kapp, J.R. (1981) Neurological response to hyperbaric oxygen — a criterion for cerebral revascularization. *Surg. Neurol.* **15,** 43.

Katz, J.A., Laverne, R.G., Fairley, H.B. and Thomas, A.N. (1982) Pulmonary oxygen exchange during endobronchial anesthesia. *Anesthesiology* **56,** 164

Katz, S. and Horres, A.D. (1972) Medullary respiratory neuron response to pulmonary emboli and pneumothorax. *J. appl. Physiol.* **33,** 390

Kaul, S.U., Heath, J.R. and Nunn, J.F. (1973) Factors influencing the development of expiratory muscle activity during anaesthesia. *Br. J. Anaesth.* **45,** 1013

Kaye, G.W.C. and Laby, T.H. (1966) *Tables of Physical and Chemical Constants,* 13th edn. London: Longman

Kelman, G.R. (1966) Digital computer subroutine for the conversion of oxygen tension into saturation. *J. appl. Physiol.* **21,** 1375

Kelman, G.R. (1971) *Applied Cardiovascular Physiology.* London and Boston, Mass: Butterworths

Kelman, G.R. and Nunn, J.F. (1966a) Clinical recognition of hypoxaemia under fluorescent lamps. *Lancet* **1,** 1400

Kelman, G.R. and Nunn, J.F. (1966b) Nomograms for correction of blood Po_2, Pco_2, pH and base excess for time and temperature. *J. appl. Physiol.* **21,** 1484

Kelman, G.R. and Nunn, J.F. (1968) *Computer Produced Physiological Tables.* London and Boston, Mass: Butterworths

Kelman, G.R. and Prys-Roberts C. (1967) Circulatory influences of artificial ventilation during nitrous oxide anaesthesia in man. I. Introduction and methods. *Br. J. Anaesth.* **39,** 523

Kelman, G.R., Coleman, A.J. and Nunn, J.F. (1966) Evaluation of a microtonometer used with a capillary glass pH electrode. *J. appl. Physiol.* **21,** 1103

Kelman, G.R., Nunn, J.F., Prys-Roberts, C. and Greenbaum, R. (1967) The influence of cardiac output on arterial oxygenation. *Br. J. Anaesth.* **39,** 450

Kelman, G.R., Swapp, G.H., Smith, I., Benzie, R.J. and Gordon, N.L.M. (1972) Cardiac output and arterial blood-gas tension during laparoscopy. *Br. J. Anaesth.* **44,** 1155

Kerr, J.H., Smith, A.C., Prys-Roberts, C., Melonche, R. and Foëx, P. (1974) Observations during endobronchial anaesthesia. II. Oxygenation. *Br. J. Anaesth.* **46,** 84

Kety, S.S. and Schmidt, C.F. (1948) The effects of altered arterial tensions of carbon dioxide and oxygen on cerebral blood flow and cerebral oxygen consumption of normal young men. *J. clin. Invest.* **27,** 500

Khanam, T. and Branthwaite, M.A. (1973) Arterial oxygenation during one-lung anaesthesia (2). *Anaesthesia* **28,** 280

Kilmartin, J.V. and Rossi-Bernardi, L. (1973) Interaction of hemoglobin with hydrogen ions, carbon dioxide, and organic phosphates. *Physiol. Rev.* **53,** 836

King, A.J., Cooke, N.J., Leitch, A.G. and Flenley, D.C. (1973) The effects of 30% oxygen on the respiratory response to treadmill exercise in chronic respiratory failure. *Clin. Sci.* **44,** 151

King, R.J. (1974) The surfactant system of the lung. *Fedn Proc.* **33,** 2238

King, R.J. and Clements, J.A. (1985) Lipid synthesis and surfactant turnover in the lungs. *Handbk Physiol. section 3,* **1,** 309

Kirby, R.R., Perry, J.C., Calderwood, H.W., Ruiz, B.C. and Lederman, D.S. (1975) Cardiorespiratory effects of high positive end-expiratory pressure. *Anesthesiology* **43,** 533

Klein, J., Trouwborst, A. and Salt, P.J. (1985) Endotoxin protection against oxygen toxicity and its reversal by acetylsalicylic acid. *Crit. Care Med.* **14,** 32

Klocke, F.J. and Rahn, H. (1959) Breath holding after breathing of oxygen. *J. appl. Physiol.* **14,** 689

Klocke, F.J. and Rahn, H. (1961) The arterial–alveolar inert gas ('N_2') difference in normal and emphysematous subjects, as indicated by the analysis of urine. *J. clin. Invest.* **40,** 286

Knill, R.L. and Clement, J.L. (1982) Variable effects of anaesthetics on the ventilatory response to hypoxaemia in man. *Can. Anaesth. Soc. J.* **29,** 93

Knill, R.L. and Clement, J.L. (1984) Site of selective action of halothane on the peripheral chemoreflex pathway in humans. *Anesthesiology* **61,** 121

Knill, R.L. and Clement, J.L. (1985) Ventilatory responses to acute metabolic acidemia in humans awake, sedated and anesthetized with halothane. *Anesthesiology* **62**, 745

Knill, R.L. and Gelb, A.W. (1978) Ventilatory responses to hypoxia and hypercapnia during halothane sedation and anesthesia in man. *Anesthesiology* **49**, 244

Koizumi, M., Frank, L. and Massaro, D. (1985) Oxygen toxicity in rats: varied effect of dexamethasone treatment depending on duration of hyperoxia. *Am. Rev. resp. Dis.* **131**, 907

Kolton, M.A. (1984) A review of high-frequency oscillation. *Can. Anaesth. Soc. J.* **31**, 416

Kolton, M., Cathran, C.B., Kent, G., Volgyesi, G., Froese, A.B. and Bryan, A.C. (1982) Oxygenation during high frequency ventilation compared with conventional mechanical ventilation in two models of lung injury. *Anesth. Analg.* **61**, 323

Krahl, V.E. (1964) Anatomy of the mammalian lung. *Handbk Physiol., section 3* **1**, 213

Kuida, H., Hinshaw, L.B., Gilbert, B.P. and Vischer, M.B. (1958) Effect of Gram-negative endotoxin on pulmonary circulation. *Am. J. Physiol.* **192**, 335

Kumar, A., Pontoppidan, H., Falke, K.J. et al. (1973) Pulmonary barotrauma during mechanical ventilation. *Crit. Care Med.* **1**, 181

Kusumi, F., Butts, W.C. and Ruff, W.L. (1973) Superior analytical performance by electrolytic cell analysis of blood oxygen content. *J. appl. Physiol.* **35**, 299

Lahiri, S. (1984) Respiratory control in Andean and Himalayan high-altitude natives. In: *High Altitude and Man,* edited by J.B. West and S. Lahiri. Bethesda, Md: American Physiological Society

Lambert, M.W. (1955) Accessory bronchiole–alveolar communications. *J. Path. Bact.* **70**, 311

Lambertsen, C.J. (1963) Factors in the stimulation of respiration by carbon dioxide. In: *The Regulation of Human Respiration,* edited by D.J.C. Cunningham and B.B. Lloyd. Oxford: Blackwell Scientific

Lambertsen, C.J. (1965) Effects of oxygen at high partial pressure. *Handbk Physiol., section 3* **2**, 1027

Lanphier, E.H. and Camporesi, E.M. (1982) Respiration and exercise. In: *The Physiology and Medicine of Diving,* edited by P.B. Bennett and D.H. Elliott. London: Baillière Tindall

Larson, C.P., Eger, E.I., Muallem, M., Buechel, D.R., Munson, E.S. and Eisele, J.H. (1969) The effects of diethyl ether and methoxyflurane on ventilation. *Anesthesiology* **30**, 174

Lassen, N.A. (1959) Cerebral blood flow and oxygen consumption in man. *Physiol. Rev.* **39**, 183

Lassen, N.A. (1966) The luxury perfusion syndrome and its possible relation to acute metabolic acidosis localized within the brain. *Lancet* **2**, 1113

Lassen, N.A. and Ingvar, D.H. (1961) The blood flow of the cerebral cortex determined by radioactive krypton-85. *Experientia* **17**, 42

Lassen, N.A. and Palvalgyi, R. (1968) Cerebral steal during hypercapnia and the inverse reaction during hypocapnia observed by the ^{133}Xe technique in man. *Scand. J. clin. Lab. Invest.* suppl. 102

Laurell, C.-B. and Eriksson, S. (1963) The electrophoretic α_1-globulin pattern of serum in α_1-antitrypsin deficiency. *Scand. J. clin. Lab. Invest.* **15**, 132

Laver, M.B. and Seifen, A. (1965) Measurement of blood oxygen tension in anesthesia. *Anesthesiology* **26**, 73

Lawler, P.G.P. (1987) Dead space/tidal volume measurements at best PEEP and at ZEEP. *Intens. Care Med.* in the press

Laws, A.K. (1968) Effects of induction of anaesthesia and muscle paralysis on functional residual capacity of the lungs. *Can. Anaesth. Soc. J.* **15**, 325

Leake, C.D. and Waters, R.M. (1928) The anesthetic properties of carbon dioxide. *J. Pharmac. exp. Ther.* **33**, 280

Leblanc, P., Ruff, F. and Milic-Emili, J. (1970) Effects of age and body position on 'airway closure' in man. *J. appl. Physiol.* **28**, 448

Ledingham, I. McA. and Norman, J.N. (1965) Metabolic effects of combined hypothermia and hyperbaric oxygen in experimental total circulatory arrest. In: *Hyperbaric Oxygenation,* edited by I. Ledingham. Edinburgh and London: Churchill Livingstone

Lee, G. de J. and DuBois, A.B. (1955) Pulmonary capillary blood flow in man. *J. clin. Invest.* **34**, 1380

Legallois, C. (1812) *Experiences sur le Principe de la Vie.* Paris: d'Hautel

Lehane, J.R., Jordan, C. and Jones, J.G. (1980) Influence of halothane and enflurane on respiratory airflow resistance and specific conductance in anaesthetized man. *Br. J. Anaesth.* **52,** 773

Lehmann, H. and Huntsman, R.G. (1966) *Man's Haemoglobin.* Amsterdam: North Holland Publ.

Leigh, J.M. (1973) Variation in performance of oxygen therapy devices. *Ann. R. Coll. Surg.* **52,** 234

Lenfant, C. and Howell, B.J. (1960) Cardiovascular adjustments in dogs during continuous pressure breathing. *J. appl. Physiol.* **15,** 425

Lenfant, C., Torrance, J., English, E., Finch, C.A., Reynafarje, C., Ramas, J. and Faura, J. (1968) Effect of altitude on oxygen binding by hemoglobin and on organic phosphate levels. *J. clin. Invest.* **47,** 2652

Leusen, I.R. (1950) Influence du pH du liquide cephalo-rachidien sur la respiration. *Experientia* **6,** 272

Leusen, I.R. (1954) Chemosensitivity of the respiratory center. *Am. J. Physiol.* **176,** 39

Liebow, A.A. (1962) Recent advances in pulmonary anatomy. In: *Pulmonary Structure and Function,* edited by A.V.S. de Reuck and M. O'Connor. Edinburgh and London: Churchill Livingstone

Linden, R.J., Ledsome, J.R. and Norman, J. (1965) Simple methods for the determination of the concentrations of carbon dioxide and oxygen in blood. *Br. J. Anaesth.* **37,** 77

Lindenberg, R. (1963) Patterns of CNS vulnerability in acute hypoxaemia including anaesthetic accidents. In: *Selective Vulnerability of the Brain in Hypoxaemia,* edited by J.P. Schade and W.H. McMenemy. Oxford: Blackwell Scientific

Llewellyn, M.A. and Swyer, P.R. (1975) Mechanical ventilation and continuous distending pressure. In: *The intensive care of the newly born. Monographs in Paediatrics, no. 6,* edited by P.R. Swyer. Basel: Karger

Lloyd, B.B. and Cunningham, D.J.C. (1963) A quantitative approach to the regulation of human respiration. In: *The Regulation of Human Respirations* edited by D.J.C. Cunningham and B.B. Lloyd. Oxford: Blackwell Scientific

Lloyd, J.E., Newman, J.H. and Brigham, K.L. (1984) Permeability pulmonary edema. *Archs intern. Med.* **144,** 143

Lloyd, B.B., Jukes, M.G.M. and Cunningham, D.J.C. (1958) The relation between alveolar oxygen pressure and the respiratory response to carbon dioxide in man. *J. exp. Physiol.* **43,** 214

Loeschcke, H.H. (1965) A concept of the role of intracranial chemosensitivity in respiratory control. In: *Cerebrospinal Fluid and the Regulation of Ventilation,* edited by C.McC. Brookes, F.F. Kao and B.B. Lloyd. Oxford: Blackwell Scientific

Loeschcke, H.H. (1983) Central chemoreceptors. In: *Control of Respiration,* edited by D.J. Pallot. London: Croom Helm

Loeschcke, H.H., Sweel, A., Kough, R.H. and Lambertsen, C.J. (1953) The effect of morphine and of meperidine (dolantin, demerol) upon the respiratory response of normal men to low concentrations of inspired carbon dioxide. *J. Pharmac. exp. Ther.* **108,** 376

Loewy, A. (1894) Ueber die Bestimmung der Gröse des 'schädlichen Luftraumes' im Thorax und der alveolaren Sauerstoffspannung. *Pflügers Arch. ges. Physiol.* **58,** 416

Longo, L.D. (1970) Carbon monoxide in the pregnant mother and fetus and its exchange across the placenta. *Ann. N.Y. Acad. Sci.* **174,** 313

Lucey, J.F. and Dangman, B. (1984) A reexamination of the role of oxygen in retrolental fibroplasia. *Pediatrics* **73,** 82

Lugaresi, E., Cirignotta, F., Coccagna, G. and Montagna, P. (1984) Clinical significance of snoring. In: *Sleep and Breathing,* edited by N.A. Saunders and C.E. Sullivan. New York: Marcel Dekker

Lumsden, T. (1923a) Observations on the respiratory centres in the cat. *J. Physiol.* **57,** 153

Lumsden, T. (1923b) Observations on the respiratory centres. *J. Physiol.* **57,** 354

Lumsden, T. (1923c) The regulation of respiration. Part 1. *J. Physiol.* **58,** 81

Lumsden, T. (1923d) The regulation of respiration. Part 2. *J. Physiol.* **58,** 111

Lundgren, C.E.G. (1984) Respiratory function during simulated wet dives. *Undersea Biomed. Res.* **11,** 139

Lundsgaard, C. and Van Slyke, D.D. (1923) *Cyanosis.* Baltimore: Williams & Wilkins

Lunn, J.N. and Mushin, W.W. (1982) *Mortality Associated with Anaesthesia.* London: Nuffield Provincial Hospitals Trust

Lurie, A.A., Jones, R.E., Linde, H.W., Price, M.L., Dripps, R.D. and Price, H.L. (1958) Cyclopropane anesthesia: cardiac rate and rhythm during steady levels of cyclopropane anesthesia in man at normal and elevated end-expiratory carbon dioxide tensions. *Anesthesiology* **19,** 457

Lynch, J.P., Mhyre, J.G. and Dantzker, D.R. (1979) Influence of cardiac output on intrapulmonary shunt. *J. appl. Physiol.* **46,** 315

Lynch, S., Brand, L. and Levy, A. (1959) Changes in lung thorax compliance during orthopedic surgery. *Anesthesiology* **20,** 278

McArdle, L. and Roddie, I.C. (1958) Vascular responses to carbon dioxide during anaesthesia in man. *Br. J. Anaesth.* **30,** 358

McConn, R. and Derrick, J.B. (1972) The respiratory function of blood: transfusion and blood storage. *Anesthesiology* **36,** 119

McCord, J.M. and Fridovich, I. (1968) The reduction of cytochrome c by milk xanthine oxidase. *J. biol. Chem.* **243,** 5753

McCord, J.M. and Roy, R.S. (1982) The pathophysiology of superoxide: roles in inflammation and ischaemia. *Can. J. Physiol. Pharmacol.* **60,** 1346

McDonald, D.M. (1981) Peripheral chemoreceptors. In: *Regulation of Breathing,* edited by T.F. Hornbein. New York: Marcel Dekker

McDonald, D.M. and Mitchell, R.A. (1975) The innervation of glomus cells, ganglion cells and blood vessels in the rat carotid body: a quantitative ultrastructural analysis. *J. Neurocytol.* **4,** 177

McDonald, R.J., Berger, E.M., White, C.W., White, J.G., Freeman, B.A. and Repine, J.E. (1985) Effect of superoxide dismutase encapsulated in liposomes or conjugated with polyethylene glycol on neutrophil bactericidal activity in vitro and bacterial clearance in vivo. *Am. Rev. resp. Dis.* **131,** 633

McDowall, D.G. (1967) The effects of clinical concentrations of halothane on the blood flow and oxygen uptake of the cerebral cortex. *Br. J. Anaesth.* **39,** 186

McEvoy, R.D. (1985) Recently developed alternatives to conventional mechanical ventilation. *Anaesth. Intens. Care* **13,** 178

McEvoy, J.D.S., Jones, N.L. and Campbell, E.J.M. (1974) Mixed venous and arterial P_{CO_2}. *Br. med. J.* **4,** 687

McHardy, G.J.R. (1972) Diffusing capacity and pulmonary gas exchange. *Br. J. Dis. Chest* **66,** 1

McIlroy, M.B., Eldridge, F.L., Thomas, J.P. and Christie, R.V. (1956) The effect of added elastic and non-elastic resistances on the pattern of breathing in normal subjects. *Clin. Sci.* **15,** 337

Mackay, A.D., Baldwin, C.J. and Tattersfield, A.E. (1983) Action of intravenously administered aminophylline on normal airways. *Am. Rev. resp. Dis.* **127,** 609

Mackie, I. (1979) Alcohol and aquatic disasters. *Practitioner* Special Report on Drowning, edited by M.G. Harries, page 9

Macklem, P.T. (1971) Airway obstruction and collateral ventilation. *Physiol. Rev.* **51,** 368

Macklem, P.T. and Mead, J. (1967) Resistance of central and peripheral airways measured by a retrograde catheter. *J. appl. Physiol.* **22,** 395

Macklem, P.T. and Wilson, N.J. (1965) Measurement of intrabronchial pressure in man. *J. appl. Physiol.* **20,** 653

Macklem, P.T., Fraser, R.G. and Bates, D.V. (1963) Bronchial pressures and dimensions in health and obstructive airway disease. *J. appl. Physiol.* **18,** 699

McNicol, M.W. and Campbell, E.J.M. (1965) Severity of respiratory failure. *Lancet,* **1,** 336

McQueen, D.S. and Pallot, D.J. (1983) Peripheral arterial chemoreceptors. In: *Control of Respiration* edited by D.J. Pallot. London: Croom Helm

Malik, A.B., Selig, W.M. and Burhop, K.E. (1985) Cellular and humoral mediators of pulmonary edema. *Lung* **163,** 193

Mansell, A., Bryan, A.C. and Levison, H. (1972) Airway closure in children. *J. appl. Physiol.* **33,** 711

Mapleson, W.W. (1954) The elimination of rebreathing in various anaesthetic systems. *Br. J. Anaesth.* **26,** 323

Marchand, P., Gilroy, J.C. and Wilson, V.H. (1950) An anatomical study of the bronchial vascular system and its variation in disease. *Thorax* **5,** 207

Maren, T.H. (1967) Carbonic anhydrase: chemistry, physiology, and inhibition. *Physiol. Rev.* **47,** 595

Marckwald, M. and Kronecker, H. (1880) Die Athembewegungen des Zwerchfells des Kaninchens. *Arch. Physiol. Leipzig,* p. 441

Marquez, J.M., Douglas, M.E., Downs, J.B., Wu, W.-H., Mantini, E.L., Kuck, E.J. and Calderwood, H.W. (1979) Renal function and cardiovascular responses during positive airway pressure. *Anesthesiology* **50**, 393

Marquez, J., Sladen, A., Gendell, H., Boehnke, M. and Medelow, H. (1981) Pardoxical cerebral air embolism without an intracardiac septal defect. *J. Neurosurg.* **55**, 997

Marrubini, M.G., Rossanda, M. and Tretola, L. (1964) The role of artificial hyperventilation in the control of brain tension during neurosurgical operations. *Br. J. Anaesth.* **36**, 415

Marshall, B.E. and Marshall, C. (1985) Anesthesia and pulmonary circulation. In: *Effects of Anesthesia*, edited by B.G. Covino, H.A. Fozzard, K. Rehder and G. Strichartz. Bethesda, Md: American Physiological Society

Marshall, B.E. and Whyche, M.Q. (1972) Hypoxemia during and after anesthesia. *Anesthesiology* **37**, 178

Marshall, B.E., Cohen, P.J., Klingenmaier, C.H. and Aukberg, S. (1969) Pulmonary venous admixture before, during, and after halothane: oxygen anesthesia in man. *J. appl. Physiol.* **27**, 653

Marshall, B.E., Marshall, C., Benumof, J. and Saidman, L.J. (1981) Hypoxic pulmonary vasoconstriction in dogs: effects of lung segment size and oxygen tension. *J. appl. Physiol.* **51**, 1543

Marshall, C. and Marshall, B. (1983) Site and sensitivity for stimulation of hypoxic pulmonary vasoconstriction. *J. appl. Physiol.* **55**, 711

Marshall, R. (1957) The physical properties of the lungs in relation to the subdivisions of lung volume. *Clin. Sci.* **16**, 507

Marshall, R. and Widdicombe, J.G. (1958) The activity of pulmonary stretch receptors during congestion of the lung. *Q. Jl Physiol.* **43**, 320

Marshall, R. and Widdicombe, J.G. (1961) Stress relaxation in the human lung. *Clin. Sci.* **20**, 19

Massaro, D. and Massaro, G.D. (1978) Biochemical and anatomical adaptation of the lung to oxygen-induced injury. *Fedn Proc.* **37**, 2485

Mattson, S.B. and Carlens, E. (1955) Lobar ventilation and oxygen uptake in man: influence of body position. *J. thorac. Surg.* **30**, 676

Mead, J. (1961) Mechanical properties of lungs. *Physiol. Rev.* **41**, 281

Mead, J. and Agostoni, E. (1964) Dynamics of breathing. *Handbk Physiol., section 3*, **1**, 1

Meade, F. and Owen-Thomas, J.B. (1975) The estimation of carbon dioxide concentration in the presence of nitrous oxide using a Lloyd–Haldane apparatus. *Br. J. Anaesth.* **47**, 22

Meldrum, N.U. and Roughton, F.J.W. (1933) Carbonic anhydrase: its preparation and properties. *J. Physiol.* **80**, 833

Mendelson, C.L. (1946) Aspiration of stomach contents into the lungs during obstetric anesthesia. *Am. J. Obstet. Gynec.* **52**, 191

Merwarth, C.R. and Sieker, H.O. (1961) Acid–base changes in blood and cerebrospinal fluid during altered ventilation. *J. appl. Physiol.* **16**, 1016

Meyer, B.J., Meyer, A. and Guyton, A.C. (1968) Interstitial fluid pressure. V. Negative pressure in the lungs. *Circulation Res.* **22**, 263

Meyer, E.C. and Ottaviano, R. (1972) Pulmonary collateral lymph flow: detection using lymph oxygen tensions. *J. appl. Physiol.* **32**, 806

Michel, C.C. and Milledge, J.S. (1963) Respiratory regulation in man during acclimatization to high altitude. *J. Physiol.* **168**, 631

Michels, D.B. and West, J.B. (1978) Distribution of pulmonary ventilation and perfusion during short periods of weightlessness. *J. appl. Physiol.* **45**, 987

Michenfelder, J.D., Fowler, W.S. and Theye, R.A. (1966) CO_2 levels and pulmonary shunting in anesthetized man. *J. appl. Physiol.* **21**, 1471

Miles, S. (1957) The effect of changes in barometric pressure on maximum breathing capacity. *J. Physiol* **137**, 85P

Milic-Emili, J., Mead, J., Turner, J.M. and Glauser, E.M. (1964) Improved technique for estimating pleural pressure from esophageal balloons. *J. appl. Physio.* **19**, 207

Millar, R.A. (1960) Plasma adrenaline and noradrenaline during diffusion respiration. *J. Physiol.* **150**, 79

Millar, R.A. and Gregory, I.C. (1972) Reduced oxygen content in equilibrated fresh heparinised and ACD-stored blood from cigarette smokers. *Br. J. Anaesth.* **44**, 1015

Millar, R.A., Beard, D.J. and Hulands, G.H. (1971) Oxyhaemoglobin dissociation curves *in vitro* with and without the anaesthetics halothane and cyclopropane. *Br. J. Anaesth.* **43**, 1003

Milledge, J.S. (1984) Renin–aldosterone system. In: *High Altitude and Man,* edited by J.B. West and S. Lahiri. Bethesda, Md: American Physiological Society

Milledge, J.S. (1985a) Acute mountain sickness: pulmonary and cerebral oedema of high altitude. *Intens. Care Med.* **11**, 110

Milledge, J.S. (1985b) The great oxygen secretion controversy. *Lancet* **2**, 1408

Milledge, J.S. and Nunn, J.F. (1975) Criteria of fitness for anaesthesia in patients with chronic obstructive lung disease. *Br. med. J.* **3**, 670

Milledge, J.S. and Stott, F.D. (1977) Inductive plethysmography — a new respiratory transducer. *J. Physiol.* **267**, 4P

Milledge, J.S., Minty, K.B. and Duncalf, D. (1974) On-line assessment of ventilatory response to carbon dioxide. *J. appl. Physiol.* **37**, 596

Miller, A.H. (1925) Ascending respiratory paralysis under general anesthesia. *J. Am. med. Assoc.* **84**, 201

Miller, W.C., Rice, D.L., Unger, K.M. and Bradley, B.L. (1981) Effect of PEEP on lung water content in experimental noncardiogenic pulmonary edema. *Crit. Care Med.* **9**, 7

Miller, W.S. (1947) *The Lung,* 2nd ed. Springfield, Ill: Thomas

Mills, E. and Jöbsis, F.F. (1972) Mitochondrial respiratory chain of carotid body and chemoreceptor response to changes in oxygen tension. *J. Neurophysiol.* **35**, 405

Mills, F.J. and Harding, R.M. (1983a) Special forms of flight. III: Supersonic transport aircraft. *Br. med. J.* **287**, 411

Mills, F.J. and Harding, R.M. (1983b) Special forms of flight. IV: Manned spacecraft. *Br. med. J.* **287**, 478

Mills, J.E., Sellick, H. and Widdicombe, J.G. (1970) Epithelial irritant receptors in the lungs. In: *Breathing: Hering–Breuer Centenary Symposium,* p. 77, edited by R. Porter. Edinburgh and London: Churchill Livingstone

Mills, R.J., Cumming, G. and Harris, P. (1963) Frequency-dependent compliance at different levels of inspiration in normal adults. *J. appl. Physiol.* **18**, 1061

Minty, B.D. and Barrett, A.M. (1978) Accuracy of automated blood-gas analyser operated by untrained staff. *Br. J. Anaesth.* **50**, 1031

Minty, B.D. and Royston, D. (1985) Cigarette smoke induced changes in rat pulmonary clearance of ^{99m}Tc DTPA. A comparison of particulate and gas phases. *Am. Rev. resp. Dis.* **132**, 1170

Minty, B.D., Jordan, C. and Jones, J.G. (1981) Rapid improvement in abnormal pulmonary epithelial permeability after stopping cigarettes. *Br. med. J.* **282**, 83

Mitchell, R.A. (1966). Cerebrospinal fluid and the regulation of respiration. In: *Advances in Respiratory Physiology,* edited by C.G. Caro. London: Edward Arnold

Mitchell, R.A. and Berger, A.J. (1975) Neural regulation of respiration. *Am. Rev. resp. Dis.* **111**, 206

Mitchell, R.A. and Berger, A.J. (1981) Neural regulation of respiration. In: *Regulation of Breathing,* Part I, edited by T.F. Hornbein. New York: Marcel Dekker

Mitchell, R.A. and Herbert, D.A. (1975) Potencies of doxapram and hypoxia in stimulating carotid-body chemoreceptors and ventilation in anesthetized cats. *Anesthesiology* **42**, 559

Mitchell, R.A., Loeschcke, H.H., Massion, W.H. and Severinghaus, J.W. (1963) Respiratory responses mediated through superficial chemosensitive areas on the medulla. *J. appl. Physiol.* **18**, 523

Mitchell, R.A., Bainton, C.R., Severinghaus, J.W. and Edelist, G. (1964) Respiratory response and CSF pH during disturbances in blood acid–base balance in awake dogs with denervated aortic and carotid bodies. *Physiologist* **7**, 208

Mitchell, R.A., Carman, C.T., Severinghaus, J.W., Richardson, B.W., Singer, M.M. and Snider, S. (1965) Stability of cerebrospinal fluid pH in chronic acid–base disturbances in blood. *J. appl. Physiol.* **20**, 443

Moote, C.A., Knill, R.L. and Clement, J. (1986) Ventilatory compensation for continuous inspiratory resistive and elastic loads during halothane anaesthesia in humans. *Anesthesiology* **64**, 582

Modell, J.H. (1984) Drowning. In: *Edema,* edited by N.C. Staub and A.E. Taylor, p. 679. New York: Raven Press

Modell, J.H. and Moya, F. (1966) Effects of volume of aspirated fluid during chlorinated water fresh water drowning. *Anesthesiology* **27**, 662

Modell, J.H., Graves, S.A. and Ketover, A. (1976) Clinical course of 91 consecutive near-drowning victims. *Chest* **70**, 231

Modell, J.H., Calderwood, H.W., Ruiz, B.C., Downs, J.B. and Chapman, R. (1974) Effects of ventilatory patterns on arterial oxygenation after near-drowning in sea water. *Anesthesiology* **40**, 376

Moote, C.A., Knill, R.L. and Clement, J. (1986) Ventilatory compensation for continuous inspiratory resistive and elastic loads during halothane anesthesia in humans. *Anesthesiology* **64**, 582

Morris, H.R., Taylor, G.W., Piper, P.J. and Tippins, J.R. (1980) Structure of slow reacting substance of anaphylaxis from guinea-pig lung. *Nature* **285**, 104

Morris, J.G. (1968) *A Biologist's Physical Chemistry*. London: Edward Arnold

Moser, K.M., Rhodes, P.G. and Kwaan, P.L. (1965) Post-hyperventilation apnea. *Fedn Proc.* **24**, 273

Moxham, J. (1984) Failure of the respiratory muscle pump. In: *Effects of anesthesia and surgery on pulmonary mechanisms and gas exchange, International Anesthesiology Clinics,* vol. 22, no. 4, edited by J.G. Jones. Boston, Mass: Little, Brown

Muller, N., Volgyesi, G., Becker, L., Bryan, M.H. and Bryan, A.C. (1979) Diaphragmatic muscle tone. *J. appl. Physiol.* **47**, 279

Munson, E.S. and Merrick, H.C. (1967) Effect of nitrous oxide on venous air embolism. *Anesthesiology* **27**, 783

Munson, E.S., Larson, C.P., Babad, A.A., Regan, M.J., Buechel, D.R. and Eger, E.I. (1966) The effects of halothane, fluroxene and cyclopropane on ventilation: a comparative study in man. *Anesthesiology* **27**, 716

Murciano, D., Aubier, M., Lecocque, Y. and Pariente, R. (1984) Effects of theophylline on diaphragmatic strength and fatigue in patients with chronic obstructive pulmonary disease. *New Engl. J. Med.* **311**, 349

Nahas, G.C., Ligou, J.C. and Mehlman, B. (1960) Effects of pH changes on O_2 uptake and plasma catecholamine levels in the dog. *J. appl. Physiol.* **198**, 60

Naito, H. and Gillis, C.N. (1973) Effects of halothane and nitrous oxide on removal of norepinephrine from the pulmonary circulation. *Anesthesiology* **39**, 575

Nash, G., Blennerhassett, J.B. and Pontoppidan, H. (1967) Pulmonary lesions associated with oxygen therapy and artificial ventilation. *New Engl. J. Med.* **276**, 368

Natelson, S. (1951) Routine use of ultramicro-methods in the clinical laboratory. *Am. J. clin. Path.* **21**, 1153

Nathan, P.W. and Sears, T.A. (1960) Effects of posterior root section on the activity of some muscles in man. *J. Neurol. Neurosurg. Psychiat.* **23**, 10

Navaratnarajah, M., Nunn, J.F., Lyons, D. and Milledge, J.S. (1984) Bronchiolectasis caused by positive end-expiratory pressure. *Crit. Care Med.* **12**, 1036

Naylor, B.A., Welch, M.H., Shafer, A.W. and Guenter, C.A. (1972) Blood affinity for oxygen in hemorrhagic shock. *J. appl. Physiol.* **32**, 829

Needham, C.D., Rogan, M.C. and McDonald, I. (1954) Normal standards for lung volumes, intrapulmonary gas-mixing, and maximum breathing capacity. *Thorax* **9**, 313

von Neergard, K. (1929) Neue Auffassungen über einen Grundbegriff der Atemmechanik. Die Retraktionskraft der Lunge, abhängig von der Oberflächenspannung in der Alveolen. *Z. ges. exp. Med.* **66**, 373

von Neergaard, K. and Wirz, K. (1927a) Ueber eine Methode zur Messung der Lungenelastizität am lebenden Menschen, inbesondere beim Emphysem. *Z. klin. Med.* **105**, 35

von Neergaard, K. and Wirz, K. (1927b) Die Messung der Strömungswiderstände in der Atemwege des Menschen inbesondere bei Asthma und Emphysem. *Z. klin. Med.* **105**, 51

Neil, E. and Joels, N. (1963) The carotid glomus sensory mechanism. In: *The Regulation of Human Respiration*, p. 163, edited by D.J.C. Cunningham and B.B. Lloyd. Oxford: Blackwell Scientific

Nelson, N.M. (1966) Neonatal lung function. *Pediat. Clins N. Am.* **13**, 769

Nemir, P., Stone, H.H., Mackrell, T.N. and Hawthorne, H.R. (1953) Studies on pulmonary function utilizing the method of controlled unilateral bronchovascular occlusion. *Surg. Forum* **4**, 234

Newberg, L.A. and Jones, J.G. (1974) A closing volume bolus method using SF$_6$ enhancement of the nitrogen glow discharge. *J. appl. Physiol.* **36,** 488

Newman, H.C., Campbell, E.J.M. and Dinnick, O.P. (1959) A simple method of measuring the compliance and the non-elastic resistance of the chest during anaesthesia. *Br. J. Anaesth.* **31,** 282

Newsom-Davis, J. (1974) Control of the muscles in breathing. In: *Respiratory Physiology,* p. 221. London: Butterworths

Newsom-Davis, J. and Plum, F. (1972) Separation of descending spinal pathways to respiratory motoneurones. *Expl Neuronol.* **34,** 78

Ng, K.K.F. and Vane, J.R. (1967) Conversion of angiotensin I to angiotensin II. *Nature* **216,** 762

Ngai, S.H., Katz, R.L. and Farhi, S.E. (1965) Respiratory effects of trichlorethylene, halothane and methoxyflurane in the cat. *J. Pharmac. exp. Ther.* **148,** 123

Niden, A.H. and Aviado, D.M. (1956) Effects of pulmonary embolus on the pulmonary circulation with special reference to arteriovenous shunts in the lung. *Circulation Res.* **6,** 67

Nielsen, H. (1932) En oplivningsmetode. *Ugeskr. Laeg.* **94,** 1201

Nims, R.G., Connor, E.H. and Comroe, J.H. (1955) Compliance of the human thorax in anesthetized patients. *J. clin. Invest.* **34,** 744

Nishino, T., Honda, Y., Kohchi, T., Shirahata, M. and Yonezawa, T. (1985) Effects of increasing depth of anaesthesia on phrenic nerve and hypoglossal nerve activity during the swallowing reflex in cats. *Br. J. Anaesth.* **57,** 208

Noble, M.I.M., Eisele, J.H., Frankel, H.L., Else, W. and Guz, A. (1971) The role of the diaphragm in the sensation of holding the breath. *Clin. Sci.* **41,** 275

Norton, P.G. and Dunn, E.V. (1985) Snoring as a risk factor for disease: an epidemiological survey. *Br. med. J.* **291,** 630

Nunn, J.F. (1956) A new method of spirometry applicable to routine anaesthesia. *Br. J. Anaesth.* **28,** 440

Nunn, J.F. (1958a) Ventilation and end-tidal carbon dioxide tension. *Anaesthesia* **13,** 124

Nunn, J.F. (1958b) Respiratory measurements in the presence of nitrous oxide. *Br. J. Anaesth.* **30,** 254

Nunn, J.F. (1960a) Prediction of carbon dioxide tension during anaesthesia. *Anaesthesia* **15,** 123

Nunn, J.F. (1960b) The solubility of volatile anaesthetics in oil. *Br. J. Anaesth.* **32,** 346

Nunn, J.F. (1961a) The distribution of inspired gas during thoracic surgery. *Ann. R. Coll. Surg.* **28,** 223

Nunn, J.F. (1961b) Portable anaesthetic apparatus for use in the Antarctic. *Br. med. J.* **1,** 1139

Nunn, J.F. (1962a) Measurement of blood oxygen tension: handling of samples. *Br. J. Anaesth.* **34,** 621

Nunn, J.F. (1962b) The effects of hypercapnia. In: *Modern Trends in Anaesthesia—2,* edited by F.T. Evans and T.C. Gray. London and Boston, Mass: Butterworths

Nunn, J.F. (1963) Indirect determination of the ideal alveolar oxygen tension during and after nitrous oxide anaesthesia. *Br. J. Anaesth.* **35,** 8

Nunn, J.F. (1964) Factors influencing the arterial oxygen tension during halothane anaesthesia with spontaneous respiration. *Br. J. Anaesth.* **36,** 327

Nunn, J.F. (1968) The evolution of atmospheric oxygen. *Ann. R. Coll. Surg.* **43,** 200

Nunn, J.F. (1972) Nomograms for calculation of oxygen consumption and respiratory exchange ratio. *Br. med. J.* **4,** 18

Nunn, J.F. (1978) Measurement of closing volume. *Acta anaesth. scand.* suppl. 70, 154

Nunn, J.F. (1983) Mandatory minute volume. *Jap. J. clin. Anaesth.* **31,** 1063

Nunn, J.F. (1984) Positive end-expiratory pressure. In: *Effects of anesthesia and surgery on pulmonary mechanisms and gas exchange, International Anesthesiology Clinics,* 224, no. 4, edited by J.G. Jones. Boston, Mass: Little, Brown

Nunn, J.F. (1985a) Oxygen — friend or foe. *Jl R. Soc. Med.* **78,** 618

Nunn, J.F. (1985b) Anesthesia and pulmonary gas exchange. In: *Effects of Anesthesia,* edited by B.G. Covino, H.A. Fazzard, K. Rehder and G. Strichartz. Bethesda, Md: American Physiological Society

Nunn, J.F. and Bergman, N.A. (1964) The effect of atropine on pulmonary gas exchange. *Br. J. Anaesth.* **36,** 68

Nunn, J.F. and Ezi-Ashi, T.I. (1961) The respiratory effects of resistance to breathing in anesthetized man. *Anesthesiology* **22**, 174

Nunn, J.F. and Ezi-Ashi, T.I. (1962) The accuracy of the respirometer and ventigrator. *Br. J. Anaesth.* **34**, 422

Nunn, J.F. and Freeman, J. (1964) Problems of oxygenation and oxygen transport during haemorrhage. *Anaesthesia* **19**, 206

Nunn, J.F. and Hill, D.W. (1960) Respiratory dead space and arterial to end-tidal CO_2 tension difference in anesthetized man. *J. appl. Physiol.* **15**, 383

Nunn, J.F. and Lyle, D.J.R. (1986) The Ohmeda CPU-1 Ventilator. *Br. J. Anaesth.* **58**, 653

Nunn, J.F. and Matthews, R.L. (1959) Gaseous exchange during halothane anaesthesia: the steady respiratory state. *Br. J. Anaesth.* **31**, 330

Nunn, J.F. and Newman, H.C. (1964) Inspired gas, rebreathing and apparatus dead space. *Br. J. Anaesth.* **36**, 5

Nunn, J.F. and Payne, J.P. (1962) Hypoxaemia after general anaesthesia. *Lancet* **2**, 631

Nunn, J.F. and Pouliot, J.C. (1962) The measurement of gaseous exchange during nitrous oxide anaesthesia. *Br. J. Anaesth.* **34**, 752

Nunn, J.F., Bergman, N.A. and Coleman, A.J. (1965) Factors influencing the arterial oxygen tension during anaesthesia with artificial ventilation. *Br. J. Anaesth.* **37**, 898

Nunn, J.F., Campbell, E.J.M. and Peckett, B.W. (1959) Anatomical subdivisions of the volume of respiratory dead space and effect of position of the jaw. *J. appl. Physiol.* **14**, 174

Nunn, J.F., Milledge, J.S. and Sigaraya, J. (1979) Survival of patients ventilated in an intensive care unit. *Br. med. J.* **1**, 1525

Nunn, J.F., Bergman, N.A., Coleman, A.J. and Casselle, D.C. (1964) Evaluation of the Servomex paramagnetic analyser. *Br. J. Anaesth.* **36**, 666

Nunn, J.F., Bergman, N.A., Bunatyan, A. and Coleman, A.J. (1965a) Temperature coefficients of P_{CO_2} and P_{O_2} of blood *in vitro*. *J. appl. Physiol.* **20**, 23

Nunn, J.F., Coleman, A.J., Sachithanandan, T., Bergman, N.A. and Laws, J.W. (1965b) Hypoxaemia and atelectasis produced by forced expiration. *Br. J. Anaesth.* **37**, 3

Nunn, J.F., Sturrock, J.E., Willis, E.J., Richmond, J.E. and McPherson, C.K. (1974) The effect of inhalational anaesthetics on the swimming velocity of *Tetrahymena pyriformis*. *J. Cell Sci.* **15**, 537

Nunn, J.F., Williams, I.P., Jones, J.G., Hewlett, A.M., Hulands, G.H. and Minty, B.D. (1978) Detection and reversal of pulmonary absorption collapse. *Br. J. Anaesth.* **50**, 91

Ogilvie, C.M., Forster, R.E., Blakemore, W.S. and Morton, J.W. (1957) A standardized breath holding technique for the clinical measurement of the diffusing capacity of the lung for carbon monoxide. *J. clin. Invest.* **36**, 1

Otis, A.B. (1954) The work of breathing. *Physiol. Rev.* **34**, 449

Otis, A.B. (1964) The work of breathing. *Handbk Physiol, section 3*, **1**, 463

Otis, A.B., Fenn, W.O. and Rahn, H. (1950) Mechanics of breathing in man. *J. appl. Physiol.* **2**, 592

Otis, A.B., Rahn, H. and Fenn, W.O. (1948) Alveolar gas changes during breath holding. *Am. J. Physiol.* **152**, 674

Otis, A.B., McKerrow, C.B., Bartlett, R.A., Mead, J., McIlroy, M.B., Selverstone, N.J. and Radford, E.P. (1956) Mechanical factors in distribution of pulmonary ventilation. *J. appl. Physiol.* **8**, 427

Ozanam, C. (1862) De l'acide carbonique en inhalations comme agent anesthésique efficace et sans danger pendant les operations chirurgicales. *C.r. Acad. Sci.* **54**, 1154

Padmanabhan, R.V., Gudapaty, R., Liener, I.E., Schwartz, B.A. and Hoidal, J.R. (1985) Protection against pulmonary oxygen toxicity in rats by the intratracheal administration of liposome-encapsulated superoxide dismutase or catalase. *Am. Rev. resp. Dis.* **132**, 164

Padmore, G.R.A. and Nunn, J.F. (1974). SI units in relation to anaesthesia. *Br. J. Anaesth.* **46**, 236

Pain, M.C.F. (1964) Digital clubbing in chronic obstructive lung disease. *Australas. Ann. Med.* **13**, 167

Paintal, A.S. (1983) Lung and airway receptors. In: *Control of Respiration*, edited by D.J. Pallot. London: Croom Helm

Palmer, K.N.V. and Diament, M.L. (1967) Effect of aerosol isoprenaline on blood-gas tensions in severe bronchial asthma. *Lancet* **2,** 1232

Panday, J. and Nunn, J.F. (1968) Failure to demonstrate progressive falls of arterial Po_2 during anaesthesia. *Anaesthesia* **23,** 38

Pappenheimer, J.R., Comroe, J.H., Cournand, A. et al. (1950) Standardization of definitions and symbols in respiratory physiology. *Fedn Proc.* **9,** 602

Pare, P.D., Warriner, B., Baile, E.M. and Hogg, J.C. (1983) Redistribution of extravascular water with positive end-expiratory pressure in canine pulmonary edema. *Am. Rev. resp. Dis.* **127,** 590

Parks, D.A., Bulkley, G.B. and Granger, D.N. (1983) Role of oxygen free radicals in shock, ischaemia and organ preservation. *Surgery* **94,** 428

Passavant, G. (1869) Ueber die Verschliessung des Schlundes beim Sprechen. *Arch. path. Anat. Physiol. klin. Med.* **46,** 1

Pattle, R.E. (1955) Properties, function and origin of the alveolar lining fluid. *Nature* **175,** 1125

Pattle, R.E., Schock, C. and Battensby, J. (1972) Some effects of anaesthetics on lung surfactant. *Br. J. Anaesth.* **44,** 1119

Pattle, R.E., Claireaux, A.E., Davies, P.A. and Cameron, A.H. (1962) Inability to form a lung lining film as a cause of the respiratory distress syndrome in newborn. *Lancet* **2,** 469

Pauling, L., Wood, R.E. and Sturdivant, J.H. (1946) Instrument for determining partial pressure of oxygen in gas. *J. Am. chem. Soc.* **68,** 795

Pavlin, E.G. and Hornbein, T.F. (1975a) Distribution of H^+ and HCO_3^- between CSF and blood during metabolic acidosis in dogs. *J. Physiol.* **228,** 1134

Pavlin, E.G. and Hornbein, T.F. (1975b) Distribution of H^+ and HCO_3^- between CSF and blood during metabolic alkalosis in dogs. *J. Physiol.* **228,** 1141

Pavlin, E.G. and Hornbein, T.F. (1975c) Distribution of H^+ and HCO_3^- between CSF and blood during respiratory acidosis in dogs. *J. Physiol.* **228,** 1145

Pavlin, E.G. and Hornbein, T.F. (1986) Anesthesia and the control of ventilation. *Handbk Physiol., section II,* **3,** part 2, 793

Pavlin, D.J., Nessly, M.L. and Cheney, F.W. (1981) Increased pulmonary vascular permeability as a cause of re-expansion edema in rabbits. *Am. Rev. resp. Dis.* **124,** 422

Payne, J.P. (1958) Hypotensive response to carbon dioxide. *Anaesthesia* **13,** 279

Payne, J.P. (1962) Apnoeic oxygenation in anaesthetized man. *Acta anaesth. scand.* **6,** 129

Peacock, A.J., Morgan, M.D.L., Turton, C., Gourlay, A.R. and Denison, D.M. (1984) Optical mapping of the thoraco-abdominal wall. *Thorax* **39,** 93

Pearce, A.C. and Jones, R.M. (1984) Smoking and anesthesia: preoperative abstinence and perioperative morbidity. *Anesthesiology* **61,** 576

Pearn, J. (1985) The management of near-drowning. *Br. med. J.* **291,** 1447

Pepe, P.E., Hudson, L.D. and Carrico, C.J. (1984) Early application of positive end-expiratory pressure in patients at risk for the adult respiratory distress syndrome. *New Engl. J. Med.* **311,** 281

Pepe, P.E., Potkin, R.T., Reus, D.H., Hudson, L.D. and Carrico, C.J. (1982) Clinical predictors of the adult respiratory distress syndrome. *Am. J. Surg.* **144,** 124

Perez-Chada, R.D., Gardaz, J.-P., Madgwick, R.G. and Sykes, M.K. (1983) Cardiorespiratory effects of an inspiratory hold and continuous positive pressure ventilation in goats. *Intens. Care Med.* **9,** 263

Perkins, N.A.K. and Bedford, R.F. (1984) Hemodynamic consequences of PEEP in seated neurological patients — implications for paradoxical air embolism. *Anesth. Analg.* **63,** 429

Perkins-Pearson, N.A.K., Marshall, W.K. and Bedford, R.F. (1982) Atrial pressures in the seated position. *Anesthesiology* **57,** 493

Permutt, S. and Riley, R.L. (1963) Hemodynamics of collapsible vessels with tone: the vascular waterfall. *J. appl. Physiol.* **18,** 924

Perutz, M.F. (1969) The haemoglobin molecule. *Proc. R. Soc. B* **173,** 113

Pesenti, A., Pelizzola, A., Mascheroni, D. et al. (1981) Low frequency positive pressure ventilation with extracorporeal CO_2 removal (LFPPV-ECCO$_2$R) in acute respiratory failure (ARF): technique. *Trans. Am. Soc. artif. intern. Organs* **27,** 263

Petheram, I.S. and Branthwaite, M.A. (1980) Mechanical ventilation for pulmonary disease. *Anaesthesia* **35,** 467

Petty, T.L. and Ashbaugh, D.G. (1971) The adult respiratory distress syndrome. *Chest* **60**, 233

Pflüger, E. (1866) Zur gasometrie des Blutes. *Zbl. med. Wiss.* **4**, 305

Pflüger, E. (1868) Ueber die Urasche der Athembewegungen, sowie der Dyspnoë und Apnoë. *Arch. ges. Physiol.* **1**, 61

Phillipson, E.A. (1977) Regulation of breathing during sleep. *Am. Rev. resp. Dis.* **155**, 217

Philpot, R.M., Anderson, M.W. and Eling, T.E. (1977) Uptake, accumulation and metabolism of chemicals by the lung. In: *Metabolic Functions of the Lung,* edited by Y.S. Bakhle and J.R. Vane. New York: Marcel Dekker

Pierce, E.C., Lambertsen, C.J., Deutsch, S., Chase, P.E., Linde, H.W., Dripps, R.D. and Price, H.L. (1962) Cerebral circulation and metabolism during thiopental anesthesia and hyperventilation in man. *J. clin. Invest.* **41**, 1664

Pietak, S., Weenig, C.S., Hickey, R.F. and Fairley, H.B. (1975) Anesthetic effects on ventilation in patients with chronic obstructive pulmonary disease. *Anesthesiology* **42**, 160

Piiper, J. (1961) Variations of ventilation and diffusing capacity to perfusion determining the alveolar–arterial O_2 difference: theory. *J. appl. Physiol.* **16**, 507

Piiper, J., Haab, P. and Rahn, H. (1961) Unequal distribution of pulmonary diffusing capacity in the anesthetized dog. *J. appl. Physiol.* **16**, 499

Piper, P.J., Samhoun, M.N., Tippins, J.R., Williams, T.J., Palmer, M.A. and Peck, M.J. (1981) Pharmacological studies on pure SRS-A and synthetic leukotrienes C_4 and D_4. In: *SRS-A and Leukotrienes,* edited by P.J. Piper. New York: Wiley

Pitts, R.F. (1946) Organization of the respiratory center. *Physiol. Rev.* **26**, 609

Pitts, R.F., Magoun, H.W. and Ranson, S.W. (1939a) Localization of the medullary respiratory centers in the cat. *Am. J. Physiol.* **126**, 673

Pitts, R.F., Magoun, H.W. and Ranson, S.W. (1939b) Interrelations of the respiratory centers in the cat. *Am. J. Physiol.* **126**, 689

Pitts, R.F., Magoun, H.W. and Ranson, S.W. (1939c) The origin of respiratory rhythmicity. *Am. J. Physiol* **127**, 654

Ponte, J. and Purves, M.J. (1974) Frequency response of carotid body chemoreceptors in the cat to changes of Pao_2, $Paco_2$ and pH. *J. appl. Physiol.* **37**, 635

Pontoppidan, H., Geffin, B. and Lowenstein, E. (1972) Acute respiratory failure in the adult. *New Engl. J. Med.* **287**, 690, 743 and 799

Potgieter, S.V. (1959) Atelectasis: its evolution during upper urinary tract surgery. *Br. J. Anaesth.* **31**, 472

Price, H.L. (1960) Effects of carbon dioxide on the cardiovascular system. *Anesthesiology* **21**, 652

Price, H.L. and Widdicombe, J. (1962) Actions of cyclopropane on carotid sinus baroreceptors and carotid body chemoreceptors. *J. Pharmac. exp. Ther.* **135**, 233

Price, H.L., Lurie, A.A. Jones, R.E. and Linde, H.W. (1958) Role of catecholamines in the initiation of arrhythmic cardiac contraction by carbon dioxide inhalation in anesthetized man. *J. Pharmac. exp. Therap.* **122**, 63A

Price, H.L., Lurie, A.A., Black, G.W., Sechzer, P.H., Linde, H.W. and Price, M.L. (1960) Modification by general anesthetics (cyclopropane and halothane) of circulatory and sympathoadrenal responses to respiratory acidosis. *Ann. Surg.* **152**, 1071

Price, H.L., Cooperman, L.H., Warden, J.C., Morris, J.J. and Smith, T.C. (1969) Pulmonary hemodynamics during general anesthesia in man. *Anesthesiology* **30**, 629

Prutow, R.J., Dueck, R., Davies, N.J.H. and Clausen, J. (1982) Shunt development in young adult surgical patients due to inhalational anesthesia. *Anesthesiology* **57**, A477

Prys-Roberts, C. (1980) Hypercapnia. In: *General Anaesthesia,* 4th edn., edited by T.C. Gray, J.F. Nunn and J.E. Utting. London: Butterworths

Prys-Roberts, C., Kelman, G.R. and Nunn, J.F. (1966) Determination of the *in vivo* carbon dioxide titration curve of anaesthetized man. *Br. J. Anaesth.* **38**, 500

Prys-Roberts, C., Smith, W.D.A. and Nunn, J.F. (1967) Accidental severe hypercapnia during anaesthesia. *Br. J. Anaesth.* **39**, 257

Prys-Roberts, C., Kelman, G.R., Greenbaum, R. and Robinson, R.H. (1967) Circulatory influences of artificial ventilation during nitrous oxide anaesthesia in man. II. Results: the relative influence of mean intrathoracic pressure and arterial carbon dioxide tension. *Br. J. Anaesth.* **39**, 533

Prys-Roberts, C., Greenbaum, R., Nunn, J.F. and Kelman, G.R. (1970) Disturbances of pulmonary function in patients with fat embolism. *J. clin. Path.* **23,** suppl. (Roy. Coll. Path.) **4,** 143

Pugh, L.G.C.E. (1962) Physiological and medical aspects of the Himalayan Scientific and Mountaineering Expedition, 1960–61, *Br. med. J.* **2,** 621

Pugh, L.G.C.E. (1964) Cardiac output in muscular exercise at 5,800 m (19,000 ft). *J. appl. Physiol.* **19,** 441

Pugh, L.G.C.E., Gill, M.B., Lahiri, S., Milledge, J.S., Ward, M.P. and West, J.B. (1964) Muscular exercise at great altitudes. *J. appl. Physiol.* **19,** 431

Radford, E.P. (1955) Ventilation standards for use in artificial respiration. *J. appl. Physiol.* **7,** 451

Rahn, H. (1964) Oxygen stores of man. In: *Oxygen in the Animal Organism,* edited by F. Dickens and E. Neil. Oxford: Pergamon

Rahn, H. and Farhi, L.E. (1964) Ventilation, perfusion, and gas exchange—the $\dot{V}A/\dot{Q}$ concept. *Handbk Physiol., section 3,* **1,** 735

Rahn, H. and Otis, A.B. (1949) Man's respiratory response during and after acclimatization to high altitude. *Am. J. Physiol.* **157,** 445

Rahn, H., Mohney, J., Otis, A.B. and Fenn, W.O. (1946) A method for the continuous analysis of alveolar air. *A. Aviat. Med.* **17,** 173

Raine, J.M. and Bishop, J.M. (1963) A–a difference in O_2 tension and physiological dead space in normal man. *J. appl. Physiol.* **18,** 284

Ramon y Cajal, S. (1909) *Histologia du systeme Nerveux de l'Homme et des Vertebres.* Paris: Moloine

Ramwell, P.W. (1958) An investigation into the changes in blood gases during anaesthesia. *PhD Thesis,* University of Leeds

Rapace, J.L. and Lowrey, A.H. (1982) Tobacco smoke, ventilation and indoor air quality. *Am. Soc. Heating, Refrigerating and Air-conditioning Engineers, Inc. Trans.* **88,** 895

Ravin, M.G., Epstein, R.M. and Malm, J.R. (1965) Contribution of thebesian veins to the physiologic shunt in anesthetized man. *J. appl. Physiol.* **20,** 1148

Raymond, L.W. and Standaert, F.G. (1967) The respiratory effects of carbon dioxide in the cat. *Anesthesiology* **28,** 974

Read, D.J.C. (1967). A clinical method for assessing the ventilatory response to carbon dioxide. *Australas. Ann. Med.* **16,** 20

Rebuck, A.S. and Campbell, E.J.M. (1974) A clinical method for assessing the ventilatory response to hypoxia. *Am. Rev. resp. Dis.* **109,** 345

Rebuck, A.S. and Slutsky, A.S. (1981) Measurement of ventilatory responses to hypercapnia and hypoxia. In: *Regulation of Breathing,* Part II, edited by T.F. Hornbein. New York: Marcel Dekker

Rees, G.J. (1980) Neonatal physiology. In: *General Anaesthesia,* 4th edition, vol. 2, edited by T.C. Gray, J.F. Nunn and J.E. Utting. London: Butterworths

Refsum, H.E. (1963) Relationship between state of consciousness and arterial hypoxaemia and hypercapnia in patients with pulmonary insufficiency, breathing air. *Clin. Sci.* **25,** 361

Rehder, K. (1985) Anesthesia and the mechanics of respiration. In: *Effects of Anesthesia,* edited by B.G. Covino, H.A. Fozzard, K. Rehder and G. Strichartz. Bethesda, Md: American Physiological Society

Rehder, K. and Marsh, H.M. (1987) Respiratory mechanics during anesthesia and mechanical ventilation. *Handbk Physiol, section 3,* **3,** part 2, 737

Rehder, K. and Sessler, A.D. (1973) Function of each lung in spontaneously breathing man anesthetized with thiopentalmeperidine. *Anesthesiology* **38,** 320

Rehder, K., Schmid, E.R. and Knopp, T.J. (1983) Long-term high-frequency ventilation in dogs. *Am. Rev. resp. Dis.* **126,** 476

Rehder, K., Sessler, A.D. and Marsh, H.M. (1975) General anesthesia and the lung. *Am. Rev. resp. Dis.* **112,** 541

Rehder, K., Theye, R.A. and Fowler, W.S. (1961) Effect of position and thoracotomy on distribution of air and blood to each lung during intermittent positive pressure breathing. *Physiologist* **4,** 93

Rehder, K., Hatch, D.J., Sessler, A.D., Marsh, H.M. and Fowler, W.S. (1971) Effects of general anesthesia, muscle paralysis, and mechanical ventilation on pulmonary nitrogen clearance. *Anesthesiology* **35,** 591

Rehder, K., Hatch, D.J., Sessler, A.D. and Fowler, W.S. (1972) The function of each lung of anesthetized and paralyzed man during mechanical ventilation. *Anesthesiology* **37,** 16

Rehder, K., Knopp, T.J., Sessler, A.D. and Didier, E.P. (1979) Ventilation–perfusion relationship in young healthy awake and anesthetized–paralyzed man. *J. appl. Physiol.* **47,** 745

Reivich, M. (1964) Arterial P_{CO_2} and cerebral hemodynamics. *Am. J. Physiol.* **206,** 25

Remmers, J.E., deGroot, W.J., Sauerland, E.K. and Anch, A.M. (1978) Pathogenesis of upper airway occlusion during sleep. *J. appl. Physiol.* **44,** 931

Report of the Surgeon General (1981) *The Health Consequences of Smoking. The Changing Cigarette.* Washington DC: US Department of Health and Human Services

Report of the Surgeon General (1984) *The Health Consequences of Smoking. Chronic Obstructive Lung Disease.* Washington DC: US Department of Health and Human Services

Richardson, F.J., Chinn, S. and Nunn, J.F. (1976) Performance and application of the Quantiflex air/oxygen mixer. *Br. J. Anaesth.* **48,** 1057

Riley, R.L., Campbell, E.J.M. and Shepard, RH. (1957) A bubble method for estimation of P_{CO_2} and P_{O_2} in whole blood. *J. appl. Physiol.* **11,** 245

Riley, R.L., Lilienthal, J.L., Proemmel, D.D. and Franke, R.E. (1946) On the determination of the physiologically effective pressures of oxygen and carbon dioxide in alveolar air. *Am. J. Physiol.* **147,** 191

Riley, R.L., Shepard, R.H., Cohn, J.E., Carroll, D.G. and Armstrong, B.W. (1954) Maximal diffusing capacity of lungs. *J. appl. Physiol.* **6,** 573

Rinaldo, J.E. and Rogers, R.M. (1982) Adult respiratory-distress syndrome: changing concepts of lung injury and repair. *New Engl. J. Med.* **306,** 900

Rizk, N.W. and Murray, J.F. (1982) PEEP and pulmonary edema. *Am. J. Med.* **72,** 381

Rizk, N.W., Luce, J.M., Hoeffel, J.M., Price, D.C. and Murray, J.F. (1984) Site of deposition and factors affecting clearance of aerosolized solute from canine lungs. *J. appl. Physiol.* **56,** 723

Robertson, J.D. and Reid, D.D. (1952) Standards for the basal metabolism of normal people in Britain. *Lancet* **1,** 940

Robertson, J.D., Swan, A.A.B. and Whitteridge, D. (1956) Effect of anaesthetics on systemic baro-receptors. *J. Physiol.* **131,** 463

Robinson, C. and Holgate, S.T. (1985) Mast cell-dependent inflammatory mediators and their putative role in bronchial asthma. *Clin. Sci.* **68,** 103

Robson, J.G. (1967) The respiratory centres and their responses. In: *Modern Trends in Anaesthesia—3,* edited by F.T. Evans and T.C. Gray. London and Boston, Mass: Butterworths

Rohrer, F. (1915) Der Strömungswiderstand in den menschlichen Atemwegen. *Plügers Arch. ges. Physiol.* **162,** 225

Romaldini, H., Rodriguez-Roisin, R., Wagner, P.D. and West, J.B. (1983) Enhancement of hypoxic pulmonary vasoconstriction by almitrine in the dog. *Am. Rev. resp. Dis.* **128,** 288

Rossier, P.H. and Méan H. (1943) L'insuffisance pulmonaire: ses diverses formes. *J. suisse Med.* **11,** 327

Rossing, T.H., Slutsky, A.S., Lehr, J.L., Drinker, P.A., Kamm, R. and Drazen, J.M. (1981) Tidal volume and frequency dependence of carbon dioxide elimination by high frequency ventilation. *New Engl. J. Med.* **305,** 1375

Roughton, F.J.W. (1964) Transport of oxygen and carbon dioxide. *Handbk Physiol., section 3,* **1,** 767

Roughton, F.J.W. and Darling, R.C. (1944) The effect of carbon monoxide on the oxyhemoglobin dissociation curve. *Am. J. Physiol.* **141,** 17

Roughton, F.J.W. and Forster, R.E. (1957) Relative importance of diffusion and chemical reaction rates in determining rate of exchange of gas in the human lung. *J. appl. Physiol.* **11,** 290

Roughton, F.J.W. and Severinghaus, J.W. (1973) Accurate determination of O_2 dissociation curve of human blood above 98.7% saturation with data on O_2 solubility in unmodified human blood from 0°C to 37°C. *J. appl. Physiol.* **35,** 861

Roussos, C. and Macklem, P.T. (1983) The respiratory muscles. *Intens. Care Dig.* **2,** 3

Roy, R., Powers, S.R., Fuestel, P.J. and Dutton, R.E. (1977) Pulmonary wedge catheterization during positive end-expiratory pressure ventilation in the dog. *Anesthesiology* **46,** 385

Russell, M.A.H., Wilson, C., Patel, U.A., Cole, P.V. and Feyeraband, C. (1975) Plasma nicotine levels after smoking cigarettes with high, medium and low nicotine yields. *Br. med. J.* **2,** 414

Ryan, U.S. (1982) Structural bases for metabolic activity. *A. Rev. Physiol.* **44,** 223

Ryan, U.S. (1985) Processing of angiotensin and other peptides by the lungs. *Handbk Physiol., section 3,* **1,** 351

Ryan, U.S. and Ryan, J.W. (1977) Correlations between the fine structure of the alveolar-capillary unit and its metabolic activities. In: *Metabolic Functions of the Lung,* edited by Y.S. Bakhle and J.R. Vane. New York: Marcel Dekker

Safar, P. (1959) Failure of manual respiration. *J. appl. Physiol.* **14,** 84

Safar, P., Escarraga, L.A. and Chang, F. (1959) Upper airway obstruction in the unconscious patient. *J. appl. Physiol.* **14,** 760

Said, S.I. (1982) Metabolic functions of the pulmonary circulation. *Circulation Res.* **50,** 325

St John, W.M., Glasser, R.L. and King, R.A. (1972) Rhythmic respiration in awake vagotomized cats with chronic pneumotaxic area lesions. *Resp. Physiol.* **15,** 233

Salmoiraghi, G.C. (1963) Functional organization of brain stem respiratory neurones. *Ann. N.Y. Acad. Sci.* **109,** 571

Salmoiraghi, G.C. and Burns, B.D. (1960) Localization and patterns of discharge of respiratory neurones in brain stem of cat. *J. Neurophysiol.* **23,** 2

Salzano, J.V., Camporesi, E.M., Stolp, B.W. and Moon, R.E. (1984) Physiological responses to exercise at 47 and 66 ATA. *J. appl. Physiol.* **57,** 1055

Sanders, R.D. (1967) Two ventilating attachments for bronchoscopes. *Delaware St. med. J.* **39,** 170

Saugstad, O.D., Hallman, M., Abraham, J.L., Epstein, B., Cochrane, C. and Gluck, L. (1984) Hypoxanthine and oxygen induced lung injury: a possible basic mechanism of tissue damage? *Pediat. Res.* **18,** 501

Schafer, E.A. (1904) Description of a simple and efficient method of performing artificial respiration in the human subject. *Trans. R. med. chir. Soc. London* **87,** 609

Scheidt, M., Hyatt, R.E. and Rehder, K. (1981) Effects of rib cage or abdominal restriction on lung mechanics. *J. appl. Physiol.* **51,** 1115

Schläfke, M.E., Pokorski, M., See, W.R., Prill, R.K. and Loeschcke, H.H. (1975) Chemosensitive neurons on the ventral medullary surface. *Bull. Physio-Pathol. Resp.* **11,** 277

Schmidt, E.R. and Rehder, K. (1981) General anesthesia and the chest wall. *Anesthesiology* **55,** 668

Schmidt, G.B., O'Neill, W.W., Koth, K., Hwang, K.K., Bennett, E.J. and Bembeck, C.T. (1976) Continuous positive airway pressure in the prophylaxis of the adult respiratory distress syndrome. *Surg. Gynec. Obst.* **143,** 613

Schofield, E.J. and Williams, N.E. (1974) Prediction of arterial carbon dioxide tension using a circle system without carbon dioxide absorption. *Br. J. Anaesth.* **46,** 442

Scholander, P.F. (1947) Analyzer for accurate estimation of respiratory gases in one-half cubic centimeter samples. *J. biol. Chem.* **167,** 235

Scott, D.B., Stephen, G.W. and Davie, I.T. (1972) Haemodynamic effects of a negative (subatmospheric) pressure expiratory phase during artificial ventilation. *Br. J. Anaesth.* **44,** 171

Scott, J. (1847) Etherisation and asphyxia. *Lancet* **1,** 355

Sechzer, P.H., Egbert, L.D., Linde, H.W., Cooper, D.Y., Dripps, R.D. and Price, H.L. (1960) Effect of CO_2 inhalation on arterial pressure, ECG and plasma catecholamines and 17-OH corticosteroids in normal man. *J. appl. Physiol.* **15,** 454

Seebohm, P.M. and Hamilton, W.K. (1958) A method for measuring nasal resistance without intranasal instrumentation. *J. Allergy* **29,** 56

Seeger, W., Stohr, G., Wolf, H.R.D. and Neufof, H. (1985) Alteration of surfactant function due to protein leakage. *J. appl. Physiol.* **58,** 326

Selman, B.J., White, Y.S. and Tait, A.R. (1975) An evaluation of the Lex-O_2-Con oxygen content analyser. *Anaesthesia* **30,** 206

Semple, S.J.G. (1965) Respiration and the cerebrospinal fluid. *Br. J. Anaesth.* **37,** 262

Senior, R.M., Griffen, G.L. and Mecham, R.P. (1980) Chemotactic activity of elastin-derived peptides. *J. clin. Invest.* **66,** 859

Servetus, M. (1553) *Christianismi Restitutio.* Vienne

Severinghaus, J.W. (1963) High temperature operation of the oxygen electrode giving fast response for respiratory gas sampling. *Clin. Chem.* **9,** 727

Severinghaus, J.W. (1965) Blood gas concentrations. *Handbk Physiol., section* 3, **2,** 1475

Severinghaus, J.W. (1966) Blood gas calculator. *J. appl. Physiol.* **21,** 1108

Severinghaus, J.W. (1981) A combined transcutaneous Po_2–Pco_2 electrode with electrochemical HCO_3^- stabilization. *J. appl. Physiol.* **51,** 1027

Severinghaus, J.W. and Astrup, P.B. (1986) History of blood gas analysis. III. Carbon dioxide tension. *J. clin. Monitor.* **2,** 60

Severinghaus, J.W. and Bradley, A.F. (1958) Electrodes for blood Po_2 and Pco_2 determination. *J. appl. Physiol.* **13,** 515

Severinghaus, J.W. and Mitchell, R.A. (1962) Ondine's curse: failure of respiratory center automaticity while awake. *Clin. Res.* **10,** 122

Severinghaus, J.W. and Stupfel, M. (1955) Respiratory dead space increase following atropine in man, and atropine, vagal or ganglionic blockade and hypothermia in dogs. *J. appl. Physiol.* **8,** 81

Severinghaus, J.W. and Stupfel, M. (1957) Alveolar dead space as an index of distribution of blood flow in pulmonary capillaries. *J. appl. Physiol.* **10,** 335

Severinghaus, J.W., Stupfel, M. and Bradley, A.F. (1956a) Accuracy of blood pH and Pco_2 determinations. *J. appl. Physiol.* **9,** 189

Severinghaus, J.W., Stupfel, M. and Bradley, A.F. (1956b) Variations of serum carbonic acid pK' with pH and temperature. *J. appl. Physiol.* **9,** 197

Severinghaus, J.W., Mitchell, R.A., Richardson, B.W. and Singer, M.M. (1963) Respiratory control at high altitude suggesting active transport regulation of CSF pH. *J. appl. Physiol.* **18,** 1153

Shafer, A.W., Tague, L.L., Welch, M.H. and Guenter, C.A. (1971) 2, 3-Diphosphoglycerate in red cells stored in acid–citrate–dextrose and citrate–phosphate–dextrose. *J. Lab. clin. Med.* **77,** 430

Shammea, M.H., Nasrallah, S.M. and Al-Khalidi, U.A.S. (1973) Serum xanthine oxidase. *Dig. Dis.* **18,** 15

Shappell, S.D. and Lenfant, C.J.M. (1972) Adaptive, genetic and iatrogenic alterations of the oxyhemoglobin-dissociation curve. *Anesthesiology* **37,** 127

Sharp, G.R., Ledingham, I. McA. and Norman, J.N. (1962) The application of oxygen at 2 atmospheres pressure in the treatment of acute anoxia. *Anaesthesia* **17,** 136

Sharpey-Schafer, E.P. (1953) Effects of coughing on intra-thoracic pressure, arterial pressure and peripheral blood flow. *J. Physiol.* **122,** 351

Shaw, L.A. and Messer, A.C. (1932) The transfer of bicarbonate ion between the blood and tissues caused by alterations of the carbon dioxide concentrations in the lungs. *Am. J. Physiol.* **100,** 122

Shenkin, H.A. and Bouzarth, W.F. (1970) Clinical methods of reducing intracranial pressure. *New Engl. J. Med.* **282,** 1465

Shepard, R.H., Campbell, E.J.M., Martin, H.B. and Enns, T. (1957) Factors affecting the pulmonary dead space as determined by single breath analysis. *J. appl. Physiol.* **11,** 241

Shepard, R.J. (1967) The maximum sustained voluntary ventilation in exercise. *Clin. Sci.* **32,** 167

Shigeoka, J.W., Colice, G.L. and Ramirez, G. (1985) Effect of normoxemic and hypoxemic exercise on renin and aldosterone. *J. appl. Physiol.* **59,** 142

Sibbald, W.I. and Dredger, A.A. (1983) Right ventricular function in acute disease states. *Crit. Care Med.* **11,** 339

Sibbald, W.J., Anderson, R.R., Reid, B., Holliday, R.L. and Driedger, A.A. (1981) Alveolo-capillary permeability in human septic ARDS. *Chest* **79,** 133

Siesjö, B.K. and Nilsson L. (1971) The influence of arterial hypoxaemia upon labile phosphates and upon extracellular and intracellular lactate and pyruvate concentrations in the rat brain. *Scand. J. clin. Lab. Invest.* **27,** 83

Siggaard-Andersen, O. (1962) The pH, log pCO_2 blood acid–base nomogram revised. *Scand. J. clin. Lab. Invest.* **14,** 598

Siggaard-Andersen, O. (1964) *The Acid–Base Status of Blood.* Copenhagen: Munksgaard

Siggaard-Andersen, O., Engel, K., Jorgensen, K. and Astrup, P. (1960) A micro-method for determination of pH, carbon dioxide tension, base excess and standard bicarbonate in capillary blood. *Scand. J. clin. Lab. Invest.* **12,** 172

Silvester, H.R. (1857) The natural method of treating asphyxia. *Med. Times Gaz.* **11,** 485

Simani, A.S., Inoue, S. and Hogg, J.C. (1974) Penetration of the respiratory epithelium of guinea pigs following exposure to cigarette smoke. *Lab. Invest.* **31,** 75

Simcock, A.D. (1986) Treatment of near drowning — a review of 130 cases. *Anaesthesia* **41,** 643

Simionescu, M. (1980) Utrastructural organization of the alveolar-capillary unit. In: *Metabolic Activities of the Lung.* Ciba Foundation Sympoisum, no. 78. Amsterdam: Excerpta Medica

Singer, M.M., Wright, F., Stanley, L.K., Roe, B.B. and Hamilton, W.K. (1970) Oxygen toxicity in man. A prospective study in patients after open-heart surgery. *New Engl. J. Med.* **283,** 1473

Sjöstrand, U. (1980) High-frequency positive-pressure ventilation (HFPPV): a review. *Crit. Care Med.* **8,** 345

Slavin, G., Nunn, J.F., Crow, J. and Dore, C.J. (1982) Bronchiolectasis — a complication of artificial ventilation. *Br. med. J.* **285,** 931

Slome, D. (1965) Physiology of respiration. In: *General Anaesthesia,* vol. 1, 2nd edn, edited by F.T. Evans and T.C. Gray. London and Boston, Mass: Butterworths

Smith, A.L. and Wollman, H. (1972) Cerebral blood flow and metabolism. *Anesthesiology* **36,** 378

Smith, B.E. and Hanning, C.D. (1986) Advances in respiratory support. *Br. J. Anaesth.* **58,** 138

Smith, G. and Lawson, D.A. (1958) Experimental coronary arterial occlusion: effects of the administration of oxygen under pressure. *Scott. med. J.* **3,** 346

Smith, G., Stevens, J., Griffiths, J.C. and Ledingham, I.McA. (1961) Near avulsion of foot treated by replacement and subsequent prolonged exposure of patient to oxygen at two atmospheres pressure. *Lancet* **2,** 1122

Smith, H. and Pask, E.A. (1959) Method for the estimation of oxygen in gas mixtures containing nitrous oxide. *Br. J. Anaesth.* **31,** 440

Smith, W.D.A. (1964) The measurement of uptake of nitrous oxide by pneumotachography. I. Apparatus, methods and accuracy. *Br. J. Anaesth.* **36,** 363

Snow, J. (1858) *On Chloroform and other Anaesthetics; their action and administration.* London: John Churchill

Sobin, S.S., Fung, Y.C., Tremer, H.M. and Rosenquist, T.H. (1972) Elasticity of the pulmonary alveolar microvascular sheet in the cat. *Circulation Res.* **30,** 440

Sole, M.J., Dobrac, M., Schwartz, L., Hussain, M.N. and Vaughan-Neil, E.F. (1979) The extraction of circulating catecholamines by the lungs in normal man and in patients with pulmonary hypertension. *Circulation* **60,** 160

Southall, D.P., Talbert, D.G., Johnson, P., Morley, C.J., Salmons, S., Miller, J. and Helms, P.J. (1985) Prolonged expiratory apnoea: a disorder resulting in episodes of severe arterial hypoxaemia in infants and young children. *Lancet* **2,** 571

Spence, A.A. and Ellis, F.R. (1971) A critical evaluation of a nitrogen rebreathing method for the estimation of $P\bar{v}_{O_2}$. *Resp. Physiol.* **10,** 313

Staněk, V., Widimisky J., Kasalicky, J., Navratil, M., Daum, S. and Levinsky, L. (1967) The pulmonary gas exchange during exercise in patients with pulmonary fibrosis. *Scand. J. resp. Dis.* **48,** 11

Stanley, T.H., Zikria, B.A. and Sullivan, S.F. (1972) The surface tension of tracheobronchial secretions during general anesthesia. *Anesthesiology* **37,** 445

Stark, D.C.C. and Smith, H. (1960) Pulmonary vascular changes during anesthesia. *Br. J. Anaesth.* **32,** 460

Starling, E.H. and Verney, E.B. (1925) The secretion of urine as studied in the isolated kidney. *Proc. R. Soc. B,* **97,** 321

Staub, N.C. (1963a) Alveolar–arterial oxygen tension gradient due to diffusion. *J. appl. Physiol.* **18,** 673

Staub, N.C. (1963b) The interdependence of pulmonary structure and function. *Anesthesiology* **24,** 831

Staub, N.C. (1974) Pulmonary edema. *Physiol. Rev.* **54,** 679

Staub, N.A. (1983) Alveolar flooding and clearance. *Am. Rev. resp. Dis.* **127,** S44

Staub, N.A. (1984) Pathophysiology of pulmonary edema. In: *Edema,* edited by N.A. Staub and A.E. Taylor. New York: Raven Press

Staub, N.C., Bishop, J.M. and Forster, R.E. (1961) Importance of diffusion and chemical blood cells. *J. appl. Physiol.* **16,** 511

Staub, N.C., Bishop, J.M. and Forster, R.E. (1962) Importance of diffusion and chemical reaction rates in O_2 uptake in the lung. *J. appl. Physiol.* **17**, 21

Stein, M., Forkner, C.E., Robin, E.D. and Wessler, S. (1961) Gas exchange after autologous pulmonary embolism in dogs. *J. appl. Physiol.* **16**, 488

Stevens, J.H. and Raffin, T.A. (1984) Adult respiratory distress syndrome — 1. Aetiology and mechanisms. *Postgrad. med. J.* **60**, 505

Strang, L.B. (1959) The ventilatory capacity of normal children. *Thorax* **14**, 305

Strang, L.B. (1965) The lungs at birth. *Archs Dis. Childh.* **40**, 575

Sturrock, J.E. and Hulands, G.H. (1980) Protective effect of steroids on cultured cells damaged by high concentrations of oxygen. *Br. J. Anaesth.* **52**, 567

Sturrock, J.E. and Nunn, J.F. (1978) Chromosomal damage and mutations after exposure of Chinese hamster cells to high concentrations of oxygen. *Mutation Res.* **57**, 27

Suggett, A.J., Barer, G.R., Mohammed, F.H. and Gill, G.W. (1982) The effects of localized hypoventilation on ventilation/perfusion ratios and gas exchange in the dog lung. *Clin. Sci.* **63**, 497

Sugihara, T., Hildebrandt, J. and Martin, C.J. (1972) Viscoelastic properties of alveolar wall. *J. appl. Physiol.* **33**, 93

Sullivan, C.E., Berton-Jones, M. and Issa, F.G. (1983) Remission of severe obesity hypoventilation syndrome following short-term treatment during sleep with nasal continuous positive airway pressure. *Am. Rev. resp. Dis.* **128**, 177

Suter, P.M., Fairley, H.B. and Isenberg, M.D. (1975) Optimum end-expiratory airway pressure in patients with acute pulmonary failure. *New Engl. J. Med.* **292**, 284

Svanberg, L. (1957) Influence of posture on lung volumes, ventilation and circulation in normals. *Scand. J. clin. Lab. Invest.* **9**, suppl. 25

Swyer, P.R. (1975) (ed.) *The Intensive Care of the Newly Born.* Monographs in Paediatrics, no. 6. Basel: Karger

Sykes, M.K. (1960) Observations on a rebreathing technique for the determination of arterial P_{CO_2} in the apnoeic patient. *Br. J. Anaesth.* **32**, 256

Sykes, M.K. (1986) Effects of anesthetics and drugs used during anesthesia on the pulmonary circulation. In: *Cardiovascular Actions of Anesthetics,* edited by B.M. Altura and S. Halevy. Basel: Karger

Sykes, M.K. and Lumley, J. (1969) The effect of varying inspiratory:expiratory ratios during anaesthesia for open-heart surgery. *Br. J. Anaesth.* **41**, 374

Sykes, M.K., Adams, A.P., Finlay, W.E.I., McCormick, P.W. and Economider, A. (1970) The effect of variations in end-expiratory inflation pressure on cardiorespiratory function in normo-, hypo-, and hyper-volaemic dogs. *Br. J. Anaesth.* **42**, 669

Sykes, M.K., Loh, L., Seed, R.F., Kafer, E.R. and Chakrabarti, M.K. (1972) The effect of inhalational anaesthetics on hypoxic pulmonary vasoconstriction and pulmonary vascular resistance in the perfused lungs of the dog and cat. *Br. J. Anaesth.* **44**, 776

Taghizadeh, A. and Reynolds, E.O.R. (1976) Pathogenesis of bronchopulmonary dysplasia following hyaline membrane disease. *Am. J. Pathol.* **82** (2), 241

Tate, R.M. and Repine, J.E. (1983) Neutrophils and the adult respiratory distress syndrome. *Am. Rev. resp. Dis.* **127**, 552

Taylor, S.H., Scott, D.B. and Donald, K.W. (1964) Respiratory effect of general anaesthesia. *Lancet* **1**, 841

Tenney, S.M. (1956) Sympatho-adrenal stimulation by carbon dioxide and the inhibitory effect of carbonic acid on epinephrine response. *Am. J. Physiol.* **187**, 341

Tenney, S.M. (1960) The effect of carbon dioxide on neurohumoral and endocrine mechanisms. *Anesthesiology* **21**, 674

Tenney, S.M. and Lamb T.W. (1965) Physiological consequences of hypoventilation and hyperventilation. *Handbk Physiol.,* section 3, **2**, 979

Thews, G. (1961) In: *Bad Oeynhausener Gespräche,* IV, edited by H. Bartels and E. Witzleb, Berlin: Springer

Theye, R.A. and Tuohy, G.F. (1964a) Oxygen uptake during light halothane anesthesia in man. *Anesthesiology* **25**, 627

Theye, R.A. and Tuohy, G.F. (1964b) Considerations in the determination of oxygen uptake and ventilatory performance during methoxyflurane anesthesia in man. *Curr. Res. Anesth. Analg.* **43**, 306

Thilenius, O.G. (1966) Effect of anesthesia on response of pulmonary circulation of dogs to acute hypoxia. *J. appl. Physiol.* **21,** 901

Thomas, D.P. and Vane, J.R. (1967) 5-Hydroxytryptamine in the circulation of the dog. *Nature* **216,** 335

Thompson, S.P. (1965) *Calculus Made Easy.* London: Macmillan

Thornton, J.A. (1960) Physiological dead space: changes during general anaesthesia. *Anaesthesia* **15,** 381

Thornton, J.A. and Nunn, J.F. (1960) Accuracy of determination of P_{CO_2} by the indirect method. *Guy's Hosp. Rep.* **109,** 203

Tibes, U. (1977) Reflex inputs to the cardiovascular and respiratory centers from dynamically working canine muscles. *Circulation Res.* **41,** 332

Tierney, D.F. and Young, S.L. (1985) Glucose and intermediary metabolism of the lungs. In: *Handbk Physiol. section 3,* **1,** 255

Timms, R.M., Khaja, F.U. and Williams, G.W. (1985) Hemodynamic response to oxygen therapy in chronic obstructive pulmonary disease. *Ann. intern. Med.* **102,** 29

Tobin, C.E. and Zariquiey, M.O. (1950) Arteriovenous shunts in the human lung. *Proc. Soc. exp. Biol. Med.* **75,** 827

Tockman, M., Menkes, H., Cohen, B., Permutt, S., Benjamin, J., Ball, W.C. and Tonascia, J. (1976) A comparison of pulmonary function in male smokers and non-smokers. *Am. Rev. resp. Dis.* **114,** 711

Torrance, J., Jacobs, P., Restrepo, A., Eschbach, J., Lenfant, C. and Finch, C.A. (1970) Intra-erythrocytic adaptation to anemia. *New Engl. J. Med.* **283,** 165

Trichet, B., Falke, K., Togut, A. and Laver, M.B. (1975). The effect of pre-existing pulmonary vascular disease on the response to mechanical ventilation with PEEP following open-heart surgery. *Anesthesiology* **42,** 56

Trinkle, J.K., Richardson, J.D., Franz, J.L., Grover, F.L., Aron, K.V. and Holmstrom, F.M.G. (1975) Management of flail chest without mechanical ventilation. *Ann. thorac. Surg.* **19,** 355

Turner, J.E., Lambertsen, C.J., Owen, S.G., Wendel, H. and Chiodi, H. (1957) Effects of 0.08 and 0.8 atmospheres of inspired P_{O_2} upon cerebral hemodynamics at a 'constant' alveolar P_{CO_2} of 43 mm Hg. *Fedn Proc.* **16,** 130

Turrens, J.F., Crapo, J.D. and Freeman, B.A. (1984) Protection against oxygen toxicity by intravenous injection of liposome-entrapped catalase and superoxide dismutase. *J. clin. Invest.* **73,** 87

Tusiewicz, K., Bryan, A.C. and Froese, A.B. (1977) Contributions of changing rib cage–diaphragm interactions to the ventilatory depression of halothane anesthesia. *Anesthesiology* **47,** 327

Ullman, E. (1970) About Hering and Breuer. In: *Breathing: Hering–Breuer Centenary Symposium,* p. 3, edited by R. Porter. Edinburgh and London: Churchill Livingstone

Utting, J.E. (1980) Hypocapnia. In: *General Anaesthesia,* 4th edn, vol. 1, edited by T.C. Gray, J.F. Nunn and J.E. Utting. London: Butterworths

Valeri, C.R. (1975) Blood components in the treatment of acute blood loss, use of freeze-preserved red cells, platelets, and the plasma proteins. *Anesth. Analg.* **54,** 1

Van Slyke, D.D. and Neill, J.M. (1924) The determination of gases in blood and other solutions by vacuum extraction and monometric measurement. *J. biol. Chem.* **61,** 523

Vance, J.P., Brown, D.M. and Smith, G. (1973) The effects of hypocapnia on myocardial blood flow and metabolism. *Br. J. Anaesth.* **45,** 455

Vane, J.R. (1969) The release and fate of vaso-active hormones in the circulation. *Br. J. Pharmac.* **35,** 209

Vann, R.D. (1982) Decompression theory and application. In: *The Physiology and Medicine of Diving,* edited by P.B. Bennett and D.H. Elliott. London: Baillière Tindall

Velasquez, T. and Farhi, L.E. (1964) Effect of negative pressure breathing on lung mechanics and venous admixture. *J. appl. Physiol.* **19,** 665

Vellody, V.P.S., Nassery, M., Balasaraswathi, K., Goldberg, N.G. and Sharp, J.T. (1978) Compliances of human rib cage and diaphragm–abdomen pathways in relaxed versus paralyzed states. *Am. Rev. resp. Dis.* **118,** 479

Verloop, M.C. (1948) The arteriae bronchiales and their anastomoses with the arteria pulmonalis in the human lung: a micro-anatomical study. *Acta anat.* **5,** 171

Virgil, Publius Vergilus Marto (19 BC) *The Aeneid,* Book II, p. 1

Wade, J.G., Larson, C.P., Hickey, R.F., Ehrenfeld, W.K. and Severinghaus, J.W. (1970) Effect of carotid endarterectomy on carotid chemoreceptor and baroreceptor function in man. *New Engl. J. Med.* **282,** 823

Wade, O.L. and Gilson, J.C. (1951) The effect of posture on diaphragmatic movement and vital capacity in normal subjects. *Thorax* **6,** 103

Wagner, P.D., Naumann, P.F. and Laravuso, R.B. (1974) Simultaneous measurements of eight foreign gases in blood by gas chromatography. *J. appl. Physiol.* **36,** 600

Wagner, P.D., Saltzman, H.A. and West, J.B. (1974) Measurement of continuous distribution of ventilation–perfusion ratios: theory. *J. appl. Physiol.* **36,** 588

Wagner, P.D., Laravuso, R.B., Uhl, R.R. and West, J.B. (1974) Continuous distributions of ventilation–perfusion ratios in normal subjects breathing air and 100% O_2. *J. clin. Invest.* **54,** 54

Wagner, P.D., Laravuso, R.B., Goldzimmer, E., Naumann, P.F. and West, J.B. (1975) Distribution of ventilation–perfusion ratios in dogs in normal and abnormal lungs. *J. appl. Physiol.* **38,** 1099

Walder, D.N. (1982) The compressed air environment. In: *The Physiology and Medicine of Diving,* edited by P.B. Bennett and D.H. Elliott. London: Baillière Tindall

Wang, S.C., Ngai, S.H. and Frumin, M.J. (1957) Organization of central respiratory mechanisms in the brain stem of the cat: genesis of normal respiratory rhythmicity. *Am. J. Physiol.* **190,** 333

Warrell, D.A., Evans, J.W., Clarke, R.O., Kingaby, G.P. and West, J.B. (1972) Pattern of filling in the pulmonary capillary bed. *J. appl. Physiol.* **32,** 346

Warren, B.A. (1963) Fibrinolytic properties of vascular endothelium. *Br. J. exp. Path.* **44,** 365

Wasserman, K. (1978) Breathing during exercise. *New Engl. J. Med.* **298,** 780

Watson, W.E. (1962a) Some observations on dynamic lung compliance during intermittent positive pressure respiration. *Br. J. Anaesth.* **34,** 153

Watson, W.E. (1962b) Observations on physiological dead space during intermittent positive pressure respiration. *Br. J. Anaesth.* **34,** 502

Wayne, D.J. and Chamney, A.R. (1969) Oxygen tents. *Anaesthesia* **24,** 591

Weatherall, D.J., Ledingham, J.G.G. and Warrell, D.A. (1983) (eds) *Oxford Textbook of Medicine.* Oxford: Oxford University Press

Webb, S.J.S. and Nunn, J.F. (1967) A comparison between the effect of nitrous oxide and nitrogen on arterial Po_2. *Anaesthesia* **22,** 69

Webb, W.R. (1984) Metabolic effects of fructose diphosphate in hypoxic and ischaemic states. *Thorac. Cardiovasc. Surg.* **88,** 863

Weibel, E.R. (1962) Morphometrische Bestimmung von Zahl, Volumen und Oberfläche der Alveolen und Kapillaren der menschlichen Lunge. *Z. Zellforsch. mikrosk. Anat.* **57,** 648

Weibel, E.R. (1963) *Morphometry of the Human Lung.* Berlin: Springer

Weibel, E.R. (1964) Morphometrics of the lung. *Handbk Physiol., section 3,* **1,** 285

Weibel, E.R. (1971) Oxygen effect on lung cells. *Archs intern. Med.* **128,** 54

Weibel, E.R. (1973) Morphological basis of alveolar–capillary gas exchange. *Physiol. Rev.* **53,** 419

Weibel, E.R. (1983) How does lung structure affect gas exchange. *Chest* **83,** 657

Weibel, E.R. (1984) *The Pathway for Oxygen.* Cambridge, Mass: Harvard University Press

Weibel, E.R. (1985) Lung cell biology. *Handbk Physiol., section 3,* **1,** 47

Weibel, E.R. and Gil, J. (1968) Electron microscopic demonstration of an extracellular duplex lining layer of alveoli. *Resp. Physiol.* **4,** 42

Weibel, E.R. and Gomez, D.M. (1962) Architecture of the human lung. *Science* **137,** 577

Weigelt, J.A., Norcross, J.F., Borman, K.R. and Snyder, W.H. (1985) Early steroid therapy for respiratory failure. *Archs Surg.* **120,** 536

Weil, J.V., Byrne-Quinn, E., Sodal, I.D., Friessen, W.O., Underhill, B., Filley, G.F. and Grover, R.F. (1970) Hypoxic ventilatory drive in normal man. *J. clin. Invest.* **49,** 1061

Weil, J.V., Byrne-Quinn, E., Sodal, I.E., Kline, J.S., McCullough, R.E. and Filley, G.F. (1972) Augmentation of chemosensitivity during mild exercise in normal man. *J. appl. Physiol.* **33,** 813

Weiskopf, R.B. and Severinghaus, J.W. (1972) Lack of effect of high altitude on hemoglobin oxygen affinity. *J. appl. Physiol.* **33,** 276

Weiskopf, R.B., Nishimura, M. and Severinghaus, J.W. (1971) The absence of an effect of halothane on blood hemoglobin O_2 equilibrium *in vitro*. *Anesthesiology* **35,** 579

Weiskopf, R.B., Raymond, L.W. and Severinghaus, J.W. (1974) Effects of halothane on canine respiratory responses to hypoxia with and without hypercarbia. *Anesthesiology* **41**, 350

Weisman, I.M., Rinaldo, J.E., Rogers, R.M. and Sanders, M.H. (1983) Intermittent mandatory ventilation. *Am. Rev. resp. Dis.* **127**, 641

West, J.B. (1962) Regional differences in gas exchange in the lung of erect man. *J. appl. Physiol.* **17**, 893

West, J.B. (1963) Distribution of gas and blood in the normal lung. *Br. med. Bull.* **19**, 53

West, J.B. (1965) *Ventilation: Blood Flow and Gas Exchange.* Oxford: Blackwell Scientific

West, J.B. (1974) Blood flow to the lung and gas exchange. *Anesthesiology* **41**, 124

West, J.B. and Dollery, C.T. (1965) Distribution of blood flow and the pressure–flow relations of the whole lung. *J. appl. Physiol.* **20**, 175

West, J.B., Dollery, C.T. and Naimark, A. (1964) Distribution of blood flow in isolated lung: relation to vascular and alveolar pressures. *J. appl. Physiol.* **19**, 713

West, J.W., Lahiri, S., Gill, M.B., Milledge, J.S., Pugh, L.G.C.E. and Ward, M.P. (1962) Arterial oxygen saturation during exercise at high altitude. *J. appl. Physiol.* **17**, 617

West, J.B., Boyer, S.J., Graber, D.J. et al. (1983a) Maximal exercise at extreme altitudes on Mount Everest. *J. appl. Physiol.* **55**, 688

West, J.B., Hackett, P.H., Maret, K.H. et al. (1983b) Pulmonary gas exchange on the summit of Mount Everest. *J. appl. Physiol.* **55**, 678

West, J.B., Peters, R.M., Aksnes, G., Maret, K.H., Milledge, J.S. and Schoene, R.B. (1987) Nocturnal periodic breathing at altitudes of 6300 and 8050 meters. *J. appl. Physiol.* **61**, in the press

Westbrook, P.R., Stubbs, S.E., Sessler, A.D., Rehder, K. and Hyatt, R.E. (1973) Effects of anesthesia and muscle paralysis on respiratory mechanics in normal man. *J. appl. Physiol.* **34**, 81

Westlake, E.K., Simpson, T. and Kaye, M. (1955) Carbon dioxide narcosis in emphysema. *Q. Jl Med.* **24**, 155

Whillis, J. (1930) A note on the muscles of the palate and the superior constrictor. *J. Anat.* **65**, 92

Whipp, B.J. (1981) The control of exercise hyperpnea. In: *Regulation of Breathing*, edited by T.F. Hornbein. New York: Marcel Dekker

Whitelaw, W.A., Derenne, J.-P. and Milic-Emilli, J. (1975) Occlusion pressure as a measure of respiratory center output in conscious man. *Resp. Physiol.* **23**, 181

Whitfield, A.G.W., Waterhouse, J.A.H. and Arnott, W.M. (1950) The total lung volume and its subdivisons. *Br. J. soc. Med.* **4**, 1

Whitteridge, D. and Bulbring, E. (1944) Changes in activity of pulmonary receptors in anaesthesia and the influence of respiratory behaviour. *J. Pharmac. exp. Ther.* **81**, 340

Whitwam, J.G., Chakrabarti, M.K., Konarzewski, W.H. and Askitopoulou, H. (1983) A new valveless all-purpose ventilator. *Br. J. Anaesth.* **55**, 1017

Widdicombe, J.G. (1961) Respiratory reflexes in man and other mammalian species. *Clin. Sci.* **21**, 163

Widdicombe, J.G. (1964) Respiratory reflexes. *Handbk Physiol., section 3*, **1**, 585

Widdicombe, J.G. (1981) Nervous receptors in the respiratory tract. In: *Regulation of Breathing*, Part I, edited by T.F. Hornbein. New York: Marcel Dekker

Wiles, C.M., Clarke, C.R.A., Irwin, H.P., Edgar, E.F. and Swan, A.V. (1986) Hyperbaric oxygen in multiple sclerosis: a double blind trial. *Br. med. J.* **292**, 367

Williams, K.G. and Hopkinson, W.I. (1965) Small chamber techniques in hyperbaric oxygen therapy. In: *Hyperbaric Oxygenation*, edited by I. Ledingham. Edinburgh and London: Churchill Livginstone

Windebank, W.J., Boyd, G. and Moran, F. (1973) Pulmonary thromboembolism presenting as asthma. *Br. med. J.* **1**, 90

Winterstein, H. (1911) Die Regulierung der Athmung durch das Blut. *Pflügers Arch. ges. Physiol.* **138**, 167

Woo, S.W., Berlin, D. and Hedley-Whyte, J. (1969) Surfactant function and anesthetic agents. *J. appl. Physiol.* **26**, 571

Wood, J.D. and Watson, W.J. (1963) Gamma-aminobutyric acid levels in the brain of rats exposed to oxygen at high pressure. *Can. J. Biochem. Physiol.* **41**, 1907

Wood, J.D., Watson, W.J. and Murray, G.W. (1969) Correlation between decreases in brain gamma-aminobutyric acid levels and susceptibility to convulsions induced by hyperbaric oxygen. *J. Neurochem.* **16,** 281

Woodbury, D.M. and Karler, R. (1960) The role of carbon dioxide in the nervous system. *Anesthesiology* **21,** 686

Woolcock, A.J., Vincent, N.J. and Macklem, P.T. (1969) Frequency dependence of compliance as a test for obstruction in the small airways. *J. clin. Invest.* **48,** 1097

Wright, B.M. (1955) A respiratory anemometer. *J. Physiol.* **127,** 25P

Wright, B.M. and McKerrow, C.B. (1959) Maximum forced expiratory flow rate as a measure of ventilatory capacity. *Br. med. J.* **2,** 1041

Wulf, R.J. and Featherstone, R.M. (1957) A correlation of Van der Waals constants with anesthetic potency. *Anesthesiology* **18,** 97

Wynne, J.W. (1984) Gas exchange during sleep in patients with chronic airway obstruction. In: *Sleep and breathing,* edited by N.A. Saunders and C.E. Sullivan. New York: Marcel Dekker

Zamel, N., Jones, J.G., Bach, S.M. and Newberg, L. (1974) Analog computation of alveolar pressure and airway resistance during maximum expiratory flow. *J. appl. Physiol.* **36,** 240

Zapol, W.M., Snider, M.T., Hill, J.D. et al. (1979) Extracorporeal membrane oxygenation in severe acute respiratory failure. *J. Am. med. Assoc.* **242,** 2193

Zechman, F., Hall, F.G. and Hull, W.E. (1957) Effects of graded resistance to tracheal air flow in man. *J. appl. Physiol.* **10,** 356

Zidulka, A., Gross, D., Minami, H., Vartian, V. and Chang, H.K. (1983) Ventilation by high frequency chest wall compression in dogs with normal lungs. *Am. Rev. resp. Dis.* **127,** 709

Zijlstra, W.G. (1958) *A Manual of Reflection Oximetry.* Assen, Netherlands: van Gorcum's Medical Library

Zuntz, N. (1882) Physiologie der Blutgase und des respiratorischen Gaswechsels. *Hermann's Handbuch Physiol.* **4,** 1

Index

567